SUSTAINABLE APPROACHES IN POSTHARVEST HANDLING AND MANAGEMENT

Postharvest Biology and Technology Series

SUSTAINABLE APPROACHES IN POSTHARVEST HANDLING AND MANAGEMENT

Pankaj B. Pathare, PhD
Editor

APPLE ACADEMIC PRESS

First edition published 2026

Apple Academic Press Inc.
1265 Goldenrod Circle, NE,
Palm Bay, FL 32905 USA

760 Laurentian Drive, Unit 19,
Burlington, ON L7N 0A4, Canada

CRC Press
2385 NW Executive Center Drive,
Suite 320, Boca Raton FL 33431

4 Park Square, Milton Park,
Abingdon, Oxon, OX14 4RN, UK

Apple Academic Press exclusively co-publishes with CRC Press, an imprint of Taylor & Francis Group, LLC

Library and Archives Canada Cataloguing in Publication

CIP data on file with Canada Library and Archives

Library of Congress Cataloging-in-Publication Data

CIP data on file with US Library of Congress

ISBN: 978-1-77964-106-9 (hbk)
ISBN: 978-1-77964-107-6 (ebk)
DOI: 10.1201/9781779641076

About the Book Series: Postharvest Biology and Technology

Editor-in-Chief

Mohammed Wasim Siddiqui, PhD
Scientist-cum-Assistant Professor, Department of Food Science and Technology, Bihar Agricultural University, Sabour, Bhagalpur, Bihar, India
AAP Acquisitions Editor | Horticultural Science
Founding/Managing Editor | *Journal of Postharvest Technology*

As we know, preserving the quality of fresh produce has long been a challenging task. In the past, several approaches were in use for the postharvest management of fresh produce, but due to continuous advancement in technology, the increased health consciousness of consumers, and environmental concerns, these approaches have been modified and enhanced to address these issues and concerns.

The Postharvest Biology and Technology series features edited books that address several aspects related to postharvest technology of fresh produce. The series presents existing and novel management systems that are in use today or that have great potential to maintain the postharvest quality of fresh produce in terms of microbiological safety, nutrition, and sensory quality.

The books are aimed at professionals, postharvest scientists, academicians researching postharvest problems, and graduate-level students. This series is intended to be a comprehensive venture that provides up-to-date scientific and technical information focusing on postharvest management for fresh produce.

Books in the series address the following themes:

- Nutritional composition and antioxidant properties of fresh produce
- Postharvest physiology and biochemistry
- Biotic and abiotic factors affecting maturity and quality
- Preharvest treatments affecting postharvest quality
- Maturity and harvesting issues
- Nondestructive quality assessment
- Physiological and biochemical changes during ripening
- Postharvest treatments and their effects on shelf life and quality

- Postharvest operations such as sorting, grading, ripening, de-greening, curing etc.
- Storage and shelf-life studies
- Packaging, transportation, and marketing
- Vase life improvement of flowers and foliage
- Postharvest management of spice, medicinal, and plantation crops
- Fruit and vegetable processing waste/byproducts: management and utilization
- Postharvest diseases and physiological disorders
- Minimal processing of fruits and vegetables
- Quarantine and phytosanitory treatments for fresh produce
- Conventional and modern breeding approaches to improve the postharvest quality
- Biotechnological approaches to improve postharvest quality of horticultural crops

BOOKS IN THE SERIES

Postharvest Biology and Technology of Horticultural Crops: Principles and Practices for Quality Maintenance
Editor: Mohammed Wasim Siddiqui, PhD

Insect Pests of Stored Grain: Biology, Behavior, and Management Strategies
Ranjeet Kumar, PhD

Postharvest Management of Horticultural Crops: Practices for Quality Preservation
Editors: Mohammed Wasim Siddiqui, PhD, and Asgar Ali, PhD

Innovative Packaging of Fruits and Vegetables: Strategies for Safety and Quality Maintenance
Editors: Mohammed Wasim Siddiqui, PhD,
Mohammad Shafiur Rahman, PhD, and Ali Abas Wani, PhD

Advances in Postharvest Technologies of Vegetable Crops
Editors: Bijendra Singh, PhD, Sudhir Singh, PhD, and
Tanmay K. Koley, PhD

Plant Food By-Products: Industrial Relevance for Food Additives and Nutraceuticals
Editors: J. Fernando Ayala-Zavala, PhD, Gustavo González-Aguilar, PhD, and Mohammed Wasim Siddiqui, PhD

Emerging Technologies for Shelf-Life Enhancement of Fruits
Editors: Basharat Nabi Dar, PhD, and Shabir Ahmad Mir, PhD

Sensor-Based Quality Assessment Systems for Fruits and Vegetables
Editors: Bambang Kuswandi, PhD, and Mohammed Wasim Siddiqui, PhD

Emerging Postharvest Treatment of Fruits and Vegetables
Editors: Kalyan Barman, PhD, Swati Sharma, PhD, and Mohammed Wasim Siddiqui, PhD

Packaging and Storage of Fruits and Vegetables: Emerging Trends
Editor: Tanweer Alam, PhD

Postharvest Physiological Disorders of Fruits
Editors: Ghulam Khaliq, PhD, and Sajid Ali, PhD

Bioengineered Fruit and Vegetables: Trends in Postharvest Quality Improvement
Editors: Mohammad Irfan, PhD, and Pankaj Kumar, PhD

Novel Packaging Systems for Fruits and Vegetables
Editors: Kirtiraj K. Gaikwad, PhD, and Suman Singh, PhD

Ozone Applications in the Food Industry: Trends and Future Prospects
Editors: Ravi Pandiselvam, PhD, Anjineyulu Kothakota, PhD, and Kaavya Rathnakumar, PhD

Nonthermal Food Processing Technologies: Impact on Color Profile
Editors: Kaavya Rathnakumar, PhD, and R. Pandiselvam, PhD

Ready-to-Eat Snacks: Emerging Technologies for Production and Safety
Editors: R. Pandiselvam, PhD and Gülşah Çalışkan Koç, PhD

Handbook of Research on Mango Fruit: Postharvest Science, Production, Nutrition, and Processing Technology
Editors: Sajjad Hussain, PhD, Kamrun Nahar, PhD, Ishtiaq A. Rajwana, PhD, Sezai Ercisli, PhD, and Shakeel Ahmad, PhD

Sustainable Approaches in Postharvest Handling and Management
Editor: Pankaj B. Pathare, PhD

Physiological Disorders of Fruits and Vegetables: Causes and Remedies
Editors: Ghulam Khaliq, PhD, Sajid Ali, PhD, and Mohammed Wasim Siddiqui, PhD

About the Series Editor

Mohammed Wasim Siddiqui, PhD
Scientist-cum-Assistant Professor, Department of Food Science and Technology, Bihar Agricultural University, Sabour, Bhagalpur, Bihar, India

Mohammed Wasim Siddiqui, PhD, is an Assistant Professor and Scientist in the Department of Food Science and Post-Harvest Technology, Bihar Agricultural University, Sabour, India, and author or co-author of peer-reviewed research articles, book chapters, two manuals, and conference papers. He has over 20 edited and an authored books to his credit, published by Elsevier, CRC Press, Springer, and Apple Academic Press. Dr. Siddiqui has established the international peer-reviewed *Journal of Postharvest Technology.* He is Editor-in-Chief of two book series *(Postharvest Biology and Technology and Innovations in Horticultural Science)*, published by Apple Academic Press. Dr. Siddiqui is also a Senior Acquisitions Editor for Apple Academic Press, USA, for Horticultural Science. He has been serving as an editorial board member and active reviewer of several international journals.

Dr. Siddiqui has received several grants and respected awards for his research work by a number of organizations. He is an active member of the organizing committees of several national and international seminars, conferences, and summits. He is one of key members in establishing the World Food Preservation Center (WFPC), LLC, USA, and is currently an active associate and supporter.

Dr. Siddiqui acquired a BSc (Agriculture) degree from Jawaharlal Nehru Krishi Vishwa Vidyalaya, Jabalpur, India. He received his MSc (Horticulture) and PhD (Horticulture) degrees from Bidhan Chandra Krishi Viswavidyalaya, Mohanpur, Nadia, India, with specialization in Postharvest Technology. He is a member of Core Research Group at the Bihar Agricultural University (BAU), which provides appropriate direction and assistance in prioritizing research.

About the Editor

Pankaj B. Pathare, PhD
Associate Professor, Department of Soils, Water and Agricultural Engineering, College of Agricultural and Marine Sciences, Sultan Qaboos University, Muscat, Oman

Pankaj Pathare, PhD, is an Associate Professor of Postharvest Technology at Sultan Qaboos University (SQU), Oman. He holds a BTech degree in Agricultural Engineering from Dr. Panjabrao Deshmukh Krishi Vidyapeeth, Akola (India); an MEngg degree from Maharana Pratap University of Agriculture and Technology, Udaipur (India); and a PhD in Process and Chemical Engineering from University College Cork, Ireland. Before joining SQU, he worked as a researcher at Newcastle University, UK, and Stellenbosch University, South Africa. Over the years, he has gained expertise in postharvest technology and food engineering, including quantification of postharvest losses during transportation, mechanical damage to perishables, food agglomeration/granulation, food drying and cooling, structural design for ventilated corrugated packaging, renewable energy in food processing for Sub-Saharan Africa, and energy-efficient production processes in the SME food and beverage industry. His research is well documented in 85 original scientific papers published in international peer-reviewed journals, along with numerous conference presentations. He has also served as supervisor or co-supervisor for 15 postgraduate research students and has examined more than 11 doctoral theses at various institutions. Dr. Pathare has been invited as a keynote or invited speaker at over 15 international conferences in the field of postharvest and food engineering. He was recognized among the World's Top 2% Scientists, as published by Stanford University, USA, in 2021 and 2022. He serves on the editorial boards of several research journals, including *PLOS ONE, Frontiers in Sustainable Food Systems, AgriEngineering, Journal of Food Quality, Journal of Food Processing and Preservation, Open Agriculture, Measurement: Food, Discover Food, Journal of Agricultural and Marine Sciences, and Current Functional Foods.*

Contents

Contributors

Mai Al-Dairi
Department of Soils, Water and Agricultural Engineering, College of Agricultural and Marine Sciences, Sultan Qaboos University, Muscat, Oman

Saadia Ambreen
University Institute of Food Science and Technology, The University of Lahore, Lahore, Punjab, Pakistan

Hudda Ayub
National Institute of Food Science and Technology, University of Agriculture, Faisalabad, Punjab, Pakistan

Zinash A. Belay
Agri-Food Systems and Omics Laboratory, Post-Harvest and Agro-Processing Technologies (PHATs), Agricultural Research Council (ARC) – Infruitec-Nietvoorbij, Stellenbosch, South Africa

Oluwafemi J. Caleb
Department of Food Science, Faculty of AgriSciences, Stellenbosch University, Stellenbosch, South Africa; Africa Institute for Postharvest Technology, Faculty of AgriSciences, Stellenbosch University, Stellenbosch, South Africa

Saowapa Chaiwong
School of Agro-Industry, Mae Fah Luang University, Chiang Rai, Thailand; Integrated Agri-Tech Ecosystem Research Group, Mae Fah Luang University, Chiang Rai, Thailand

Ajay Chinchkar
Department of Food Science and Technology, National Institute of Food Technology Entrepreneurship and Management (NIFTEM), Sonipat, Haryana, India

Amit Baran Das
Department of Food Engineering and Technology, Tezpur University, Napaam, Sonitpur, Assam, India

Rohini Dhenge
Department of Food and Drug, University of Parma, Parma, Italy

Olaniyi Amos Fawole
Department of Botany and Plant Biotechnology, South African Research Chairs Initiative in Sustainable Preservation and Agroprocessing Research, Postharvest and Agroprocessing Research Centre, University of Johannesburg, Auckland Park, Gauteng, South Africa; UNESCO International Centre for Biotechnology, Nsukka, Enugu, Nigeria

Tommaso Ganino
Department of Food and Drug, University of Parma, Parma, Italy

Guillermo Garcia-Garcia
Department of Chemical Engineering, Faculty of Sciences, University of Granada, Granada, Spain

Sumit Gupta
Department of Mechanical Engineering, Amity School of Engineering and Technology, Amity University, Noida, Uttar Pradesh, India

Nasser Al Habsi
Department of Food Science and Nutrition, College of Agricultural and Marine Sciences, Sultan Qaboos University, Al-Khod, Muscat, Oman

Norhashila Hashim
Department of Biological and Agricultural Engineering, Faculty of Engineering, Universiti Putra Malaysia, Selangor, Malaysia; SMART Farming Technology Research Centre (SFTRC), Faculty of Engineering, Universiti Putra Malaysia, Selangor, Malaysia

Abdo Hassoun
Faculty of Agricultural Engineering, University of Aleppo, Aleppo, Syria; Sustainable AgriFoodtech Innovation & Research (SAFIR), Arras, France

Imtiaz Hussain
Department of Food Science and Technology, University of Poonch, Rawalakot, Pakistan

Sandeep Jagtap
Sustainable Manufacturing Systems Centre, Cranfield University, Cranfield, United Kingdom; Division of Engineering Logistics, Lund University, Lund, Sweden

Abhimanyu Kalne
Department of Agricultural Process and Food Engineering, Indira Gandhi Agricultural University (IGAU), Raipur, Chhattisgarh, India

Gaganjyot Kaur
Department of Processing and Food Engineering, Punjab Agricultural University, Ludhiana, Punjab, India

Gurjeet Kaur
Department of Processing and Food Engineering, Punjab Agricultural University, Ludhiana, Punjab, India

Preetinder Kaur
Department of Processing and Food Engineering, Punjab Agricultural University, Ludhiana, Punjab, India

Maha Al Khalili
Department of Food Science and Nutrition, College of Agricultural and Marine Sciences, Sultan Qaboos University, Al-Khod, Muscat, Oman

Faima Atta Khan
Department of Food Science, Faculty of Life Sciences, Government College University, Faisalabad, Punjab, Pakistan

Rasaq O. Lamidi
Centre for Sustainable Cooling, School of Chemical Engineering, University of Birmingham, Birmingham, United Kingdom

Yang Luo
School of Intelligent Manufacturing Ecosystem, Xi'an Jiaotong-Liverpool University, Suzhou, Jiangsu, China

Naveen Kumar Mahanti
Post Harvest Technology Research Station, Dr. Y. S. R. Horticultural University, Tadepalligudem, Andhra Pradesh, India

Hameed B. Mahood
Centre for Sustainable Cooling, School of Chemical Engineering, University of Birmingham, Birmingham, United Kingdom

Harold K. Malahlela
Department of Food Science, Faculty of AgriSciences, Stellenbosch University, Stellenbosch, South Africa; Africa Institute for Postharvest Technology, Faculty of AgriSciences, Stellenbosch University, Stellenbosch, South Africa

Bernard Maringgal
Faculty of Resource Science and Technology, Universiti Malaysia Sarawak, Sarawak, Malaysia

Wayne Martindale
MPC Research Ltd, DMC, County Way, Barnsley, United Kingdom

Arjun Mohanakumar
Department of Food and Drug, University of Parma, Parma, Italy

Dababandya Mohapatra
Automation and Plant Engineering Division, ICAR–National Institute of Secondary Agriculture, Ranchi, Jharkhand, India

Rebogile R. Mphahlele
Department of Agriculture, Private Bag, Pretoria, South Africa

C. Nickhil
Department of Food Engineering and Technology, Tezpur University, Napaam, Sonitpur, Assam, India

Ikechukwu Kingsley Opara
Faculty of AgriSciences, Africa Institute for Postharvest Technology, South African Research Chair in Postharvest Technology, Stellenbosch University, Stellenbosch, Western Cape, South Africa

Umezuruike Linus Opara
Faculty of AgriSciences, Africa Institute for Postharvest Technology, South African Research Chair in Postharvest Technology, Stellenbosch University, Stellenbosch, Western Cape, South Africa; UNESCO International Centre for Biotechnology, Nsukka, Enugu, Nigeria

Krishna Kumar Patel
Department of Food Processing and Agricultural Structure, Baba Saheb Dr. Bhim Rao Ambedkar College of Agricultural Engineering and Technology (Etawah), Chandra Shekhar Azad University of Agriculture and Technology, Kanpur, Uttar Pradesh, India

Pankaj B. Pathare
Department of Soils, Water and Agricultural Engineering, College of Agricultural and Marine Sciences, Sultan Qaboos University, Muscat, Oman

Dilip Pawar
Agro Produce Processing Division, ICAR–Central Institute of Agricultural Engineering, Bhopal, Madhya Pradesh, India

Chureerat Prahsarn
National Metal and Materials Technology Center, National Science and Technology Development Agency, Pathum Thani, Thailand

Muhammad Abdul Rahim
Department of Food Science, Faculty of Life Sciences, Government College University, Faisalabad, Punjab, Pakistan

Jutarat Rattanakaran
Integrated Agri-Tech Ecosystem Research Group, Mae Fah Luang University, Chiang Rai, Thailand

Laxmi Kant Rawat
Department of Food Engineering and Technology, Tezpur University, Napaam, Sonitpur, Assam, India

Jagbir Rehal
Department of Food Science and Technology, Punjab Agricultural University, Ludhiana, Punjab, India

Massimiliano Rinaldi
Department of Food and Drug, University of Parma, Parma, Italy

Rattapon Saengrayap
School of Agro-Industry, Mae Fah Luang University, Chiang Rai, Thailand; Integrated Agri-Tech Ecosystem Research Group, Mae Fah Luang University, Chiang Rai, Thailand

Ravinun Saengwong-Ngam
Integrated Agri-Tech Ecosystem Research Group, Mae Fah Luang University, Chiang Rai, Thailand

Aurbab Shoukat
National Institute of Food Science and Technology, University of Agriculture, Faisalabad, Punjab, Pakistan

Laraib Shoukat
Department of Biochemistry, Faculty of Life Sciences, Government College University, Faisalabad, Punjab, Pakistan

Gunnar O. Sigge
Department of Food Science, Faculty of AgriSciences, Stellenbosch University, Stellenbosch, South Africa

Hana Trollman
School of Management, College of Business, University of Leicester, Leicester, United Kingdom

Tatiya Trongsatitkul
School of Polymer Engineering, Institute of Engineering, Suranaree University of Technology, Nakhon Ratchasima, Thailand

Loriane A. Yanclo
Department of Food Science, Faculty of AgriSciences, Stellenbosch University, Stellenbosch, South Africa; Agri-Food Systems and Omics Laboratory, Post-Harvest and Agro-Processing Technologies, Agricultural Research Council (ARC) – Infruitec-Nietvoorbij, Stellenbosch, South Africa; Africa Institute for Postharvest Technology, Faculty of AgriSciences, Stellenbosch University, Stellenbosch, South Africa

Abbreviations

ACP	atmospheric cold plasma
AEW	acidic electrolyzed water
AEW	alkaline electrolyzed water
ALF	aluminum foil
ATP	adenosine triphosphate
BCT	box compression test
BOPP	biaxially oriented polypropylene
CA	controlled atmosphere
CAC	Codex Alimentarius Commission
$CaCl^2$	calcium chloride
CAP	cold atmospheric plasma
CCF	corrugated common footprint
CD	celiac disease
CFB	corrugated fiberboard box
CFC	corrugated fiberboard cartons
CFD	computational fluid dynamics
CR	computed radiography
CRM	confocal Raman microspectroscopy
CV	computer vision
DBD	dielectric barrier discharge
ECT	edge crush test
EPE	expanded polyethylene
EPRI	Electric Power Research Institute
EU	European Union
EW	electrolyzed water
FAC	free available chlorine
FAO	Food and Agriculture Organization
FC	fresh cut
FDA	Food and Drug Administration
FEFCO	European Federation of Corrugated Board Manufacturers

FFV	fresh fruits and vegetables
FID	free induction decay
FSP	fig seed powder
FTD	full telescope design
FTHS	full telescope Hak slotted
GDP	gross domestic product
GHG	greenhouse gas
GPS	global positioning system
GRAS	generally recognized as safe
GSHP	ground source heat pump
H2O2	hydrogen peroxide
HDPE	high-density polyethylene
HPP	high hydrostatic pressure
IAEA	International Atomic Energy Agency
INDEX	inside-needle dynamic extraction
IPFI	International Project in the field of Food Irradiation
ISO	International Organization for Standardization
KCl	potassium chloride
LAC	linear attenuation coefficient
LDA	linear discriminant analysis
MAP	modified atmosphere packaging
MASLT	multivariate accelerated shelf-life testing
MDS	molecular dynamics simulation
MgCl2	magnesium chloride
MIMS	membrane introduction mass spectrometry
MPa	megapascals
MRI	magnetic resonance imaging
MSI	multispectral imaging
NEW	neutral electrolyzed water
NHB	National Horticultural Board
NIR	near infrared
NIRS	near-infrared spectroscopy
NMR	nuclear magnetic resonance
NMRI	nuclear magnetic resonance imaging
NRL	natural rubber latex
NSP	Na^2CO^3-soluble pectin

O^2	oxygen
O^3	ozone
OHC	oil holding capacities
ORP	oxidation-reduction potential
P&T	purge and trap
PD	power density
PDCAAS	protein digestibility-corrected amino acid score
PE	polyethylene
PG	polygalacturonase
PHL	Postharvest loss
PIR	polyisocyanurate
PL	pulsed light
PO	polyolefin
POD	peroxidase
PP	polypropylene
PPO	polyphenol oxidase
PS	polystyrene
PSK	pumpkin seed kernel
PU	polyurethane
PVA	polyvinyl alcohol
QR	quick response
RF	radio frequency
RFID	radio frequency identification
ROS	reactive oxygen species
RPC	reusable plastic container
RSC	regular slotted carton
RSC	regular slotted container
RSM	response surface methodology
SBSE	stir bar sportive extraction
SCF	Scientific Committee on Food
SD	Sprague-Dawley
SHS	static headspace
SNR	signal-to-noise ratio
SOD	superoxide dismutase
SPME	solid-phase microextraction
SSC	soluble solid content

SVM	support vector machine
TA	titratable acidity
TKP	tamarind kernel powder
TSS	total soluble solid
UV	ultraviolet
WHO	World Health Organization
WSF	watermelon seed flour
WSN	wireless sensor networks

Acknowledgments

As the editor of this book, I am grateful to all of my research collaborators for their invaluable contributions. I wish to express my sincere gratitude to Sultan Qaboos University, Muscat, Oman, for providing the opportunity, facilities, and support to execute such an exciting book project. I sincerely acknowledge my parents and teachers for their unconditional contributions to our educational progress and support in life. I acknowledge my wife, Sneha, my two lovely daughters, Parvi and Shaarvi, and my siblings for their kind support, encouragement, and patience throughout the project. Special thanks to my colleagues and other research team members for their support and encouragement.

Foreword

One of the most important fronts in our quest for a more sustainable food system is reducing postharvest losses. An enormous quantity of fruits, vegetables, and other agricultural products perishes every year due to spoilage after harvest. In addition to being a massive waste of resources, this contributes to food insecurity for millions of people worldwide.

This book, *Sustainable Approaches in Postharvest Handling and Management*, offers a beacon of hope in this fight. It delves into the exciting realm of sustainable postharvest practices, illuminating a path toward a future where we can minimize losses and ensure that fresh, nutritious produce reaches consumers.

Once harvest is complete, a new challenge arises: preserving the quality and freshness of produce. This book serves as a guide to postharvest handling and the sustainable practices that ensure perishables reach consumers in optimal condition.

The book is distinct in a number of ways. It includes contributions from world-renowned experts who have devoted their professional lives to researching the postharvest handling and management of fresh food produce. There are numerous ways to reduce losses and enhance food safety, including handling procedures to stop the spread of pathogens, cold storage, and refrigerated transportation. Sustainable postharvest handling practices reduce losses and contamination while maximizing productivity and minimizing the use of energy and non-renewable resources.

However, this book offers more than just technical justifications. It highlights the significance of sustainability and promotes actions that are not only resource-efficient but also environmentally friendly. Readers will learn about the applications of cold plasma, ozone, irradiation, electrolyzed water, edible coatings, and packaging for quality and safety. It also explores the integration of sustainable practices across the entire postharvest chain and the potential use of sustainable energy sources to power storage facilities.

This book is further distinguished by its coverage of advanced and highly relevant topics, including non-destructive techniques, electronic noses (e-nose), and the Internet of Things (IoT) in fresh produce handling.

It also addresses postharvest loss quantification and sustainability through postharvest value addition.

A wide range of users can benefit from sustainable postharvest handling practices. This book is a vital resource for farmers, scientists, students, and anyone else committed to developing a more sustainable food system. It provides the knowledge and motivation needed to put these practices into action and help create a future in which food waste is reduced and everyone has access to fresh, wholesome products.

This is not just a guidebook—it is a call to action. To ensure a more stable and abundant food supply for future generations, it urges us to embrace innovation and adopt sustainable practices. Together, let us embark on this journey and realize the full potential of sustainable postharvest handling and management.

I congratulate all the authors and editors for bringing forth a remarkable volume with the right content at the right time.

Dr. S. N. Jha
Deputy Director General (Agricultural Engineering),
Indian Council of Agricultural Research,
New Delhi, India

Preface

Increased urbanization, changing dietary preferences, and population growth are putting unprecedented strain on the world's food systems. The safety and quality of fruits and vegetables have become major concerns for consumers in recent times. Consequently, the fresh produce industry must ensure that its output is of the highest quality. As a result, guaranteeing the availability of fresh produce that is healthy, affordable, and safe has become a top priority. A key factor in addressing this issue is postharvest handling, which refers to the crucial time frame between harvest and consumption. Because of its significant scale, reducing postharvest losses will help create more resilient and sustainable food systems while also lowering greenhouse gas emissions. Various postharvest treatments are employed to minimize food loss; however, due to their high energy inefficiency and carbon footprint, some of these technologies are not sustainable. Immediate attention is needed to develop sustainable postharvest systems for fresh horticultural crops.

Sustainable postharvest handling and management techniques for fresh produce quality, safety, and shelf-life extension are covered in this book. A thorough review of sustainable postharvest methods is provided, along with information on the newest techniques, inventions, and technologies that can reduce food waste and loss while maintaining the freshness and nutritional content of produce. We can improve food security and make the agriculture industry more robust and ecologically friendly by using sustainable postharvest practices.

This book covers a wide range of topics related to sustainable postharvest handling, including sustainable postharvest methods such as edible coatings, irradiation, ozone, and cold plasma for quality, safety, and shelf-life extension. Quality detection through non-destructive techniques and electronic nose is also included. Opportunities to integrate Blockchain and the Internet of Things (IoT) in the fresh food supply chain to regain public trust by improving transparency and real-time visibility are discussed. It also covers the socioeconomic and environmental impacts of postharvest losses. Due to numerous countries' developing economies and rising energy demands, the amount of energy needed is increasing dramatically. Reducing fossil energy consumption and improving product quality through the use of sustainable energy as the primary or supplemental energy for postharvest operations could lessen the environmental effect of these activities. Moreover, technologies and methods for protein extraction from food processing waste are included in order to maximize sustainability.

We believe that this book will serve as a valuable resource for researchers, students, farmers, food processors, and policymakers who are committed to building a more sustainable and equitable food system. By working together, we can create a future where fresh produce is accessible to all and its production and consumption have a minimal negative impact on our planet. The editor is confident that readers will find this book informative and interesting.

We are grateful to all the authors for contributing chapters to this book. We are also thankful to the staff of the editorial and production departments of Apple Academic Press for their support and efforts in bringing this book to publication.

CHAPTER 1

Overview of Sustainable Approaches to Reduce Postharvest Losses

PANKAJ B. PATHARE* and MAI AL-DAIRI

Department of Soils, Water and Agricultural Engineering, College of Agricultural and Marine Sciences, Sultan Qaboos University, Muscat, Oman

*Corresponding author

ABSTRACT

Fruit and vegetables are very important for human diets, and their consumption has increased in recent years. Fruit and vegetables show numerous beneficial effects, as they help to decrease susceptibility to cardiovascular diseases, cancer, diabetes, high blood pressure, and other chronic diseases. Fruit and vegetables are highly prone to a high occurrence of postharvest loss during the postharvest supply chain processes (sorting, storing, packaging, transporting, handling, and marketing). Losses in fresh produce include damage, decay, weight reduction, senescence, discoloration, and so forth, which make them not acceptable for consumption by consumers. Hence, reducing postharvest losses in fresh produce by using sustainable, eco-friendly, and cost-effective approaches and technologies is very important to reach sustainable development goals. Developing these technologies will allow wholesalers, warehouses, retailers, packaging, and transportation companies along the fresh produce supply chain to guarantee the ideal quality and prolonged shelf life of fresh produce. These technologies include irradiation, cold plasma, ozone, electrolyte water, ethylene management, edible coating, packaging, non-destructive methods, biosensors, and value addition. Measuring loss quantities during

Sustainable Approaches in Postharvest Handling and Management: Pankaj B. Pathare (Ed.)

DOI: 10.1201/9781779641076-1

the postharvest supply chain of fresh produce can help to estimate the magnitude of loss and will provide sufficient strategies for reducing such loss. Ideal postharvest treatments for fresh produce seek to delay/slow down the physiological processes of senescence and maturation, inhibit the development of physiological disorders, and decrease the risk of contamination and microbial growth.

1.1 INTRODUCTION

Fruit and vegetables are a significant portion of the food supply chain, where both are depended on globally for good nutrition and health. Fresh fruit and vegetables are rich in nutrients, bright in color, and highly beneficial to human health (Zhang et al., 2021). In the daily diet, fruit and vegetables have been strongly linked with reducing the risk for some types of cancer, stroke, heart disease, and other chronic diseases. Some elements of fruit and vegetables are considered strong antioxidants, and they function to modify the metabolic activation or even impact processes that change the course of the tumor cell (Hailu and Derbew, 2015). Demands for fruit and vegetables are increasing in parallel with the worldwide population growth. In 2016, 1.07 billion tons of fresh vegetables were produced globally from more than 57 million hectares of land. Besides, from 65 million hectares of land, 865 million tons of fresh fruit were produced (Elik et al., 2019).

Despite all the benefits obtained from fruits and vegetables, fresh produce easily and quickly deteriorates in quality during the postharvest supply chain processes like handling, transportation, storage, and retail, resulting in high losses and showing a huge economic value reduction (Zhang et al., 2021). The rate of postharvest losses is highly occurring in developing and underdeveloped countries (Elik et al., 2019). Postharvest losses mainly result from biological spoilage because of inappropriate postharvest management practices, including improper handling systems of storage or packaging, inadequate transportation facilities, and unfavorable climatic conditions of low relative humidity and high temperatures. Thus, significant environmental and economic losses are caused by the failure to delay ripening and excessive softening of fruits between harvesting and marketing, while reduction of water from fresh fruit and vegetables negatively affects their quality (Kalaïtzis and Craita, 2016). The occurrence of postharvest losses in the fresh fruit and vegetable value chain is a worldwide concern challenging food safety, security, and sustainability.

Mechanical damage to agricultural products is one of the key issues during harvest and postharvest supply chain, resulting in shelf-life reduction (Al-Dairi et al., 2022). Due to inappropriate management of postharvest operations, 50% of cultivated fruits and vegetables are lost (Elik et al., 2019) with an estimated economic loss of $750 billion per annum (Opara, Fawole, and Opara, 2021). In other words, half of the cultivated fresh fruits and vegetables (FFVs) are lost before reaching the stage of consumption (Elik et al., 2019).

In recent years, delivering secure, quality, and safe edible fresh fruit and vegetables for consumers has become an important issue in the food supply chain (Al-Dairi et al., 2022). Postharvest loss reduction plays a vital role in sustainably feeding the population in the future. Thus, improving postharvest technologies like good harvesting, packaging, sorting, storing, and transporting systems are very essential in minimizing and preventing fresh produce postharvest losses as well as improving the quality attributes of fruit and vegetables so that more produce is actually consumed (Porat et al., 2018). Developing such postharvest technologies will permit warehouses, wholesalers, retailers, and transportation companies along the fresh produce value chain to ensure ideal quality and prolonged shelf life (Kalaïtzis and Craita, 2016). Ideal postharvest treatments for fresh fruit and vegetables seek to delay the physiological processes of maturation and senescence, inhibit/decrease the development of physiological disorders, and minimize the risk of contamination and microbial growth (Al-Dairi et al., 2023b).

Recently, many researchers have developed several postharvest preservation techniques to extend the shelf life and decrease postharvest losses of fresh fruit and vegetables (Zhang et al., 2020). Currently, some chemical preservatives like 1-methylcyclopropene (1-MCP, which has been fully commercialized) are frequently utilized (Zhang et al., 2020). Besides, several natural chemical preservatives in their development stage have attracted the attention of many researchers, like methyl jasmonate (Seo et al., 2020), calcium chloride (Gharezi, Joshi, and Sadeghian, 2012), methyl salicylate (Ge et al., 2020), melatonin (Aghdam et al., 2020), and nitric oxide. Also, cold storage is considered the most common and effective preservation method and is highly used for postharvest storage and preservation of the majority of fresh fruit and vegetables. Cold storage could decline the metabolic activity of plant cells, slow down senescence, and maintain the quality of fresh produce (Rajapaksha et al., 2021).

Cold storages are essentially built to control the respiration and transpiration rate, microorganism growth, and to preserve the fresh produce in the most useable form for the consumer. However, for tropical and subtropical fruit and vegetables, cold storage could cause chilling injuries, therefore leading to quality deterioration (Zhang et al., 2020). Hot water treatment, controlled atmosphere storage and modified atmosphere storage (Rai, Kumari, and Vashistha, 2022), low oxygen storage (Affandi et al., 2021), and solar drying (Hailu and Derbew, 2015) are some other technologies used to minimize postharvest losses.

Many studies have investigated the use of alternative sustainable treatments that are cost-effective and environmentally friendly. This chapter provides an overview of the most innovative sustainable approaches that are practiced to reduce postharvest losses in the value chain, including nonthermal (irradiation, cold plasma, ozone), electrolyte water, ethylene management, edible coating, packaging, nondestructive methods, biosensors, and value addition. Besides, loss quantification is also mentioned, as it assesses the loss during the supply chain, which can determine the magnitude of loss, and subsequently helps to identify the strategies to reduce it.

1.2 DIFFERENT SUSTAINABLE APPROACHES TO REDUCE POSTHARVEST LOSSES

1.2.1 NONTHERMAL

1.2.1.1 IRRADIATION

In postharvest treatment of fresh fruit and vegetables, irradiation has been utilized for decades. The irradiation is used to: (1) defect sorting, where defected fruit is separated from healthy fruit; (2) control of pathogenic microorganisms and spoilage; (3) enhance bioactive compounds; (4) delay fresh produce senescence and ripening; and (5) control human pathogens that can contaminate fresh produce (Zulkifli et al., 2019). Ultraviolet (UV) irradiation emerged as an alternative technique used as postharvest phytosanitary treatment (Mditshwa et al., 2017). UV irradiation has been used to maintain and preserve the nutritional quality attributes of fresh produce by decreasing the chilling symptoms (Rai, Kumari, and Vashistha, 2022). UV irradiation is used to enhance the lycopene content and other nutritional qualities in tomatoes without changing the physical attributes of the fruit (Liu, Jahangir, and Ying, 2012).

There are three types of UV irradiation, including UV-A (400–315 nm – high level), UV-B (315–280 nm – medium level), and UV-C (280–100 nm – low level). Medium and high-level doses are not suitable for fresh fruit and vegetables due to their ability to cause some sensory defects (flavor, visual, and texture) and expedited senescence because of the irreparable damage to proteins and DNA (Mahajan et al., 2014).

UV-C irradiation is frequently utilized in sterilizing food products to control foodborne diseases (Mditshwa et al., 2017). Ultraviolet (UV-C) irradiation has been reported to be successful in slowing down fruit and vegetable ripening. Exposure to low doses of UV-C delayed chlorophyll degradation, senescence, and ripening of many produce like tomatoes, apples, strawberries, mango, and broccoli (Sripong et al., 2015). UV-C-treated produce like tomatoes has recorded resistance to decay and microbial growth, reduced the loss of vitamins C and E, and led to higher content of phenolic compounds, flavonoids, and antioxidant capacity (Mditshwa et al., 2017). The study by George and Razali (George et al., 2015) supported the use of UV-C treatment for better retention of mango fruit quality, promoting compounds for the benefit of consumers, and efficient microbial inactivation.

1.2.1.2 COLD PLASMA

Plasma technology is a novel approach to maintaining quality and inactivating spoilage microorganisms and pathogens of processed and fresh produce. It is an accepted technology for industry, and this is because of its relatively low input cost. Plasma is generally known as the fourth state of matter, after gases, liquids, and solids. Plasma is more gaseous than a liquid or solid, but its property differs from liquid, solid, and gas. There are two major types of plasma distinguished based on thermodynamics: thermal plasma and non-thermal plasma (cold plasma, temperature $< 60°C$). Hence, cold plasma is chosen to be applied to various foods involving fruit and vegetables to prevent the loss of sensory and nutritional contributions (Uthairatanakij et al., 2023).

Cold plasma is one of the important non-thermal food preservation technologies and is considered a new intervention for food safety improvement (Niemira, 2012). The application of cold plasma technology has been reported to be extremely effective in the sanitation of fruits and vegetables and prolongs their shelf life. Cold plasma can be generated by a combination of electrical discharge and atmospheric gas under atmospheric or lower pressure and vacuum conditions as well. This technology can provide safe fresh produce without affecting its nutrient and sensory qualities. The effectiveness of the various cold plasma application techniques highly depends on produce type, surface area properties, the initial microbial load, and several other operational parameters that need optimization to accomplish desirable results (Pathare et al., 2023).

For dielectric barrier discharge (DBD) cold plasma, both low and atmospheric pressure are used. The DBD cold plasma has been performed to enhance several agricultural products (Rashvand et al., 2022) like fresh-cut apples (Ramazzina et al., 2016), mushrooms (Gavahian, and Khaneghah, 2020), kiwifruit (Figure 1.1A) (Ramazzina et al., 2015), tomato (Ali, Cheng, and Sun, 2021), pear (Berardinelli et al., 2011), and strawberry (Figure 1.1B) (Ahmadnia et al., 2021). Cold plasma technology is not only influencing the chemical quality attributes of fresh produce but also can influence the mechanical properties. Rashvand, Hajizadeh (2022) investigated the influence of the DBD cold plasma technology on the mechanical attributes of plums during storage for 20 days. Their study reported that treating the fruit with DBD cold plasma technology for 10 minutes had an acceptable effect on the bio yield stress, Young's modulus, and tangent modulus trends during the 20 days of storage. This emphasized the DBD cold plasma method can enhance plums' resistance to deformation and decrease the bruise volume and bruise susceptibility resulted from impact damage.

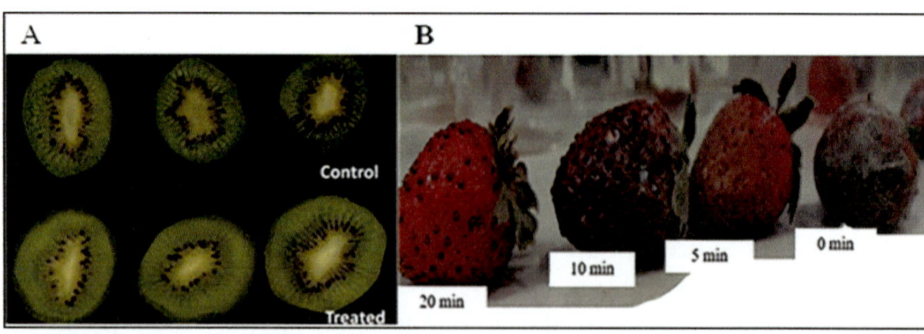

FIGURE 1.1 Kiwifruit slices subjected to 20 + 20 min DBD gas plasma treatment and control ones obtained after 4 days of storage in controlled conditions (A); and strawberry samples treated by 14% duty cycle dielectric barrier discharge plasma at different durations after 12 days of storage at 6°C (B).

1.2.1.3 OZONE

Ozone (O_3) is a triatomic oxygen molecule with a high oxidative reduction potential. It is unstable, and when it decomposes, it develops radicals like water, hydrogen, carbon dioxide, as well as carbon monoxide (Bambalele et al., 2021). In liquid form, ozone can be utilized to disinfect processing water and vegetables, and in its gaseous form, ozone assists in sanitizing, controlling, and preserving the quality of FFVs during storage (Sarron, Gadonna-Widehem, and Aussenac, 2021). The utilization of ozone to maintain the quality of fresh produce and prolong the shelf-life of horticultural commodities has been widely used and documented (Shezi et al., 2020). Emerging evidence found that ozone is a very effective way of maintaining firmness, reducing weight loss, and extending the shelf-life of produce (Minas et al., 2014; Tran et al., 2013). Tran, Aimla-Or (2013) recorded a reduction in respiration rate in mango fruit fumigated with 10 $\mu L\ L^{-1}\ O_3$ for 10 minutes during six days of storage at 25°C.

Toti and Carboni (2018) found that gaseous ozone treatment decreased the activity of cell wall enzymes such as polygalacturonase, α-arabinopyranosidase, and β-galactopyranosidase, which slow down fruit softening and preserve the quality of cantaloupe melon. Chen et al. (2016) concluded that ozone treatment (6.42 mg cm^{-3} for 15 min) improved the effectiveness of the antioxidant defense system of fresh-cut green peppers. The results of Chen et al. (2020) reported that cantaloupe subjected to the proper dose of ozone showed a lower ethylene production rate and respiration rate and higher levels of pectin content, firmness, titratable acidity, and reducing sugar of exocarp and sarcocarp. Horvitz and Cantalejo (2014) observed that papaya fruit exposed to 2.5 ppm ozone included higher levels of β-carotene content, total soluble solids (TSS), ascorbic acid content, and antioxidant activity. Besides, ozone decreased weight loss at day 10 of storage compared with untreated papaya fruit. They also observed that the sensory attributes of papaya fruit treated with ozone were also superior in sweetness and other overall acceptability, which endorses ozone as a safe and non-thermal food and quality preservation technique for fresh fruit and vegetables.

1.2.2 ELECTROLYTE WATER

Electrolyte water (EW) treatment is an emerging, cost-effective, and environmentally friendly hurdle technique. It has a very strong antibacterial impact and has been revealed to be a scavenger of free radicals (Nyamende et al., 2021). EW is produced via electrolysis of tap water in the presence of a dilute salt (NaCl) solution, and it is safe for human contact (Kim and Hung, 2014). Postharvest application of electrolyte water has been shown to effectively and successfully manage microbial contaminations in pears (Al-Haq et al., 2002), citrus (Fallanaj et al., 2016), spinach, grapes, snap beans (Qi, Huang, and Hung, 2018), and apples (Nyamende et al., 2021).

Ferri, Yaseen (2015) studied the effect of 400 mg L^{-1} electrolyte water treatment on 'Cripps Pink' apple fruit during 4 months of storage at 1°C. It has been observed that EW treatment improved shelf life and storage quality and reduced the pesticide concentration in apple fruit. Besides, Nyamende, Belay (2022) found that EW maintained the capacity of antioxidants of apples compared to the non-treated fruit. They also demonstrated that EW treatment is considered an alternative approach to pack-house practices for apples. Li et al. (2020) recorded that EW maintained the phenolic content at a higher level and preserved glucosinolates in fresh-cut eggplants. Nutritional components such as carotenoids, vitamin C, and phenolics were maintained by EW treatment on fresh-cut mango as reported by de Almeida et al. (2021). It was also observed by Liu et al. (2021) that the browning degree of sweet potato slices of electrolyzed water treatment (55.98 mg/L) during 8 days of storage differed significantly. Browning-related enzymes polyphenol oxidase (PPO) and peroxidase activities of sweet potato were significantly inhibited by EW ($p < 0.05$).

1.2.3 ETHYLENE MANAGEMENT

Ethylene plays a very important role in the postharvest quality and life of many fruits and vegetables. Ethylene is a colorless gas with a faint sweetish smell that is the inherently produced ripening hormone of some fruits (Jobling, 2000). Exposing harvested horticultural crops to ethylene has been shown to have a beneficial or detrimental effect on FFVs, depending on its initial concentration, functional role, and extent of exposure. If ethylene exposure is not well managed, it can induce many physiological processes in fresh produce like softening, senescence, discoloration (Mabusela et al., 2021), shorter storage life, yellowing of leafy vegetables, russet spotting, and increased susceptibility to decay (Wills, 2005). Endogenous ethylene production and its exogenous application showed both deleterious and beneficial impacts on horticultural fresh produce. The beneficial consequences of exogenously applied ethylene involve improving the produce color, triggering ripening, and maintaining the quality of some horticultural crops like avocado, bananas, persimmon, kiwifruit, mangoes, tomatoes, and citrus (Mahajan et al., 2014).

Ethylene management plays a critical role in maintaining postharvest life and quality of climacteric as well as non-climacteric fresh produce. The most common commercial strategies for preserving horticultural crops include storing at lower temperatures, decreasing produce exposure to ethylene during ripening, blocking ethylene biosynthesis and its action, and controlling atmospheric gas composition and temperature during transportation and storage (Watkins, 2002).

1.2.4 EDIBLE COATING

Edible coating is a thin layer (< 0.3 mm) of biodegradable material coated or wrapped around the surface of fresh fruit and vegetables, which acts as a barrier for moisture content and gas exchange between the fresh produce and the surrounding environment (Uthairatanakij et al., 2023). Edible coatings are natural and comprised of antioxidants and vitamins, which are highly beneficial to the consumers. Edible coatings are mainly categorized into three main groups, including lipid-based materials (waxes and fatty acids), protein-based materials (soy protein, zein, whey protein, casein, gelatin, and albumin), and polysaccharide-based materials (cellulose, starch, alginate, chitosan, and gums) (Pascall and Lin, 2013). Besides, edible coatings are considered 'green technologies' because they are simple, eco-friendly, safe, and can be applied in liquid form by spraying, dipping, and brushing. The core characteristics of edible coatings are that they must be tasteless, food-safe, flexible, and odorless (Uthairatanakij et al., 2023).

Edible coatings possess anti-microbial and anti-browning characteristics that maintain the quality of fresh horticultural commodities (Bambalele et al., 2021), preserve color, maintain texture, retain natural aroma (Mahajan et al., 2014), slow down fruit respiration and ethylene production rate, and delay microbial growth (Kahramanoğlu et al., 2020). Edible coatings can also control many postharvest diseases and disorders like stem-end rot, anthracnose, and black spots in fresh produce (Gava et al., 2018). Hong and Xie (2012) reported that the application of 2%

chitosan in guava fruit stored at 11°C can maintain firmness, reduce weight loss, and slow down changes in sugar and acidity content during 12 days of storage. Numerous examples display the application of 'green' edible coatings to minimize postharvest losses and improve the shelf life of fresh produce shown in Table 1.1.

TABLE 1.1 Green Edible Coatings Used to Minimize Postharvest Losses and Improve Shelf Life of Fresh Produce

Fresh Produce	Type of Edible Coating	Major Outcomes	References
Rose apple	Sodium alginate solution mixed with 40 mL L^{-1} calcium chloride ($CaCl_2$)	Decreased the weight loss and respiration rate for 10 days at 13°C.	Duong et al. (2022)
Cherry tomatoes	1% peach gum polysaccharides	Decreased weight loss and respiration rate, maintained firmness, and extended the shelf.	Li, Tao, and Zhang (2017)
Banana	50% Aloe vera gel	Reduced weight loss, lowered the respiration rate, and increased the shelf life	Ratra, Kaur, and Thukral (2016)
Sweet cherry	5% Alginate	Decreased respiration rate and control fruit firmness and acidity compared to untreated fruit.	Díaz-Mula, Serrano, and Valero (2012)
Tomato	3% Carboxymethyl cellulose blended with 2% chitosan and wax	Extended the shelf life of tomato stored at 20–25°C for 24 days by delaying the ripening process.	Mandal et al. (2017)

1.2.5 PACKAGING

Packaging plays a vital role in maintaining fresh produce as it moves during the supply chain from farm to consumer (Porat et al., 2018). The critical advantages of packaging are to provide protection against harmful external factors that cause physical damage, to maintain fresh produce safety, to make the fresh produce clean from dirt, dust, and microbial contamination, to facilitate the display of fresh fruit and vegetable information including the identification and instructions of storage, to allow extension of the produce' shelf life by creating an environment with high-humidity (help to reduce shrinkage and water loss), low O_2, and high CO_2 concentrations that slow down senescence and ripening processes (Verghese et al., 2015). Thus, it is very important to design suitable packaging systems for the many types of fruit and vegetables. The package unit must permit proper ventilation and cooling and must match the respiratory behavior of the produce and its acceptances to low O_2 and high CO_2 environments, and storage and transportation temperatures as well (Porat et al., 2018).

Modified atmosphere packaging (MAP) contributed to increasing the shelf-life and preserving the quality of horticultural commodities (Bambalele et al., 2021). The beneficial influence of MAP in controlling the quality of fresh produce during transport and retail markets has been reported for many types of fresh produce (Porat et al., 2018). MAP includes the packaging of whole or fresh-cut fruit and vegetables in plastic film bags, which can be either passive or active (Mahajan et al., 2014). In passive MAP, the equilibrium concentrations of O_2 and CO_2 are a function of the product respiration rate and its weight, which is influenced by the temperature, surface area, thickness, perforations, and gas permeability of films utilized in packaging. In active MAP, the required atmosphere is provided in the package headspace before heat sealing; however, the final atmosphere will finally be a function of the same factors that impact passive MAP. Active modified atmospheric packaging involves some technologies that are used to adsorb substances, such as flavors/odors, ethylene, O_2, CO_2, and moisture, and release substances like CO_2, antioxidants, antimicrobial agents, and flavors (Mahajan et al., 2014; Minas et al., 2014).

1.2.6 NONDESTRUCTIVE

Among all mentioned emerging technologies, non-destructive techniques (computer vision, near-infrared spectroscopy (NIRS), electronic noses, thermal imaging, etc.) present many advantages over destructive and traditional methods (Al-Dairi et al., 2023b). There is an increasing interest in using non-destructive methods that provide rapid monitoring of fresh produce quality without any losses. Consumer interest in food safety and quality is increasing, mainly due to the international food trade, and this needs rapid and non-destructive inspection techniques (Ferreira et al., 2022). Non-destructive techniques are chemical-free analytical procedures that can measure the quality and do early detection of damage to fresh fruit and vegetables without destroying their system characteristics as well as functionality (Du et al., 2020).

There are many non-destructive techniques used to measure quality attributes and identify the quantitative degree of damage to reduce fresh produce losses and economical value, such as bio-speckle imaging for potatoes (Gao and Rao, 2019), computer vision systems for bananas (Al-Dairi et al., 2023a), hyperspectral imaging techniques for pears (Fu and Wang, 2021), and structured-illumination reflectance imaging for peaches (Sun et al., 2019), and so forth.

1.2.7 BIOSENSORS

Postharvest agriculture operations like harvesting, sorting, grading, storage, packaging, and transporting are complex. The demand for inexpensive and reliable techniques for the evaluation of fresh produce quality during the supply chain is expanding. Biosensors are among all emerging trends that can enhance the productivity and sustainability of fresh produce. Recently, biosensors are gaining popularity in all sectors from farms to consumers (Kundu et al., 2019). A biosensor is known as a combined receptor transducer system, with the capability of providing discriminative semi-quantitative or quantitative analytical description by means of a bio-recognition unit. It could also be described as an analytical system combining a bio-substance, a bio-derived substance, or a bio-mimic well linked with or within a physiochemical transducer, that might be electrochemical, optical, thermometric, magnetic, or piezoelectric (Shams et al., 2020).

Biosensors are used to enhance food quality, as these biosensors can identify contaminants like gases, metal ions, organic molecules, vapors, biomolecules, and other microbes. Besides, a biosensor includes a sensor component, which can measure electric potential and electric current, and it involves enzymes, antibodies, tissue, and living cells that act as bio-elements (Shams et al., 2020). Overall, biosensors immobilized with enzymes such as alcohol oxidase, alcohol peroxidase, and a chromogen can be utilized to recognize injuries resulting from less oxygen in broccoli, lettuce, cabbage, and cauliflower, which are lightly processed and packed in a modified atmosphere. They can also be used to identify ethanol in apples during storage in a controlled atmosphere and determine decay in potato tubers (Castillo et al., 2003).

1.2.8 VALUE ADDITION

Adding value to many horticultural products can enhance quality, improve farmers' income, reduce waste, and address food security concerns towards sustainability by reducing postharvest losses, improving production, reaching food security, and so forth (Al-Hinai, Jayasuriya and Pathare, 2022). Adding value to the initial/original crops can also help farmers overcome losses and spoilage and get high returns on the newly added technology. Value addition businesses are aimed at providing value to the raw commodities into multiple food products such as jam, fruit candies, fruit nectars, jellies, juices, marmalade, dehydrated products, semi-processed food, and so forth. Value addition can provide safe and convenient food to consumers (Parveen et al., 2014). Abdullah (2010) stated that the main reason for the value addition of fruit and vegetables is to prolong the shelf life of fresh produce away from the season period. For example, when a specific fresh produce comes in season, there may be loads of them, and if the extra is not conserved, it will decay and go to waste. Thus, supply outweighs demand, and products fetch less money.

1.2.9 LOSS QUANTIFICATION

While there is a growing body of scientific research and knowledge on improved technologies and procedures for fresh produce production and handling to meet market demand, little is known regarding the magnitude of loss that happens at the farm and post-farmgate. Quantification of fresh fruit and vegetable losses at the packhouse, identifying the main causes, and estimating the impacts of losses are very critical (Opara, Fawole, and Opara, 2021). Discussions on postharvest causes and losses are mostly based on estimates that are conducted without site-level measurements, which are known to be costly and difficult. Researchers globally agree on the requirements for more research and studies to immediately quantify postharvest loss amount to recognize the site-specific contributing factors along the value chain (Opara et al., 2021).

Opara, Fawole (2021) evaluate the magnitude of the postharvest losses of pomegranate fruit at the packhouse level to find out the causes and estimate the environmental and socio-economic impacts of the losses. Loss quantification measurements involved the calculations of fruit loss proportional to the amount put in the packhouse processing line. They recorded 6.74 to 7.69% losses (328.79 tons) of pomegranate fruit which were removed during packhouse operation per production season at the examined packhouse. Also, Schneider, Part (2019) conducted on-site measurements to determine potato losses which were carried out directly on the field at five different locations in Austria and Germany. Their method enables the quantification of potato losses based on defined areas along the harvested potato rows, where the analyzer collects potatoes during their harvest manually. As stated by Opara, Fawole (2021), loss quantification is very important to provide strategies to control and reduce fruit and vegetable losses in the farm and during the supply chain. This will ensure increased revenue for farmers, sustainable utilization of natural resources, a decrease in the environmental impacts of the fruit industry, and extra availability of quality fresh produce for nutritional security.

1.3 CONCLUSION

Harvested fruit and vegetables are metabolically active, experiencing senescence and ripening processes that must be controlled to extend postharvest quality. Inappropriate management of these processes can lead to nutritional, physiological, and quality attribute losses, release pathogens, and cause financial loss along the supply chain from growers to consumers. Ideal postharvest treatments for fresh fruit and vegetables maintain the quality of fresh produce and prolong their shelf-life. Thus, sustainable technologies that are non-thermal, environment-friendly, and cost-effective have been approached to reduce postharvest loss and quality damage in fresh produce. Several emerging technologies have been utilized, like irradiation, ozone, electrolyte water, edible coating, proper packaging (MAP), cold plasma, biosensors, non-destructive methods, and value addition. Many studies stated that these techniques helped to maintain the physiological attributes, control color change, delay ripening, reduce microbial growth, preserve flavor, and so forth, during the postharvest supply chain. Besides, the losses must be well assessed and quantified to provide sufficient suggestions that help to determine the cause and find solutions to avoid and prevent such losses during the supply chain of fruits and vegetables.

ACKNOWLEDGMENTS

We would like to thank Sultan Qaboos University, Oman, for their financial support under the project codes: CL\SQU\QU\AGR\23\02. The research leading to these results received funding from the Ministry of Higher Education, Research and Innovation (MOHERI) of the Sultanate of Oman under Block Funding Program No. RC/RG-AGR/SWAE/22/01.

KEYWORDS

- **emerging preservation methods**
- **fresh produce**
- **non-thermal treatments**
- **postharvest losses**
- **shelf life extension**
- **sustainable technologies**

REFERENCES

Abdullah, A. (2010). Global ARD future direction on value addition of fruits and vegetables. *Universiti Kebangsaan Malaysia (UKM). APCoAB. Asia Pacific Consortium on Agricultural Biotechnology. Malaysia.*

Affandi, F. Y., et al. (2021). Low oxygen storage improves tomato postharvest cold tolerance, especially for tomatoes cultivated with far-red LED light. *Foods, 10*(8), 1699.

Aghdam, M. S., et al. (2020). Melatonin treatment maintains nutraceutical properties of pomegranate fruits during cold storage. *Food Chemistry, 303*, 125385.

Ahmadnia, M., et al. (2021). Decontamination of whole strawberry via dielectric barrier discharge cold plasma and effects on quality attributes. *Journal of Food Processing and Preservation, 45*(1), e15019.

Al-Dairi, M., et al. (2022). Mechanical damage of fresh produce in postharvest transportation: Current status and future prospects. *Trends in Food Science & Technology, 124*(1), 195–207.

Al-Dairi, M., et al. (2023a). Effect on physiological properties of banana fruit based on pendulum impact test and storage. *Current Research in Food Science*, 100640.

Al-Dairi, M., et al. (2023b). Postharvest quality, technologies, and strategies to reduce losses along the supply chain of banana: A review. *Trends in Food Science & Technology*.

Al-Haq, M. I., et al. (2002). Disinfection effects of electrolyzed oxidizing water on suppressing fruit rot of pear caused by *Botryosphaeria berengeriana. Food Research International, 35*(7), 657–664.

Al-Hinai, A., Jayasuriya, H., & Pathare, P. B. (2022). Development of guidelines and procedures for value addition to improve productivity and sustainability: Case of dates in Oman. *Sustainability, 18*, 13378.

Ali, M., Cheng, J. H., & Sun, D. W. (2021). Effects of dielectric barrier discharge cold plasma treatments on degradation of anilazine fungicide and quality of tomato (*Lycopersicon esculentum* Mill) juice. *International Journal of Food Science & Technology, 56*(1), 69–75.

Bambalele, N. L., et al. (2021). Recent advances on postharvest technologies of mango fruit: A review. *International Journal of Fruit Science, 21*(1), 565–586.

Berardinelli, A., et al. (2011). Impact of atmospheric plasma generated by a DBD device on quality-related attributes of "Abate Fetel" pear fruit. In *Plasma for Bio-Decontamination, Medicine and Food Security* (pp. 457–467). Springer.

Castillo, J., et al. (2003). Bienzyme biosensors for glucose, ethanol and putrescine built on oxidase and sweet potato peroxidase. *Biosensors and Bioelectronics, 18*(5–6), 705–714.

Chen, C., et al. (2020). The effect of different doses of ozone treatments on the postharvest quality and biodiversity of cantaloupes. *Postharvest Biology and Technology, 163*, 111124.

Chen, J., et al. (2016). Combined effect of ozone treatment and modified atmosphere packaging on antioxidant defense system of fresh-cut green peppers. *Journal of Food Processing and Preservation, 40*(5), 1145–1150.

de Almeida Lopes, M. M., et al. (2021). The use of electrolyzed water as a disinfectant for fresh cut mango. *Scientia Horticultural, 287*, 110227.

Díaz-Mula, H. M., Serrano, M., & Valero, D. (2012). Alginate coatings preserve fruit quality and bioactive compounds during storage of sweet cherry fruit. *Food and Bioprocess Technology, 5*, 2990–2997.

Du, Z., et al. (2020). Recent advances in imaging techniques for bruise detection in fruits and vegetables. *Trends in Food Science & Technology, 99*, 133–141.

Duong, N. T. C., et al. (2022). An innovative single step of cross-linked alginate-based edible coating for maintaining postharvest quality and reducing chilling injury in rose apple cv. 'Tabtimchan' (*Syzygium samarangenese*). *Scientia Horticultural, 292*, 110648.

Elik, A., et al. (2019). Strategies to reduce post-harvest losses for fruits and vegetables. *Strategies, 5*(3), 29–39.

Fallanaj, F., et al. (2016). Electrolyzed sodium bicarbonate inhibits *Penicillium digitatum* and induces defense responses against green mold in citrus fruit. *Postharvest Biology and Technology, 115*, 18–29.

Ferreira, I. J., et al. (2022). Determination of quality and ripening stages of 'Pacovan' bananas using Vis-NIR spectroscopy and machine learning. *Engenharia Agrícola, 42*.

Ferri, V., et al. (2015). Effects of electrolyzed water on apples: Field treatment and postharvest application. In *III International Symposium on Postharvest Pathology: Using Science to Increase Food Availability, 1144*.

Fu, X., & Wang, M. (2021). Detection of early bruises on pears using fluorescence hyperspectral imaging technique. *Food Analytical Methods*, 1–9.

Gao, Y., & Rao, X. (2019). Blackspot bruise in potatoes: Susceptibility and biospeckle activity response analysis. *Journal of Food Measurement and Characterization, 13*(1), 444–453.

Gava, C. A. T., et al. (2018). Isolation of fruit colonizer yeasts and screening against mango decay caused by multiple pathogens. *Biological Control, 117*, 137–146.

Gavahian, M., & Khaneghah, A. M. (2020). Cold plasma as a tool for the elimination of food contaminants: Recent advances and future trends. *Critical Reviews in Food Science and Nutrition, 60*(9), 1581–1592.

Ge, W., et al. (2020). Combining salicylic acid and trisodium phosphate alleviates chilling injury in bell pepper (*Capsicum annuum* L.) through enhancing fatty-acid desaturation efficiency and water retention. *Food Chemistry, 327*, 127057.

George, D. S., et al. (2015). Effects of ultraviolet light (UV-C) and heat treatment on the quality of fresh-cut Chokanan mango and Josephine pineapple. *Journal of Food Science, 80*(2), S426–S434.

Gharezi, M., Joshi, N., & Sadeghian, E. (2012). Effect of postharvest treatment on stored cherry tomatoes. *Journal of Nutrition & Food Sciences, 2*(8), 1–10.

Hailu, G., & Derbew, B. (2015). Extent, causes and reduction strategies of postharvest losses of fresh fruits and vegetables– A review. *Journal of Biology, Agriculture and Healthcare, 5*(5), 49–64.

Hong, K., et al. (2012). Effects of chitosan coating on postharvest life and quality of guava (*Psidium guajava* L.) fruit during cold storage. *Scientia Horticultural, 144*, 172–178.

Horvitz, S., & Cantalejo, M. (2014). Application of ozone for the postharvest treatment of fruits and vegetables. *Critical Reviews in Food Science and Nutrition, 54*(3), 312–339.

Jobling, J. (2000). Postharvest ethylene: A critical factor in quality management. *Sydney Postharvest Laboratory Information Sheet*. Sydney, Australia.

Kahramanoğlu, İ., et al. (2020). The effects of edible coatings on the postharvest quality of citrus fruits as affected by granulation. *Journal of Food Quality, 2020*, 1–8.

Kalaïtzis, P., & Craita, E. (2016). Innovative postharvest technologies for sustainable value chain. In *Mediterra 2016. Zero Waste in the Mediterranean. Natural Resources, Food and Knowledge/International Centre for Advanced Mediterranean Agronomic Studies (CIHEAM) and Food and Agriculture Organization of the United Nations (FAO)* (p. 263). Paris: Presses de Sciences Po.

Kim, M. J., & Hung, Y. C. (2014). Effect of alkaline electrolyzed water as an inhibitor of enzymatic browning in Red Delicious apples. *Journal of Food Biochemistry, 38*(6), 542–550.

Kundu, M., et al. (2019). Recent developments in biosensors to combat agricultural challenges and their future prospects. *Trends in Food Science & Technology, 88*, 157–178.

Li, C., Tao, J., & Zhang, H. (2017). Peach gum polysaccharides-based edible coatings extend shelf life of cherry tomatoes. *3 Biotech, 7*, 1–5.

Li, X., et al. (2020). The effect of electrolyzed water on fresh-cut eggplant in storage period. *LWT, 123*, 109080.

Liu, C., Jahangir, M. M., & Ying, T. (2012). Alleviation of chilling injury in postharvest tomato fruit by preconditioning with ultraviolet irradiation. *Journal of the Science of Food and Agriculture, 92*(15), 3016–3022.

Liu, R., et al. (2021). The enzymatic browning reaction inhibition effect of strong acidic electrolyzed water on different parts of sweet potato slices. *Food Bioscience, 43*, 101252.

Mabusela, B. P., et al. (2021). Trends in ethylene management strategies: Towards mitigating postharvest losses along the South African value chain of fresh produce – A review. *South African Journal of Plant and Soil, 38*(5), 347–360.

Mahajan, P. V., et al. (2014). Postharvest treatments of fresh produce. *Philosophical Transactions of the Royal Society A: Mathematical, Physical and Engineering Sciences, 372*(2017), 20130309.

Mandal, D., et al. (2017). Bilayer edible coating with chitosan and wax extended shelf life and maintained quality of tomatoes at ambient storage. *Research on Crops, 18*(4), 662–667.

Mditshwa, A., et al. (2017). Effect of ultraviolet irradiation on postharvest quality and composition of tomatoes: A review. *Journal of Food Science and Technology, 54*, 3025–3035.

Minas, I. S., et al. (2014). Ozone-induced kiwifruit ripening delay is mediated by ethylene biosynthesis inhibition and cell wall dismantling regulation. *Plant Science, 229*, 76–85.

Niemira, B. A. (2012). Cold plasma decontamination of foods. *Annual Review of Food Science and Technology, 3*, 125–142.

Nyamende, N. E., et al. (2021). Alternative postharvest pre-treatment strategies for quality and microbial safety of 'Granny Smith' apple. *Helion, 7*(5).

Nyamende, N. E., et al. (2022). Impacts of alkaline-electrolyzed water treatment on physicochemical, phytochemical, antioxidant properties and natural microbial load on 'Granny Smith' apples during storage. *International Journal of Food Science & Technology, 57*(1), 447–456.

Opara, I. K., et al. (2021). Quantification of on-farm pomegranate fruit postharvest losses and waste, and implications on sustainability indicators: South African case study. *Sustainability, 13*(9), 5168.

Opara, I. K., Fawole, O. A., & Opara, U. L. (2021). Postharvest losses of pomegranate fruit at the packhouse and implications for sustainability indicators. *Sustainability, 13*(9), 5187.

Parveen, S., et al. (2014). Value addition: A tool to minimize the post-harvest losses in horticultural crops. *Greener Journal of Agricultural Sciences, 4*(5), 195–195.

Pascall, M. A., & Lin, S. J. (2013). The application of edible polymeric films and coatings in the food industry. *Food Processing & Technology*.

Pathare, P. B., et al. (2023). Application of cold plasma for fresh produce quality and shelf-life extension. In *Postharvest Management of Fresh Produce* (pp. 165–194). Elsevier.

Porat, R., et al. (2018). Postharvest losses of fruit and vegetables during retail and in consumers' homes: Quantifications, causes, and means of prevention. *Postharvest Biology and Technology, 139*, 135–149.

Qi, H., Huang, Q., & Hung, Y. C. (2018). Effectiveness of electrolyzed oxidizing water treatment in removing pesticide residues and its effect on produce quality. *Food Chemistry, 239*, 561–568.

Rai, A., Kumari, K., & Vashistha, P. (2022). Umbrella review on chilling injuries: post-harvest issue, cause, and treatment in tomato. *Scientia Horticultural, 293*, 110710.

Rajapaksha, L., et al. (2021). Reducing post-harvest losses in fruits and vegetables for ensuring food security—Case of Sri Lanka. *MOJ Food Processing & Technology, 9*(1), 7–16.

Ramazzina, I., et al. (2015). Effect of cold plasma treatment on physio-chemical parameters and antioxidant activity of minimally processed kiwifruit. *Postharvest Biology and Technology, 107*, 55–65.

Ramazzina, I., et al. (2016). Effect of cold plasma treatment on the functional properties of fresh-cut apples. *Journal of Agricultural and Food Chemistry, 64*(42), 8010–8018.

Rashvand, M., et al. (2022). Effect of dielectric barrier discharge cold plasma on the bruise susceptibility of plum fruit. *Journal of Food Process Engineering, 45*(12), e14182.

Ratra, S., Kaur, L., & Thukral, B. (2016). Effect of *Aloe vera* and wheat grass juice as an edible coating to prolong the shelf life of bananas. *International Journal of Engineering Research and Technology, 3*, 2648–2655.

Sarron, E., Gadonna-Widehem, P., & Aussenac, T. (2021). Ozone treatments for preserving fresh vegetables quality: A critical review. *Foods, 10*(3), 605.

Schneider, F., et al. (2019). A methodological approach for the on-site quantification of food losses in primary production: Austrian and German case studies using the example of potato harvest. *Waste Management, 86*, 106–113.

Seo, J., et al. (2020). Seed browning in pepper (*Capsicum annuum* L.) fruit during cold storage is inhibited by methyl jasmonate or induced by methyl salicylate. *Postharvest Biology and Technology, 166*, 111210.

Shams, R., et al. (2020). Application of biosensors in food quality control. *Journal of Postharvest Technology, 8*(1), 53–74.

Shezi, S., et al. (2020). Changes in biochemistry of fresh produce in response to ozone postharvest treatment. *Scientia Horticultural, 269*, 109397.

Sripong, K., et al. (2015). Combined treatment with hot water and UV-C elicits disease resistance against anthracnose and improves the quality of harvested mangoes. *Crop Protection, 77*, 1–8.

Sun, Y., et al. (2019). Detection of early decay in peaches by structured-illumination reflectance imaging. *Postharvest Biology and Technology, 151*, 68–78.

Toti, M., Carboni, C., & Botondi, R. (2018). Postharvest gaseous ozone treatment enhances quality parameters and delays softening in cantaloupe melon during storage at 6°C. *Journal of the Science of Food and Agriculture, 98*(2), 487–494.

Tran, T., et al. (2013). Fumigation with ozone to extend the storage life of mango fruit cv. Nam Dok Mai No. 4. *Agricultural Science Journal, 44*(2), 663–672.

Uthairatanakij, A., et al. (2023). Green technology for reducing postharvest losses and improving the nutritional quality of fresh horticultural produce.

Verghese, K., et al. (2015). Packaging's role in minimizing food loss and waste across the supply chain. *Packaging Technology and Science, 28*(7), 603–620.

Watkins, C. B. (2002). Ethylene synthesis, mode of action, consequences and control. In *Fruit Quality and Its Biological Basis* (pp. 180–224).

Wills, R. (2005). Minimizing the harmful effects of ethylene on the quality of fruit and vegetables. In S. Ben-Yehoshua (Ed.), *Environmentally Friendly Technologies for Agricultural Produce Quality* (pp. 133–148).

Zhang, W., et al. (2020). Applications of nitric oxide and melatonin in improving postharvest fruit quality and the separate and crosstalk biochemical mechanisms. *Trends in Food Science & Technology, 99*, 531–541.

Zhang, W., et al. (2020). Multiple 1-MCP treatment more effectively alleviated postharvest nectarine chilling injury than conventional one-time 1-MCP treatment by regulating ROS and energy metabolism. *Food Chemistry, 330*, 127256.

Zhang, W., et al. (2021). Advances in biochemical mechanisms and control technologies to treat chilling injury in postharvest fruits and vegetables. *Trends in Food Science & Technology, 113*, 355–365.

Zulkifli, N., et al. (2019). Application of laser-induced backscattering imaging for predicting and classifying ripening stages of "Berangan" bananas. *Computers and Electronics in Agriculture, 160*, 100–107.

CHAPTER 2

Non-Thermal Techniques for Fresh Produce Quality and Safety

PANKAJ B. PATHARE,[1*] DABABANDYA MOHAPATRA,[2] C. NICKHIL,[3] DILIP PAWAR,[4] and NAVEEN KUMAR MAHANTI[5]

[1]*Department of Soils, Water and Agricultural Engineering, College of Agricultural and Marine Sciences, Sultan Qaboos University, Muscat, Oman*

[2]*Automation and Plant Engineering Division, ICAR–National Institute of Secondary Agriculture, Ranchi, Jharkhand, India*

[3]*Department of Food Engineering and Technology, Tezpur University, Napaam, Sonitpur, Assam, India*

[4]*Agro Produce Processing Division, ICAR–Central Institute of Agricultural Engineering, Bhopal, Madhya Pradesh, India*

[5]*Post Harvest Technology Research Station, Dr. Y. S. R. Horticultural University, Tadepalligudem, Andhra Pradesh, India*

*Corresponding author

ABSTRACT

In recent years, consumers have preferred convenient and healthy foods that have 'fresh-like' characteristics while still being safe and having an extended shelf life. The modern consumer's interest has increased due to the new global trend towards the use of natural products rich in phytochemicals that promote health and bioactive compounds. However, the current technologies based on thermal treatments reduce the nutritional

Sustainable Approaches in Postharvest Handling and Management: Pankaj B. Pathare (Ed.)

DOI: 10.1201/9781779641076-2

value and degrade the sensory attributes of these products in relation to the fresh produce. Hence, non-thermal food processing can be a good substitute for conventional thermal processing that can satisfy consumer demands for wholesome, convenient, and minimally processed meals. Since these processing technologies do not require longer treatment times or higher temperatures compared to traditional thermal processing, this implies that food's nutritious components are better preserved and its sensory qualities are less affected. The current state of knowledge and developments on the effects of non-thermal technologies—such as cold plasma, irradiation, high-pressure processing, ozone treatment, and supercritical carbon dioxide technology—on the safety and quality of fresh produce are discussed in this chapter.

2.1 INTRODUCTION

Foods are a complex mixture of moisture, carbohydrates, lipids, proteins, and other organic and mineral substances. After harvest, metabolic changes carry on, including the enzymatic activities and biosynthetic pathways, causing the biomolecules to degrade and form different unwanted metabolites in the food. The activities of microbes and other pests further add to the deterioration process. Hence, the food needs to be processed and preserved to arrest food spoilage and prevent food borne illness while retaining the nutritional value. Food processing is the transformation of raw material into final or intermediate products by using various techniques and methods. It includes chemical, mechanical, and thermal methods to increase the palatability and shelf life of the product. The goal of food processing has evolved continuously to achieve food security, food safety, and nutritional security. Various food processing methods such as sun drying, salting, fermentation, and smoking have been used since prehistoric times to preserve food and make it palatable. Food processing methods have undergone several transformations to render harmful substances, poisons, and pathogenic microorganisms inactive, ensuring that processed foods fulfill consumer standards for shelf life, safety, and nutritional value.

In general, food processing techniques are categorized into thermal and non-thermal. For many years, heat was used as a tool for microbial stability and the preservation of nutritional and sensory quality of food.

In thermal processing, food was exposed to very high temperatures for a long period of time. This technique has been used for many years because of its ability to inactivate microorganisms and enzymes and improve product stability. However, thermal treatment brings numerous physicochemical, textural, and organoleptic changes, and it can develop harmful compounds such as keto-aldehydes, glyoxal, heterocyclic amines, methylglyoxal, glycation end products, 3-deoxyglucosone, and acrylamides resulted from heat-induced Maillard reaction (Zhang et al., 2019). The type and amount of these compounds depends on the type of thermal method used. The functional quality of thermally processed food is also uncertain because the thermal treatment causes significant changes in nutritional attributes of foods. Advanced thermal processing techniques such as ohmic, radio frequency, and microwave heating are alternatives to the traditional thermal processing techniques; they offer rapid heating, thereby the nutrient degradation rate and adverse reactions can be minimized.

Nowadays, consumers are more concerned about food quality and safety, especially after the COVID-19 pandemic. Due to the media-created awareness in the public related to food issues, particularly how processing affects the functional components of various food products, the public demands food with high quality, a long shelf life, nutritious and good sensory qualities, and an optimal calorific value that can be incorporated into their regular diet in order to balance their daily diet. Hence, food processing industries always look for the best technologies that can meet consumer demands. This gap has driven researchers and academicians to explore novel technologies that can meet industrial and consumer demands. As a result, numerous non-thermal food processing techniques have evolved in a few decades, such as cold plasma, ozone, UV radiation, high hydrostatic pressure (HPP), ultrasonication, pulsed light (PL), pulsed electric field, and so forth. The effect of non-thermal techniques on food quality is less because they generally target the non-covalent bonds of food, whereas thermal treatment damages both covalent and non-covalent bonds (Liu et al., 2020). Hence, non-thermal techniques have less effect on the quality attributes of food. In non-thermal technologies, heat may be generated in some techniques due to the generation of internal heat, such as microwave heating, infrared, irradiation, and radio frequency. However, these technologies were classified as mild heat treatments as compared to thermal techniques.

These non-thermal technologies are gaining more attention from food processing industries due to the advantages of maximum quality retention, lower processing time, energy efficiency, high microbial inactivation efficiency, and no risk of formation of any toxic or undesirable compounds. Extensive research has been carried out on the application of these non-thermal technologies for food quality and safety. Maintenance of quality while processing is a great concern; therefore, selection of a suitable food processing technique is of the utmost importance. In this chapter, we discuss briefly various non-thermal techniques used for the shelf-life enhancement of various food commodities, the inactivation mechanism of microorganisms, and the effect of treatments.

2.2 COLD PLASMA TECHNOLOGY

In general, matter exists in solid, liquid, or gaseous states, but cold plasma is the fourth state of matter. When the kinetic energy of solids increases, the molecules get heated up, and a phase change occurs from solid to liquid. With a further increase in energy, the liquid converts into gas. The further increase in energy results in the disintegration of intermolecular structure; when this energy reaches a certain limit, the ionization of gas molecules takes place, which gives rise to plasma. Therefore, it is designated as the fourth state of matter or quasineutral gas, which comprises ions, atoms, or molecules in the excited state. Gases such as argon, helium, oxygen, nitrogen, and air, or a combination of these gases in an adequate ratio, can be used for plasma generation. These gases are excited to an ionization state with thermal, electrical, or mechanical energy to generate plasma containing negative and positive ions and reactive species such as ozone and singlet ozone. The composition of gas used for plasma generation decides the composition of reactive species (Alves et al., 2019). The net electric charge of plasma is zero (Misra et al., 2016). The reactive species generated by using oxygen gas has a more lethal effect towards microbial cells (Alves et al., 2019). Cold plasma is a completely or partly ionized gas mixture that contains free radicals, photons, electrons, positive and negative ions, or excited or non-excited molecules (Mandal et al., 2018).

In general, plasma is categorized into thermal and non-thermal plasma (cold plasma) (Zhang et al., 2019). Non-thermal cold plasma is further classified into non-equilibrium (<60 °C) and quasi-equilibrium plasma (100–150°C). Thermal plasma consists of electrons and ionized gases; at a temperature of 20,000 K, thermodynamic equilibrium occurs between charges and neutral species. Cold plasma is also referred to as atmospheric cold plasma (ACP) or non-equilibrium plasma, which is suitable for heat-sensitive food products because it is generated at ambient temperature and low or ambient pressure. The efficiency of low-pressure CP against microbial load is more effective, but the process is cost-intensive due to the vacuum system. Hence, ACP is suitable for application in the food processing sector.

ACP ensures complete decontamination at detoxification; therefore, there is no scope for thermal damage of heat-sensitive compounds in food products (Jadhav et al., 2021). Cold plasma generation utilizes most of its energy in terms of electrons, not for heating the whole gas system. The microbe's inactivation in cold plasma takes place due to the damage caused by reactive species of cell DNA, microbes' cellular components, and protein induce oxidation, finally leading to cell death (Phan et al., 2017). Plasma technology has a wide range of applications based on the nature of plasma, such as food, chemical engineering, pharmaceuticals, chemistry, electronics, and textile sectors (Lajnaf, 2023). Cold plasma is suitable in the food sector for the inactivation of microbes in food (Misra et al., 2016), equipment sterilization, inactivation of food spoilage enzymes, wastewater treatment (Puligundla et al., 2016), treatment of food packaging material (Ekezie et al., 2017), and for desired textural and cooking characteristics (Thirumdas et al., 2017).

Several methods to develop plasma include radio frequency, dielectric barrier discharge (DBD), gliding arc discharge, and microwave corona discharge (Pipliya et al., 2023). Numerous factors affect the effectiveness of cold plasma on microbial inactivation, such as type of electrode, voltage intensity, type of microorganism, properties of microorganism cell membrane, and composition of food commodity (Mandal et al., 2018).

2.2.1 APPLICATIONS

Researchers have unveiled the various applications of cold plasma in food processing sector, such as inactivation of microorganisms in various food commodities such as agriculture and horticulture produce, meat and poultry products, marine products, and dairy products and enhancing physiochemical properties foods.

In a recent study, the effect of cold plasma treatment on *Escherichia coli* O157:H7, *Salmonella*, *Listeria monocytogenes*, and Tulane virus in whey protein-coated boiled chicken breast cubes was investigated (Roh et al., 2020). The optimal treatment voltage and time were 39 kV and 3.5 min, respectively. At these optimal conditions, they achieved 3.7 log CFU/cube, 3.9 log CFU/cube, 3.5 log CFU/cube, and 2.2 PFU/cube reduction in *Salmonella*, *E. coli* O157:H7, *L. monocytogenes*, and TV, respectively. They concluded that cold plasma can be used to inactivate the surface microorganisms of chicken without affecting its quality. In another study, the effect of vacuum packing and non-packaging on the microbial, physiochemical, and sensory quality of cold plasma treated (20.7–29.9 W) beef loin was evaluated (Bauer et al., 2017). The high-power levels had a significant effect on the chromatic properties of unpacked beef loins; on the other hand, a non-significant effect on color, lipid peroxidation, sarcoplasmic protein denaturation, nitrate/nitrite uptake, or myoglobin isoform distribution was observed in packed beef loin. Exposing the poly-amide film inoculated with *Staphylococcus aureus*, *Listeria monocytogenes*, and two *Escherichia coli* strains to cold plasma resulted in 2 log reduction without affecting the packaging film integrity. Similarly, Roh et al. (2019) explored the effect of atmospheric DBD cold plasma (38.7 kV) on in-package boiled chicken breast against *Salmonella*. They also studied the influence of surface coating, concentration of microbes, shaking of samples, sample stacking, and surface to volume ratio on *Salmonella* inactivation. The results revealed that the coating of whey protein isolate enhanced the inactivation efficiency due to the smoothing effect. The maximum inactivation efficiency of *Salmonella* was observed in sample treated with 20.5%, 68.9%, and 10.6% of chicken protein isolate, water, and soybean oil, respectively. The initial microbial load had a negative effect, and surface-to-volume ratio had a non-significant effect on *Salmonella* inactivation during cold plasma treatment. The D value rose from 0.2 to 1.3 min when the inoculum concentration increased from 3.8 to 5.7 log CFU/sample, the highest. However, shaking had a significant positive effect on the inactivation efficiency. In another study, the efficacy of radio-frequency atmospheric pressure plasma was evaluated against *Staphylococcus aureus* on the surface of polystyrene, agar, and beef jerky (Kim et al., 2014). They observed that within 2 min, the population of

Staphylococcus aureus was reduced by 3–4 log on agar and polystyrene; however, the same level of inactivation was observed on beef jerky after 10 min. The inactivation efficiency was influenced by the surface condition of sample and matrix. The decimal reduction time of *Staphylococcus aureus* on polystyrene plates, agar plates, and beef jerky was 39 s, 29 s, and 3 min, respectively. The treatment had a non-significant effect on the fatty acid composition, while color and shear forces remained unaltered.

2.3 OZONE IN FOOD PROCESSING

Ozone, in its gaseous or aqueous form, is widely applied in food industries. It is a powerful oxidant, second only to elemental fluorine in oxidizing power (Pandiselvam et al., 2017). Instant decomposition and nil hazardous residuals have popularized ozone as a "green" technology (Tiwari et al., 2008). The general applications of ozone are disinfection of water, surfaces, production areas, fumigation, and sterilization (Nickhil et al., 2021; Pandiselvam et al., 2017). Microbial inactivation, pathogen control, mycotoxin degradation, and pesticide degradation are the potential applications of ozone in food preservation. The US Food and Drug Administration (FDA) has approved ozone for various food applications (Priyanka et al., 2014). It is generally recognized as safe (GRAS) by the United States for various applications, such as bottled water disinfection, to remove strains from processing in water bottle plants (FDA, 1995). Ozone has stronger antimicrobial activity than chlorine, and it also controls foodborne pathogens.

Chlorine and its derivatives, hydrogen peroxide, ozone, iodine derivatives, and quaternary amines are the commonly used sanitizing agents. Commercially, chlorine is used as a disinfectant, but it triggers food safety issues due to the formation of carcinogenic products (Priyanka et al., 2014). Therefore, non-thermal and green ozone technology is the best alternative to chlorine in food processing.

2.3.1 OZONE GENERATION AND ITS PROPERTIES

Ozone is also a naturally occurring substance available in the troposphere of the environment and produced by interaction between hydrocarbons and solar radiation. A fresh, characteristic smell after a thunderstorm indicates the presence of ozone in nature. Ozone can be produced artificially through any of the three methods: electrical discharge, ultraviolet (UV) light, and electrochemical method. The electrical discharge method is commercially used for the production of ozone. In this method, properly dried air or oxygen is passed between the high-voltage electrodes. The two electrodes are separated by a dielectric material, which is generally glass. When an oxygen (O_2) molecule is broken by means of high energy input in the form of UV irradiation or corona discharge (high-voltage electrical discharge), the separated single oxygen molecule again combines with oxygen in the air and forms ozone (O_3) (Karaca and Velioglu, 2007; Mahapatra et al., 2005; Suslow, 2004). The gas mixture coming out from the ozone generator has about 1–3% ozone concentration.

Ozone has a more substantial oxidizing potential (2.07 V) than chlorine (1.36 V), which leverages its strong bactericidal, viricidal, and sporicidal properties (Khadre et al., 2001). It is a colorless gas when produced from pure oxygen, whereas it is blue in color when generated from dried air. Ozone (2.14 g/L) is denser than air (1.28 g/L) at 0°C. It is unstable and dissociates at a faster rate; the free radicals O- thus produced react with contact surfaces and, hence, are difficult to store (Cullen et al., 2007). Ozone is generally nontoxic in nature and safe to handle, but inhalation at higher concentrations (0.1–1.0 ppm) may lead to symptoms like throat drying, coughing, headache, eye irritation, and respiratory issues (Pascual et al., 2007).

2.3.2 MICROBIAL INACTIVATION WITH OZONE

The effectiveness of ozone in microbial inactivation is a testament to its unique properties. When cells are diseased due to bacterial, viral, or fungal attacks, they lose energy through the release of electrons, becoming electropositive. Simultaneously, the third oxygen molecule of ozone, which is electrophilic and always unstable, seeks balance with electrically charged substances. Diseased cells and pathogens are also attracted to ozone, attempting to achieve electrical balance. Another theory is that ozone, in action or its decomposition, releases hydroxyl radicals, which act upon the nucleic material such as cytosine and thymine of microorganisms. It damages the cell envelope material such as polysaccharides, intracellular enzymes, polyunsaturated fatty acids, amino acids, and viral capsids (Khadre et al., 2001). While reacting with polysaccharides, ozone breaks the glycoside bonds and leads to the formation of aliphatic acid and aldehydes. This process ultimately results in the disintegration and damage of the cell wall, rendering the microbes inactive (Mahapatra et al., 2005).

Ozone in action or its decomposition releases hydroxyl radicals, which act upon the nucleic material such as cytosine and thymine of microorganisms. It damages the cell envelope material such as polysaccharides, intracellular enzymes, polyunsaturated fatty acids, amino acids, and viral capsids (Khadre et al., 2001). While reacting with polysaccharides, ozone breaks the glycoside bonds and leads to the formation of aliphatic acid and aldehydes.

2.3.3 APPLICATIONS

Ozone is a strong oxidizing agent, with proven applications in wastewater treatment, pulp bleaching, control of odor, disinfection of medical utensils, water cooling towers, and sanitization of swimming pool water (Loeb et al., 2011). Because of its residue-free nature, ozone has been quite popular in recent decades for its several applications in food processing (Tiwari et al., 2008).

2.3.3.1 FRUIT AND VEGETABLE

Ozone has been proven to be a very promising technology in shelf-life enhancement of fruits and vegetables with control of decay by microbial inactivation. The shelf life of fresh (whole and cut) fruits and vegetables has been found to increase considerably with appropriate treatment of ozone concentrations and time. The gaseous or aqueous form of ozone is applied as pre-storage treatment, during storage, or transportation (Palou et al., 2002). Ozone in aqueous form is preferred for its applications for sterilizing whole or cut fruits and vegetables.

Some studies on the application of ozone for shelf-life enhancement of fresh fruits and vegetables (FFVs) have been summarized in Table 2.1.

TABLE 2.1 Applications of Ozone to Shelf-Life Enhancement of Fresh Fruits and Vegetables

Fruit/Vegetable	Treatment Method	Major Findings	References
Lychee fruit, Cv. Chakapat (*Litchi chinensis Sonn.*)	Ozone treatment: Gaseous form/fumigation: 80, 160, 200, 240 mg/L Aqueous form: 2.2, 2.4, 3.2, 3.4 mg/L Treatment time: 10, 20, 30, 60 min	• Ozone fumigation for 60 min found suitable to reduce the *Chlorpyrifos* by 45%. • Aqueous ozone treatment reduced only 10.3% *Chlorpyrifos*. • Sensory quality of aqueous treated Lychee sample decreased significantly compared to control and fumigation treatment. • Quality retention up to 6 days when stored at 25°C.	Whangchai et al. (2011)
Papaya (*Carica Papaya L.*), Cv. Maradol-red	Gaseous ozone: 500 mg/m^3 for 2 hour per day. Ozone containing water: 1 ppm for 30 min per day Storage: at 25°C & 65% RH, for 10 days	• Delayed ripening • Effect on soluble solid was non-significant • Ozone treatment was good alternative to Amitsar fungicide.	Bataller et al. (2012)
Kiwi fruit, (*Actinidia deliciosa*) Cv. Hayward	Effect was studied on development of stem-end rot diseases caused by caused by *Botrytis cinerea.* Storage: Conventional cold storage (0°C & 95% RH) for 4 months. Continuous supply of gaseous ozone at 0.3 μL/L, Catalytic application of ethylene as control	• Ozone treatment delayed and decreased disease by 56%. • Induced resistance in kiwi fruit to pathogenic diseases. • Ozone did not affect antioxidant substances, antioxidant activity and phenolic content.	Minas et al. (2010).
Carrot, *Cv. Carandai*	Ozone treatment: Gaseous: 0–5 mg/L Dissolved in water: 0–10 mg/L Storage: Temperature: 18±2°C, RH: 80±5%	• Weight loss, firmness and color did not get altered by both the treatments. • Gaseous treatment of ozone did not affect the pH, but aqueous ozone treatment reduced the pH with increased concentration. • O_3 gas treatment retarded sharp increase of soluble solids. • Shelf life increased by 5 days.	De Souza et al. (2018)

TABLE 2.1 *(Continued)*

Fruit/Vegetable	Treatment Method	Major Findings	References
Tomato, (*Lycopersicon esculentum Mill*) cultivar FA-180	Ozone concentrations: Gaseous form: 25 & 45 mg/m^3, for 2 hours per day during 16 days. Storage at non-controlled storage and humidity conditions. Aqueous form: 0.5–1.0 ppm for 15–20 min	• Extended shelf life with retention of sensory quality. • Effective disinfection with aqueous O_3 at 1 ppm for 15 min treatment	Venta et al. (2010)

2.3.3.2 MINIMALLY PROCESSED FRUITS AND VEGETABLES

Minimal processing of fruits and vegetables has been a growing area in recent years in the food processing sector (Ali et al., 2018). Retention of quality and obtaining extended shelf life of minimally processed fruits and vegetables is the key challenge; for that, different chemical and physical treatments are used. Sodium hypochlorite, citric acid, calcium chloride, and ascorbic acid are the different chemicals used for the treatment of cut fruits and vegetables. However, the use of chemicals is being discouraged nowadays due to their adverse effects on human health, triggering food safety issues. Ozone has been found to be very effective in the shelf-life extension of cut perishable fruits by controlling the spoilage microorganisms (Venta et al., 2010). It is also effective in the removal of pesticide and fungicides from the processed products (Ikeura et al., 2011). Ozone, in both gaseous and aqueous forms, is used in the treatment of cut fruits and vegetables. Ozone has been used in minimal processing of lettuce (2 μL/L for 2 min; Olmez and Akbas, 2009), tomato slices (0.4 mg/L for 3 min; Aguayo et al., 2014); carrot sticks (10 mg/L for 10 min; Chauhan et al., 2011); pineapple (gaseous ozone, 0.73 mMol for 20 min; Alothman et al., 2010), Carrot and Cauliflower (1 ppm for 10 min; Giri et al., 2021). Control of spoilage causing bacteria, retention of firmness, inhibition of browning, and improved antioxidant capacity are the key positive effects of ozone treatment to cut fruits and vegetables.

2.3.3.3 STORAGE OF FARM PRODUCE

Organophosphate insecticides like Malathion and Dichlorvos, methyl bromide, and phosphine are the generally used fumigants for the storage of grains. Resistance to phosphine has been a serious problem, and there is a high demand for alternative fumigants to phosphine (Benhalima et al., 2004). Ozone is emerging as the best alternative to phosphine, as it is highly reactive, has strong oxidizing properties, and hence, bears insecticidal properties. For storage applications, ozone is preferred in gaseous form. Ozone has shown a promising effect on the control of insects like *Tribolium castaneum*, *Sitophilus oryzae*, *Rhizopertha dominica*, *Oryzaephilus surinamenis* (Pandiselvam et al., 2017). Different concentrations of ozone ranging from 45 ppmv to 1800 ppm have been used for the storage of different food grains (Pandiselvam et al., 2017). The exposure time varied from a few minutes in an intermittent manner to about 12 days. Pulse bruchids could be eliminated from infested chickpea samples through ozone application in pulse mode for 5 consecutive days at a concentration of 1000 ppmv (Nickhil et al., 2021). The majority of studies have obtained about 95–100% insect mortality using ozone as a fumigant.

Apart from grain storage, ozone also has applications for storing semi-perishables, such as onions (Shelake et al., 2022). Results revealed that pulsed mode ozone application is quite promising. Ozone was found effective in disrupting *Aspergillus Niger* mycelia and conidiophore. The effect of ozone fumigation on the quality parameters of stored onions was examined (Shelake et al., 2023) at different concentrations ranging from 100–300 ppm in a pulsed manner. Results showed that the content of ascorbic acid and pyruvic acid, which is responsible for imparting the pungency to the onions, decreased with increasing the concentrations of ozone. On the other hand, the content of total phenol and flavonoids increased at higher ozone concentrations. Scanning electron microscopy images revealed structural breakdown in the outer surface of onion, particularly in the first scale of the bulb.

An ozone fumigation coupled with cold storage effectively controlled the spoilage-causing and pathogenic bacteria (Bigi et al., 2021). The effect of 0.5 ppm ozone exposure for 30 and 60 minutes on internal surface contaminations and air in the cold chamber was examined. Ozone treatment for 60 minutes significantly reduced the bacterial load by 1.35 log on internal surfaces, whereas the airborne load was undetectable after 60 minutes of ozone treatment in a cold chamber.

2.3.3.4 MILK AND MEAT PROCESSING

Ozone has also found applications in microbial inactivation of milk and meat products. Different microbes such as *Listeria monocytogenes, Staphylococcus* sp, *Enterobacteriaceae,* molds, and yeasts are the main targets for preserving perishable milk and meat products. Several studies have been carried out on the ozone treatment in the milk and meat industry. Complete inactivation of bacteria and improved quality of products have been achieved with ozone treatment (Khanashyam et al., 2022). Milk (raw and processed) and milk products like yogurts, cheese, butter, and milk powder were treated with different ozone concentrations (0.5 mg to 2 g/L for 1 min to hours, depending upon the products) (Khanashyam et al., 2022). In the case of meat, the target microorganisms such as L. monocytogenes, *Pseudomonas* spp., LAB, yeasts and molds, Coliform, *Salmonellae*, *Escherichia coli*, and so forth, were controlled with exposure of either gaseous or aqueous ozone. Ozone has been found effective for raw chicken, beef, meat, pork, chicken legs, and so forth, with control of associated microorganisms and improved quality in nutritional and physiochemical terms (Khanashyam et al., 2022).

Ozone demonstrates its versatility as a promising oxidant, emerging with a multitude of applications in food processing. Unlike other chemicals, ozone leaves no residual effects, making it a compelling choice for various food processing needs.

2.4 HIGH HYDROSTATIC PRESSURE (HHP)

HHP processing is an innovative method for pasteurizing food that does not rely on heat. It has already found applications in the food industry, ensuring food safety and maintaining quality (Wang et al., 2016). HHP also offers exciting possibilities for enhancing the health benefits of food products. HHP has demonstrated its ability to improve or preserve the nutritional value of the food products. This process promotes the synthesis of g-aminobutyric acid in food materials, preserves immunoglobulin constituents in dairy products, increases resistant starch content in cereals, and reduces the glycemic index of fruits and vegetables (Huang et al., 2020). These benefits help regulate blood glucose levels, facilitate better control of calorie intake, and contribute to overall health. Furthermore, HHP serves as a complementary technology that can be combined with existing processing methods. It can be used to develop low-sodium food products and maintains microbial safety, thereby reducing the risk of cardiovascular diseases (Roobab et al., 2021). Moreover, HHP broadens the range of probiotic food products by enabling the addition of appropriate sporogenous probiotics, which remain viable even after HHP treatment (Huang et al., 2020). Despite causing physical damage to food product structures, HHP acts as a synergistic extraction technology. It enhances the efficiency of extracting functional components from food waste, effectively reducing production costs and extraction time (Kamal et al., 2021).

2.4.1 PRINCIPLE OF HIGH HYDROSTATIC PRESSURE (HHP)

The principle of HHP involves subjecting food, beverages, or other substances to intense hydrostatic pressure to achieve preservation, pasteurization, or extraction (Aganovic et al., 2021). By applying pressures greater than atmospheric pressure, typically in the range of 100 to 1000 megapascals (MPa), HHP can inactivate microorganisms, enzymes, and other biological agents without the need for high temperatures (Morris et al., 2007). Figure 2.1 illustrates the schematic diagram of the HHP process. This non-thermal preservation method helps retain the sensory attributes, nutritional quality, and freshness of the treated products, making it a promising technology for enhancing safety and quality in various industries (Zhao et al., 2019).

2.4.1.1 PROCESS DESCRIPTION OF HHP

The process of HHP involves several steps to subject materials to intense pressure for preservation, pasteurization, or extraction purposes. Here is a general description of the HHP process: loading, pressurization, soaking, pressure release, and unloading (Khurana, 2012).

In the high-pressure treatment, meticulous preparation of the material is crucial to ensure effective results. The specific requirements for preparation depend on the desired outcome and the nature of the material being treated. For instance, in food preservation, fruits, vegetables, or other perishable products undergo various preparation steps such as washing, peeling, slicing, or dicing to meet desired specifications. This preparation helps remove any impurities, enhances surface area exposure, and facilitates uniform penetration of pressure during the treatment. Once the material is properly prepared, it is loaded into a specialized pressure vessel.

These vessels are designed to withstand high pressure and are constructed using sturdy materials that can safely contain the intense forces exerted during the treatment. The loaded material fills the vessel, and the vessel is sealed securely to create a closed system that ensures no pressure is lost during the treatment. The next step is pressurization, where a high-pressure medium, commonly water, is introduced into the vessel. The pressure medium serves as a transmission medium to evenly distribute the pressure throughout the vessel, ensuring uniform treatment of the material (Muntean et al., 2016). The introduction of the pressure medium is carried out gradually, allowing the pressure to increase steadily to the desired level. To achieve the desired pressure level, hydraulic systems or pressure intensifiers are employed, which control and regulate the pressure buildup within the vessel. By gradually increasing the pressure, the high-pressure treatment achieves its objective of altering the material characteristics or achieving desired effects. The pressure medium plays a crucial role in transmitting pressure uniformly, allowing it to penetrate the material effectively. This controlled pressurization process ensures that the material is subjected to the desired level of pressure for the required duration, ensuring optimal treatment outcomes. The steps mentioned above, namely preparation, loading, and pressurization, lay the foundation for the high-pressure treatment process (Permanye et al., 2010). They set the stage for the subsequent stages, which involve soaking the material in a high-pressure environment, gradually releasing the pressure, and unloading the treated material. The desired pressure is achieved and maintained during the soaking period; the material undergoes a thorough treatment in a high-pressure environment. The soaking time is determined based on factors such as the type of material being treated and the desired outcome. This step allows the pressure to exert its effects on the material, leading to desirable changes in its structure, texture, or other properties. Throughout the soaking process, the pressure is consistently maintained to ensure a uniform treatment. Following the completion of the soaking period, the pressure within the vessel needs to be gradually released. This step is critical to prevent any sudden changes in pressure that could adversely affect the treated material. To achieve a controlled release, there are different methods employed. One approach is to slowly vent the pressure medium from the vessel, allowing the pressure to dissipate gradually. Alternatively, a controlled depressurization system can be used, carefully regulating the release of pressure. This cautious approach ensures that the material is not subjected to abrupt changes that could compromise its quality or integrity. Once the pressure is fully released and the vessel is safe to open, the treated material is unloaded from the pressure vessel. In the context of food applications, the treated products may undergo further processing steps depending on the desired end product. This could involve packaging the treated food items to maintain their freshness and extend their shelf life. Alternatively, additional processing steps like cooking, freezing, or other preservation techniques may be employed to achieve the desired final product characteristics. The high-pressure treatment process involves a sequence of steps that include soaking the material in the high-pressure environment, gradually releasing the pressure, and finally unloading the treated material. These steps are designed to ensure optimal results and maintain the quality of the treated material throughout the process. By following a controlled and systematic approach, high-pressure treatment can effectively alter the properties of various materials, ranging from food products to industrial components, opening up a wide range of applications and benefits. The important parameters of the HHP process, including pressure level, soaking time, and temperature, are determined based on the material being treated and the desired outcome (Poojary et al., 2017). Optimization of these parameters is crucial to achieving the desired preservation, pasteurization, or extraction effects while maintaining product quality. Overall, the process of HHP involves loading the material into a pressure vessel, pressurizing it with a high-pressure medium, soaking it for a specified time, releasing the pressure, and unloading the treated material. By utilizing the principles of pressure, HHP offers a non-thermal technology for various applications in industries such as food, beverages, pharmaceuticals, and cosmetics.

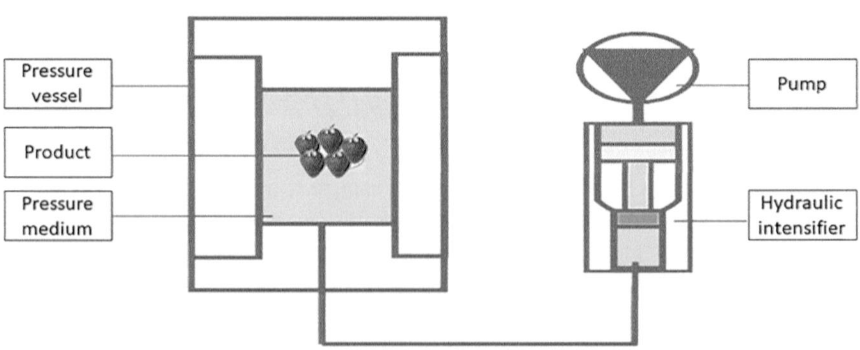

FIGURE 2.1 Different components that are involved in high hydrostatic pressure.

2.4.1.2 EFFECT OF HPP ON QUALITY AND SAFETY

HPP has significant effects on the quality and safety of treated materials. Here are the key impacts of HHP on quality and safety: microbial inactivation, preservation of nutritional quality, retention of fresh-like attributes, elimination of the need for chemical additives, minimal impact on texture, and increased food safety assurance (Barba et al., 2015).

- **Microbial Inactivation: HHP** is highly effective in inactivating or reducing the activity of microorganisms (bacteria, viruses, molds, and yeasts). This helps extend the shelf life of the perishable products and enhances their safety. By reducing or eliminating harmful pathogens, HHP can significantly reduce the risk of foodborne illnesses (Bermúdez-Aguirre and Barbosa-Cánovas, 2011).
- **Preservation of Nutritional Quality:** HHP offers a non-thermal preservation method that helps retain the nutritional quality of treated materials. Unlike traditional thermal processing, which can cause nutrient loss, HHP allows for the preservation of vitamins, enzymes, antioxidants, and other sensitive nutritional components. This helps in maintaining the nutritional value of foods and beverages (Jan et al., 2017).
- **Retention of Fresh-Like Attributes:** HHP preserves the sensory attributes of treated products, including color, taste, texture, and aroma. By minimizing the use of high temperatures, HHP helps retain the natural appearance and organoleptic properties of food and beverages. The treated products often maintain a fresh-like quality, which is desirable to consumers (Wang et al., 2016).
- **Elimination of Chemical Additives and Enzyme Inactivation:** HHP can reduce the need for chemical preservatives and additives in food and beverage products. By effectively inactivating microorganisms and enzymes, HHP can extend the shelf life. Enzymes play a significant role in food deterioration, such as browning, flavor changes, and texture degradation. HHP effectively inactivates enzymes, thereby slowing down enzymatic reactions and preserving the quality of the treated materials. This can result in improved product stability and sensory characteristics, a reduction in the use of artificial preservatives, leading to cleaner-label products (Wang et al., 2016).

- **Minimal Impact on Texture:** Unlike thermal processing methods, HHP minimally affects the texture of treated materials. This is particularly important for delicate products that are sensitive to heat. HHP can help maintain the texture and integrity of fruits, vegetables, seafood, and meats while achieving microbial inactivation (Rastogi et al., 2008).
- **Increased Food Safety Assurance:** HHP provides an additional layer of food safety assurance by effectively reducing the microbial load in treated products. This can be particularly valuable for high-risk foods, such as raw seafood or fresh juices, where pathogens are a concern. HHP helps enhance consumer confidence in the safety of treated products (Roobab et al., 2022).

It is important to note that the specific effects of HHP on quality and safety can vary depending on the material being treated, process parameters, and other factors. Optimization of HHP conditions is crucial to achieve the desired outcomes while ensuring product safety and quality.

2.5 IRRADIATION

Food irradiation, a process that exposes food products to ionizing radiation like gamma rays, X-rays, or electron beams (Ashraf et al., 2019), is a widely recognized food preservation method. It is used for eliminating harmful bacteria, parasites, and insects and controlling the ripening and sprouting of fresh produce (Prakash et al., 2020). Importantly, this technology has been extensively studied and approved by regulatory authorities worldwide, including the World Health Organization (WHO) and the Food and Agriculture Organization (FAO). Food irradiation offers numerous benefits, such as extended shelf life, reduced foodborne illnesses, and enhanced food safety. However, it's crucial to note that irradiation is part of a comprehensive food safety system and should be used in conjunction with good manufacturing practices and proper food handling. This non-thermal technique utilizes specific doses of non-ionizing or ionizing radiation to eliminate microbes, such as bacteria and viruses, in food and agricultural commodities, thereby enhancing their hygiene, safety, and storage and distribution capabilities. Despite its antimicrobial effects, food irradiation has minimal impact on the treated food's color, taste, flavor, and nutritional value. Fruits and vegetables, essential nutrient sources, can benefit from UV light treatment post-harvest. Studies have shown positive outcomes in various fruits and vegetables, such as mango, pineapple, grapes, broccoli, and strawberries (Bhatnagar et al., 2022). Gamma radiation has also proven effective in microbial inactivation and extending the shelf life of food products. Moreover, UV-C and UV-B irradiation are used in the food industry to disinfect food surfaces and delay fungal growth during post-harvest treatment (Abdipour et al., 2019). These methods offer promising solutions for improving food safety and quality.

2.5.1 PRINCIPLE

The principle of irradiation revolves around ionizing radiation to induce specific changes in materials. Ionizing radiation, including gamma rays, X-rays, and electron beams, can penetrate substances and interact with their components (Silindir and Özer, 2009). This interaction alters molecular and cellular structure by breaking chemical bonds or generating reactive species (Juan et al., 2021). The principle of irradiation is based on the understanding that these radiation-induced changes can have desired effects, such as sterilization, preservation, or modification of the material's properties. This principle finds application in various fields, including food processing, medical sterilization, and industrial applications, where controlled exposure to ionizing radiation offers valuable benefits. Figure 2.2 illustrates the schematic diagram of the irradiation process.

2.5.2 PROCESS DESCRIPTION OF IRRADIATION

The irradiation process is a series of steps designed to effectively treat materials using ionizing radiation. The process begins with preparation, where the material to be treated is carefully handled, which may include cleaning, trimming, or packaging, especially in food irradiation, to ensure proper handling and effective irradiation. Next, an appropriate source of ionizing radiation is selected based on the nature of the material and the desired treatment outcome. Common radiation sources include gamma rays from Cobalt-60 or Cesium-137, as well as X-ray machines or electron beam accelerators (Ashraf et al., 2019). The prepared material is then loaded onto conveyors, trays, or containers suitable for irradiation, with care taken to arrange it in a way that ensures uniform exposure to the radiation source. The radiation source is housed in a suitably sealed structure, so as to prevent leakage of radiation. The loaded material is exposed to the chosen ionizing radiation as it passes through the radiation field. The ionizing radiation effectively penetrates the material, interacting with its components and bringing about the desired effects, such as sterilization or extended shelf life. In addition to these steps, there are several other crucial aspects involved in the irradiation process. Dose measurement is an important step in which absorbed radiation by the material is carefully monitored and controlled. Dosimeters, specialized devices that measure radiation dose, are placed within or alongside the material to ensure accurate dosage. The desired dose of radiation is calculated based on factors such as the material type, desired treatment outcome, and regulatory requirements (Kuntz and Strasser, 2016). The radiation source is adjusted, and the exposure time is controlled to achieve the specified dose accurately. Radiation safety is of the utmost importance throughout the irradiation process. Strict protocols and measures are followed to safeguard the safety of operators, the environment, and the treated material. Shielding and containment systems are in place to minimize radiation exposure to personnel and prevent the release of radiation into the surroundings. Once the irradiation process is complete, post-irradiation handling takes place. The material is unloaded from the irradiation area and undergoes necessary post-processing steps. These may include cooling, packaging, labeling, or other procedures to maintain the integrity and safety of the irradiated product. It is crucial to follow appropriate handling and quality control measures during this stage to ensure compliance with safety standards and regulatory requirements (Hallman, 2017).

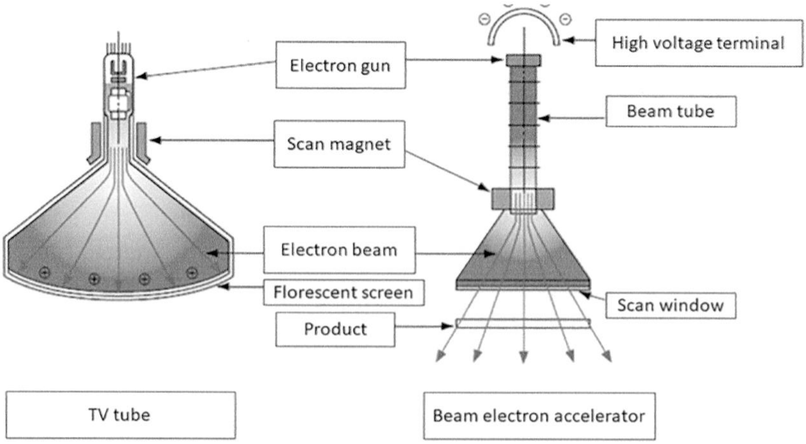

FIGURE 2.2 Different components that are involved in irradiation.

2.5.3 EFFECT ON QUALITY AND SAFETY OF IRRADIATION

Irradiation exerts significant effects on the quality and safety of treated materials, leading to the following key impacts:

- **Microbial Inactivation:** Irradiation effectively kills or inactivates microorganisms (bacteria, viruses, parasites, and molds) by damaging their DNA or cellular components. This helps in extending the shelf life of food and reducing the risk of foodborne illnesses. By reducing or eliminating pathogens, irradiation enhances the safety of treated products (Shahi et al., 2021).
- **Insect Control:** Irradiation can control insects and pests in agricultural commodities. The radiation disrupts their reproductive cycles, sterilizing them or preventing their development. This reduces infestations and the need for chemical insecticides, thereby improving the safety and quality of the treated materials (Follett et al., 2007).
- **Delayed Ripening and Spoilage:** This slows down the ripening process of fruits and vegetables by inhibiting the activity of enzymes responsible for ripening and spoilage. This extends the shelf life of the fresh produce, maintaining its quality during storage and transportation (Lacroix and Ouattara, 2000).
- **Reduction of Foodborne Pathogens:** Irradiation significantly reduces the levels of foodborne pathogens, such as *Salmonella*, *E. coli*, and *Listeria*, in various food products. This enhances the safety of these foods, particularly those consumed raw or minimally processed (Begum et al., 2020).
- **Sterilization and Decontamination:** Irradiation achieves sterilization or significant reduction of microorganisms on medical products, pharmaceuticals, and certain packaging materials. This ensures the safety and integrity of these products by preventing microbial contamination (Silindir and Özer, 2009).
- **Minimal Effect on Nutritional Quality:** Irradiation has a negligible impact on the nutritional quality of treated materials. It does not significantly affect the nutrient content, vitamins, or minerals. This helps in preserving the nutritional value of

irradiated food and ensuring its contribution to a healthy diet (Pasha et al., 2014).

- **Preservation of Sensory Attributes:** Irradiation preserves the sensory attributes of treated materials, such as color, taste, texture, and aroma. It minimizes the changes in sensory properties, ensuring that the irradiated products retain their desired characteristics (Prakash et al., 2000).
- **Enhanced Product Stability:** By reducing microbial load and delaying spoilage, irradiation enhances the stability of treated materials. It extends their shelf life, allowing for longer storage and distribution periods without compromising safety or quality (Pasha et al., 2014).

It's important to note that irradiation is a controlled process, following strict regulatory guidelines and dose limits to ensure safety. Irradiated products must adhere to labeling requirements to inform consumers about the treatment they have undergone. Overall, irradiation offers significant benefits in terms of microbial control, insect control, delayed ripening, pathogen reduction, sterilization, and preservation of sensory attributes. It provides a valuable tool for increasing the safety and quality of various materials, including food, medical products, and pharmaceuticals.

2.6 CONCLUSIONS

Non-thermal processing technologies refer to methods of inactivating microorganisms and enzymes in food products without the primary use of heating. Consequently, non-thermal processing ensures high standards of food safety conditions. It complies with customer demands for "minimally processed foods" while having little impact on the color, aroma, taste, and nutritional content of food products. Because consumers want safe, wholesome food that is free of microbes, non-thermal treatments are one of the food industry's most targeted research topics. There is no risk of heat-related damage to food's heat-sensitive nutritional components, food texture, or creation of any harmful compounds in food because of the brief exposure period and low temperature.

ACKNOWLEDGMENT

The authors would like to express their deep appreciation for the Ministry of Higher Education, Research and Innovation (MoHERI) for their financial support under the project code: RC/RG-AGR/SWAE/22/01.

KEYWORDS

- **emerging food technologies**
- **food safety**
- **fresh produce**
- **minimally processed foods**
- **non-thermal processing**
- **sensory quality**

REFERENCES

Abdipour, M., Hosseinifarahi, M., & Naseri, N. (2019). Combination method of UV-B and UV-C prevents post-harvest decay and improves organoleptic quality of peach fruit. *Scientia Horticultural, 256*, 108564.

Aganovic, K., Hertel, C., Vogel, R. F., Johne, R., Schlüter, O., Schwarzenbolz, U., & Heinz, V. (2021). Aspects of high hydrostatic pressure food processing: Perspectives on technology and food safety. *Comprehensive Reviews in Food Science and Food Safety, 20*(4), 3225–3266.

Aguayo, E., Escalona, V., Silveira, A. C., & Artés, F. (2014). Quality of tomato slices disinfected with ozonated water. *Food Science and Technology International, 20*(3), 227–235.

Ali, A., Yeoh, W. K., Forney, C., & Siddiqui, M. W. (2018). Advances in postharvest technologies to extend the storage life of minimally processed fruits and vegetables. *Critical Reviews in Food Science and Nutrition, 58*(15), 2632–2649.

Alothman, M., Kaur, B., Fazilah, A., Bhat, R., & Karim, A. A. (2010). Ozone-induced changes of antioxidant capacity of fresh-cut tropical fruits. *Innovative Food Science & Emerging Technologies, 11*(4), 666–671.

Alves Filho, E. G., de Brito, E. S., & Rodrigues, S. (2019). Effects of cold plasma processing in food components. In D. Bermudez-Aguirre (Ed.), *Advances in Cold Plasma Applications for Food Safety and Preservation* (pp. 253–268). Elsevier Inc. https://doi.org/10.1016/B978-0-12-814921-8.00008-6 (accessed on 9th July 2025).

Ashraf, S., Sood, M., Bandral, J. D., Trilokia, M., & Manzoor, M. (2019). Food irradiation: A review. *International Journal of Chemical Studies, 7*(2), 131–136.

Barba, F. J., Terefe, N. S., Buckow, R., Knorr, D., & Orlien, V. (2015). New opportunities and perspectives of high-pressure treatment to improve health and safety attributes of foods: A review. *Food Research International, 77*, 725–742.

Bataller, M., Gonzalez, J. E., Veliz, E., & Fernandez, L. A. (2012). Ozone applications in the post-harvest of papaya (*Carica papaya* L.): An alternative to Amistar fungicide. *Ozone: Science & Engineering, 34*(3), 151–155.

Begum, T., Follett, P. A., Hossain, F., Christopher, L., Salmieri, S., & Lacroix, M. (2020). Microbicidal effectiveness of irradiation from Gamma and X-ray sources at different dose rates against the foodborne illness pathogens *Escherichia coli, Salmonella Typhimurium* and *Listeria monocytogenes* in rice. *LWT, 132*, 109841.

Benhalima, H., Chaudhry, M. Q., Mills, K. A., & Price, N. R. (2004). Phosphine resistance in stored-product insects collected from various grain storage facilities in Morocco. *Journal of Stored Products Research, 40*(3), 241–249.

Bermúdez-Aguirre, D., & Barbosa-Cánovas, G. V. (2011). An update on high hydrostatic pressure, from the laboratory to industrial applications. *Food Engineering Reviews, 3*, 44–61.

Bhatnagar, P., Gururani, P., Bisht, B., Kumar, V., Kumar, N., Joshi, R., & Vlaskin, M. S. (2022). Impact of irradiation on physico-chemical and nutritional properties of fruits and vegetables: A mini review. *Heliyon*, e10918.

Bigi, F., Haghighi, H., Quartieri, A., De Leo, R., & Pulvirenti, A. (2021). Impact of low-dose gaseous ozone treatment to reduce the growth of *in vitro* broth cultures of foodborne pathogenic/spoilage bacteria in a food storage cold chamber. *Journal of Food Safety, 41*(3), e12892.

Chauhan, O. P., Raju, P. S., Ravi, N., Singh, A., & Bawa, A. S. (2011). Effectiveness of ozone in combination with controlled atmosphere on quality characteristics including lignification of carrot sticks. *Journal of Food Engineering, 102*(1), 43–48.

Cullen, P. J., Valdramidis, V. P., Tiwari, B. K., Patil, S., Bourke, P., & O'Donnell, C. P. (2010). Ozone processing for food preservation: An overview on fruit juice treatments. *Ozone: Science & Engineering, 32*(3), 166–179.

da Silva Aquino, K. A. (2012). Sterilization by gamma irradiation. *Gamma Radiation, 9*, 172–202.

De Souza, L. P., Faroni, L. R. D. A., Heleno, F. F., Cecon, P. R., Gonçalves, T. D. C., da Silva, G. J., & Prates, L. H. F. (2018). Effects of ozone treatment on postharvest carrot quality. *LWT, 90*, 53–60.

FDA. (1995). Beverages: Bottled water; final rule. Food and Drug Administration. *Federal Register, 60*, 57075–57130. https://www.federalregister.gov/documents/1995/11/13/95-27888/beverages-bottled-water-final-rule (accessed on 9th July 2025).

Follett, P. A., Yang, M. M., Lu, K. H., & Chen, T. W. (2007). Irradiation for postharvest control of quarantine insects. *Formosan Entomologist, 27*, 1–15.

Giri, S. K., Sadvatha, R. H., Tripathi, M. K., & Pawar, D. A. (2020). Enhancing shelf-life of fresh-cut carrot and cauliflower floret with combined ozone and ultraviolet-C radiation treatment. *Journal of Agricultural Engineering (India), 57*, 210–225.

Hallman, G. J. (2017). Process control in phytosanitary irradiation of fresh fruits and vegetables as a model for other phytosanitary treatment processes. *Food Control, 72*, 372–377.

Huang, H. W., Hsu, C. P., & Wang, C. Y. (2020). Healthy expectations of high hydrostatic pressure treatment in food processing industry. *Journal of Food and Drug Analysis, 28*(1), 1–13.

Ikeura, H., Kobayashi, F., & Tamaki, M. (2011). Removal of residual pesticide, fenitrothion, in vegetables by using ozone microbubbles generated by different methods. *Journal of Food Engineering, 103*(3), 345–349.

Jadhav, H. B., Annapure, U. S., & Deshmukh, R. R. (2021). Non-thermal technologies for food processing. *Frontiers in Nutrition, 8*, 657090.

Jan, A., Sood, M., Sofi, S. A., & Norzom, T. (2017). Non-thermal processing in food applications: A review. *International Journal of Food Science and Nutrition, 2*(6), 171–180.

Juan, C. A., Pérez de la Lastra, J. M., Plou, F. J., & Pérez-Lebeña, E. (2021). The chemistry of reactive oxygen species (ROS) revisited: Outlining their role in biological macromolecules (DNA, lipids and proteins) and induced pathologies. *International Journal of Molecular Sciences, 22*(9), 4642.

Kamal, H., Le, C. F., Salter, A. M., & Ali, A. (2021). Extraction of protein from food waste: An overview of current status and opportunities. *Comprehensive Reviews in Food Science and Food Safety, 20*(3), 2455–2475.

Khadre, M. A., Yousef, A. E., & Kim, J. G. (2001). Microbiological aspects of ozone applications in food: A review. *Journal of Food Science, 66*(9), 1242–1252.

Khanashyam, A. C., Shanker, M. A., Kothakota, A., Mahanti, N. K., & Pandiselvam, R. (2022). Ozone applications in milk and meat industry. *Ozone: Science & Engineering, 44*(1), 50–65.

Khurana, M. (2012). Temperature distribution in vertical and horizontal high-pressure vessels and its impact on food safety. *Rutgers The State University of New Jersey, School of Graduate Studies*.

Kuntz, F., & Strasser, A. (2016). The specifics of dosimetry for food irradiation applications. *Radiation Physics and Chemistry, 129*, 46–49.

Lacroix, M., & Ouattara, B. (2000). Combined industrial processes with irradiation to assure innocuity and preservation of food products—A review. *Food Research International, 33*(9), 719–724.

Lajnaf, R. (2023). Introductory chapter: Novel thermal and non-thermal technologies for food processing. In *Food Processing and Preservation*. IntechOpen. https://doi.org/10.5772/intechopen.110433 (accessed on 9th July 2025).

Loeb, B. L. (2011). *Ozone: Science & Engineering*: Thirty-three years and growing. *Ozone: Science & Engineering, 33*(4), 329–342.

Mahapatra, A. K., Muthukumarappan, K., & Julson, J. L. (2005). Applications of ozone, bacteriocins and irradiation in food processing: A review. *Critical Reviews in Food Science and Nutrition, 45*(6), 447–461.

Mandal, R., Singh, A., & Singh, A. P. (2018). Recent developments in cold plasma decontamination technology in the food industry. *Trends in Food Science & Technology, 80*, 93–103.

Minas, I. S., Karaoglanidis, G. S., Manganaris, G. A., & Vasilakakis, M. (2010). Effect of ozone application during cold storage of kiwifruit on the development of stem-end rot caused by *Botrytis cinerea*. *Postharvest Biology and Technology, 58*(3), 203–210.

Morris, C., Brody, A. L., & Wicker, L. (2007). Non-thermal food processing/preservation technologies: A review with packaging implications. *Packaging Technology and Science: An International Journal, 20*(4), 275–286.

Mostafavi, H. A., Fathollahi, H., & Motamedi, F. (2010). Food irradiation: Applications, public acceptance and global trade. *African Journal of Biotechnology, 9*(20).

Muntean, M. V., Marian, O., Barbieru, V., Cătunescu, G. M., Ranta, O., Drocas, I., & Terhes, S. (2016). High pressure processing in food industry–Characteristics and applications. *Agriculture and Agricultural Science Procedia, 10*, 377–383.

Nickhil, C., Mohapatra, D., Kar, A., Giri, S. K., Verma, U. S., Sharma, Y., & Singh, K. K. (2021). Delineating the effect of gaseous ozone on disinfestation efficacy, protein quality, dehulling efficiency, cooking time and surface morphology of chickpea grains during storage. *Journal of Stored Products Research, 93*, 101823. https://doi.org/10.1016/j.jspr.2021.101823 (accessed on 9th July 2025).

Ölmez, H., & Akbas, M. Y. (2009). Optimization of ozone treatment of fresh-cut green leaf lettuce. *Journal of Food Engineering, 90*(4), 487–494.

Palou, L., Crisosto, C. H., Smilanick, J. L., Adaskaveg, J. E., & Zoffoli, J. P. (2002). Effects of continuous 0.3 ppm ozone exposure on decay development and physiological responses of peaches and table grapes in cold storage. *Postharvest Biology and Technology, 24*(1), 39–48.

Pandiselvam, R., Sunoj, S., Manikantan, M. R., Kothakota, A., & Hebbar, K. B. (2017). Application and kinetics of ozone in food preservation. *Ozone: Science & Engineering, 39*(2), 115–126.

Pascual, A., Llorca, I., & Canut, A. (2007). Use of ozone in food industries for reducing the environmental impact of cleaning and disinfection activities. *Trends in Food Science & Technology, 18*, S29–S35.

Pasha, I., Saeed, F., Sultan, M. T., Khan, M. R., & Rohi, M. (2014). Recent developments in minimal processing: A tool to retain nutritional quality of food. *Critical Reviews in Food Science and Nutrition, 54*(3), 340–351.

Permanyer, M., Castellote, C., Ramírez-Santana, C., Audí, C., Pérez-Cano, F. J., Castell, M., & Franch, A. (2010). Maintenance of breast milk immunoglobulin A after high-pressure processing. *Journal of Dairy Science, 93*(3), 877–883.

Phan, K. T. K., Phan, H. T., Brennan, C. S., & Phimolsiripol, Y. (2017). Nonthermal plasma for pesticide and microbial elimination on fruits and vegetables: An overview. *International Journal of Food Science and Technology, 52*, 2127–2137. https://doi.org/10.1111/ijfs.13509 (accessed on 9th July 2025).

Pipliya, S., Kumar, S., Babar, N., & Srivastav, P. P. (2023). Recent trends in non-thermal plasma and plasma activated water: Effect on quality attributes, mechanism of interaction and potential application in food & agriculture. *Food Chemistry Advances*, 100249.

Poojary, M. M., Dellarosa, N., Roohinejad, S., Koubaa, M., Tylewicz, U., Gómez-Galindo, F., & Barba, F. J. (2017). Influence of innovative processing on γ-aminobutyric acid (GABA) contents in plant food materials. *Comprehensive Reviews in Food Science and Food Safety, 16*(5), 895–905.

Prakash, A. (2020). What is the benefit of irradiation compared to other methods of food preservation? In *Genetically Modified and Irradiated Food* (pp. 217–231). Academic Press.

Prakash, A., Guner, A. R., Caporaso, F., & Foley, D. M. (2000). Effects of low-dose gamma irradiation on the shelf life and quality characteristics of cut romaine lettuce packaged under modified atmosphere. *Journal of Food Science, 65*(3), 549–553.

Priyanka, B. S., Rastogi, N. K., & Tiwari, B. K. (2014). Opportunities and challenges in the application of ozone in food processing. In *Emerging Technologies for Food Processing* (pp. 335–358). Academic Press.

Rastogi, N. K., Nguyen, L. T., & Balasubramaniam, V. M. (2008). Effect of pretreatments on carrot texture after thermal and pressure-assisted thermal processing. *Journal of Food Engineering, 88*(4), 541–547.

Roobab, U., Inam-Ur-Raheem, M., Khan, A. W., Arshad, R. N., Zeng, X. A., & Aadil, R. M. (2022). Innovations in high-pressure technologies for the development of clean label dairy products: A review. *Food Reviews International*, 1–22.

Roobab, U., Khan, A. W., Lorenzo, J. M., Arshad, R. N., Chen, B. R., Zeng, X. A., & Aadil, R. M. (2021). A systematic review of clean-label alternatives to synthetic additives in raw and processed meat with a special emphasis on high-pressure processing (2018–2021). *Food Research International, 150*, 110792.

Shahi, S., Khorvash, R., Goli, M., Ranjbaran, S. M., Najarian, A., & Mohammadi Nafchi, A. (2021). Review of proposed different irradiation methods to inactivate food-processing viruses and microorganisms. *Food Science & Nutrition, 9*(10), 5883–5896.

Shelake, P. S., Mohapatra, D., Tripathi, M. K., & Giri, S. K. (2023). Explicating the effect of the ozonation on quality parameters of onion (*Allium cepa* L.) in terms of pungency, phenolics, antioxidant activity, color, and microstructure. *Ozone: Science & Engineering, 45*(1), 75–88.

Shelake, P. S., Mohapatra, D., Tripathi, M. K., Giri, S. K., Kate, A., & Kumar, M. (2022). Inactivation of *Aspergillus niger* and *Erwinia carotovora* in onion (*Allium cepa* L.) bulbs subjected to pulsed ozone treatment. *Postharvest Biology & Technology, 192*, 111998. https://doi.org/10.1016/j.postharvbio.2022.111998 (accessed on 9th July 2025).

Silindir, M., & Özer, A. Y. (2009). Sterilization methods and the comparison of E-beam sterilization with gamma radiation sterilization. *FABAD Journal of Pharmaceutical Sciences, 34*(1), 43.

Tiwari, B. K., Muthukumarappan, K., O'Donnell, C. P., & Cullen, P. J. (2008). Modelling color degradation of orange juice by ozone treatment using response surface methodology. *Journal of Food Engineering, 88*(4), 553–560.

Venta, M. B., Broche, S. S. C., Torres, I. F., Pérez, M. G., Lorenzo, E. V., Rodriguez, Y. R., & Cepero, S. M. (2010). Ozone application for postharvest disinfection of tomatoes. *Ozone: Science & Engineering, 32*(5), 361–371.

Wang, C. Y., Huang, H. W., Hsu, C. P., & Yang, B. B. (2016). Recent advances in food processing using high hydrostatic pressure technology. *Critical Reviews in Food Science and Nutrition, 56*(4), 527–540.

Whangchai, K., Uthaibutra, J., Phiyanalinmat, S., Pengphol, S., & Nomura, N. (2011). Effect of ozone treatment on the reduction of chlorpyrifos residues in fresh lychee fruits. *Ozone: Science & Engineering, 33*(3), 232–235.

Zhao, Y. M., de Alba, M., Sun, D. W., & Tiwari, B. (2019). Principles and recent applications of novel non-thermal processing technologies for the fish industry—A review. *Critical Reviews in Food Science and Nutrition, 59*(5), 728–742.

CHAPTER 3

Irradiation Techniques for Fresh Produce Quality and Safety

ROHINI DHENGE,[1,*] ARJUN MOHANAKUMAR,[1] AJAY CHINCHKAR,[2] MASSIMILIANO RINALDI,[1] and TOMMASO GANINO[1]

[1]*Department of Food and Drug, University of Parma, Parma, Italy*

[2]*Department of Food Science and Technology, National Institute of Food Technology Entrepreneurship and Management (NIFTEM), Sonipat, Haryana, India*

*Corresponding author

ABSTRACT

Thermal processing has long been the go-to method in the food industry for ensuring safety and prolonging shelf life. However, in response to growing consumer demand for natural, healthier, and safer products, nonthermal technologies have garnered significant attention. One such promising method for ensuring future food safety is ionizing radiation treatment, particularly for fresh produce like fruits and vegetables. Irradiation is a nonthermal food processing technique known for its safety, effectiveness in preventing microbial growth, preservation of quality, and minimal impact on food properties. It is also used as a phytosanitary treatment. Generally, food irradiation involves subjecting food to ionizing radiation, which possesses sufficient energy to remove electrons from atoms and ionize molecules. This includes high-energy photons such as gamma rays or X-rays and accelerated electrons from electron beams. When applied to fresh fruits and vegetables (FFVs), irradiation can act as

Sustainable Approaches in Postharvest Handling and Management: Pankaj B. Pathare (Ed.)

DOI: 10.1201/9781779641076-3

a postharvest fungistatic treatment, preventing spoilage without leaving any harmful residues in the edible parts. Furthermore, it can extend the shelf life of these fresh products by slowing down their natural processes. In the current research, the potential of food irradiation technology is explored in addressing various critical issues. These include addressing short shelf life, reducing initial microbial loads, and preventing the oxidation, polymerization, decarboxylation, and dehydration of fatty acids and lipids. Additionally, food irradiation can bring about changes in the antioxidant profile and result in the release of various compounds depending on the food's composition. It is worth noting that irradiating food at an optimal dose can be considered safe, as some food samples can withstand high doses without sacrificing sensory qualities. However, it's essential to be aware that reactive radicals generated during food irradiation can interact with chemical components, leading to the formation of radiolytic compounds like formaldehyde and short-chain hydrocarbons. Consumer acceptance of irradiated foods largely depends on product availability and satisfaction with quality and safety. Over time, with the support and confidence of governments and international agencies such as the World Health Organization (WHO), the Food and Drug Administration (FDA), and the International Atomic Energy Agency (IAEA), irradiation technology is gaining wider acceptance in modern society, albeit with both advantages and disadvantages.

3.1 INTRODUCTION

Food safety significantly affects people's health, even in developed countries with advanced food processing and distribution systems. Foodborne infections remain a substantial threat to human health and contribute to reduced economic productivity (Mostafavi et al., 2010). Global public health is greatly concerned about food contamination, particularly involving harmful microorganisms like pathogenic non-spore-forming bacteria, parasitic helminths, and protozoa. It's particularly vital to eliminate or reduce foodborne pathogens for individuals with weakened immune systems or immune-related illnesses (Farkas, 1998). In the interest of safety and health, risk assessment plays a pivotal role. Certain foods and food products are considered regulated items, requiring authorization before they can be sold, regardless of their safety.

Various methods have been developed to address food deterioration, enhance safety, and meet consumer demands for nutritious and flavorful foods without chemical preservatives, among other factors like pricing, and so forth. Preservation techniques extend the shelf life of food while maintaining its safety and sensory attributes. These methods encompass the necessary steps to maintain food quality for a specific duration. Over time, advances in scientific knowledge have led to improved food preservation techniques (Ahmad et al., 2014; Rahman, 2012). Conventional preservation methods include pasteurization, drying, canning, freezing, refrigeration, chemical treatments, and others, each affecting food quality in different ways, both positively and negatively. However, there is a growing demand for wholesome, fresh-tasting food products with excellent sensory qualities, improved safety, and longer shelf life (Ahmad et al., 2014; Junqueira-Goncalves et al., 2011). The aim of this book chapter is to provide an overview of the use of ionizing radiation in preserving fresh produce and food processing, with a specific focus on its effects on microbiological contamination, food nutritional properties, as well as the safety and quality of fruits and vegetables.

The use of irradiation on harvested fruits and vegetables is effective only within specific dosage ranges that extend the postharvest lifespan or enhance quality and safety, without causing harm to the crop. Research has shown that the natural disease resistance in fruits and vegetables may decline after harvest or during the early stages of ripening. This decline can lead to the activation of dormant infections due to a reduction in the levels of pre-existing or inducible antifungal chemicals (Terry and Joyce, 2004). Fresh fruits and vegetables (FFVs) are evaluated for various attributes, including appearance, texture, flavor, and taste, to determine their quality.

To enhance product safety and shelf life, food irradiation technology is increasingly employed in numerous countries for decontaminating and sterilizing dried fruits, vegetables, meats, poultry, fish, and seafood (Ahmad et al., 2014). Food irradiation is a non-thermal preservation method that involves exposing food to a specific level of energy in the form of radiation or high-speed particles. This technique is employed in the food processing industry to prevent food spoilage and the growth of pathogenic microorganisms while preserving other quality characteristics. Food is subjected to a precise dose of ionizing radiation, and this method is applied to over 60 different types of foods in more than 40 countries.

3.2 FOOD IRRADIATION

Food irradiation, a technology that employs ionizing radiation or electron beams to enhance food safety and extend shelf life by reducing bacteria and insects, is a safe method for processing food. When food is exposed to radiation, it gains a longer shelf life, and the growth of microbes and insects, and the ripening and sprouting of produce are delayed. This technology, similar to pasteurization for milk and preserving fruits and vegetables, has the potential to make food safer for consumers. Importantly, food irradiation does not render foods radioactive, nor does it significantly affect their nutritional value, flavor, texture, or appearance. In fact, the changes induced by irradiation are so subtle that it's challenging to discern whether a food has undergone this process. Food irradiation utilizes low-energy radiation.

In the 1950s, research programs on food irradiation were initiated in Western Europe to investigate the effects of radiation on food safety and nutritional content. The International Project in the field of Food Irradiation (IPFI) was launched in 1970 to further explore these aspects. A joint committee comprising the World Health Organization (WHO), the Food and Agriculture Organization (FAO), and the International Atomic Energy Agency (IAEA) reviewed the findings of this project (WHO). The committee concluded that exposing food to ionizing radiation at levels below 10 kGy did not pose any toxicological, nutritional, or microbiological risks (Diehl, 2002). One significant advantage of ionizing radiation is its non-residual nature, reducing the need for extensive pesticide use on fruits and vegetables. The FAO, the World Health Organization (WHO), and the International Atomic Energy Agency in Vienna all regard food irradiation as a globally safe and effective method (El-Samahy et al., 2000).

Food irradiation has proven to be a safe and effective non-thermal technology for improving food safety and extending the shelf life of various foods. While the types of foods and permissible radiation levels may vary from one country to another, nearly 50 countries have allowed or approved food irradiation. Gamma irradiation technology, which was initially developed in 1906, has undergone extensive testing, validation, and adoption by the medical and food industries over the past 60 years. It stands as one of the earliest non-thermal technologies.

3.3 FOOD IRRADIATION WORLDWIDE

Around 380,000 tons of food intended for human and animal consumption were radioactively treated in 2009.

3.3.1 EU

In 2011, the European Union (EU) employed food irradiation for approximately 8100 tons of food intended for human consumption. This usage remained fairly consistent from 2007 to 2011 (EU, 2012). However, in earlier years, the anticipated quantity of irradiated food was higher, reaching 20,000 tons in 2002 but decreasing to 15,000 tons in 2006. In a survey conducted by the EU in 2011, 130 food samples from the United Kingdom underwent analysis using CEN analytical methods (EU, 2012). These samples comprised a range of food categories, including soups and sauces, noodles, dehydrated Asian meals, fresh and dried herbs and spices, food supplements, as well as dried fish and seafood. The survey results indicated that six samples (4.6%) were non-compliant, primarily due to issues such as incorrect labeling or the absence of evidence confirming that the irradiation had been conducted in a licensed facility. Conversely, 117 samples (90%) adhered to compliance standards. In the case of seven samples (5.4%), the results were inconclusive or unclear. Across the EU, a total of 5397 samples were analyzed, with 5232 (97%) meeting compliance requirements, 105 (2%) failing to do so, and 60 (1%) yielding inconclusive results.

3.3.2 THE AMERICAS

In 2010, Mexico exported over 7500 tons of peppers, mangoes, and guavas that had undergone irradiation treatment to the United States (Eustice, 2011).

Canada has granted authorization for the irradiation of items like potatoes, onions, wheat, flour, whole wheat flour, spices (whole or crushed), and dehydrated seasoning preparations. However, despite concerns among the Canadian public related to foodborne illnesses, the practical application of irradiation in these cases has faced challenges.

In 2009, Brazil utilized irradiation to treat 25,000 tons of products, including pet supplies, animal feed, dried goods, and spices.

3.3.3 ASIA PACIFIC

China holds the position of the largest producer of irradiated food in Asia, with a total of 200,000 tons irradiated in 2009. This primarily included garlic, spices, dried vegetables, and cooked meats. In the same year, India irradiated 10,000 tons of products, including spices, spice blends, dried vegetable seasonings, and mangoes. Several other countries also employed irradiation on a smaller scale. Vietnam, for instance, irradiated 5300 tons of spices, frozen foods, and dragon fruit. South Korea treated 2500 tons of dried vegetables and spices using irradiation. Indonesia used irradiation on 2265 tons of spices, dehydrated goods, and frozen shrimp, fish, and frog legs. In Thailand, 2100 tons of products, including fermented sausage (ham), spices, herbs, vegetable seasonings, sweet tamarind, and mangoes, underwent irradiation. In Australia, the amount of mangoes, papayas, and lychees that were irradiated and then imported into New Zealand experienced a significant increase, rising from 256 tons in 2004 to 1205 tons in 2010.

3.4 SOURCES OF FOOD IRRADIATION

However, there is a significant amount of misinformation and apprehension concerning consumer acceptance, transportation, storage, occupational hazards, and the disposal of radiation sources. All three of these sources of ionizing energy can have a similar effect on any material they come into contact with, making gamma rays from radioactive elements, high-energy electrons from particle accelerators, and X-rays generated by high-energy electrons suitable forms of radiant energy. High-energy electrons, gamma rays, and X-rays can eliminate or render inactive bacteria, spores, fungi, and insects by breaking the molecular bonds in their DNA. This ability of radiation to generate powerful rays or particles capable of displacing electrons from atoms and molecules, resulting in electrically charged ions, is why it is sometimes referred to as "ionizing radiation." "Cold pasteurization" and "irradiation therapy" are also terms commonly used to describe irradiation. For e-beam and X-ray methods, which have the added benefit of ceasing radiation emission when turned off, the term "electronic pasteurization" has been coined.

There are three radiation sources utilized in food irradiation facilities: gamma radiation, X-rays (with energy levels of ≤ 7.5 MeV in some countries and ≤ 5 MeV in others), and electron beams (with energy levels of ≤ 10 MeV). Radionuclides such as ^{137}Cs and ^{60}Co are employed to produce gamma radiation (Figure 3.1).

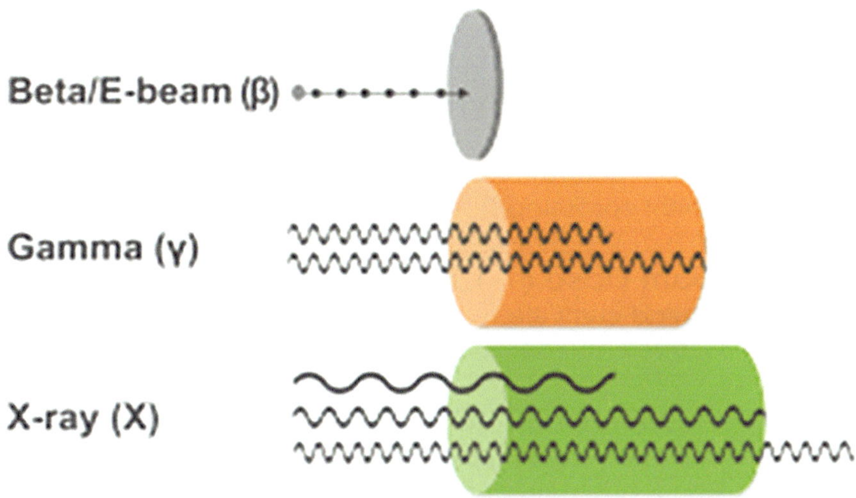

FIGURE 3.1 Doses of irradiation typically applied in food.

The FDA recommends food irradiation as a safe process. When ionizing radiation is applied to irradiated food, it leads to the breakdown of triglycerides containing palmitic acid, resulting in the formation of 2-DCB. Additionally, 2-DCB reacts with HA to produce a ketoxime (with permission). The authorization for the use of irradiation was granted by R. Ravindran and A.K. Jaiswal in Food Chemistry 285 (2019) 363–368. For various purposes, such as controlling or eliminating insects, pests, and other arthropods, as well as preventing sprouting and ripening to maintain freshness, fruits and vegetables can be exposed to radiation doses not exceeding 1 kGy. In the case of poultry, irradiation at a maximum dose of 3 kGy is recommended to control microorganisms associated with food contamination. Frozen meat is advised to be irradiated at 4.5 kGy, while chilled meat should not exceed 7.0 kGy to effectively eliminate microorganisms. Dehydrated enzymes can be treated with doses of up to 10 kGy to control microorganisms. Spices and seasonings can also be irradiated to manage germs, with recommended doses not exceeding 30 kGy.

For instance, gamma irradiation has been utilized to modify certain ingredients, prevent the sprouting of potatoes, eliminate insects in grains, alter the physical chemistry of food, and enhance its sensitivity (Wang and Chao, 2002).

TYPES OF IRRADIATION

- Low Dose (<1 kGy)
  - Control insects
  - Inhibit maturation
  - Inhibit sprouting
- Medium Dose (1-10 kGy)
  - Extend shelf life
  - Reduce microorganism level
- High Dose (> 30 kGy)
  - Sterilize - analogous to canning
  - Decontaminate certain food additives, e.g., spices

As per FDA regulations, food that has been subjected to radiation treatment must bear the official irradiation symbol. Food labels must include phrases such as "Treated with radiation" or "Treated by irradiation," along with the Radura symbol. For bulk commodities like fruits and vegetables, the selling container should either have a label adjacent to it or individual labeling. It's worth noting that FDA regulations do not mandate labeling for foods with multiple ingredients, such as spices.

3.5 QUALITY OF IRRADIATED FOODS

3.5.1 NUTRITIONAL QUALITY OF IRRADIATED FOOD

Irradiation has a minimal impact on the loss of macronutrients, particularly when dealing with living organisms that contain DNA and/or RNA.

Even when subjected to doses exceeding 10 kGy, proteins, lipids, and carbohydrates experience only slight nutritional changes, although there may be some sensory alterations. Similarly, minerals, trace elements, important fatty acids, amino acids, and minerals remain unaffected. While certain vitamins, especially thiamine, can be reduced, this occurs to a similar extent as in other industrial processes like drying or canning (thermal sterilization). For example, calculations indicate that irradiating chops and roast pork at 1 kGy would result in a 1.5% thiamine loss in the American diet (Wilkinson and Gould, 1996). Additional information can be found in WHO (1994) and FAO/IAEA/WHO (1999).

In contrast, bread made from irradiated flour displayed a 17% higher niacin concentration compared to control flour that was not irradiated (Diehl, 1991). Another study revealed that pork chops had increased niacin content (24%) and riboflavin levels (15%) after irradiation (Fox et al., 1989).

3.5.2 SENSORY QUALITY OF IRRADIATED FOODS

Irradiation isn't suitable for all food products. Foods with high-fat content, like fatty fish and certain dairy items, can develop undesirable odors and flavors due to accelerated rancidity even at very low doses. Some fruits and vegetables may also experience a loss of their natural firmness. High-protein foods, such as meat and poultry, can undergo flavor and odor changes when irradiated at room temperature. These changes can be mitigated by subjecting the food to radiation at freezing or refrigerated temperatures.

To prevent rancidity, the maximum dose for fatty pork products and high-fat fresh ground beef should not exceed 2.5 kGy. Shell eggs can tolerate doses of up to 2 kGy without affecting the yolk sac membrane, while liquid and dry eggs have a maximum tolerance of 3 kGy. Different cheeses can withstand doses up to 3 kGy without issues, but milk can develop an unpleasant flavor at relatively low concentrations (Diehl, 1983). These changes can be minimized by irradiating the food at refrigerated or frozen temperatures, and careful selection of appropriate packaging methods along with controlled gas atmospheres can further reduce these effects.

3.6 EFFECTS OF FOOD IRRADIATION ON FOOD PRODUCTS

Irradiation can have both positive and negative impacts on the nutritional value and shelf life of food. It extends the shelf life of fresh, high-quality food by preventing sprouting, deactivating microorganisms, eliminating inherent bacterial populations, and removing contaminants. The underlying principle of how ionizing radiation deactivates microorganisms is by disrupting normal cellular function through the destruction of nucleic acids, employing both "direct" and "indirect" mechanisms (Pillai, 2004). The primary targets of irradiation are cell membrane lipids and nucleic acids. Ionizing radiation causes damage to cell membranes and other structures, resulting in sublethal injury. Changes in membrane lipid composition, particularly involving polyunsaturated fatty acids, lead to membrane disruption, affecting various membrane functions, including permeability. Additionally, it can impact the activity of membrane enzymes (Erkmen and Bozoglu, 2016).

The effects of radiation become evident through the generation of genomic, biochemical, physiological, and morphogenetic changes in living cells such as yeasts, molds, and bacteria when microorganisms are inactivated by radiation. Several factors are critical in the inactivation of microorganisms by radiation, including the type of radiation, the type of microorganisms, the food composition, the oxygen content, the physical state of the food, and the physiological state of the microorganisms (Erkmen and Bozoglu, 2016; Pillai, 2004). However, high-dose irradiation, especially at doses exceeding 10 kGy, can lead to physicochemical changes and significantly impair the sensory qualities of food (Kim et al., 2006; Miller, 2005). Radiation doses exceeding 10 kGy can harm the structural characteristics of fibrous carbohydrates (Crawford and Ruff, 1996; Dionísio et al., 2009; Miller, 2005) (Table 3.1).

3.6.1 MACRONUTRIENTS

Radioactive treatment can bring about significant changes in the constituents of food. Among the macronutrients, carbohydrates are the least sensitive to radiation. Exposure to radiation can cause the breakdown of some glycosidic bonds that link monosaccharides, leading to reduced polymerization and an increase in the viscosity of polysaccharide solutions.

When it comes to proteins, their amino acid chains can undergo alterations in the presence of water due to an electron transfer process, potentially accelerating denaturation by initially affecting secondary and tertiary structures. However, compared to thermal processing, this denaturation is milder.

In the case of lipids, radiation processes can expedite oxidation and various other reactions, including the formation of free radicals, the production of hydrogen peroxides, and the degradation of molecules such as carboxylic acids and antioxidants. Consequently, radiation-based processes are not recommended for products with high fat content (Harder et al., 2016; Woodside et al., 2015).

3.6.2 MICRONUTRIENTS

Any food processing method has the potential to affect the stability of vitamins (Woodside, 2015). While certain vitamins like riboflavin (B2), pyridoxine (B6), and biotin typically remain stable when food is subjected to irradiation, others such as thiamine (B1) and vitamins A, C, and E are more sensitive to it. Among these, thiamine and vitamin C are particularly susceptible to radiation. The sensitivity of vitamin C is influenced by various factors, including exposure to oxygen, temperature changes, and alterations in pH levels (Dionsio et al., 2009).

3.7 SAFETY ASPECTS OF IRRADIATION IN THE FOOD INDUSTRY

"Wholesomeness" is a term associated with food additives, suggesting that their inclusion in food products makes them safe in terms of microbiological, nutritional, and toxicological aspects. While not all radiolytic products pose health risks, they are typically consumed in concentrations too low to harm biological systems. It's important to consider safety alongside toxicological studies when assessing irradiated foods. In food irradiation facilities, the amount of energy or radiation absorbed by a food product is determined by a set speed, and the food itself never directly contacts the radiation source. Higher radiation doses can potentially make some components of food radioactive. According to the US FDA, irradiated foods are safe, free from parasites, pests, and disease-causing microbes, and they do not become radioactive as a result of the process. As awareness of the technique grows, irradiated foods are gaining acceptance in society.

TABLE 3.1 Summary of the Advantages and Impacts of Irradiation (Type/Dose) on the Shelf Life, Quality, Sensory Attributes, Microflora, and Physical Characteristics of Fruits and Vegetables

Products	Dose	Benefits/Loss/Quality-Shelf-Life Extension	Irradiation Effects on Microflora and Sensory Properties	References
Onion, Garlic, Potato, sugar beet, ginger, carrot	0.05–0.15 kGY	Low-dose (up to 1 kGy) Inhibition of sprouting	–	Kader (1986), Prakash (2016)
Mature green and pink tomato (*Lycopersicon esculentum* Mill.)	0.7–2.2 kGy Gamma or X-rays	Polygalacturonase activity in mature-green stage tomatoes appeared to be permanently inhibited, remaining at less than 10% of the activity observed in non-irradiated fruit during storage at 20°C. However, the texture of these tomatoes did become softer over time. In contrast, pink tomatoes exposed to radiation experienced a milder effect on polygalacturonase activity compared to the mature green ones, although their activity remained lower than that of the control group.	–	Assi et al., (1997)
lettuce (*Lactuca sativa*), cabbage (*Brassica oleracea*), and celery (*Apium graveolens*).	0.50, 0.75, and 1.00 kGy	The initial levels of natural total ascorbic acid in the different vegetables varied significantly, and cabbage had the highest amount. Importantly, the irradiation process did not decrease these initial concentrations; in fact, it led to an increase in the case of cabbage.	–	Rubio et al., (2001)
Broccoli, corn, lima beans, and peas	2.5 to 3.1 kGy at −5°C	Did not cause significant changes in texture	–	Niemira et al. (2002)
Broccoli, corn, lima beans, and peas	3.9 to 4.6 kGy at –20°C	Resulted in substantial tenderness in peas and broccoli stems but had no such effect on corn or lima beans.	–	Niemira et al. (2002)

TABLE 3.1 *(Continued)*

Products	Dose	Benefits/Loss/Quality-Shelf-Life Extension	Irradiation Effects on Microflora and Sensory Properties	References
Coriander leaves (*Coriandrum sativum* L.)	Gamma irradiation 1 kGy (Packaged in polyethylene sachets) at 8–10°C	–	After exposing the leaves to 1 kGy of radiation and preserving them for two weeks, they exhibited 7–8% yellowing, whereas the unirradiated leaves showed 12–15% yellowing. The radiation reduced bacteria by 3 log cycles, eliminated yeast and mold by 1 log, and brought coliform levels down to 43 cfu/g. This relatively low dose of radiation effectively eliminated Listeria and Yersinia that were initially present in the product. The initial bacterial and mold counts in coriander leaves ranged from 106 to 108 cfu/g and 103 to 104 cfu/g, respectively. Importantly, exposure to a 1 kGy dose of radiation did not impact the levels of total carotenoid in the leaves.	Kamat et al. (2003)
Parsley (*Petroselinum crispum*)	0.5 to 2 kGy Packed in polymeric film bags at 4°C	–	A decrease in mesophilic and psychrotrophic counts by 3 to 4 log cycles occurred.	Trigo et al. (2004)
Broccoli and Peas	0.505 kGy Irradiated at 5°C and for peas 0.916 kGy at Irradiated at 20°C	–	To achieve a 90% reduction in the bacterial population of Listeria monocytogenes, specific D10-values need to be met.	Niemira et al. (2002)

TABLE 3.1 *(Continued)*

Products	Dose	Benefits/Loss/Quality-Shelf-Life Extension	Irradiation Effects on Microflora and Sensory Properties	References
Kimchi (Korean fermented vegetables)	0.38 kGy 0.54 kGy 0.47 kGy 0.32 kGy 0.87 kGy	–	The D_{10} value, which indicates the radiation dose required to reduce the populations of *Enterobacter agglomerans, Salmonella typhimurium, Alcaligenes xylosoxydans*, the total enteric group, and Latobacillus spp.	Kim et al. (2004)
Okra, baby corn, chaom, bird pepper, goat pepper, brinjal, eggplant, bitter cucumber, asparagus, and basil	Gamma irradiation 0.3, 0.6, 0.9 kGy at 10 ± 1°C	–	After being stored for seven days, it remained acceptable in terms of sensory qualities.	Segsarnviriya et al. (2005)
Broccoli and mung bean sprouts	1 kGy at 4°C	–	Following seven days of storage after irradiation, there were no significant alterations in the product's appearance, color, texture, flavor, and overall acceptability.	Bari et al. (2005)
Red cabbage, broccoli, and endive	Gamma irradiation 0.48,0.98, 1.46, 1.94, 2.49, 2.90 kGy	These plants exhibited the greatest resistance to radiation, and as the radiation dose increased, there was a linear increase in electrolyte leakage for all of them.	–	Fan and Sokorai (2005)
Celery, carrot and green onion	Gamma irradiation 0.48, 0.98, 1.46, 1.94, 2.49, 2.90 kGy	These plants were sensitive to radiation, and as the radiation dose increased, there was a consistent linear increase in electrolyte leakage for all of them.	–	Fan and Sokorai (2005)
Sliced tomatoes (*Lycopersicon syn. L esculentum)*	1 kGy	There was no notable impact on the overall carotenoid and vitamin C levels in sliced tomatoes (*Lycopersicon* syn. L. esculentum). However, there was an approximate 40% reduction in α-tocopherol due to irradiation.	–	Mohacsi-Farkas et al. (2006)

TABLE 3.1 *(Continued)*

Products	Dose	Benefits/Loss/Quality-Shelf-Life Extension	Irradiation Effects on Microflora and Sensory Properties	References
Carrot (*Daucus carota L.*) and Cucumber (*Cucumis sativus L)*	1 and 2 kGy at 4°C	The levels of total carotenoids and vitamin C in the irradiated samples were not significantly different from those in the control samples. Additionally, the changes in vitamin C and carotene concentrations during storage were statistically similar to those observed in the control samples. Qualified panelists could not discern any difference between the samples that had been exposed to radiation and those that had not.	–	Bandekar et al. (2006)
Carrot	<2.0 kGy at Room temperature	–	The color, lightness, flavor, sweetness, odor, and taste of the samples were not significantly affected. However, samples irradiated with doses below 2.0 kGy had lower overall acceptability during storage compared to the control samples.	Shurong et al. (2006)
Carrot	<2.0 kGy at Room temperature	–	There was no noticeable distinction in terms of taste, aroma, sweetness, brightness, flavor, or color. Moreover, products exposed to radiation levels below 2.0 kGy were better received in terms of overall acceptability compared to non-irradiated samples.	Shurong et al. (2006)
Tomato	>1 to >1.5 kGy at 4–7°C	Negative effect on the taste, sweetness and flavor	Adverse impact on the product's color and brightness.	Shurong et al. (2006)

TABLE 3.1 *(Continued)*

Products	Dose	Benefits/Loss/Quality-Shelf-Life Extension	Irradiation Effects on Microflora and Sensory Properties	References
Tomato	>1 kGy at Room temperature	–	Considerably less satisfactory than the control samples concerning attributes such as color, taste, sweetness, and notably, taste and flavor.	Shurong et al. (2006)
Tomato	>2 kGy at Room temperature	Samples not accepted	–	Shurong et al. (2006)
Tomato (*lycopersicon syn. L. esculentum*)	>1 kGy at Room temperature	Statistically significant alterations in color, aroma, flavor, and texture were observed only in the case of watermelon. There were no substantial differences in the rank sums of pre-cut cantaloupe and tomato cubes.	–	Mohacsi-Farkas et al. (2006)
Tomatoes (*lycopersicon syn.L. esculentum*)	2 kGy	The firmness of the samples significantly decreased, particularly in the case of watermelon cubes, indicating that they became noticeably softer or more tender.	–	Mohacsi-Farkas et al. (2006)
Cucumber (*Cucumis sativus L.*)	2 kGy	There were no alterations observed in the sensory characteristics or the texture of the samples.	–	Bandekar et al. (2006)
Cabbage (*Lactuca sativa var. capitata*)	0.5 up to 3.0 kGy at 5°C for 14 days	Cabbage did not experience significant changes.	–	Bibi et al. (2006)
Cucumber, blanched and seasoned spinach, and seasoned burdock	Gamma irradiation 1 kGy	–	A decrease of about 3 log CFU/g of *Salmonella* Typhimurium	Lee et al. (2006)
Blanched and seasoned spinach	Gamma irradiation 2 kGy	–	3 log CFU/g reduction of the *L. ivanovii* and by about 4 log cfu/g reduction of the *L. ivanovii*	Lee et al. (2006)

TABLE 3.1 *(Continued)*

Products	Dose	Benefits/Loss/Quality-Shelf-Life Extension	Irradiation Effects on Microflora and Sensory Properties	References
Mixed salad composed of cherry tomatoes (*Solanum spp.*)	1.2 kGy	–	5 log cycles decrease of *S. aureus*	Horak et al. (2006)
Celery (*Apium, graveolens*) and Cabbage (*Lactuca sativa var. capitata*)	0.18 ± 0.01 kGy and 0.22 ± 0.03 kGy at 4°C	–	D_{10} value for *E. coli* ATCC	Lopez et al. (2006)
Spinach (*Spinacia oleracea*)	0.32 ± 0.01 kGy at 4°C	–	D_{10} value for *L. innocua*	Lopez et al. (2006)
Cherry tomato	0.08 kGy	–	D_{10}-value of *E. coli* O157:H7	Shurong et al. (2006)
Carrot	0.24 kGy to 0.33 kGy	–	D_{10}-values of *Salmonella* Enteritidis	Shurong et al. (2006)
Tomato (*Lycopersicon syn. L. esculentum*	1 kGy	–	A decrease in the quantity of viable cells of more than 5 log-cycles	Mohacsi-Farkas et al. (2006)
Carrot samples (*Daucus carota*	2 kGy at 5°C for 14 days	–	To completely eradicate all fungi during storage, the control samples' fungal levels were 2.7 10CFU/g.	Bibi et al. (2006)
Cabbage (*Lactuca sativa var. capitata*	2.5 kGy at 5°C for 14 days		Free of viable fungal colonies during storage	Bibi et al. (2006)
Onion (*Allium cepa*)	0.23 kGy Aerobically packaged 5°C–2°C	Hardness not affected by doses up to 3 kGy	*Listeria monocytogenes* (D10 = 0.23 kGy)	Faridah et al. (2006)
Carrot	0.1 kGy	50% loss of beta-carotene	–	Hajare et al. (2006)
Mushrooms	2kGy	Reduction in sugar content	–	Fernandes et al. (2016)
Spinach leaf	Combination of 0.3 kGy, 1% citric acid	The treatment's combined impacts did not lead to a reduction in quality.	The inclusion of 1% citric acid alongside X-ray irradiation enhanced the bactericidal effectiveness.	Jeon et al. (2020)
Three-quarter ripe and fully ripe pineapple fruit (*Ananas comosus*)	0.05, 0.1, and 0.15 kGy	They preserved their texture more effectively in comparison to the control group. The maximum permissible dose was approximately 0.25 kiloGrays (kGy).	–	Susheela et al. (1997)

TABLE 3.1 *(Continued)*

Products	Dose	Benefits/Loss/Quality-Shelf-Life Extension	Irradiation Effects on Microflora and Sensory Properties	References
Papaya	Gamma irradiation 0.5 kGy	The onset of the ripening phase was postponed by a 48-hour delay due to irradiation. However, irradiation did not impact the total soluble solids (measured in Brix), which increased from 8% to 12% in both the treated and untreated fruits.	–	D'innocenzo and Lajolo (2001)
Watermelon (*Citrullus lanatus*)	Fruits were exposed to two different radiation doses (0.5 and 1 kiloGray) and then packed in Nutrip-PS (polystyrene) trays, followed by polymeric film bags. They were stored at 4°C for 9 days in the case of the 0.5 kGy treatment (comprising 4 days for the control group and 3 days for the 1 kGy treatment).	On the initial day post-irradiation, there was a minor darkening in color. However, as storage progressed, this distinction became less noticeable. The texture analysis results demonstrated no discernible alterations as a result of irradiation.	1–2 log reduction in the total aerobic mesophilic counts and total aerobic psychrotrophic counts	Trigo et al. (2004)
Jackfruit (*Artocarpus heterophyllus*)	Aerobically packaged– 0.4 kGy	Listeria monocytogenes (D10 = 0.4 kGy)	–	Faridah et al. (2006)
Jackfruit (*Artocarpus heterophyllus*)	Aerobically packaged- 0.16 kGy– 5°C ± 2°C at least 8 days	*E. coli* O157 (D10 = 0.16 kGy)	–	Faridah et al. (2006)

TABLE 3.1 *(Continued)*

Products	Dose	Benefits/Loss/Quality-Shelf-Life Extension	Irradiation Effects on Microflora and Sensory Properties	References
Grapefruits (*Citrus paradisi* c.v. Rio Red)	Fruits were exposed to radiation at three different doses: 0, 0.15, and 0.3 kiloGray (kGy), and subsequently, they were stored at 10°C for 36 days, followed by an additional 20 days at 20°C.	The overall soluble solids content in grapefruits remained largely unaffected by both irradiation and storage. However, there was a notable decrease in acidity during storage. In comparison to the control group (0 Gy), fruits subjected to 0.3 kGy of radiation exhibited higher acidity levels. Furthermore, their results suggest that low-dose irradiation at 0.3 kGy either increased or, at the very least, maintained the concentration of flavonoids.		Vanamala et al. (2007)
Fresh blueberries (*Vaccinium corymbosum* L.	Electron beam 1.1, 1.6, 3.2 kGy	The findings indicate that blueberries exposed to radiation levels as high as 3.2 kiloGrays (kGy) do not experience a loss in their juiciness. Additionally, the blueberries maintained suitable acidity levels that remained consistent throughout storage, even when exposed to radiation up to 3.2 kGy.	Fruits retained their desired texture (i.e., remained firm) unless exposed to irradiation doses exceeding 1.6 kiloGrays (kGy). Panelists found blueberries subjected to radiation up to 1.6 kGy to have an acceptable overall quality, color, texture, and aroma.	Moreno et al. (2007)
Pineapple (*Citrullus vulgaris*) in cubes and Watermelon (*Citrullus vulgaris*) in cubes	1 and 2.5 kGy at 4°C	Irradiation had no impact on the tartness of the pineapple.	–	Landgraf et al. (2006)
Strawberry	0–1 kGy	The onset of fruit browning can be postponed, and the reduction in fruit weight and spoilage can be mitigated by applying a 1 kiloGray (kGy) dose during storage.	increase sensory characteristics during storage	Yoon et al. (2020)
Cereals, pulses, fruits (fresh and dried), fish, meat and pork etc.	0.15–0.5	Phyto sanitation	–	Al-Kahtani et al. (1998), Cornwell (2013), McDonald et al. (2012), Pillai and Shayanfar (2017)

TABLE 3.1 *(Continued)*

Products	Dose	Benefits/Loss/Quality-Shelf-Life Extension	Irradiation Effects on Microflora and Sensory Properties	References
Meat, poultry, seafood, Spices, natural gum et	20–40	Intensive levels of radiation exposure ranging from 10 to 50 kiloGrays (kGy) are employed for industrial sterilization and decontamination of food additives.	–	Dionísio, Gomes, and Oetterer (2009), SádECká (2007)
Fish, meat, corn, celery, meat	1.0–3.0	Moderate levels of radiation exposure, ranging from 1 to 10 kiloGrays (kGy), are used to extend the shelf life of products.	–	Fadhel et al. (2016), Kumar, Gautam, and Sharma (2015), Lefebvre, Thibault, Charbonneau, and Piette (1994), Prakash, Inthajak, Huibregtse, Caporaso, and Foley (2000), Yang et al. (2014)
Fresh fruits and vegetables	0.25–1.0	Slowing down natural processes like ripening.	–	Hossain, Parvez, Munshi, Khalil, and Huque (2014), Sea, Rakovski, and Prakash (2015), Surendranathan and Nair (2013), Yadav and Patel (2014)

In recent years, consumers have been purchasing irradiated foods due to their satisfaction with the product's quality and safety. Irradiation has also made it possible for certain fruits and vegetables, previously restricted from entering the US due to the risk of carrying pests, to be legally imported. Some tropical Asian produce, like specialty mangoes, which cannot undergo conventional pest treatment methods, are now being irradiated to ensure pest eradication. Educating consumers is crucial for the public's acceptance of food irradiation. When provided with reliable information, consumers are more likely to choose irradiated food over conventionally treated options. Market research surveys have shown that 80–90% of consumers would purchase irradiated food products after learning about their benefits and safety. For example, a 10-minute educational video led to a significant increase in consumers' interest in purchasing irradiated food.

The European Commission's Scientific Committee on Food (SCF) examined the toxicity of the 2-alkylcyclobutanone group of radiolytic compounds and issued a statement in July 2002 based on their evaluation. In 2004, a review of toxicological food safety issues related to food irradiation was released. The European Food Safety Authority reexamined the evidence in 2011 and reaffirmed the safety of food irradiation. It was also noted that alkylcyclobutanones were not unique radiolytic products as they had been found in commercial, non-irradiated fresh cashew nut and nutmeg samples.

3.8 LEGISLATION RELATED TO FOOD IRRADIATION

3.8.1 EU LEGISLATION RELATED TO FOOD IRRADIATION-CONT'D

The various types and functions of radiation are distinguished by the frequency or wavelength of the energy waves they emit. Among these, high-frequency radiation such as UV, X, and gamma rays poses the greatest risk to human health (FSAI, 2005). The legal framework for food irradiation is outlined in specific circumstances, governed by European Union Directives 1999/2/EC and 1999/3/EC (EU, 2007). The European Union has established rigorous regulations for irradiated foods. The European Parliament approved the framework directive 1999/2/EC, which addresses all essential aspects of food subjected to ionizing radiation treatment.

According to EU law, any irradiated food product (or one containing irradiated components) must be clearly labeled as "irradiated" or "processed by ionizing radiation" to enable consumers to make informed choices. Furthermore, each EU member state is required to forward the results of inspections conducted at irradiation facilities. The EU has established validated and standardized analytical methods that member states must use and adhere to. The second directive, 1999/3/EC, provides member states with guidelines regarding which foods and food components can be irradiated. Consequently, in EU member states, only three food categories—dried aromatic herbs, spices, and vegetable seasonings—can undergo irradiation and be sold (Parliament, 1999).

Regulation (EEC) No. 3954/87, which came into effect on January 2, 1988, outlines the process for establishing the maximum allowable levels of radioactive contamination in food and feed that may be placed on the market following a nuclear accident or any other radiological emergency. "Foodstuffs" in this context refer to items intended for human consumption either immediately after processing or at a later time, while "feeding stuffs" are products exclusively meant for animal nutrition. If the Commission, based on official sources, determines that the maximum permissible levels have been reached or are likely to be reached in the event of an accident or radiological emergency, it will promptly adopt regulations to apply these maximum levels. The validity period of any regulation must be as short as possible and cannot exceed three months. The regulation covers baby foods, liquid foods, dairy products, and feeds.

Regulation (EEC) No. 2219/89, effective from July 25, 1989, imposes special requirements for exporting foods and feeds following a nuclear disaster or radiation emergency. It prohibits the export of any food or feed that exceeds the maximum allowable amounts.

Regulation (EEC) No. 737/90, effective from April 1, 1990, sets conditions for importing agricultural products from third countries following the Chernobyl nuclear power station accident. It establishes rules for products originating from other nations, determining the maximum radioactivity levels for ^{134}Cs and ^{137}Cs. Non-compliance triggers control measures. This regulation underwent several modifications, with the last one being Regulation (EC) No. 806/2003, effective from June 5, 2003.

Decision 87/600/EC, effective from March 21, 1988, outlines community plans for early information exchange in the event of a radiological emergency. This decision introduced the "Ecurie" system, allowing the

Commission to receive information from Member States. The designated point of contact and Commission service must be available 24 hours a day for transmitting this information.

3.8.2 U.S. LEGISLATION RELATED TO FOOD IRRADIATION

U.S. regulatory requirements for food irradiation were established and enforced starting in 1986. These regulations encompass legal mandates and safety considerations related to radiological, toxicological, microbiological, and nutritional aspects of irradiated foods. They also cover the labeling requirements for irradiated food products. Notable changes to these standards were documented in Federal Register entries 62 (1997) and 64 (1999). The practice of irradiating food in the production, processing, and handling of food became enforceable starting in 1997. For the irradiation of fresh meat (chilled but not frozen), a maximum dose of 4.5 kiloGrays (kGy) was requested in the petition. Additionally, a maximum dose of 7.0 kGy was determined for irradiating frozen meat.

Food irradiation, which became enforceable in 1999, involves subjecting food to ionizing radiation. This technique is utilized to prevent food spoilage and eliminate harmful microorganisms such as *Salmonella*. The FDA granted approval for the use of irradiation to control pathogenic bacteria in red meat. Furthermore, in the context of the Production, Processing, and Handling of Food, regulations that took effect in 2000 allowed for the safe use of ionizing radiation to reduce the levels of *Salmonella* in fresh shell eggs. The macronutrient composition of fresh shell eggs exposed to an absorbed dosage of 3 kGy is only minimally altered.

3.8.3 CANADIAN LEGISLATION RELATED TO FOOD IRRADIATION

The Food and Drug Act, which became enforceable in 2008, addresses the handling of foods that have been subjected to irradiation. It prohibits the sale of certain products that have had their vitamin content increased through either irradiation or supplementation. Importers of irradiated food for sale in Canada are mandated to maintain records containing property-related information.

3.8.4 AUSTRALIAN LEGISLATION RELATED TO FOOD IRRADIATION

The implementation of Food Irradiation regulations in 2003 allows for the use of radiation in the form of electrically generated electron beams, machine-generated X-rays, or gamma rays from ^{60}Co for treating food in Australia and New Zealand. This process extends the shelf life of fruits such as strawberries by eliminating molds at low radiation doses and prevents sprouting in vegetables like potatoes. Furthermore, irradiation is effective in eradicating harmful bacteria and pathogens that can cause foodborne illnesses when applied at higher levels.

Irradiation of Tropical Fruits, also enforced in 2003, pertains to the treatment of tropical fruits like rambutan, breadfruit, carambola, custard apple, lychee, longan, and mangosteen with radiation. In Australia and New Zealand, it is considered safe for consumers to irradiate tropical fruits up to a maximum dose of 1 kiloGray (kGy) when using approved manufacturing and irradiation methods.

3.9 CONCLUSION

In recent years, the practice of irradiating food has gained traction as a viable processing technique, with more countries utilizing it to sanitize and eliminate pests in agricultural products. This has sparked renewed interest in the scientific community regarding the chemistry behind the production of radiolytic products resulting from the irradiation of various food components. Southeast Asian developing nations and the European Union are supportive of using food irradiation to extend the shelf life of products and enhance phytosanitization. However, the average consumer, often viewing irradiation as a risky food processing method, may not share this perspective. Nonetheless, this approach is gaining acceptance in modern culture as governments demonstrate increased confidence in irradiated food products.

The effects and advantages of food irradiation on the safety and wholesomeness of food are detailed in Table 3.1. Various outcomes, such as reduced storage losses, prolonged shelf life, and improved microbiological safety, can be achieved depending on the radiation dose applied. Ionizing radiation has potential applications ranging from preventing the sprouting of tubers and bulbs to creating commercially sterile food products. Notably, the chemical changes induced by irradiation in food are typically minimal. There is no significant loss of macronutrients due to irradiation, and the impact on the nutritional value of proteins, lipids, and carbohydrates is negligible compared to conventional food preservation methods. Food irradiation has the capacity to enhance food quality and safety by extending its shelf life.

This chapter aims to provide an overview of the effects of ionizing radiation on fresh products, their quality, and safety. It briefly discusses the fundamental concepts of food irradiation, how ionizing radiation affects bacteria, and its impact on the nutritional value of irradiated food. Ionizing radiation is recognized as a safe, extensively researched method applicable in various ways to eliminate harmful biological organisms in food. Multiple health organizations endorse it, and governments worldwide have granted approval for various uses. With its potential to prolong shelf life, food irradiation can enhance microbiological safety and quality. When compared to other food processing techniques like heat and chemical methods, it is considered a more suitable and effective approach to enhance food stability and safety, while having minimal effects on sensory and nutritional attributes.

KEYWORDS

- **food irradiation**
- **ionizing radiation**
- **fresh produce**
- **shelf life extension**
- **microbial safety**
- **radiolytic compounds**

REFERENCES

Ahmad Shah, M., Ahmad Mir, S., & Ahmad Pala, S. (2014). Enhancing food safety and stability through irradiation: A review. *Journal of Microbiology, Biotechnology and Food Sciences, 3*(5), 371–378.

Al-Kahtani, H. A., Abu-Tarboush, H. M., Al-Dryhim, Y. N., Ahmed, M. A., Bajaber, A. S., Adam, E. S. E., & El-Mojaddidi, M. A. (1998). Irradiation of dates: Insect disinfestation, microbial and chemical assessments, and use of thermoluminescence technique. *Radiation Physics and Chemistry, 53*(2), 181–187.

Assi, N. E., Huber, D. J., & Brecht, J. K. (1997). Irradiation-induced changes in tomato fruit and pericarp firmness, electrolyte efflux, and cell wall enzyme activity as influenced by ripening stage. *Journal of the American Society for Horticultural Science, 122*(1), 100–106.

Bandekar, J. R., Dhokane, V. S., Shashidhar, R., Hajare, S., Saroj, S., & Sharma, A. (2006). Use of irradiation to ensure hygienic quality of fresh, pre-cut fruits and vegetables and other minimally processed foods of plant origin. In *Use of Irradiation to Ensure the Hygienic Quality of Fresh, Pre-Cut Fruits and Vegetables and Other Minimally Processed Food of Plant Origin* (pp. 170–187). Proceedings of a final research coordination meeting organized by the Joint FAO/IAEA Programmed of Nuclear Techniques in Food and Agriculture, Islamabad, Pakistan, 22–30 July 2005.

Bari, M. L., Nakauma, M., Todoriki, S., Juneja, V. K., Isshiki, K., & Kawamoto, S. (2005). Effectiveness of irradiation treatments in inactivating *Listeria monocytogenes* on fresh vegetables at refrigeration temperature. *Journal of Food Protection, 68*(2), 318–323.

Bibi, N., Khattak, M. K., Badshah, A., & Chaudry, M. A. (2006). Radiation treatment of minimally processed fruits and vegetables for ensuring hygienic quality. In *Use of Irradiation to Ensure the Hygienic Quality of Fresh, Pre-Cut Fruits and Vegetables and Other Minimally Processed Food of Plant Origin* (pp. 205–224). Proceedings of a final research coordination meeting organized by the Joint FAO/IAEA Programmed of Nuclear Techniques in Food and Agriculture, Islamabad, Pakistan, 22–30 July 2005.

Cornwell, P. B. (2013). *The Entomology of Radiation Disinfestation of Grain: A Collection of Original Research Papers*. Elsevier.

Crawford, L. M., & Ruff, E. H. (1996). A review of the safety of cold pasteurization through irradiation. *Food Control, 7*, 87–97.

D'Innocenzo, M., & Lajolo, F. M. (2001). Effect of gamma irradiation on softening changes and enzyme activities during ripening of papaya fruit. *Journal of Food Biochemistry, 25*(55), 425–438.

Diehl, J. F. (1983). Radiolytic effects on foods. In E. S. Josephson & M. S. Peterson (Eds.), *Preservation of Foods by Ionizing Radiation* (Vol. 1, pp. 279–357). CRC Press Inc.

Diehl, J. F. (1991). Nutritional effects of combining irradiation with other treatments. *Food Control, 2*(1), 20–25.

Diehl, J. F. (2002). Food irradiation—Past, present and future. *Radiation Physics and Chemistry, 63*(3–6), 211–215.

Dionísio, A. P., Gomes, R. T., & Oetterer, M. (2009). Ionizing radiation effects on food vitamins: A review. *Brazilian Archives of Biology and Technology, 52*, 1267–1278.

EFSA. (2011). EFSA statement on the safety of irradiation of food. *EFSA Journal, 9*(4), 2107.

El-Samahy, S. K., Youssef, B. M., Aaskar, A. A., & Swailam, H. M. M. (2000). Microbiological and chemical properties of irradiated mango. *Journal of Food Safety, 20*, 139–156.

Erkmen, O., & Bozoglu, F. (2016). Food preservation by irradiation. In *Food Microbiology: Principles into Practice* (Vol. 2, pp. 106–127). John Wiley & Sons, Ltd.

EU. (2012). Report from the Commission to the European Parliament and the Council on food and food ingredients treated with ionizing radiation for the year

2011, COM(2012) 659 final. http://eur-lex.europa.eu/LexUriServ/LexUriServ.do?uri=COM:2012:0659:FIN:EN:PDF (accessed on 9th July 2025).

European Union. (2007). Food irradiation: Community legislation. http://ec.europa.eu/food/food/biosafety/irradiation/comm_legisl_en.htm (accessed on 9th July 2025).

Eustice, R. F. (2011). Food irradiation: A global perspective and future prospects. http://www.cirms.org/pdf/2011_conference_pdf/2011_10_18_CIRMS_Eustice.pdf (accessed on 9th July 2025).

Fadhel, Y. B., Leroy, V., Dussault, D., St-Yves, F., Lauzon, M., Salmieri, S., & Lacroix, M. (2016). Combined effects of marinating and γ-irradiation in ensuring safety, protection of nutritional value and increase in shelf-life of ready-to-cook meat for immunocompromised patients. *Meat Science, 118*, 43–51.

Fan, X., & Sokorai, K. J. B. (2005). Assessment of radiation sensitivity of fresh-cut vegetables using electrolyte leakage measurement. *Postharvest Biology and Technology, 36*, 191–197.

Faridah, M. S., Nur Ilida, M., Asiah, A. S., & Mahmud, M. (2006). Effect of gamma irradiation on the safety and quality of minimally processed fruits and vegetables. In *Use of Irradiation to Ensure the Hygienic Quality of Fresh, Pre-Cut Fruits and Vegetables and Other Minimally Processed Food of Plant Origin* (pp. 188–224). Proceedings of a final research coordination meeting organized by the Joint FAO/IAEA Programmed of Nuclear Techniques in Food and Agriculture and held in Islamabad, Pakistan, 22–30 July 2005.

Farkas, J. (1998). Irradiation as a method for decontaminating food: A review. *International Journal of Food Microbiology, 44*, 189–204.

Fernandes, Â., Barreira, J. C. M., Antonio, A. L., Oliveira, M. B. P. P., Martins, A., & Ferreira, I. C. F. R. (2016). Extended use of gamma irradiation in wild mushrooms conservation: Validation of 2 kGy dose to preserve their chemical characteristics. *LWT–Food Science and Technology, 67*, 99–105.

Food Safety Authority of Ireland. (2005). Food irradiation: Information document. http://www.piwet.pulawy.pl/irradiacja/food%20irradiation%20-%20information%20document.pdf (accessed on 9th July 2025).

Fox, J. B., Thayer, D. W., Jenkins, R. K., et al. (1989). Effect of gamma irradiation on the B vitamins of pork chops and chicken breasts. *International Journal of Radiation Biology, 55*, 689–703.

Hajare, S. N., Dhokane, V. S., Shashidhar, R., Sharma, A., & Bandekar, J. R. (2006). Radiation processing of minimally processed carrot (*Daucus carota*) and cucumber (*Cucumis sativus*) to ensure safety: Effect on nutritional and sensory quality. *Journal of Food Science, 71*(3).

Harder, M. N. C., Arthur, V., & Arthur, P. B. (2016). Irradiation of food: Processing technology and effects on nutrients: Effect of ionizing radiation on food components. In *Encyclopedia of Food and Health* (pp. 476–481). Elsevier. https://doi.org/10.1016/B978-0-12-384947-2.00405-0 (accessed on 9th July 2025).

Horak, C. I., Pietranera, M. A., Malvicini, M., Narvaiz, P., Gonzalez, M., & Kairiyama, E. (2006). Improvement of hygienic quality of fresh, pre-cut, ready-to-eat vegetables using gamma irradiation. In *Use of Irradiation to Ensure the Hygienic Quality of Fresh, Pre-Cut Fruits and Vegetables and Other Minimally Processed Food of Plant Origin* (pp. 23–40). Proceedings of a final research coordination meeting organized by the Joint

FAO/IAEA Programmed of Nuclear Techniques in Food and Agriculture and held in Islamabad, Pakistan, 22–30 July 2005.

Hossain, F., Parvez, A. K., Munshi, M. K., Khalil, I., & Huque, R. (2014). Post-harvest treatments of radiation and chemical on organoleptic and biochemical properties of mango (*Mangifera indica*) in relation to delay. *American-Eurasian Journal of Agricultural and Environmental Sciences, 14*(6), 555–564.

IFT Scientific Status Summary. (2004). *Food Technology, 58*(11), 48–55.

Jeon, M. J., & Ha, J. W. (2020). Synergistic bactericidal effect and mechanism of X-ray irradiation and citric acid combination against foodborne pathogens on spinach leaves. *Food Microbiology, 91*, 103543.

Junqueira-Goncalves, M. P., Galotto, M. J., Valenzuela, X., Dinten, C. M., Aguirre, P., & Miltz, J. (2011). Perception and view of consumers on food irradiation and the radura symbol. *Radiation Physics and Chemistry, 80*, 119–122.

Kader, A. A. (1986). Potential applications of ionizing radiation in postharvest handling of fresh fruits and vegetables. *Food Technology, 40*(6), 117–121.

Kamat, A., Pingulkar, K., Bhushan, B., Gholap, A., & Thomas, P. (2003). Potential application of low dose gamma irradiation to improve the microbiological safety of fresh coriander leaves. *Food Control, 14*, 529–537.

Kim, D. H., Song, H. P., Yook, H. S., Ryu, Y., & Byun, M. W. (2004). Isolation of enteric pathogens in the fermentation process of kimchi (Korean fermented vegetables) and its rededication by gamma irradiation. *Food Control, 15*(6), 441–445.

Kim, J., Rivadeneira, R. G., Castell-Perez, R., Rosana, M. L., & Moreira, G. (2006). Development and validation of a methodology for dose calculation in electron beam irradiation of complex-shaped foods. *Journal of Food Engineering, 74*, 359–369.

Kumar, S., Gautam, S., & Sharma, A. (2015). Hurdle technology including chlorination, blanching, packaging and irradiation to ensure safety and extend shelf life of shelled sweet corn kernels. *Journal of Food Processing and Preservation, 39*(6), 2340–2347.

Landgraf, M., Goularte, L., Martins, C., Cestari, J. R. A., Nunes, T., Aragonalegro, L., Destro, M., Behrens, J., Vizeu, D., & Hutzler, B. (2006). Use of irradiation to improve the microbiological safety of minimally processed fruits and vegetables. In *Use of Irradiation to Ensure the Hygienic Quality of Fresh, Pre-Cut Fruits and Vegetables and Other Minimally Processed Food of Plant Origin* (pp. 41–59). Proceedings of a final research coordination meeting organized by the Joint FAO/IAEA Programme of Nuclear Techniques in Food and Agriculture and held in Islamabad, Pakistan, 22–30 July 2005.

Lee, N. Y., Jo, C., Shin, D. H., Kim, W. G., & Byun, M. W. (2006). Effect of γ-irradiation on pathogens inoculated into ready-to-use vegetables. *Food Microbiology, 23*, 649–656.

Lefebvre, N., Thibault, C., Charbonneau, R., & Piette, J. P. (1994). Improvement of shelf-life and wholesomeness of ground beef by irradiation—2. Chemical analysis and sensory evaluation. *Meat Science, 36*(3), 371–380.

Lopez, L., Avendano, S., Romero, J., Wittig, E., Garrido, S., Solis, L., Thumann, K., Acevedo, C., Espinoza, J., & Vargas, M. (2006). Use of ionizing radiation to ensure the safety of pre-cut fresh vegetables. In *Use of Irradiation to Ensure the Hygienic Quality of Fresh, Pre-Cut Fruits and Vegetables and Other Minimally Processed Food of Plant Origin* (pp. 69–86). Proceedings of a final research coordination meeting organized by the Joint FAO/IAEA Programme of Nuclear Techniques in Food and Agriculture and held in Islamabad, Pakistan, 22–30 July 2005.

McDonald, H., McCulloch, M., Caporaso, F., Winborne, I., Oubichon, M., Rakovski, C., & Prakash, A. (2012). Commercial scale irradiation for insect disinfestation preserves peach quality. *Radiation Physics and Chemistry, 81*(6), 697–704.

Miller, R. B. (2005). *Electronic Irradiation of Foods: An Introduction to the Technology*. Springer.

Mohacsi-Farkas, C. S., Farkas, J., Andrassy, E., Polyak-Feher, K., Bruckner, A., Kisko, G., & Agoston, R. (2006). Improving the microbiological safety of some fresh pre-cut and prepackaged chilled produce by low-dose gamma irradiation. In *Use of Irradiation to Ensure the Hygienic Quality of Fresh, Pre-Cut Fruits and Vegetables and Other Minimally Processed Food of Plant Origin* (pp. 130–169). Proceedings of a final research coordination meeting organized by the Joint FAO/IAEA Programmed of Nuclear Techniques in Food and Agriculture and held in Islamabad, Pakistan, 22–30 July 2005.

Moreno, M. A., Castell-Perez, M. E., Gomes, C., Da Silva, P. F., & Moreira, R. G. (2007). Quality of electron beam irradiation of blueberries (*Vaccinium corymbosum* L.) at medium dose levels (1.0–3.2 kGy). *LWT, 40*, 1123–1132.

Mostafavi, H. A., Mirmajlessi, S. M., & Fathollahi, H. (2012). The potential of food irradiation: Benefits and limitations. In A. A. Eissa (Ed.), *Trends in Vital Food and Control Engineering* (pp. 43–68). IntechOpen Limited.

Niemira, B. A., Fan, X., & Sommers, C. H. (2002). Irradiation temperature influences product quality factors of frozen vegetables and radiation sensitivity of inoculated *Listeria monocytogenes*. *Journal of Food Protection, 65*(9), 1406–1410.

Pillai, S. D. (2004). Food irradiation. In Ross et al. (Eds.), *Preharvest and Postharvest Food Safety: Contemporary Issues and Future Directions*. Blackwell Publishing and the Institute of Food Technologists.

Pillai, S. D., & Shayanfar, S. (2017). Electron beam technology and other irradiation technology applications in the food industry. *Topics in Current Chemistry, 375*(1), 6.

Rahman, M. S. (2012). Food preservation and processing methods. In J. Ahmed & M. S. Rahman (Eds.), *Handbook of Food Process Design*. Blackwell Publishing.

Rubio, T., Araya, E., Avendano, S., Lopez, L., Espinoza, J., & Vargas, M. (2001). Effect of ionizing radiation on fresh vegetables artificially contaminated with *Vibrio cholerae*. *IAEA-TECDOC-1213*. Irradiation to control *Vibrio* infection from consumption of raw seafood and fresh produce. Results of a coordinated research project organized by the Pan American Health Organization and the Joint FAO/IAEA Division of Nuclear Techniques in Food and Agriculture.

Sádecká, J. (2007). Irradiation of spices—A review. *Czech Journal of Food Science, 25*(5), 231–242.

Sea, S., Rakovski, C., & Prakash, A. (2015). Ripening quality of 'Bartlett' pears (*Pyrus communis* L.) subjected to phytosanitary X-ray irradiation treatment followed by simulated retail display.

Segsarnviriya, S., Malakrong, A., & Kongratarpon, T. (2005). The effect of gamma radiation on quality of fresh vegetables. In *International Symposium "New Frontier of Irradiated Food and Non-Food Products,"* 22–23 September 2005, KMUTT, Bangkok, Thailand.

Shurong, L., Meixu, G., & Chuanyao, W. (2006). Use of irradiation to ensure hygienic quality of fresh pre-cut and blanched vegetables and tofu. In *Use of Irradiation to Ensure the Hygienic Quality of Fresh, Pre-Cut Fruits and Vegetables and Other Minimally*

Processed Food of Plant Origin (pp. 87–105). Proceedings of a final research coordination meeting organized by the Joint FAO/IAEA Programmed of Nuclear Techniques in Food and Agriculture and held in Islamabad, Pakistan, 22–30 July 2005.

Stewart, E. M. (2004). Food irradiation: More pros than cons? Part 2. *Biologist, 51*(2), 141–144.

Surendranathan, K., & Nair, P. (2013). Carbohydrate metabolism in ripening banana and its alteration on gamma irradiation in relation to delay in ripening. *Journal of the Indian Institute of Science, 62*(8), 63.

Susheela, K., Damayanti, M., & Sharma, G. J. (1997). Irradiation of *Ananas comosus*: Shelf-life improvement, nutritional quality and assessment of genotoxicity. *Biomedical Letters, 56*(223–224), 135–144.

Terry, L. A., & Joyce, D. C. (2004). Elicitors of induced disease resistance in postharvest horticultural crops: A brief review. *Postharvest Biology and Technology, 32*(1), 1–13.

Vanamala, J., Cobb, G., Loaiza, J., Yoo, K., Pike, L. M., & Patil, B. S. (2007). Ionizing radiation and marketing simulation on bioactive compounds and quality of grapefruit (*Citrus paradisi* cv. Rio Red). *Food Chemistry, 105*, 1404–1411.

Wang, J., & Chao, Y. (2002). Drying characteristics of irradiated apple slices. *Journal of Food Engineering, 52*, 83–88.

Wilkinson, V. M., & Gould, G. W. (1996). *Food Irradiation: A Reference Guide.* Butterworth Heinemann.

Woodside, J. V. (2015). Nutritional aspects of irradiated food. *Stewart Postharvest Review, 3*, 1–6. https://doi.org/10.2212/spr.2015.3.2 (accessed on 9th July 2025).

World Health Organization. (1994). *Safety and Nutritional Adequacy of Irradiated Food.* WHO, Geneva.

World Health Organization. (1999). *High-Dose Irradiation: Wholesomeness of Food Irradiated with Doses Above 10 kGy.* Report of a FAO/IAEA/WHO Study Group. *WHO Technical Report Series No. 890.* WHO, Geneva.

Yadav, M., & Patel, N. (2014). Optimization of irradiation and storage temperature for delaying ripening process and maintaining quality of Alphonso mango fruit (*Mangifera indica* L.). *African Journal of Agricultural Research, 9*(5), 562–571.

Yoon, Y. S., et al. (2020). Effects of X-ray irradiation on the post-harvest quality characteristics of 'Maehyang' strawberry (*Fragaria × ananassa*). *Food Chemistry, 325*, 126817.

LEGISLATIONS

1. Directive 1999/2/EC. Available at: http://eur-lex.europa.eu/LexUriServ/LexUriServ.do?uri=CELEX:31999L0002:EN:HTML (accessed on 9th July 2025).
2. Directive 1999/3/EC. Available at: http://eur-lex.europa.eu/LexUriServ/LexUriServ.do?uri=OJ:L:1999:066:0024:0025:EN:PDF (accessed on 9th July 2025).
3. Regulation (EEC) No. 3954/87. Available at: http://eur-lex.europa.eu/LexUriServ/LexUriServ.do?uri=CELEX:31987R3954:EN:HTML (accessed on 9th July 2025).
4. Regulation (EEC) No. 2219/89. Available at: http://eur-lex.europa.eu/LexUriServ/LexUriServ.do?uri=CELEX:31989R2219:EN:HTML (accessed on 9th July 2025).

5. Regulation (EEC) No. 737/90. Available at: http://eur-lex.europa.eu/LexUriServ/LexUriServ.do?uri=CELEX:31990R0737:EN:HTML (accessed on 9th July 2025).
6. Food and Drug Act. (2008). Available at: http://laws.justice.gc.ca/en/ShowTdm/cs/f-27///en (accessed on 9th July 2025).
7. Food Irradiation. (1999). Available at: http://www.foodstandards.gov.au/foodmatters/foodirradiation.cfm (accessed on 9th July 2025).
8. Food Irradiation. (2003). Available at: http://www.ific.org/publications/brochures/upload/FoodIrradiation-A-Global-Food-Safety-Tool.pdf (accessed on 9th July 2025).
9. Irradiation in the Production, Processing and Handling of Food. (1997). Available at: http://ecfr.gpoaccess.gov/cgi/t/text/textidx?c=ecfr&tpl=/ecfrbrowse/Title21/21cfr179_main_02.tpl (accessed on 9th July 2025).
10. Irradiation in the Production, Processing, and Handling of Food. (2000). Available at: http://www.epa.gov/EPA-IMPACT/2004/December/Day-21/i27868.htm (accessed on 9th July 2025).
11. Irradiation of Tropical Fruit. (2003). Available at: http://www.foodstandards.gov.au/newsroom/factsheets/factsheets2003/irradiationoftropica1944.cfm (accessed on 9th July 2025).
12. USDA. (1990). Issues final rule on meat and poultry irradiation. Available at: http://www.fsis.usda.gov/Oa/background/irrad_final.htm (accessed on 9th July 2025).
13. U.S. Regulatory Requirements for Irradiating Foods. (1986). Available at: http://www.fda.gov/Food/FoodIngredientsPackaging/IrradiatedFoodPackaging/ucm110730.htm (accessed on 9th July 2025).

CHAPTER 4

Cold Atmospheric Plasma-Mediated Treatments: Impact on Physical, Biochemical, and Phytonutrient Quality Attributes of Fresh and Minimally Processed Fruit

LORIANE A. YANCLO,[1,2,3] GUNNAR O. SIGGE,[1] ZINASH A. BELAY,[2] and OLUWAFEMI J. CALEB[1,3,*]

[1]*Department of Food Science, Faculty of AgriSciences, Stellenbosch University, Stellenbosch, South Africa*

[2]*Agri-Food Systems and Omics Laboratory, Post-Harvest and Agro-Processing Technologies (PHATs), Agricultural Research Council (ARC) – Infruitec-Nietvoorbij, Stellenbosch, South Africa*

[3]*Africa Institute for Postharvest Technology, Faculty of AgriSciences, Stellenbosch University, Stellenbosch, South Africa*

*Corresponding author

ABSTRACT

The quality and safety of fresh, whole, and minimally processed fruit along the value chains remains at imminent risk due to natural spoilage microorganisms and/or food-borne pathogens' cross-contamination. This risk has both local and global food security implications. Over the last two decades, cold atmospheric plasma (CAP) technology has been demonstrated as an effective and efficient alternative for microbial inactivation and/or surface decontamination of fresh and minimally processed fruit.

Sustainable Approaches in Postharvest Handling and Management: Pankaj B. Pathare (Ed.)

DOI: 10.1201/9781779641076-4

The efficacy of CAP treatment at low temperature (non-thermal) has been shown as a positive attribute for its application on fresh produce. It has a minimal negative impact on quality attributes and organoleptic properties of fresh and fresh-cut produce. Extensive reviews on the basic application principles, mechanism of microbial inactivation, and degradation of chemical residues of CAP on fresh produce have been published. Hence, this review critically assessed the status of CAP with emphasis on its impact on physical, biochemical, and phytonutrient (bioactive compounds and macro/micro-nutrients) properties of fresh and minimally processed fruit. This article highlighted challenges of CAP technology and future research needs for the successful adoption by the Agri-food industry. The conclusion emphasizes the need for a balanced optimization process that is focused both on preservation of essential bioactive components and reducing microbial load on fresh and minimally processed fruit.

4.1 INTRODUCTION

Cold atmospheric plasma (CAP) is a non-thermal technology that has been adapted by the Agri-food industry for the surface decontamination of food products to ensure safety and extend storage life (Misra et al., 2015a, b). Atmospheric plasma is described as ionized or energetic gas, and it is considered the fourth state of matter after solids, liquid, and gas (De Corato, 2020; Mir et al., 2016). The non-thermal nature of CAP is of great benefit to the fresh commodity industries, due to minimal fruit tissue disruption. In addition, the treatment can be applied at room temperature for a short duration, and it is relatively cost-effective and efficient (Stoica et al., 2014).

Therefore, over the past two decades, the interest in and application of CAP for food processing and preservation has gained momentum (Ekezie et al., 2017). This includes extensive studies on microbial inactivation (Muhammad et al., 2018; Scholtz et al., 2015); degradation of agrochemicals (Misra, 2015; Sarangapani et al., 2017); enzyme inactivation (Han et al., 2019); starch modification (Banura et al., 2018; Chang et al., 2020; Okyere et al., 2019; Thirumdas et al., 2017a, b), and enhancing protein properties (Moosavi et al., 2020; Terpiłowski et al., 2017). In addition, the effectiveness of CAP treatments for aflatoxin disintegration (Devi et al., 2017), meat curing and impact on cooking properties of sausages (Jung et al., 2015; Sarangapani et al., 2015), as well as sterilization of food packages and contacting surfaces, especially stainless steel, and polyethylene surfaces (Pankaj et al., 2014), have been investigated.

Fruit can be consumed as fresh or minimally processed, as it attracts consumers due to its flavor, nutritious value, and mostly ready-to-eat nature. However, active degradation of biochemical properties, physiological changes, and microbial growth during postharvest handling and storage limit its storage/shelf life (Chen et al., 2020). Hence, maintaining the quality of fresh and minimally processed fruit using appropriate and optimized postharvest technologies is crucial for better quality and longer shelf life. Application of chemical and thermal techniques has been in use for decades in the Agri-food industry (Nyamende et al., 2021). The use of synthetic chemicals in the Agri-food industry could be linked to the accumulation of toxic residues on the produce and/or development of acquired resistance by pathogens (Matrose et al., 2021). On the other hand, the application of heat treatment could lead to undesirable effects such as loss of functional/bioactive compounds and organoleptic properties (Caleb et al., 2016).

However, the CAP technology has shown a significant potential to retain color change (Ramazzina et al., 2015; Tappi et al., 2014), retard enzymatic activity (Han et al., 2019), enhance antioxidant activity (Won et al., 2017), and reduce the natural microbial load (Berardinelli et al., 2012). Additionally, the efficacy of CAP towards inactivation of microorganisms such as *Salmonella Typhimurium, Staphylococcus aureus, Aspergillus brasiliensis, Escherichia coli,* and *Listeria monocytogenes* on surfaces of cabbage, lettuce, dried figs, and other commodities has been reported (Fernandez et al., 2013; Lee et al., 2015). On the contrary, few studies have reported on the impact of CAP on the overall quality (phytonutrient, biochemical, and physical) of fresh and minimally processed fruit. According to Surowsky et al. (2015), the efficiency of CAP depends on the depth of the plasma penetration and the type of active species produced.

Misra et al. (2018) provided an extensive review of the basic principles and application of CAP. Most recently, Chen et al. (2020) reviewed the effects of CAP treatments on the quality of fruit and vegetables, and Han et al. (2019) provided an in-depth analysis of the CAP technology's endogenous enzyme inactivation mechanism. Pan et al. (2021) discussed the effects of CAP treatments on fruit texture and biochemistry during storage, and Mir et al. (2020) presented the most recent understanding of the role of CAP technology in reducing microbial contamination and enhancing the quality attributes of various fruits. However, despite numerous review articles on the application of CAP treatments for fresh commodities, the effects of this technology on fruit tissue microstructural and biochemical changes, as well as phytonutrients, have not been fully addressed. Therefore, this review provides critical insights into the impact of CAP pre-treatments on fruit tissue microstructure based on available studies. In addition, the impacts of various CAP treatments on the physical, biochemical, and phytonutrient attributes, as well as safety, were critically examined.

4.2 OVERVIEW OF CAP TECHNOLOGY

4.2.1 PROCESS GASES AND REACTIVE SPECIES

Figure 4.1 presents the applicable process gases and the associated particulates, reactive species, and free radicals generated when these process gases are ionized. Plasma contains charged particles and different reactive species such as charged or neutral molecules, atoms, ions, and electrons, as well as free radicals (Figure 4.1). This occurs when chemical reactions and ultraviolet (UV) radiation result in the formation of active volatile compounds with anti-microbial efficacy (Muhammad et al., 2018; Scholtz et al., 2015). Various types of gases are used for plasma operation, and the choice of gas has a crucial influence on the efficiency of the plasma system. These gases include the simple use of natural air or pure nitrogen, or the use of a mixture of helium, argon, neon as di-nitrogen and nitrous oxide (N_2/N_2O), or dinitrogen and dioxygen (N_2/O_2), or argon and dioxygen (Ar/O_2), or helium and dioxygen (He/O_2), or helium and dinitrogen (He/N_2), or $He/O_2/H_2O$ gas mixture (Guo et al., 2015).

Studies have shown that the selected operating gas becomes more efficient when oxygen is added (Scholtz et al., 2015). When using an ionized-He and atmospheric-He mixture as operating gas with elevated voltage and increased electron energy and density, a variety of reactive oxygen species (ROS) are produced downstream. This excitation and increase in ROS production enhances microbial inactivation (Pathare et al., 2023). Likewise, the use of nitrogen as working gas leads to the production of reactive nitrogen species (RNS), nitric oxide (NO•) being the principal reacting nitrogen species, which react with almost all cell components through charge exchanges known as oligomerization (Mir et al., 2016). The excess of NO• modifies peroxyl and alkoxyl radicals and decreases the opposing effects of plasma in produce containing high contents of oils and lipids. The use of air as gas with the DBD plasma produces reactive oxygen and nitrogen species, the latter presiding plasma composition. While using glow discharge plasma, RNS are dominating species, whereas OH radicals and nitric oxide concentration are predominant compared to DBD plasma. This implies that RNS is proficiently stabilized in organic materials compared to ROS (Fernandes and Rodrigues, 2021).

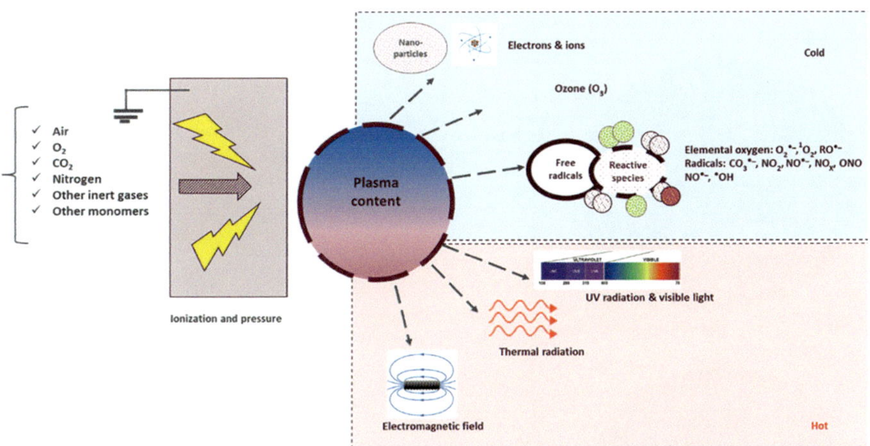

FIGURE 4.1 Basic description of cold plasma content and the gas temperatures.

4.2.2 CLASSIFICATION AND MODE OF APPLICATION

Plasma is described as a charged gas that contains ions, photons, free electrons, and atoms in their excited states and where the charges are both positively and negatively equivalent (Pankaj et al., 2013). It is generally described as the fourth state of matter, the others being solids, liquids, and gases (Pathare et al., 2023). It is commonly found in stars, lightning, or plasma televisions (Mandal et al., 2018).

Plasma can be classified into two categories: high-temperature plasma and low-temperature plasma. In high-temperature plasma, the charged and/or neutral ions, electrons, and gas molecules are in a state of thermodynamic equilibrium, with temperatures ranging between 106 and

108 Kelvin (Pathare et al., 2023). High-temperature plasma is generated with high-pressure power and has been successfully applied in the aeronautic field (Francioso et al., 2016) or in the metal industry for welding (Pathare et al., 2023). On the other hand, low-temperature plasma is divided into quasi-equilibrium plasma (100–150°C) and non-equilibrium plasma (< 60°C), also known as cold plasma (Pathare et al., 2023). Non-thermal plasma can be generated at low pressure using discharged gas under reduced atmospheric pressures (vacuum) and near ambient temperature (30–60°C) for the sterilization of heat-sensible materials (Misra et al., 2011).

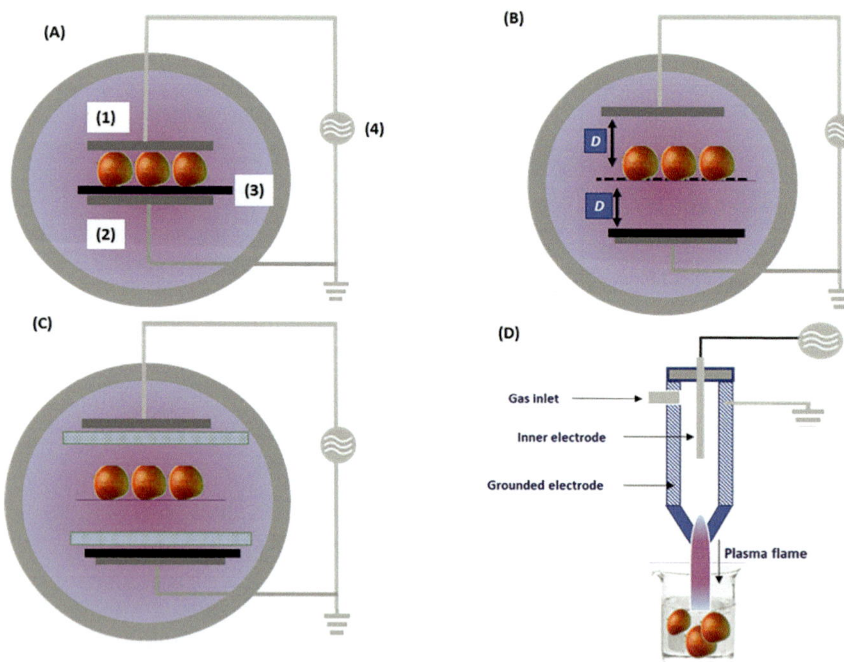

FIGURE 4.2 Description of the different modes of cold plasma application in the treatment of fresh fruit with their mechanisms of action. (A) Direct plasma treatment: samples have direct contact with all reactive species; (B) Semi-direct plasma treatment: Plasma treatment to either prevent UV effects or to select UV effects with *D* as distance (cm/m); (C) Semi-direct plasma treatment: samples have contact with only selected reactive species; and (D) Indirect plasma treatment: samples have contact with reactive species through a channel. (1) electrode(s); (2) sample in chamber (where plasma in generated); (3) sample holder; and (4) high-frequency generator.

Over the years, the methods of cold plasma generation have been extensively reviewed and annotated by Misra et al. (2018), Han et al. (2019), Chen et al. (2020), Mir et al. (2020), and Pan et al. (2021). Therefore, this review will not be revisiting this subject matter, but it will emphasize the plasma application approach (Figure 4.2). The application approach could have direct/indirect implications on the quality attributes of fresh and minimally processed fruit because it determines the main reactive species and particles in contact with the produce. The mode of application could be described as direct, semi-direct, or indirect, as annotated in Figure 4.2 (Bovi et al., 2016; Schottroff et al., 2018).

Under the direct application mode, treated samples are in direct contact with all excited plasma discharge, including the charged particles, radicals, and reactive species, as well as UV and thermal radiation (Figure 4.2A). For the semi-direct mode, the samples do not have access to the total plasma discharge, either by the function of distance from the discharge source (Figure 4.2B) or the use of selective optical filters (Figure 4.2C). On the other hand, for indirect plasma treatment, direct UV lights are excluded, and plasma reactive species are suspended or dissolved in a transmitting media (Figure 4.2D), such as plasma-processed water, which is a new alternative for the treatment of fresh produce on a pilot scale (Andrasch et al., 2017; Schottroff et al., 2018).

4.3 IMPACTS OF CAP ON PHYSICAL QUALITY ATTRIBUTES

4.3.1 COLOR

Table 4.1 presents an extensive summary of investigations within the last decade on the effects of various cold plasma treatments on the physical and chemical quality attributes of horticultural commodities. Color is an essential quality attribute for consumer acceptability of fresh fruits (Ma et al., 2015). Studies reporting on different effects of CAP treatments on color attributes of fresh and minimally processed fruit are summarized in Table 4.1. For instance, Ramazzina et al. (2015) reported that the CAP treatment of the pericarp for fresh cut (FC) 'Hayward' kiwifruit improved the lightness (*L*), which resulted in a less darkened product at the end of storage.

Similarly, Misra et al. (2014c) investigated the effect of CAP (voltage 60 kV and frequency 50 Hz) on the color of 'Elsanta' strawberries treated for 5 min and stored at 10°C and 90% relative humidity after 24h of storage. The authors reported a significant increase in the **L* of both treated and untreated strawberry samples. On the contrary, Lacombe et al. (2015) investigated the effect of CAP (frequency 47 kHz and power 549 W) on fresh blueberries (cv. not specified) stored at 4°C storage and found a significant decrease on the color parameters after 120 s for **L* value, indicating a darkening of the blueberry surface color, and resulting in the melting of the blueberries' cutaneous wax. Furthermore, a significant increase was observed for **a* and **b* values, indicating respectively the red surface and the blue color of the sample. These results suggest that CAP can easily affect the materials without a thick peel. This was further explained by the oxidation of pigments due to the radicals in plasma, leading to a negative impact on the color (Lacombe et al., 2015).

Furthermore, a correlation study was done by Paixão et al. (2019) for CAP (80 W power supply, frequency 50 kHz) treated Siriguela fruit (cv. not specified). The authors positively associated the increase in fruit redness **a* to the increase in the lightness **L*. The darkening in samples was associated with oxidative reactions catalyzed by peroxidase and polyphenoloxidase, which transform quinones to a dark-colored pigment called melanin (Hamdan et al., 2022). Generally, a decrease in fruit lightness value and an increase in the redness value is characterized by browning (Hamdan et al., 2022; Paixão et al., 2019).

4.3.2 MOISTURE

Fresh and minimally processed fruit are subjected to a rapid rate of moisture loss during storage. Available literature has provided diverse outcomes on the role played by CAP treatments in moisture transfer in minimally processed fruit (Bao et al., 2020; Zhang et al., 2019). Table 4.1 includes selected reports on the influence of CAP treatment on moisture content of horticultural commodities. For instance, Bao et al. (2020) reported that CAP pre-treatment (voltage of 5 kV, frequency of 40 kHz) at 50, 60, 70°C for 15 s led to a decrease in the moisture ratio for sliced 'Junzao' jujube fruit during drying. Moreover, a slight reduction was observed in the moisture ratio of CAP-treated 'Junzao' jujube samples compared to the control when the fruits were subjected to a drying temperature of 50°C. An increase of the drying temperature to 60°C and 70°C led to a faster change in moisture content after CAP treatment for 15 s. They suggested that CAP for a short duration of 15 s on jujube 'Junzao' fruit slices could alter the microstructure through etching the fruit surface, leading to fissures, and facilitating moisture transfer during the drying process.

It has been suggested that an increase in CAP pre-treatment duration leaves irregular micro-holes on the surfaces of commodities, which increases the moisture transfer rate and consequently reduces the drying time (Nishime et al., 2017). In addition, Zhang et al. (2019) showed that extending the duration of the CAP treatment could lead to a disruption of the fruit cell wall, the collapse of cell structure, and consequently increase the resistance of moisture movement. Additionally, Wang et al. (2012) reported that a moisture loss lower than 5% does not generally affect the hardness of the tissue of fruit such as pears. They further reported that moisture loss during CAP treatment might be attributed to the air flow from the plasma device. Overall, and based on existing literature stated above and in Table 4.1, exposure of fresh and FC produce to CAP treatment enhances moisture transfer by acting upon the fruit tissue surface through etching, leading to a fissure on the cell.

TABLE 4.1 Effects of Cold Plasma Application on Physical Quality Attributes of Fresh and Minimally Processed Produce There Were Reported Within the Last 10 Years

Produce	Plasma Treatment Conditions	Key Findings	References
Mango ∞	DBD, voltage 50 V, frequency 10 kHz exposed to treated water (tap, distilled and ultrapure) PAW	• PAW treated samples best maintained color attributes of mangoes fruit	Wu et al. (2023)
*Blueberries 'Emerald'	DBD, voltage 45 kV, treatment time 50 s	• Suppressed the reduction in firmness after 20 or 25 d storage • Increase in soluble sugar content after 25 d storage • Decrease in TA content after 15 and 25 d storage • No significant differences in L^* • Increase in a^* and b^* values	Zhou et al. (2023)
*Wolfberry	DBD, voltage 700 V, treatment time 480s	• Increase in firmness by 11.07% • Increase in TSS by 5.88%	Du et al. (2023)
*Cucamelons	DBD diffusor, PAW, power 1500 Hz, voltage 120 v, 60 kHz resonance frequency, NaOCl 100 ppm total chlorine, treatment time	• Increase firmness in PAW-treated Cucamelons • DBDD-PAW treatment extended shelf life and maintained high the quality of the produce	Rothwell et al. (2023)
Mango ∞	DBD plasma system, 50 V input voltage and a 10 kHz frequency	• Increase in hardness • Decrease in TSS	Wu et al. (2022)
*Banana	DBD, voltage 6.9 kV, treatment time 46 s	• Slight decrease in hardness	Pour et al. (2022)
*Mango 'Hongyu'	Dielectric barrier discharge, voltage 75 kV, treatment time 3 min	• Higher retentions of chromaticity (L^*, a^* and b^*) • Increase in firmness • Increase in soluble solids content, titratable acidity, and SSC/TA ratio	Yi et al. (2022)

TABLE 4.1 *(Continued)*

Produce	Plasma Treatment Conditions	Key Findings	References
*Apricots	DBD, voltage 1320 J, vibration intensity of 10%, a frequency of 16 Hz, and a frequency slope of 1 Hz, treatment time 60 s	• Inhibited adverse physiological changes in apricot fruit • Maintained sensory and nutritional quality • Delayed the decrease of firmness and TSS	Hua et al. (2022)
* Sour Cherry ∞	New system cold atmospheric pressure plasma, voltage 10, 15, 20 kV, frequency 10, 15, 20 kHz, gas flow rate 3, 5, 7 L min^{-1}, oxygen 0%, 0.5%, 1%	• No effect on color of samples • No effect on pH of samples	Hosseini et al. (2021)
Kiwi	DBD, voltage –15, 25, 35 kV, power 13, 22, 31 W, Freq. 60 kHz, treatment time 1–5 min	• No changes in Color • Increase flavor • Increase texture	Liu et al. (2021)
DR 'Junzao' Jujube slices	CAP, voltage – 5 kV, Freq. – 40 kHz, and treatment time 15 s	• Significant decrease in the value of red/green color substances • No effect on the soluble solid contents after 15 s • Reduced moisture	Bao et al. (2020)
* 'Duch' Strawberries	CAP, voltage – 260 V, Freq. – 50 Hz, and treatment time 30 min	• No effect on moisture content and total soluble solids • Decrease in the pH content	Rana et al. (2020)
DR Wolfberry ∞	Atmospheric pressure plasma, 3 L/min flow, Freq. – 20 kHz, 750 W, treatment time 5, 30, 45, 60 s	• Total color difference declined by 18–27%	Zhou et al. (2020)
Blueberry	Jet plasma, voltage – 11 kV, Freq. 1000 kHz, treatment time 2–6 min	• No changes in color • Decrease in anthocyanin and antioxidants	Hou et al. (2019)
* Siriguela ∞	Glow discharge plasma, 80 W, Freq. – 50 kHz, and treatment time 5 to 15 min	• Slight change in the chroma and hue values • No adverse change observed in *L**, *a**, and *b** • Decrease in pH value	Paixão et al. (2019)
Chili pepper ∞	Gliding arc discharge, Pulse freq. – 20 kHz, 750 W, and treatment time 5, 30, 45, 60 s	• Increase in *L**, *a**, and *b** values	Zhang et al. (2019)
Apple	DBD, power 90 W, Freq. 60 kHz, treatment time 0–140 s	• Decrease in pH • No changes in TSS	Xiang et al. (2018)
* Mango 'Nam Dok Mai'	Gliding arc discharge (non-thermal plasma), 600 W, Ar gas flow rate of 2, 5 and 8 L/min, treatment time 5 or 10 min	• Significant differences in *L** and *a** values • No significant differences in *b** values and mango color change • No significant changes in hardness, cohesiveness, and springiness • Titratable acidity significantly declined, but no change in TSS	Phan et al. (2018)

TABLE 4.1 *(Continued)*

Produce	Plasma Treatment Conditions	Key Findings	References
* kumquats ∞	Intermittent corona discharge plasma jet, voltage – 8 kV DC, Freq. – 20 kHz, power 2.0, 3.0 & 4.0 A, treatment time 10 s off and on	• No significant change in the firmness after 120 s • Significant positive effect on the storage quality • No change in total sugars after 15 d storage with 3 and 4 A power	Puligundla et al. (2018)
* Apples 'Granny Smith'	Microwave-driven plasma torch, Freq. – 2.45 GHz, power – 1.2 kW, gas flow of 20 L min^{-1}, treatment time 10 min	• Increase in color • Decreased pH value • No impact on the dry matter content and no changes in the firmness	Bußler et al. (2017)
* Blueberries ∞	Dielectric barrier discharge, voltage of 60, 80 kV and frequency of 50 Hz, treatment time 0–5 min	• No significant difference in color and titratable acidity • Significant decrease in the firmness • Significant increase in TSS	Sarangapani et al. (2017)
* Grapes ∞	PAW, flow rate of 1.2 L/min, power 1.1 to 1.3 mA, voltage – 8.2 kV, treatment time 30 and 60 min	• Significant decrease in pH after 60 min • No significant changes in color after 30 min of Plasma activated water	Guo et al. (2017)
* Cantaloupe ∞	Plasma activated Hydrogen Peroxide system, dist. – 9 mm, voltage – 17 kV, flow rate 9.7 mL/min, pressure 15 psi, treatment time 45 s, 30 min	• No significant change in L^* (luminosity or level of light or darkness) • No significant change in a^* (on a green negative to red positive number and on a blue negative to yellow positive number)	Jiang et al. (2017)
* 'Raptor' Melon	DBD, voltage – 19 V and about 3 A, high voltage – 15 kV, Freq. – 12.5 kHz, treatment time 15 + 15 min and 30 + 30 min on each side of fruit	• Higher water loss observed during storage • Firmness declined for samples treated for 15 + 15 min • Significant decline in L^*, a^*, and b^* on 2 and 4 days for 15 + 15 min • Significant increase in CO_2 production after 22 h in the 15 + 15 sample • Significant decrease in soluble solids and in titratable acidity	Tappi et al. (2016)
* Blueberries ∞	Cold atmospheric plasma jet, Freq. – 47 kHz, 549 W, and treatment time 0, 15, 30, 45, 60, 90, 120 s	• Significant reduction in firmness • Significant increase in L^* and a^* after 120 s and b^* after 45 s	Lacombe et al. (2015)
*Kiwifruit 'Hayward'	DBD, 15 kV, wavelength 200 – 450 nm, treatment time 20 min (10 + 10 min for each side) and 40 min (20 + 20 min for each side)	• Increase in water loss during storage • Significant decrease in lightness during storage • No effect on colour Hue angle and Chroma, and texture • Significant increase in soluble solids and titratable acidity	Ramazzina et al. (2015)

TABLE 4.1 *(Continued)*

Produce	Plasma Treatment Conditions	Key Findings	References
*Apple 'Granny Smith'	Microwave-driven atmospheric pressure plasma, power 1.2 kW, frequency 2.45 GHz, gas flow of 20 L min^{-1}, treatment time 2.5, 5 or 10 min	• Oxidation of superficial tissue • Decrease in L^* and b^* • No significant changes in firmness	Baier et al. (2015)
*Strawberry 'Elsanta'	Atmospheric cold plasma, voltage – 60 kV rms, Freq. – 50 Hz, treatment time 5 min	• Decrease in respiration rate • Significant increase in lightness (L^*) (when oxygen used as gas) • Significant decrease in lightness (L^*) (when nitrogen used as gas) • Decrease firmness after 24 h of storage	Misra et al. (2014c)
*Strawberries 'Elsanta'	In-package DBD, voltage – 60 kV_{RMS}, Freq. – 50 Hz, and treatment time 5 min	• No significant increase in respiration rate • No significant effect on color • Significant decrease in firmness after 24 h	Misra et al. (2014b)
*Apple 'Pink Lady®'	DBD, voltage – 9 V, and treatment time 10, 20, 30 min	• Significant reduction in the brown area after 4 h of storage • Slight but significant increase in soluble solids and titratable acidity • Significant increase in firmness immediately after the treatment	Tappi et al. (2014)
* Pear ∞	Atmospheric pressure microjet, power 30 mA, voltage – 500 V, and treatment time 1 – 4 s	• No effect in color • Decrease in moisture after 8 min	Wang et al. (2012)

*FC = Fresh cut; DR = dried; ∞ = No cultivar name given/provided; freq. = frequency, TSS = total soluble solids, DBD = Dielectric barrier discharge, PAW = Plasma activated water.

4.3.3 TEXTURE PROFILE

Textural properties play an important role in consumers' choice of fresh commodities, due to their impact on the organoleptic perception of flavor quality and the shelf life (Pathare et al., 2023). The effects of CAP treatments on the textural properties of fresh commodities are summarized in Table 4.1. For example, FC 'Pink Lady' apples were exposed to a DBD plasma discharge of 150 W and 15 kV for 10, 20, and 30 min. Treated samples resulted in a decline in the crunchiness of the fruit slices (Tappi et al., 2014). The authors related the visual remark to the fruit being covered by a biofilm issued from the destruction of superficial cells during CAP treatment.

In another study, Wu et al. (2020) showed that the 60 kV CAP treatment of cherries 'Hongdeng' for 60, 80, 100, and 140 s, respectively, was able to retain fruit firmness during short-term storage at 0°C in comparison to the control. Moreover, Sarangapani et al. (2017) reported that a decrease in firmness is related to the damage of outer cells, which result from internal structure degradation, leading to the softening of the produce. According to Sudheesh and Sunooj (2020), the reduction in firmness is associated with loss of moisture. In conclusion, these articles reveal that the degradation of firmness in fruit is generally associated with the loss in moisture content and the various enzymes responsible for cellular structural breakdown. Hence, the application of CAP has been shown to contribute to the maintenance of the cell structure and the overall firmness in fruit.

4.3.4 MICROSTRUCTURE

Cold plasma generates reactive species, which, when applied as a pretreatment step, diffuse from the surface of fruit cells into the tissues, resulting in modification of cellular microstructures. Recently, a study by Bao et al. (2020) subjected 'Junzao' jujube fruit to CAP treatment for 15 s prior to hot air drying at 50, 60, and 70°C. Based on a comparison of the microstructure of the control and treated samples, the authors demonstrated that the non-treated sample revealed a compact structure with few intracellular spaces and small cavities, while the treated samples presented a deformation in the cell followed by shrinkages. The authors concluded that the application of CAP before drying changed the microstructure of the fruit. The observed change included etching of larger cavities on the fruit surface due to the impact of reactive species produced during the treatment, and as a result, facilitated moisture transfer during the drying process (Figure 4.3), thus enhancing the drying rate.

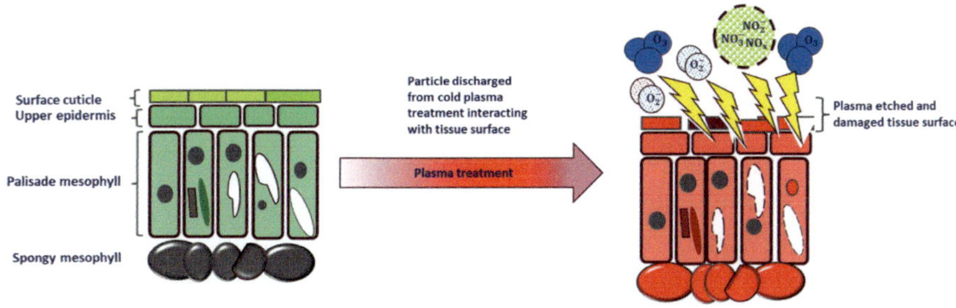

FIGURE 4.3 Annotated description of the impact of reactive species generated via cold plasma of plant and fruit tissues during treatment.

Zhang et al. (2019) observed that the application of CAP before drying shortened the drying time for chili peppers. The authors explained this phenomenon by the fact that micro-holes were created during CAP treatment, resulting from the etching effects of the reactive species. Furthermore, Zhang et al. (2019) elucidated that the reactive species produced during treatments, especially electrons and ions, could possibly destroy non-covalent bonds between cell wall polymers, leading to more intracellular spaces and cavities in the dried product. Similarly, pretreatment of wolfberry fruit with cold plasma of 3 L/min plasma flow, 20 kHz pulse frequency, and 750 W power consumption treated for 15, 30, 45, and 60 s, followed by drying at 50°C, was found to shorten the drying time by 50% (Zhou et al., 2020). The authors observed irregular etched micro-holes in the cuticle of the dried wolfberry samples pretreated for 15 s compared to the control and suggested that the micro-holes observed obstructed water migration from the interior of wolfberry's wax layer, thus facilitating the moisture transfer and the evaporation during the drying process.

Ashtiani et al. (2020) also observed the same phenomenon in 'Asgari' grapes after pretreating the samples with CAP of 10 L/min flow rate, 50 Hz of pulse frequency, 300 W of applied power, and a peak-to-peak voltage of 27 kV treated for 10 s and 60 s, followed by hot air drying under a constant temperature of 60°C and air velocity of 1.5 m/s. The authors noticed that gliding arc plasma treatment was responsible for micron-scale irregular holes in the skin surface of the grapes. They further reported an increase in the diameter of the holes by increasing the pretreatment time from 10 to 60 s. They credited the observed changes in the microstructures to the etching produced by the reactive species during the pre-treatment (notably nitric oxide radicals and nitrogen) observed in the range of 337–380 nm.

Shishir et al. (2020) explained that the penetration of the reactive species on the surface of the fresh Shiitake mushrooms occurred during cold plasma treatment. The mushrooms were exposed to CAP for 1 min (each side 30 s) using a power consumption of 650 W and compressor airflow of 0.2 MPa. The authors reported a decrease in the strength of the cell wall, and fissures and intracellular spaces were created, which degraded the non-covalent bonds between the polymers of cell walls. The authors also revealed that more intracellular spaces and larger cavities were observed in Shiitake mushroom samples pretreated with cold plasma followed by hot air drying at 50 ± 2, 60 ± 2, and 70 ± 2°C. In addition, samples treated with CP showed a greater range of cellular deformation, shrinkages, disruption or breakdown of cell walls, and irregular structures. The electrons and ions produced during CP pretreatment might disrupt hydrogen and other noncovalent bonds between cell wall polymers and led to a decrease in the strength of the cell wall network, generating more intracellular spaces and cavities (Liao et al., 2017).

Furthermore, available literature has demonstrated that the size of the microstructural deformation created by exposure of fruit tissue to CAP could also depend on the degree of fruit ripeness or cell wall firmness prior to treatment (Bao et al., 2021; Zhang et al., 2019). Thus, it could be concluded that CAP modifies the surface topography of fruit by creating intracellular spaces on the fruit surface, disrupting the cellular bonds, shrinking the contours of the cell wall, producing intracellular spaces, and creating micro-holes in the cellular structure due to reactive species generated.

4.4 IMPACTS OF CAP ON BIOCHEMICALS IN FRUIT

4.4.1 TITRATABLE ACIDITY AND PH

Titratable acidity (TA) is an important parameter used to evaluate the characteristics of fruits during storage. The effects of CAP on the acidity of various fruits have been reported. A study done for mango (cv. Nam Dok Mai) fruit treated for 2 min with CAP at 50 kHz by Phan et al. (2017) reported a decrease in the TA associated with advancing fruit ripening. Moreover, the TA of 'Nam Dok Mai' mango decreased significantly ($p \leq 0.05$) after application of CAP treatment at 600 W at 5 L/ min and 8 L/ min argon flow rates as compared to the control. According to Misra et al. (2015b), the reduction of TA after CAP treatment at voltages of 60 and 80 kV for 1 and 5 min could be attributed to the reaction with the ROS generated during the treatment on the cell structure of fresh strawberry fruit (cv. Elsanta). In a study conducted by Rana et al. (2020), atmospheric CAP dielectric barrier discharge (DBD) at 60 kV with an input voltage of 260 V at 50 Hz applied to strawberries (*Fragaria ananassa* Duch.) for 10 min and 15 min led to a non-significant decrease in the pH. Liao et al. (2018) observed similar results for apple treated for 0 to 40 s with DBD atmospheric CAP with an input power intensity of 30, 40, and 50 W and attributed this decrease to the active species generated during CAP treatment. Likewise, Bußler et al. (2017) also stated a significant decrease in the pH of 'Granny Smith' apples treated with CAP processed air at a frequency of 2.45 GHz, a supplied power of approx. 1.2 kW, and a gas flow of 20 L/min. Further explanation by Misra et al. (2016) and Schnabel et al. (2015) revealed that pH decreases due to the reactive nitrogen species produced during CP treatment in the abundant moisture of the tissue.

On the other hand, the increase of pH due to CAP treatment was also reported by various studies. Won et al. (2017) treated 'Satsuma' mandarin with CAP at 0.7 kPa for 10 min and observed an increase in the TA as the treatment time increased. Similarly, significant increases in TA affected by the storage and treatment time, and their interactions in 'Hayward' kiwi fruit treated with CAP at 19 V for 1, 5, and 10 min has also been reported by Ramazzina et al. (2015). Likewise, Rana et al. (2020) observed an increase of 16.4%, 18%, and 14% in the pH in the strawberries fruit (*Fragaria ananassa* Duch.) after 9 days of storage at 4°C after 10, 15, and 30 min, respectively. Misra et al. (2014a) attributed the increase in the pH of cherry tomato treated with CP of an input voltage of 120 V during 30 s, 60 s, 180 s, and 300 s, to the alteration of metabolism, followed by water loss of the samples during storage. Misra et al. (2016) reported that generally, a slight change in the pH of fresh produce after application of CP treatment does not have an apparent effect on further biochemical reactions. The pH was significantly increased in Siriguela fruit treated with CP of 80 W and 50 kHz power supply for 5 to 15 min; however, the CP treatment did not affect the quality of the product (Paixão et al., 2019). In conclusion, the reactive species that are produced during cold plasma treatment react on the cell structure, leading to a decrease in the pH; however, an alteration of the metabolism of fresh produce could also induce an increase in the pH.

4.4.2 TOTAL SOLUBLE SOLID (TSS)

TSS is one of the attributes used to evaluate the aroma characteristics of fruits during storage. Atmospheric CP DBD at 60 kV with an input voltage of 260 V at 50 Hz, applied to strawberries (*Fragaria ananassa Duch.*) for 10 min and 15 min led to an insignificant effect on the TSS value (Rana et al., 2020). However, in the same study, increasing the treatment exposure time for 30 min led to an increase in the TSS. Similarly, jujube slices CP treated for 30 or 60 s and dried at 70°C presented a significant increase in the TSS value (Bao et al., 2020). The authors associated this with the formation of a thick layer on the surface of jujube fruit slices, which prevented the TSS from leaving the interior of jujube slices. In a separate study conducted by Tappi et al. (2014), an increase in the TSS (from 0.4 to 0.8°Brix) was observed in fresh-cut apples (cv. Pink Lady) treated with a DBD CAP for 10 min with an input voltage of 19 V. Moreover, the increase observed was correlated with a slight increase in the conversion rate of starch to glucose in the fresh-cut apples 'Pink Lady' tissue.

The increase in the TSS in kiwi fruit (cv. Hayward) treated with CAP at 19 V for 1, 5, and 10 min was attributed to starch conversion to sugars (Ramazzina et al., 2015). The authors also reported a significant interactive effect between the treatment time and storage time, emphasizing that the longer the exposure to CAP treatment, the higher the increase in the TSS. Upon investigation of the effect of non-thermal plasma on the TSS of 'Nam Dok Mai' mango fruit, Phan et al. (2017) observed that plasma treatment of high-voltage power ranging from 800 to 1500 V during 2, 4, 6, and 10 min had a significantly higher TSS content ($p < 0.05$) compared to the control. Phan et al. (2017) concluded that sugars and acids are consumed as the main substrates of respiratory metabolism and are responsible for the changes in TSS of fruits. Ma et al. (2016) reported that higher contents of TSS in cold plasma-treated mangoes may be because of the respiratory rate of mango, which consequently increased the consumption of sugars and acids of this fruit. Contrary to the above-mentioned studies, a significant reduction in the TSS was observed in jujube fruits treated with CP for 15 s and dried at 60 and 70°C when compared to the control ($p < 0.05$) and was linked to the oxidation reaction that arises during the drying process (Bao et al., 2020). Applying CAP treatment on fruit plays a significant role in the TSS content by preventing the TSS from leaving the interior of the fruit.

4.4.3 PHYTONUTRIENTS AND BIOACTIVE COMPOUNDS

The term phytonutrient is a general name for a wide variety of compounds produced by plants, including minerals, vitamins, and dietary fiber available in vegetables and fruits (Bule et al., 2020). Phytonutrients are categorized into various classes by their chemical structure and functional attributes (Belwal et al., 2020). Cold plasma treatment has shown a beneficial effect towards the phytonutrient capacity of fruit (Bao et al., 2020; Sudheesh and Sunooj, 2020). For instance, Zhou et al. (2020) showed that

CAP treatment time significantly enhanced the phytochemical contents of dried wolfberries. A similar observation was reported for banana slices (Pour et al., 2022), fresh-cut pitaya fruit (Li, et al., 2019), pomegranate juice (Herceg et al., 2016), and blueberries (Sarangapani et al., 2017). In contrast, Amini and Ghoranneviss (2016) demonstrated that CP treatment had no significant effect on fresh and dried walnuts treated for 11 min. The effects of CAP on the phytonutrient content of some fresh and minimally processed fruits have been summarized in Table 4.2.

4.4.3.1 ANTIOXIDANTS

Antioxidants have recently attracted the attention of many researchers and consumers due to their pharmacological and health benefits (Lourenço et al., 2019). Contradictory reports are available on the effects of CAP treatment on the antioxidant capacity of various fruits. For example, according to Ramazzina et al. (2015), atmospheric double barrier discharge plasma (19 V) treatment for 1, 5, and 10 min provided no significant changes in the antioxidant content and antioxidant activity of FC 'Hayward' kiwifruit. The authors suggested that double barrier discharge plasma-induced reactive species could have caused the oxidation of single phenolic compounds responsible for the antioxidant activity of minimally processed kiwifruit. The results obtained were explained by the fact that the effect of the treatment was counteracted by tissue response mechanisms (Ramazzina et al., 2015). Similarly, investigation by Chen et al. (2020) revealed that antioxidant compounds could be degraded or oxidized by active species generated from cold plasma.

Contrary to the above studies, Kim et al. (2019) showed that CAP treatment enhanced antioxidant activity of 'Mill' prickly pear cactus fruit. Fruit samples were treated with CAP at 750 W for 40 min, and at 856 W for 36 min, resulting in increased antioxidant activity by 1.8% and 1.7%, respectively. In addition, CAP treatment at 60 kV for 5 min enhanced the antioxidant activity in fresh-cut pitaya fruit (Li et al., 2019). Similarly, the effect of atmospheric CP DBD at 60 kV with an input voltage of 260 V at 50 Hz on strawberries was investigated by Rana et al. (2020), and an increase of 14.5% was observed in the antioxidant activity after 10 min. However, a decrease of 7.2% was observed after 30 min of exposure. The authors suggested that the extended exposure time from 10 to 30 min led to lower antioxidant activity due to the formation of large-charged gas species.

TABLE 4.2 Effects of Cold Plasma Application on Phytonutrients, Antioxidant Activity and Other Attributes of Fresh and Fresh-Cut Fruits That Were Reported Within the Last 10 Years

Produce	Description of Plasma Treatment(s)	Key Findings/ Salient Results	References
Mango ∞	DBD, voltage – 50 V, frequency 10 kHz exposed to treated water (tap, distilled and ultrapure) PAW, PAW+MAP,	• PAW+MAP significantly delayed fruit decay and accumulation of malondialdehyde • PAW treated samples best maintained color attributes of mangoes	Wu et al. (2023)
*Blueberries 'Emerald'	DBD, voltage –45 kV, treatment time 50 s	• Increase in total phenols to 2.55 $g\,kg^{-1}$ on day 10 • Increase in anthocyanin levels • Decrease in ascorbic acid after 25 d storage • Increase in procyanidin B2 and procyanidin A2 on day 10 • Increase in cyanin chloride, cyanidin-3-o-glucoside, cyanidin, delphinidin 3-sophoroside-5-rhamnoside, and albiflorin	Zhou et al. (2023)
* Wolfberry	DBD, voltage 300–700 V, treatment time 480s	• Increase in DPPH free radical scavenging by 19.20% • Inhibition of antioxidant enzyme activity	Du et al. (2023)
Mango ∞	DBD, 50 V input voltage and a 10 kHz frequency	• Increase in antioxidant enzyme activity	Wu et al. (2022)
*Mango 'Hongyu'	Dielectric barrier discharge, voltage 75 kV, treatment time 3 min	• Increase in total phenolics and flavonoids ascorbic acid • Lower activities of polyphenol oxidase and peroxidase • Inhibition of browning-related phenolic oxidation • Maintained antioxidant capacity	Yi et al. (2022)
*Apricots	DBD	• Increased the accumulation of antioxidants • Improved the activity of antioxidant enzymes	Hua et al. (2022)

TABLE 4.2 *(Continued)*

Produce	Description of Plasma Treatment(s)	Key Findings/ Salient Results	References
Blueberries	Diffuse coplanar surface barrier discharge 400 (DCSBD) plasma	• Anthocyanin was not significantly affected by treatments	Pathak et al. (2022)
*Banana	DBD, voltage 6.9 kV treatment time 46 s	• Decreased in PPO and POD activity • Increase in antioxidant, total phenol, and flavonoid content	Pour et al. (2022)
*Kiwi	DBD, voltage –15, 25, 35 kV, power 13, 22, 31 W, Freq. 60 kHz, treatment time 1–5 min	• Decrease total phenols content	Liu et al. (2021)
*Cashew apple ∞	Atmospheric cold plasma, voltage 20 kV, frequencies 200 and 700 Hz, time 15 min	• Decrease in glucose and fructose • Increase in vitamin C and malic acid, but no effect on total phenolics	Leite et al. (2021)
*Sour Cherry ∞	Cold atmospheric pressure plasma, voltage 10, 15, 20 kV, frequency 10, 15, 20 kHz, gas flow rate 3, 5, 7 L min−1, oxygen 0%, 0.5%, 1%	• Increase in total phenol content from 277 to 279 GAE/100 g after plasma treatment	Hosseini et al. (2021)
DR Wolfberry ∞	Atmospheric plasma, frequency of 20 kHz, power 750 W, treatment time 15, 30, 45, 60 s	• Significantly decreased the total phenolic content after 30 s • Significantly increased the total phenolic content after 45 s	Zhou et al. (2020)
*Strawberries 'Duch'	Atmospheric cold plasma dielectric barrier discharge at 60 kV with an input voltage of 260 V at 50 Hz, treatment time 15 min	• Increased total phenolic and antioxidant activity • Enhanced the concentration of chlorogenic acid, hyprin, phloretin, vanillin, gallic acid, 4-hydroxybenzaldehyde and rutin	Rana et al. (2020)
DR Jujube 'Junzao'	Cold plasma at voltage 5 kV, frequency 40 kHz, treatment time 15, 30, 60s	• Increased antioxidant by 36.85%, procyanidins by 53.81%, flavonoids by 33.89%, phenolics by 13.85%	Bao et al. (2020)

TABLE 4.2 *(Continued)*

Produce	Description of Plasma Treatment(s)	Key Findings/ Salient Results	References
*Pitaya 'Shuijing'	DBD cold plasma, voltage 60 kV, treatment time 5 min	• Increased cutting-induced phenolic accumulation • Enhanced antioxidant activity • Promoted the consumption of main sugars • Accelerated generation of reactive oxygen species at earlier storage • Increased gene expression and activity of crucial enzymes in phenylpropanoid pathway	Li et al. (2019)
Siriguela ∞	Glow discharge plasma generator, 80 W power supply, frequency 50 kHz, treatment time 5, 10 min	• No significant changes in vitamin C • Increased pigments, total phenolics, antioxidant activity, and Vit. B • Increased antioxidant activity and peroxidase about 6% • Decreased polyphenol oxidase activity about 20%	Paixão et al. (2019)
DR Chili pepper ∞	Gliding arc discharge, frequency 20 kHz, power 750 W, treatment time 15, 30, 45, 60 s	• Retention of carotenoids red pigment content after 30 s • Increased antioxidant activity of samples	Zhang et al. (2019)
*kumquat ∞	Intermittent corona discharge plasma jet, voltage 8 kV DC, frequency 20 kHz, power 2.0, 3.0 & 4.0 A, treatment time 10 s (on and off)	• No change in DPPH radical scavenging activity of samples treated at 3 and 4 A after day 12 • Significant reduction in DPPH radical scavenging activity generated at 2 A after day 12	Puligundla et al. (2018)
*Apple	DBD, power 90 W, Freq. 60 kHz, treatment time 0–140 s	• No changes in total phenols, increased antioxidant activity	Xiang et al. (2018)
*Mango 'Nam Dok Mai'	Gliding arc discharge non-thermal plasma at 600 W, Ar gas flow rates: 2, 5 and 8 L/min, treatment time 5 or 10 min	• Decreased chorpyrifos by 74% and cypermetrin by 63% • Decreased significantly total phenolic content • Significantly increased carotenoid content	Phan et al. (2018)

TABLE 4.2 *(Continued)*

Produce	Description of Plasma Treatment(s)	Key Findings/ Salient Results	References
*Goji berry ∞	Gas phase discharge plasma with voltages of 5, 8, 10, 12 and 15 kV, treatment time 0.5 s to 30 min	• No significant changes in vitamin C from 0 to 30 min • No significant changes in beta-carotene from 0 to 30 min	Zhou et al. (2018)
*Apple 'Granny Smith'	Microwave-driven plasma torch of 2.45 GHz at 1.2 kW, time 10 min	• Reduced polyphenol oxidase activity by about 62%	Bußler et al. (2017)
*Grape ∞	PAW, flow rate of 1.2 L/min, power 1.1 to 1.3 mA, voltage 8.2 kV, time 30 and 60 min	• No significant change in total anthocyanin content after 30 min of PAW treatment	Guo et al. (2017)
*White grape	DBD, voltage – 80 kV, treatment time 4 min	• Decrease in antioxidants, total phenols • Decrease in flavonoids and Scavenging potential	Pankaj et al. (2017)
*Melon 'Raptor'	Dielectric barrier discharge, power supplies at 19 V and about 3 A, high voltage of 15 kV and frequency of 12.5 kHz, treatment time 15+15 min & 30+30 min	• Significant reduction in peroxidase • No effect in pectin methylesterase after 15 + 15 min • Increase in pectin methylesterase 30 + 30 min • Reduction in polyphenoloxidase	Tappi et al. (2016)
*Apple 'Pink Lady'	Dielectric barrier discharge plasma, frequency 12.7 kHz, power supply 150 W, time 30 min	• Significant reduction of procyanidins – B1 dimer (56%), trimer (59%), and trimer 4 (62%) • Significant decline in polyphenols and reduced antioxidant activity	Ramazzina et al. (2016)
*Chokeberry	Jet plasma, power 4 W, Freq. 25 kHz, treatment time 3,5 min	• Increase in hydroxycinnamic acids • Decrease in total flavanols and anthocyanins content	Kovačević et al. (2016)
*Orange	DBD, voltage –70 kV, Freq. 50 kHz, treatment time 5 –60 s	• Increase in ascorbic acid • Decrease in total phenols, flavonoids, antioxidants	Almeida et al. (2015)

TABLE 4.2 *(Continued)*

Produce	Description of Plasma Treatment(s)	Key Findings/ Salient Results	References
*Apple 'Granny Smith'	Microwave-driven atmospheric pressure plasma, power 1.2 kW, frequency 2.45 GHz, gas flow of 20 L/min, treatment time 2.5 min, 5 min or 10 min	• Significant decline in photochemical photosynthetic efficiency after • 48 h	Baier et al. (2015)
*Blueberry ∞	Cold atmospheric plasma jet, frequency 47 kHz, power 549 W, treatment time 0, 15, 30, 45, 60, 90, 120 s	• Significant reduction in anthocyanins after 90 s • Significant increase in ascorbic acid, total phenolics and flavonoids • Significant decrease in anthocyanin	Lacombe et al. (2015)
*Kiwifruit 'Hayward'	Atmospheric double barrier discharge plasma 15 kV frequency, voltage of 19 V, wavelength 200–450 nm, treatment time 20 min (10 + 10) & 40 min (20 + 20)	• Reduced the formation of darkened area • Significant decrease in chlorophyll and carotenoids • No effect on ascorbic acid immediately after treatment until day 4	Ramazzina et al. (2015)
*Apple 'Pink Lady®'	Dielectric barrier discharge atmospheric plasma, voltage of 9 V, treatment time 10, 20, 30 min	• Decrease in polyphenol oxidase activity • Slow down the metabolic activity of the tissue	Tappi et al. (2014)
*Pear ∞	Atmospheric pressure air cold plasma microjet, power 30 mA, voltage 500 V; treatment time 1–4 s	• Decrease in vitamin C by 2.8%	Wang et al. (2012)

*FC = Fresh cut; DR=dried, ∞ = No cultivar name given/provided, DBD = Dielectric barrier discharge, PAW = Plasma activated water, MAP = Modified atmosphere packaging.

Pankaj et al. (2017) observed a decrease in the antioxidant capacity for 'Thompson seedless' grapes after an increase in the cold plasma treatment duration (1, 2, 3, and 4 min) using a voltage of 80 kV (peak-to-peak); an input of 230 V and 60 Hz from the mains supply. The authors concluded that the longer the treatment, the lesser the antioxidant capacity due to the formation of charged gas species from the reactive species produced during the treatment. It has been demonstrated that CAP has a positive effect on red pigment content in fresh produce (Zhang et al., 2019). However, the extension of CAP treatment duration led to pigment loss. Zhang et al. (2019) explained that the cell wall of a fruit can be damaged by CAP application due to accumulation of pigments. Pigments are associated with vitamins and antioxidant compounds, and their degradation designates a loss in the product quality (Paixão et al., 2019). According to Lacombe et al. (2015), the exposure of a sample to ozone and other free radical compounds produced by CAP led to the degradation of bioactive compounds in fruit. Antioxidants have been reported to protect cells against the damaging effects of ROS, which include singlet oxygen, superoxide, peroxyl radicals, hydroxyl ions, and peroxynitrite (Thirumdas et al., 2015). In conclusion, CAP treatment for a short duration could enhance the antioxidant capacity of fruit; however, the effect of CAP varies with fruit type, treatment duration, and the CAP intensity.

4.4.3.2 PHENOLICS

Table 4.2 presents the effects of CAP treatments on the phenolic compounds of fruit. For instance, the application of CAP generated by a DBD at 80 kV on 'Elsanta' strawberries for 1 and 5 min did not influence the phenolic content (Misra et al., 2015b). The authors reported that the phenolics were not influenced by either the treatment time or the intensity of the voltage discharge. A similar outcome was observed for 'Satsuma' mandarin flesh treated with nitrogen (N_2) plasma at 900 W for 10 min (Won et al., 2017). On the contrary, a study by Lacombe et al. (2015) revealed that CAP treatment of a frequency of 47 kHz and a power of 549 W, applied to blueberries for 15, 30, 45, 60, 90, and 120 s showed a decrease in the phenolic content treated for a longer time, due to the longer exposure to radical species produced which led to the degradation of phenolic compounds. Dong and Yang (2019) evaluated the application of CP at input voltage of 36 V on blueberries for 0, 2, 4, 6, 8, and 10 min, and observed an increase in the polyphenols content. The authors reported that an increase in the treatment time up to 10 min led to an induction of polyphenol synthesis in the first days of storage, but prolonged storage reduced the phenolic contents.

An increase in the cutting-induced phenolic accumulation was observed in fresh-cut 'Shuijing' pitaya fruit treated with CP treatment at 60 kV for 5 min (Li et al., 2019). The authors reported that UV radiation formed during plasma generation may be responsible for the formation of phenolic compounds, which are extracted from the cells of fruit. Studies by Jacobo-Velázquez et al. (2015) revealed that ROS produced during CP treatment are demonstrated as signaling molecules and play an important role in cutting-induced phenolic accumulation; they could thus effectively mediate the phenolic content in wounded produce. In addition, the accumulation of phenolic compounds, which are secondary metabolites, is considered one of the most important defense mechanism responses in biological tissues elicited by UV irradiation (Yang et al., 2018).

Studies by Jacobo-Velázquez et al. (2015) reported that the first step of biosynthesis of phenolic compounds in fruit is the conversion of carbohydrates. In addition, the hexoses are converted respectively to phosphoenolpyruvate through glycolysis and to erythrose-4-P through the pentose phosphate pathway, which are essential substrates (Jacobo-Velázquez et al., 2015). Furthermore, these substrates participate in the shikimate pathway and are gradually converted to L-phenylalanine, which is the precursor of the phenylpropanoid metabolism (Jacobo-Velázquez et al., 2015). It is worth noting that treating FC 'Shuijing' pitaya fruit with CP treatment at 60 kV for 5 min partly facilitated the utilization of fructose and glucose, which were used as essential precursors for the biosynthesis of phenolics (Li et al., 2019). In conclusion, according to the above-mentioned studies, CP treatment induced the accumulation of phenolic compounds in fruit by using the ROS generated as signaling molecules, triggering the conversion of carbohydrate, and the longer the CP treatment, the higher the reduction of phenolic compounds.

4.4.3.3 VITAMINS

Various studies reported the effect of CP treatment to enhance the vitamin content of fruit (Table 4.2). Camu-Camu fruit (cv. not specified) treated with CP at 960 Hz showed an increase in vitamin C concentration (de Castro et al., 2020). Similarly, Paixão et al. (2019) reported that the application of CP to Siriguela (cv. not specified) increased the concentration of vitamins (B3, B6, and C). On the contrary, other studies reported the reduction of vitamins due to CP treatments. For instance, Hosseini et al. (2020) reported a significant decrease in vitamin C of sour cherry (cv. not specified) treated with DBD CP (power supply varying between 0 and 20 kV, and frequency of 20 kHz), and they attributed the reduction observed to the increased oxygen content in argon. Moreover, Ashtiani et al. (2020) attributed elevated temperature and oxygen during drying as the cause of oxidation and degradation in vitamin C content of dried seedless 'Asgari' grapes pre-treated with cold plasma (gas flow of 10 L/min, frequency of 50 Hz, power supply of 300 W, and voltage of 27 kV). It was concluded that a shorter drying time would mitigate vitamin C oxidation and degradation. Therefore, this implies that a short exposure time to drying can alleviate vitamin C oxidation and degradation. Misra et al. (2015b) suggested that oxygen radicals led to oxidation of vitamin C. In conclusion, it was established that CP pretreatment can successfully improve the retention rate of ascorbic acid or vitamin C in fruits during drying. Furthermore, plasma type and long exposure to oxygen during CP treatment can lead to vitamin C oxidation because of the reactive species in the fruit. Additionally, vitamin C is light-sensitive and can therefore be adversely affected by the UV produced during plasma treatment.

4.4.3.4 ENZYMATIC BROWNING

One of the main effects related to the application of CAP treatment is the reduction of enzymatic browning linked to the phenolic compounds in fresh and minimally processed fruit (Sudheesh and Sunooj, 2020). Development of brown coloration on the fruit skin or flesh could be due to enzymatic browning because of the fusion of PPO with phenolic substrate (Sudheesh and Sunooj, 2020). CAP treatment for 20 min using DBD approach at 19 V was shown to reduce darkened area of 'Hayward' kiwifruits during storage for four days at 10°C and 95% relative humidity (Ramazzina et al., 2015). Likewise, DBD treatment after 30 min with an input voltage of 19 V decreased the brown area on 'Pink Lady' FC apples by 65% (Tappi et al., 2014). These studies suggested that the active species generated by CAP play an important role by making a breakage in peptide bonds and damaging the 3D structure of proteins. Studies by Pankaj et al. (2018) and Zhang et al. (2019) also revealed that CAP modifies the properties of fruit by releasing the reactive species on their surfaces.

Bao et al. (2020) treated jujube slices with CP treatment at a voltage of 5 kV and a frequency of 40 kHz for 15 s and hot air dried the samples at 70°C. The results showed a higher browning index in the CP treated fruit, which they attributed to the increase in the drying temperature (54.2°C). They concluded in their study that a short exposure of 15 s of jujube slices to CP treatment increased the fruit drying rate and attributed the decrease of 5-hydroxymethylfurfural production to the inhibition of enzymatic browning. Studies by Bußler et al. (2017) also concurred with the same findings by reporting a possible induction in the browning index values of apples cubes (cv. Granny Smith) treated with CP treatment (frequency of 2.45 GHz, power of 1.2 kW and a gas flow of 20 L/min). After storing the apples slices at 20°C for 19 days, Bußler et al. (2017) attributed the increase in browning index to the enzymatic browning caused during cold plasma treatment.

Furthermore, the non-enzymatic reactions of secondary plant metabolites could have been induced by reactive species triggered by cold plasma treatment (Lee et al., 2023). Cold plasma is suggested to have a significant effect in inactivating enzymes responsible for browning in fruit (Han et al., 2019). In conclusion, as can be observed from the above discussion, CP has a beneficial effect to control browning in fresh fruit regardless of treatment time and intensity. However, its effect would be limited for dried fruit at longer treatment exposure. In addition, the process conditions, including treatment time, have a significant impact on the success of enzyme inactivation and the product quality parameters.

4.5 MICROBIAL DECONTAMINATION

Several studies are being carried out to understand the impact of CAP treatment on the microbial safety of fresh and minimally processed fruit (Sudheesh and Sunooj, 2020; Wang et al., 2016). Table 4.3 presents an extensive summary of investigations within the last decade on the effects of various cold plasma treatments on the microbial safety of horticultural commodities. Application of a plasma jet for 10 min on fresh walnuts (cvs. Taleghan, Mazandaran, Toyeserkan, and Shahmirzad) was less efficient in reducing *Aspergillus flavus* cells compared to the dried fruit due to properties such as water activity and moisture (Amini and Ghorannevis, 2016). Other studies reported the increase of microbial inactivation with increasing water activity when using high pressure (Podolak et al., 2020; Sehrawat et al., 2020) or pulsed electric fields (Kantala et al., 2022; Puligundla et al., 2018). In literature, microbial resistance could be attributed to microbial inactivation at low water activity values to cell shrinkage, which led to a thickening of the cell membrane and hindering the reactive species from accessing the cells (Farag et al., 2021; Perinban et al., 2019). At low water activity values, there is an increase in the amino acids and polyols contained in the cells to prevent water loss caused by osmotic pressure and, on the other hand, avoid other types of stresses (Erkmen and Bozoglu, 2016). Consequently, any cells that survived at low water activity might possibly be resistant to cold plasma.

A similar trend on the microbial inactivation efficacy of CP on dried fruit has been reported by Lee et al. (2015). In this study, the application of CP (wave discharge of 2.45 GHz and power supply between 50 and 1000 W, pressure between 500 and 30 000 Pa, gas flow of 20 standard L/min for the plasma-forming gas: nitrogen or the mixture of helium and oxygen) on dried figs (cv. not specified) was not as effective at decontaminating microorganisms compared to fresh figs. This was justified by the rise in the solutes (amino acids and polyols) in the cells at low water activity values, to prevent water loss caused by osmotic pressure. The authors concluded that free water molecules on the food product surface could contribute to CP microbial inactivation.

Once the reactive species diffuse into the bacterial cell membranes, it can lead to severe injury by reacting with macromolecules, which include the membrane lipids, the proteins, and the nucleic acids (Juan et al., 2021). Furthermore, the presence of free radicals in cold plasma forms lesions on the membrane surface by direct bombardment of the cell wall or by impression, which can lead to a breaking of chemical bonds, erosion, and localized lesions in the membrane with further penetration of toxic reactive plasma species into the cell (Dobslaw and Glocker, 2020). In addition, these free radicals' presence in cold plasma treatment could be adsorbed on the surfaces of microorganisms, which leads to the formation of carbon dioxide, volatile compounds that are further eliminated from the cell (Hage et al., 2022). The accumulation of plasma electrons and ions on the cell surface may result in the disruption of the cell membrane. To inactivate microorganisms, the electrons and the positively and negatively charged ions act in sync with reactive species (Huang et al., 2018; Małajowicz et al., 2022). A detailed description of microbial inactivation mechanisms by cold plasma and their interaction with food components has been extensively covered by Schottroff et al. (2018), Surowsky et al. (2015), and Bourke et al. (2017) in their review papers. Thus, this article will exclude this subject area and focus on the critical impact of cold plasma treatments on fruit quality attributes and bioactive compounds.

According to Surowsky et al. (2014), who treated apple juice (cv. not specified) with CP (frequency of 1.1 MHz, process gases: argon and oxygen, gas flow rate 5 L/min, voltage of 65 V, treatment time 0 and 480 s), cold argon/O_2 plasma is a great source of bacteria inactivation compared to oxygen. The authors corroborate these findings by mentioning that there was no relevant antimicrobial potential behavior in the sample treated with pure argon compared to the use of oxygen gas. Where there was an increased antimicrobial behavior, it was attributed to the increased amounts of atomic oxygen in the plasma, which leads to the formation of H_2O_2 (Figure 4.4). Plasma-generated compounds such as hydrogen peroxide (H_2O_2) and hydroperoxyl radicals (OOH), OH and O radicals lead to cell permeabilization and possible nucleic acid damage due to the breakdown of the cytoplasmic membrane of bacterial cells and therefore a degradation of proteins and lipids which are susceptible to oxidation (Pathare et al., 2023). Further literature by Frandsen et al. (2020), Gan et al. (2021), Hou et al. (2019), Liao et al. (2018), Han et al. (2016a), Lunov et al. (2015), and (2016) extensively discussed the mechanisms and effects of cold plasma on the microbial safety of fruit. These articles are recommended for further reading.

4.6 CHALLENGES AND FUTURE WORK

Extensive investigations have been devoted to the antimicrobial efficacy of CAP technology in food science research (Du et al., 2023; Wu et al., 2022, 2023). Reports on the impact of CAP treatments on fresh produce quality (physical, biochemical, phytonutrients/bioactives, and enzymes) and the ability to promote effective drying have relatively increased within the last decade (Ashtiani et al., 2020; Ekezie et al., 2017; Onal-Ulusoy et al., 2019). Generally, the effectiveness of plasma treatment

TABLE 4.3 Effects of Cold Plasma Application on Microbial Activity on Fresh and Minimally Processed Fruits, Which Were Reported Within the Last 10 Years

Produce	Description of Plasma Treatment(s)	Key Findings/ Salient Results	References
Mango ∞	DBD at 50 V, frequency 10 kHz exposed to treated water (tap, distilled and ultrapure) PAW	• PAW down-regulated pathogenic genes • Inhibited the effect on *C. asianum* pathogenic enzymes, and effectively realized the retardation of mango anthracnose	Wu et al. (2023)
*Blueberry 'Emerald'	DBD at 45 kV, treatment time 50 s	• Reduced bacterial counts from 5.12 log CFU kg^{-1} to 0.33 log CFU kg^{-1} • Reduced yeasts and molds with the lowest value of 0.93 log CFU kg^{-1}	Zhou et al. (2023)
*Wolfberry	DBD, voltage 300–700 V, treatment time 480s	• At 300 V, decrease by up to 4 log CFU/mL of *A. alternata* by 0.29–1.52 log CFU/mL • At 700 V, decrease by up to 2.26 log CFU/mL of *A. alternata*	Du et al. (2023)
*Cuca-melons	DBD diffusor, PAW, NaOCl, power 1500 Hz, voltage 120 v, 60 kHz resonance frequency, treatment time 2 min	• Reduced pathogens with a 1–1.5 log CFU g^{-1} at 2 min PAW treatment • PAW Reduced total viable mesophilic bacteria counts by 1.7 log CFU g^{-1} • PAW treatment reduced yeast and moulds counts by 2 log CFU g^{-1} • Reduced *E. coli, S. enterica* and *L. monocytogenes* by 3 log CFU g^{-1} with DBDD-PAW	Rothwell et al. (2023)
Mango ∞	DBD plasma system, 50 V input voltage and a 10 kHz frequency	• Inhibited the growth of *C. asianum in vitro* and *in vivo* • Decrease in germination rate by 13% after 1 min treatment	Wu et al. (2022)
*Mango 'Hongyu'	Dielectric barrier discharge, voltage 75 kV, treatment time 3 min	• Inhibited growth of total microbial counts by 1.04 log red at 2 d • Inhibited growth of total microbial counts by 0.61 log red at 4 d	Yi et al. (2022)

TABLE 4.3 *(Continued)*

Produce	Description of Plasma Treatment(s)	Key Findings/ Salient Results	References
*Sour Cherry ∞	New system cold atmospheric pressure plasma, voltage 10, 15, 20 kV, frequency 10, 15, 20 kHz, gas flow rate 3, 5, 7 L min^{-1}, oxygen 0%, 0.5%, 1%	• Reduction of *Escherichia coli* • Enhanced inactivation of *Escherichia coli* • Decrease in *Escherichia coli* at 19.6 kV voltage, 1% oxygen, 4.5 L/min gas flow rate	Hosseini et al. (2021)
Blueberries	Diffuse coplanar surface barrier discharge 400 (DCSBD) plasma	• Longer treatment time with N-generated CAP resulted in higher reduction in the population of native microflora on fresh blueberries	Pathak et al. (2022)
*Strawberry 'Duch'	DBD at 60 kV power, 260 V, 50 Hz; and 15 min	• ≈2 log reduction of microbial load (yeast/mold)	Rana et al. (2020)
*Strawberry ∞	In-package DBD, voltage 60 kV, pulsed frequency at 50 Hz treatment time 5 min	• Reduction of mesophilic count: 3.7 log CFU/sample • Reduction of yeast and mold: 3.3 log CFU/sample	Lafarga et al. (2019)
*Pitayas 'Shuijing'	DBD, voltage 60 kV, treatment time 5 min	• Significant inhibition of growth of total aerobic bacterial counts	Li et al. (2019)
*Siriguela ∞	Glow discharge plasma generator, 80 W power, frequency 50 kHz, treatment time 5, 10 min	• No microbial contamination found in Siriguela	Paixão et al. (2019)
*Mango 'Nam Dok Mai'	Gliding arc discharge at 600 W power supply, time 7 min	• Inhibition of *Colletotrichum gloeosporioides* mold growth	Phan et al. (2019)
*Strawberry ∞	98% Ag – 2% O_2 plasma jet, frequency 10-kHz, 18-kV voltage, time 10 and 20 min	• Reduction of *S. aureus*: 1.6 to 2.3 log CFU/g after day 0 • Reduction of *S. aureus*: 1.7 to 3.4 log CFU/g after 4 days	Kumar et al. (2018)

TABLE 4.3 *(Continued)*

Produce	Description of Plasma Treatment(s)	Key Findings/ Salient Results	References
*kumquat ∞	Intermittent corona discharge plasma jet, voltage 8 kV DC, frequency 20 kHz, power 2–4 A, time 10 s	• Drastically reduced aerobic bacteria, yeasts and molds in 90 s at 4.0 A • Reduced microbial load by ≈1.0 log CFU/g in 0–120 s, 2 A	Puligundla et al. (2018)
*Grape ∞	PWA, flow rate of 1.2 L/min, power 1.1 to 1.3 mA, voltage 8.2 kV, time 30 and 60 min	• Significant reduction of *S. cerevisiae* to 0.53 Log CFU/mL	Guo et al. (2017)
*Cantaloupe ∞	Activated ionized H_2O_2 system, distance 9 mm, voltage 17 kV, flow rate for H_2O_2 9.7 mL/min, air pressure of 15 psi, time 45 s, 30 min	• Reduced populations of *E. coli* O157:H7 by 4.9 log CFU/piece • Reduced populations of *S. Typhimurium* by 1.3 log CFU/piece • Reduced populations of *L. innocua* by 3.0 log CFU/piece	Jiang et al. (2017)
*Melon 'Raptor'	DBD, power supplies at 19 V and about 3 A, high voltage 15 kV, frequency of 12.5 kHz, time 15+15 min and 30+30 min	• Reduced cell viability of the indigenous bacteria • Inhibited yeasts 3.5 log CFU/g compared to control 7.5 log CFU/g • Negligible effect on microbial shelf-life	Tappi et al. (2016)
*Apple 'Granny Smith'	Microwave- APP, power 1.2 kW, frequency 2.45 GHz, gas flow 20 L/min, time 2.5 min, 5/10 min	• Reduction of total mesophilic counts by 3.4 log cycles after 5 min • Reduction of *Escherichia coli* by 4.6 log cycles after 10 min	Baier et al. (2015)
*Blueberry ∞	Plasma jet, at 47 kHz using 549 W, time 0, 15, 30, 45, 60, 90, and 120 s	• Significant reduction of aerobic plate count from 0.8 to 1.6 log CFU/g after 1 day and 1.5 to 2.0 log CFU/g after 7 days	Lacombe et al. (2015)
*Strawberry ∞	In-package DBD, voltage 60 kV, frequency 50 Hz, time 5 min	• Reduction of mesophilic count: 2.4 log CFU/sample • Reduction of yeast and mold: 3.4 log CFU/sample	Liu et al. (2015)

TABLE 4.3 *(Continued)*

Produce	Description of Plasma Treatment(s)	Key Findings/ Salient Results	References
*Blueberry ∞	MW Ag plasma torch; frequency 2.45 GHz; power 9, 7 and 5 W, Ag at 7 L/min, time 15, 30, 60 s	• Antimicrobial effect observed for blueberries	Bernard et al. (2014)
*Strawberry 'Elsanta'	In-package DBD, voltage 60 kV, 50 Hz for 5 min	• Reduced aerobic mesophilic bacteria, yeast and mold by 2 log in 24 h	Misra et al. (2014b)
	Atmospheric cold plasma, voltage of 60 kV RMS, and frequency of 50 Hz, time 5 min	• Reduced total mesophilic by 3.7 log cycles (N_2 gas) • Reduced yeasts/molds by 3.3 log cycles (N_2 gas) • Reduced total mesophilic by 3.1 log cycles (O_2 gas) • Reduced total mesophilic, yeasts/molds by 3.4 log cycles (O_2 gas)	Misra et al. (2014c)
*Strawberry ∞	Air plasma jet, frequency 47 kHz, power consumption 549 W, time 0 to 120 s	• Reduced total aerobic plate count: 0.8 to 1.6 log CFU/g after 1 day • Reduced total aerobic plate count: 1.5 to 2.0 log CFU/g after 7 days	Jensen et al. (2013)
*Pear ∞	APP microjet at 30 mA, voltage 500 V; time 1–4 s	• Inactivated 40% *Salmonella* in half a second, and 80% in a second	Wang et al. (2012)
*Strawberry ∞	Air in-package DBD, voltage 70 kV, frequency 50 Hz, time 30 to 300 s	• Reduction of *Escherichia coli*: 3.5 log CFU/sample • Reduction of *Salmonella Typhimurium*: 3.8 log CFU/sample • Reduction of *Listeria monocytogenes*: 4.2 log CFU/sample	Sarvikivi et al. (2012)

*FC = Fresh cut; DR=dried, ∞ = No cultivar name given/provided, DBD = Dielectric barrier discharge, MW = Microwave, APP = Atmospheric pressure plasma.

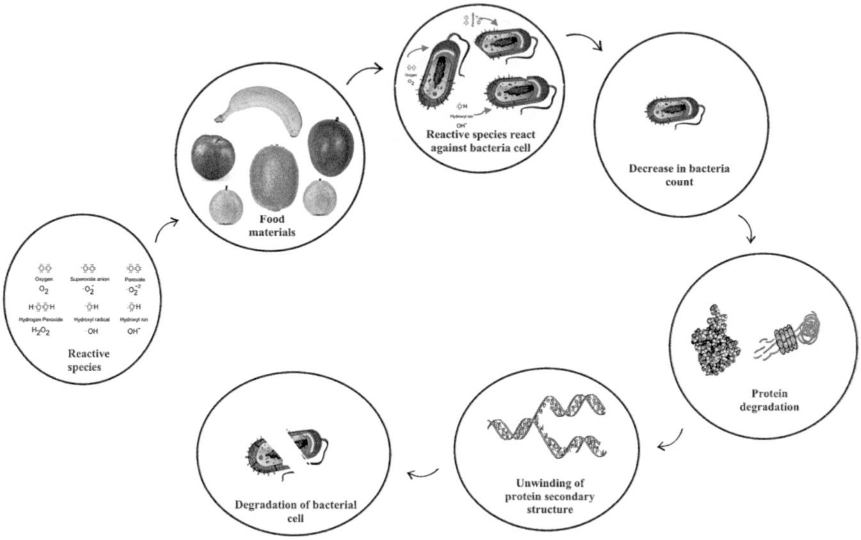

FIGURE 4.4 Mechanisms of degradation of bacteria cell after cold plasma application.

is first measured/established based on microbial safety. However, such plasma processing parameters may not be optimal for the enhancement of phytochemical contents. Several factors, such as process gas, generator power or voltage, commodity types, and duration of exposure to CAP treatments, could impact phytochemical contents. For example, longer exposure time to CAP treatments has been established to ensure optimal produce surface decontamination. However, such treatment duration could induce surface discoloration, tissue etching or rupturing, and increase surface temperature (Mao et al., 2021). These induced effects would lead to an increase in respiration rate, accelerated metabolic processes, and enhanced natural senescence of fresh produce. Therefore, the complexities of these factors would necessitate further studies that are either focused on i) the application of high intensity/frequency CP treatments with very short exposure time, or ii) the optimization of indirect plasma treatments (such as plasma-activated water) that will optimally inhibit spoilage and pathogenic microbes and effectively maintain quality attributes of fresh produce.

Furthermore, one of the benefits of CAP treatment is the limited depth penetration capability, which makes it applicable for surface decontamination of fruit and vegetables. However, this advantage could limit its application and efficacy against eukaryotic microbes such as fungal pathogens with a thicker cell wall than bacteria. As demonstrated in previous studies, CAP treatments were not fungicidal and could not effectively inactivate fungal pathogens *Colletotrichum alienum* and *C. fioriniae* (Siddique et al., 2019), *C. gloeosporioides* (Phan et al., 2019), and *C. asianum* (Wu et al., 2022). For instance, an *in vivo* study by Wu et al. (2022) showed that DBD plasma treatment exhibited inhibitory activity against the growth of *C. asianum* on mango fruit. After 9 min of treatment, the spore germination rate and spore viability of *C. asianum* were decreased by 95.48% and 98.82%, respectively. The treatment effectively controlled the growth of the fungal spore, delayed the disease incidence, and enhanced measured quality attributes during storage (Wu et al., 2022). Similarly, using a gliding arc plasma flame treatment, an *in vitro* study of *C. alienum* and *C. fioriniae* (fungal pathogens isolated from avocados) by Siddique et al. (2019). The authors showed that CAP treatment for 360 s at 5 cm (from the discharge source) in an open environment reduced the colony growth of fresh cultured plates and 2-day-old cultures to approximately < 2 mm/day and 5 mm/day, respectively. Furthermore, under the same conditions, CAP treatment for 180 s had no significant inhibitory impact on colony growth. Overall, the reduction in colony growth rate by CAP treatment was established to be a function of the fungal pathogen growth stage, and effective control was achieved during early growth stages. Similarly, Gram-positive bacteria have been established to have a thicker membrane compared to Gram-negative bacteria. Therefore, careful consideration should be given to plasma process optimization when investigating microorganisms that can develop recalcitrant biofilms and/or hardened cell wall structures. In addition, the impact of the initial growth stage of the microorganisms and inoculum load should be further studied to fully establish the efficacy of CAP treatments.

Generally, the application of CAP technology in agri-food processing has been regarded as a safe approach and a novel alternative that does not induce the biosynthesis of toxic compounds. The non-toxic and safe declaration was further emphasized in recent investigations by Han et al. (2016b) and Nastasa et al. (2021). For instance, Han et al. (2016b) orally administered a single-dose acute (5000 mg/kg body weight) or 14-day subacute (1000 mg/kg body weight/day) edible films subjected to CAP treatment to Sprague-Dawley (SD) rats. The authors demonstrated with their study that the administered CAP-treated edible film did not result in acute toxicity. Similarly, long-term administration of plasma-activated water in CD1 mice showed that the consumption of the plasma-activated water had no negative impact on the mice's homeostasis (Nastasa et al., 2021). Furthermore, long-term consumption of plasma-activated water did not induce functional and histological changes in the digestive systems and all body organs. Although these studies demonstrated that CAP treatments are non-toxic, a full evaluation of the effects of cold plasma in the food matrix should be undertaken to provide more information. This should include: i) understanding the persistence of reactive species generated by CAP treatment in the food matrix, including their concentration, migration, and oral toxicity; and ii) evaluation of chemical modifications in the food matrix, such as the effects of plasma on volatile organic compounds, lipids, and amino acids. Overall, more studies are required to establish the non-toxic status of cold plasma treatment on food products.

Based on established literature, the reactiveness of plasma particles is dependent on the types, concentration, and exposure time to the plasma. Therefore, when investigating plasma treatment in future foods, it is crucial to evaluate in detail the dynamics of the type of reactive species, the reactions involved in the process, and their migration through the food matrix. Furthermore, the influence of these reactive species on the food matrix with complex biochemicals and biomolecules, as well as the surrounding environment, is hard to predict. Elucidating these interactions will provide vital information on the chemistry of plasma-induced food products. Computational modeling and simulation of plasma reactive species in the food matrix is a relatively new research area, and only limited studies applying computational tools are available in the literature. Tools such as computational fluid dynamics (CFD) and classical molecular dynamics simulation (MDS) would be useful in food biosystems. They would help in understanding the discharged plasma particles at the supramolecular level (based on the examination of weaker and reversible noncovalent interactions between plasma species and food product) and the interaction of reactive species with biomolecules on the atomic scale, respectively (Dharini et al., 2023). The most important contribution needed for the reactive molecular simulation is the interatomic interaction of plasma species with food constituents (biomolecules) such as proteins, lipids, and polysaccharides. This future study would enable a better understanding of the impact of plasma treatments in food systems.

4.7 CONCLUSION

Our extensive literature review shows that CAP technology is an efficient postharvest hurdle technique with numerous advantages. It is also of interest in the technical and commercial aspects to the Agri-food industries because of its applicability at room temperature, rapid performance, increased treatment speed, and ease of use at the industrial level. With its sterilization and decontamination effects, CAP treatment is proven efficient in extending the shelf life of fruit. The efficiency of CAP technology in fruit is dependent on the initial microbial load of the fruit surface, treatment time, and equipment configurations. However, the major limitations attributed to the use of this technology include the changes in the quality attributes of the final product after treatment. This observation highlights the need for treatment optimization that combines antimicrobial efficiency with maintaining quality attributes of horticultural commodities.

Currently, as a novel technology, the application of CAP on fresh fruit is still limited to laboratory scale. One of the drawbacks is the gas use during treatment and the fact that different gas systems produce a unique plasma. Hence, it is crucial to understand the impact of all gas types on fresh and minimally processed fruit to ensure quality and safety is maintained. Studies available on the quality changes based on CAP treatments of fruit are progressively accumulating. However, it is necessary to explore the underpinning mechanisms that can provide deeper insight into the effects CP on fresh and minimally processed fruit. Furthermore, the efficiency of CAP as pre-treatment is dependent on factors such as treatment time and the gas used to generate plasma. More research focusing on the optimization of CAP treatments will be of great benefit in understanding the resistance of microorganisms for the Agri-food industry.

AUTHOR CONTRIBUTION STATEMENT

Loriane A. Yanclo: Conceptualization, data curation, formal analysis, writing-original draft. Zinash A. Belay: Methodology, visualization, validation, writing-review and editing. Gunnar O. Sigge: Conceptualization, visualization, formal analysis, writing-review and editing. Oluwafemi J. Caleb: Conceptualization, validation, project administration, supervision, and writing-reviewing and editing.

FUNDING DECLARATION

This work is based upon research supported by the National Research Foundation (NRF) of South Africa (Grant Nos. 137990 and 146360) awarded to Dr. OJ Caleb. The HORTGRO science project (Grant No. NF8-2021) awarded to Dr. ZA Belay is also gratefully acknowledged.

ACKNOWLEDGMENTS

The PhD Fellowship awarded to Ms. Loriane A. Yanclo by the Organization for Women in Science for the Developing World (OWSD, Rev. No. 3240309373) is gratefully acknowledged. We are grateful for the comments provided by four anonymous reviewers and the guidance provided by the editor.

DATA AVAILABILITY STATEMENTS

Data sharing not applicable to this article as no datasets were generated or analyzed during the current study.

DECLARATIONS

Competing Interests: The authors declare no competing interests.

Conflict of Interest: The authors declare no competing interests.

KEYWORDS

- **cold atmospheric plasma**
- **fresh and minimally processed fruit**
- **microbial decontamination**
- **postharvest technology**
- **quality preservation**
- **shelf life extension**

REFERENCES

Almeida, F. D. L., Cavalcante, R. S., Cullen, P. J., Frias, J. M., Bourke, P., Fernandes, F. A. N., & Rodrigues, S. (2015). Effects of atmospheric cold plasma and ozone on prebiotic orange juice. *Innovative Food Science & Emerging Technologies, 32*, 127–135. https://doi.org/10.1016/j.ifset.2015.09.001 (accessed on 9th July 2025).

Amini, M., & Ghoranneviss, M. (2016). Effects of cold plasma treatment on antioxidants activity, phenolic contents, and shelf life of fresh and dried walnut (*Juglans regia* L.) cultivars during storage. *LWT–Food Science and Technology, 73*, 178–184. https://doi.org/10.1016/j.lwt.2016.06.014 (accessed on 9th July 2025).

Andrasch, M., Stachowiak, J., Schlüter, O., Schnabel, U., & Ehlbeck, J. (2017). Scale-up to pilot plant dimensions of plasma processed water generation for fresh-cut lettuce treatment. *Food Packaging and Shelf Life, 14*, 40–45. https://doi.org/10.1016/j.fpsl.2017.08.007 (accessed on 9th July 2025).

Ashtiani, S. H. M., Rafiee, M., Morad, M. M., Khojastehpour, M., Khani, M., Rohani, A., & Martynenko, A. (2020). Impact of gliding arc plasma pretreatment on drying efficiency and physicochemical properties of grape. *Innovative Food Science & Emerging Technologies, 63*, 102381. https://doi.org/10.1016/j.ifset.2020.102381 (accessed on 9th July 2025).

Baier, M., Ehlbeck, J., Knorr, D., Herppich, W. B., & Schlüter, O. (2015). Impact of plasma processed air (PPA) on quality parameters of fresh produce. *Postharvest Biology and Technology, 100*, 120–126. https://doi.org/10.1016/j.postharvbio.2014.09.015 (accessed on 9th July 2025).

Banura, S., Thirumda, R., Kaur, A., Deshmukh, R. R., & Annapure, U. S. (2018). Modification of starch using low pressure radio frequency air plasma. *LWT–Food Science and Technology, 89*, 719–724. https://doi.org/10.1016/j.lwt.2017.11.056 (accessed on 9th July 2025).

Bao, T., Hao, X., Shishir, M. R. I., Karim, N., & Chen, W. (2020). Cold plasma: An emerging pretreatment technology for the drying of jujube slices. *Food Chemistry, 337*, 127783. https://doi.org/10.1016/j.foodchem.2020.127783 (accessed on 9th July 2025).

Belwal, T., Devkota, H. P., Ramola, S., Andola, H. C., & Bhatt, I. D. (2020). Optimization of extraction methodologies and purification technologies to recover phytonutrients from food. In *Phytonutrients in Food* (pp. 217–235). Woodhead Publishing. https://doi.org/10.1016/B978-0-12-815354-3.00007-1 (accessed on 9th July 2025).

Berardinelli, A., Vannini, L., Ragni, L., & Guerzoni, M. E. (2012). Impact of atmospheric plasma generated by a DBD device on quality-related attributes of "Abate Fetel" pear fruit. In *Plasma for Bio-Decontamination, Medicine and Food Security* (pp. 457–467). Springer. https://doi.org/10.1007/978-94-007-2852-3_35 (accessed on 9th July 2025).

Bernard, H., Faber, M., Wilking, H., Haller, S., Höhle, M., Schielke, A., & Werber, D. (2014). Large multistate outbreak of norovirus gastroenteritis associated with frozen strawberries, Germany, 2012. *Eurosurveillance, 19*(8), 20719. http://www.eurosurveillance.org/ViewArticle.aspx?ArticleId=20719 (accessed on 9th July 2025).

Bourke, P., Ziuzina, D., Han, L., Cullen, P. J., & Gilmore, B. F. (2017). Microbiological interactions with cold plasma. *Journal of Applied Microbiology, 123*(2), 308–324. https://doi.org/10.1111/jam.13429 (accessed on 9th July 2025).

Bovi, G. G., Caleb, O. J., Linke, M., Rauh, C., & Mahajan, P. V. (2016). Transpiration and moisture evolution in packaged fresh horticultural produce and the role of integrated mathematical models: A review. *Biosystems Engineering, 150*, 24–39. https://doi.org/10.1016/j.biosystemseng.2016.07.013 (accessed on 9th July 2025).

Bule, M., Issa, I. A., Khan, F., Shah, M. A., & Niaz, K. (2020). Development of new food products based on phytonutrients. In *Phytonutrients in Food* (pp. 197–216). Woodhead Publishing. https://doi.org/10.1016/B978-0-12-815354-3.00008-3 (accessed on 9th July 2025).

Bußler, S., Ehlbeck, J., & Schlüter, O. K. (2017). Pre-drying treatment of plant related tissues using plasma processed air: Impact on enzyme activity and quality attributes of cut apple and potato. *Innovative Food Science & Emerging Technologies, 40*, 78–86. https://doi.org/10.1016/j.ifset.2016.05.007 (accessed on 9th July 2025).

Caleb, O. J., Wegner, G., Rolleczek, C., Herppich, W. B., Geyer, M., & Mahajan, P. V. (2016). Hot water dipping: Impact on postharvest quality, individual sugars, and bioactive compounds during storage of 'Sonata' strawberry. *Scientia Horticultural, 210*, 150–157. https://doi.org/10.1016/j.scienta.2016.07.021 (accessed on 9th July 2025).

Chang, R., Lu, H., Tian, Y., Li, H., Wang, J., & Jin, Z. (2020). Structural modification and functional improvement of starch nanoparticles using vacuum cold plasma. *International Journal of Biological Macromolecules, 145*, 197–206. https://doi.org/10.1016/j.ijbiomac.2019.12.167 (accessed on 9th July 2025).

Chen, Y. Q., Cheng, J. H., & Sun, D. W. (2020). Chemical, physical, and physiological quality attributes of fruit and vegetables induced by cold plasma treatment: Mechanisms and application advances. *Critical Reviews in Food Science and Nutrition, 60*(16), 2676–2690. https://doi.org/10.1080/10408398.2019.1654429 (accessed on 9th July 2025).

De Castro, D. R. G., Mar, J. M., da Silva, L. S., da Silva, K. A., Sanches, E. A., de Araújo Bezerra, J., & Campelo, P. H. (2020). Dielectric barrier atmospheric cold plasma applied on camu-camu juice processing: Effect of the excitation frequency. *Food Research International, 131*, 109044. https://doi.org/10.1016/j.foodres.2020.109044 (accessed on 9th July 2025).

De Corato, U. (2020). Improving the shelf-life and quality of fresh and minimally processed fruits and vegetables for a modern food industry: A comprehensive critical review from the traditional technologies into the most promising advancements. *Critical Reviews in Food Science and Nutrition, 60*(6), 940–975. https://doi.org/10.1080/10408398.2018.1553025 (accessed on 9th July 2025).

Dharini, M., Jaspin, S., & Mahendran, R. (2023). Cold plasma reactive species: Generation, properties, and interaction with food biomolecules. *Food Chemistry, 405*(Part A), 134746. https://doi.org/10.1016/j.foodchem.2022.134746 (accessed on 9th July 2025).

Dobslaw, C., & Glocker, B. (2020). Plasma technology and its relevance in waste air and waste gas treatment. *Sustainability, 12*(21), 8981. https://doi.org/10.3390/su12218981 (accessed on 9th July 2025).

Dong, X. Y., & Yang, Y. L. (2019). A novel approach to enhance blueberry quality during storage using cold plasma at atmospheric air pressure. *Food and Bioprocess Technology, 12*(8), 1409–1421. https://doi.org/10.1007/s11947-019-02305-y (accessed on 9th July 2025).

Du, Y., Mi, S., Wang, H., Yang, F., Yu, H., Xie, Y., & Yao, W. (2023). Inactivation mechanism of *Alternaria alternata* by dielectric barrier discharge plasma and its quality control on fresh wolfberries. *Food Control*, 109620. https://doi.org/10.1016/j.foodcont.2023.109620 (accessed on 9th July 2025).

Ekezie, F. G. C., Sun, D. W., & Cheng, J. H. (2017). A review on recent advances in cold plasma technology for the food industry: Current applications and future trends. *Trends in Food Science & Technology, 69*, 46–58. https://doi.org/10.1016/j.tifs.2017.08.007 (accessed on 9th July 2025).

Erkmen, O., & Bozoglu, T. F. (2016). Food preservation by reducing water activity. In *Food Microbiology: Principles into Practice*. https://doi.org/10.1002/9781119237860.ch30 (accessed on 9th July 2025).

Fang, Z., Qiu, Y., Sun, Y., Wang, H., & Edmund, K. (2008). Experimental study on discharge characteristics and ozone generation of dielectric barrier discharge in a cylinder–cylinder reactor and a wire–cylinder reactor. *Journal of Electrostatics, 66*(7, 8), 421–426. https://doi.org/10.1016/j.elstat.2008.04.007 (accessed on 9th July 2025).

Farag, M. A., Mesak, M. A., Saied, D. B., & Ezzelarab, N. M. (2021). Uncovering the dormant food hazards: A review of foodborne microbial spores' detection and inactivation methods with emphasis on their application in the food industry. *Trends in Food Science & Technology, 107*, 252–267. https://doi.org/10.1016/j.tifs.2020.10.037 (accessed on 9th July 2025).

Fernandez, A., Noriega, E., & Thompson, A. (2013). Inactivation of *Salmonella enterica* serovar Typhimurium on fresh produce by cold atmospheric gas plasma technology. *Food Microbiology, 33*, 24–29. https://doi.org/10.1016/j.fm.2012.08.007 (accessed on 9th July 2025).

Francioso, L., De Pascali, C., Pescini, E., De Giorgi, M. G., & Siciliano, P. (2016). Modeling, fabrication, and plasma actuator coupling of flexible pressure sensors for flow separation detection and control in aeronautical applications. *Journal of Physics D: Applied Physics, 49*(23), 235201. https://doi.org/10.1088/0022-3727/49/23/235201 (accessed on 9th July 2025).

Frandsen, S. K., Vissing, M., & Gehl, J. (2020). A comprehensive review of calcium electroporation—A novel cancer treatment modality. *Cancers, 12*(2), 290. https://doi.org/10.3390/cancers12020290 (accessed on 9th July 2025).

Gan, Z., Feng, X., Hou, Y., Sun, A., & Wang, R. (2021). Cold plasma jet with dielectric barrier configuration: Investigating its effect on the cell membrane of *E. coli* and *S. cerevisiae* and its impact on the quality of chokeberry juice. *LWT–Food Science and Technology, 136*(Part 1), 110223. https://doi.org/10.1016/j.lwt.2020.110223 (accessed on 9th July 2025).

Guo, J., Huang, K., & Wang, J. (2015). Bactericidal effect of various non-thermal plasma agents and the influence of experimental conditions in microbial inactivation: A review. *Food Control, 50*, 482–490. https://doi.org/10.1016/j.foodcont.2014.09.037 (accessed on 9th July 2025).

Guo, J., Huang, K., Wang, X., Lyu, C., Yang, N., Li, Y., & Wang, J. (2017). Inactivation of yeast on grapes by plasma-activated water and its effects on quality attributes. *Journal of Food Protection, 80*(2), 225–230. https://doi.org/10.4315/0362-028X.JFP-16-116 (accessed on 9th July 2025).

Hage, M., Khelissa, S., Akoum, H., Chihib, N. E., & Jama, C. (2022). Cold plasma surface treatments to prevent biofilm formation in food industries and medical sectors. *Applied Microbiology and Biotechnology, 106*(1), 81–100. https://doi.org/10.1007/s00253-021-11715-y (accessed on 9th July 2025).

Hamdan, N., Lee, C. H., Wong, S. L., Fauzi, C. E. N. C. A., Zamri, N. M. A., & Lee, T. H. (2022). Prevention of enzymatic browning by natural extracts and genome-editing: A review on recent progress. *Molecules, 27*(3), 1101. https://doi.org/10.3390/molecules27031101 (accessed on 9th July 2025).

Han, L., Patil, S., Boehm, D., Milosavljević, V., Cullen, P. J., & Bourke, P. (2016a). Mechanisms of inactivation by high-voltage atmospheric cold plasma differ for *Escherichia coli* and *Staphylococcus aureus*. *Applied and Environmental Microbiology, 82*(2), 450–458. https://doi.org/10.1128/AEM.02660-15 (accessed on 9th July 2025).

Han, S. H., Suh, H. J., Hong, K. B., Kim, S. Y., & Min, S. C. (2016b). Oral toxicity of cold plasma-treated edible films for food coating. *Journal of Food Science, 81*(12), T3052–T3057. https://doi.org/10.1111/1750-3841.13551 (accessed on 9th July 2025).

Han, Y., Cheng, J. H., & Sun, D. W. (2019). Activities and conformation changes of food enzymes induced by cold plasma: A review. *Critical Reviews in Food Science and Nutrition, 59*(5), 794–811. https://doi.org/10.1080/10408398.2018.1555131 (accessed on 9th July 2025).

Hosseini, S. M., Hosseinzadeh Samani, B., Rostami, S., & Lorigooini, Z. (2021). Design and characterization of jet cold atmospheric pressure plasma and its effect on *Escherichia coli*, color, pH, and bioactive compounds of sour cherry juice. *International Journal of Food Science & Technology, 56*(10), 4883–4892. https://doi.org/10.1111/ijfs.15220 (accessed on 9th July 2025).

Hosseini, S. M., Rostami, S., Hosseinzadeh Samani, B., & Lorigooini, Z. (2020). The effect of atmospheric pressure cold plasma on the inactivation of *Escherichia coli* in sour cherry juice and its qualitative properties. *Food Science & Nutrition, 8*(2), 870–883. https://doi.org/10.1002/fsn3.1364 (accessed on 9th July 2025).

Hou, Y., Wang, R., Gan, Z., Shao, T., Zhang, X., He, M., & Sun, A. (2019). Effect of cold plasma on blueberry juice quality. *Food Chemistry, 290*, 79–86. https://doi.org/10.1016/j.foodchem.2019.03.123 (accessed on 9th July 2025).

Hua, X., Li, T., Wu, C., Zhou, D., Fan, G., Li, X., et al. (2022). Novel physical treatments (Pulsed light and cold plasma) improve the quality of postharvest apricots after long-distance simulated transportation. *Postharvest Biology and Technology, 194*, 112098. https://doi.org/10.1016/j.postharvbio.2022.112098 (accessed on 9th July 2025).

Huang, M., Zhuang, H., Wang, J., Yan, W., Zhao, J., & Zhang, J. (2018). Inactivation kinetics of *Salmonella typhimurium* and *Staphylococcus aureus* in different media by dielectric barrier discharge non-thermal plasma. *Applied Sciences, 8*(11), 2087. https://doi.org/10.3390/app8112087 (accessed on 9th July 2025).

Jensen, B., Knudsen, I. M., Andersen, B., Nielsen, K. F., Thrane, U., Jensen, D. F., & Larsen, J. (2013). Characterization of microbial communities and fungal metabolites on field grown strawberries from organic and conventional production. *International Journal of Food Microbiology, 160*(3), 313–322. https://doi.org/10.1016/j.ijfoodmicro.2012.11.005 (accessed on 9th July 2025).

Juan, C. A., Pérez de la Lastra, J. M., Plou, F. J., & Pérez-Lebeña, E. (2021). The chemistry of reactive oxygen species (ROS) revisited: Outlining their role in biological macromolecules (DNA, lipids and proteins) and induced pathologies. *International Journal of Molecular Science, 22*(9), 4642. https://doi.org/10.3390/ijms22094642 (accessed on 9th July 2025).

Jung, S., Kim, H. J., Park, S., Yong, H. I., Choe, J. H., Jeon, H. J., et al. (2015). The use of atmospheric pressure plasma-treated water as a source of nitrite for emulsion-type sausage. *Meat Science, 108*, 132–137. https://doi.org/10.1016/j.meatsci.2015.06.009 (accessed on 9th July 2025).

Kantala, C., Supasin, S., Intra, P., & Rattanadecho, P. (2022). Evaluation of pulsed electric field and conventional thermal processing for microbial inactivation in Thai orange juice. *Foods, 11*(8), 1102. https://doi.org/10.3390/foods11081102 (accessed on 9th July 2025).

Kim, S. Y., Lee, S. Y., & Min, S. C. (2019). Improvement of the antioxidant activity, water solubility, and dispersion stability of prickly pear cactus fruit extracts using argon cold plasma treatment. *Journal of Food Science, 84*(10), 2876–2882. https://doi.org/10.1111/1750-3841.14791 (accessed on 9th July 2025).

Kovačević, D. B., Brdar, D., Fabečić, P., Barba, F. J., Lorenzo, J. M., & Putnik, P. (2020). Strategies to achieve a healthy and balanced diet: Fruits and vegetables as a natural source of bioactive compounds. In *Agri-Food Industry Strategies for Healthy Diets and Sustainability* (pp. 51–88). Academic Press. https://doi.org/10.1016/B978-0-12-817226-1.00002-3 (accessed on 9th July 2025).

Kovačević, D. B., Kljusurić, J. G., Putnik, P., Vukušić, T., Herceg, Z., & Dragović-Uzelac, V. (2016). Stability of polyphenols in chokeberry juice treated with gas phase plasma. *Food Chemistry, 212*, 323–331. https://doi.org/10.1016/j.foodchem.2016.05.192 (accessed on 9th July 2025).

Kumar, S., Baghel, M., Yadav, A., & Dhakar, M. K. (2018). Postharvest biology and technology of berries. In *Postharvest Biology and Technology of Temperate Fruits* (pp. 349–370). Springer, Cham. https://doi.org/10.1007/978-3-319-76843-4_15 (accessed on 9th July 2025).

Lacombe, A., Niemira, B. A., Gurtler, J. B., Fan, X., Sites, J., Boyd, G., & Chen, H. (2015). Atmospheric cold plasma inactivation of aerobic microorganisms on blueberries and effects on quality attributes. *Food Microbiology, 46*, 479–484. https://doi.org/10.1016/j.fm.2014.09.010 (accessed on 9th July 2025).

Lafarga, T., Colás-Medà, P., Abadias, M., Aguiló-Aguayo, I., Bobo, G., & Viñas, I. (2019). Strategies to reduce microbial risk and improve quality of fresh and processed strawberries: A review. *Innovative Food Science & Emerging Technologies, 52*, 197–212. https://doi.org/10.1016/j.ifset.2018.12.012 (accessed on 9th July 2025).

Lee, H., Kim, J. E., Chung, M. S., & Min, S. C. (2015). Cold plasma treatment for the microbiological safety of cabbage, lettuce, and dried figs. *Food Microbiology, 51*, 74–80. https://doi.org/10.1016/j.fm.2015.05.004 (accessed on 9th July 2025).

Lee, M. J., Lee, H. J., Lee, Y., Yang, J. Y., & Song, J. S. (2023). Cold plasma treatment increases bioactive metabolites in oat (*Avena sativa* L.) sprouts and enhances *in vitro* osteogenic activity of their extracts. *Plant Foods for Human Nutrition, 78*, 146–153. https://doi.org/10.1007/s11130-022-01029-3 (accessed on 9th July 2025).

Leite, A. K., Fonteles, T. V., Miguel, T. B., da Silva, G. S., de Brito, E. S., Alves Filho, E. G., & Rodrigues, S. (2021). Atmospheric cold plasma frequency imparts changes on cashew apple juice composition and improves vitamin C bio-accessibility. *Food*

Research International, 147, 110479. https://doi.org/10.1016/j.foodres.2021.110479 (accessed on 9th July 2025).

Li, X., Li, M., Ji, N., Jin, P., Zhang, J., Zheng, Y., & Li, F. (2019). Cold plasma treatment induces phenolic accumulation and enhances antioxidant activity in fresh-cut pitaya (*Hylocereus undatus*) fruit. *LWT–Food Science and Technology, 115*, 108447. https://doi.org/10.1016/j.lwt.2019.108447 (accessed on 9th July 2025).

Liao, X., Li, J., Muhammad, A. I., Suo, Y., Chen, S., Ye, X., & Ding, T. (2018). Application of a dielectric barrier discharge atmospheric cold plasma (DBD-ACP) for *Escherichia coli* inactivation in apple juice. *Journal of Food Science, 83*(2), 401–408. https://doi.org/10.1111/1750-3841.14045 (accessed on 9th July 2025).

Liao, X., Liu, D., Xiang, Q., Ahn, J., Chen, S., Ye, X., & Ding, T. (2017). Inactivation mechanisms of non-thermal plasma on microbes: A review. *Food Control, 75*, 83–91. https://doi.org/10.1016/j.foodcont.2016.12.021 (accessed on 9th July 2025).

Liu, C., Li, X., & Chen, H. (2015). Application of water-assisted ultraviolet light processing on the inactivation of murine norovirus on blueberries. *International Journal of Food Microbiology, 214*, 18–23. https://doi.org/10.1016/j.ijfoodmicro.2015.07.023 (accessed on 9th July 2025).

Lourenço, S. C., Moldão-Martins, M., & Alves, V. D. (2019). Antioxidants of natural plant origins: From sources to food industry applications. *Molecules, 24*(22), 4132. https://doi.org/10.3390/molecules24224132 (accessed on 9th July 2025).

Lunov, O., Churpita, O., Zablotskii, V., Deyneka, I. G., Meshkovskii, I. K., Jäger, A., & Dejneka, A. (2015). Non-thermal plasma mills bacteria: Scanning electron microscopy observations. *Applied Physics Letters, 106*(5), 053703. https://doi.org/10.1063/1.4907624 (accessed on 9th July 2025).

Lunov, O., Zablotskii, V., Churpita, O., Jäger, A., Polívka, L., Syková, E., & Kubinová, Š. (2016). The interplay between biological and physical scenarios of bacterial death induced by non-thermal plasma. *Biomaterials, 82*, 71–83. https://doi.org/10.1016/j.biomaterials.2015.12.027 (accessed on 9th July 2025).

Ma, R., Wang, G., Tian, Y., Wang, K., Zhang, J., & Fang, J. (2015). Non-thermal plasma-activated water inactivation of food-borne pathogen on fresh produce. *Journal of Hazardous Materials, 300*, 643–651. https://doi.org/10.1016/j.jhazmat.2015.07.061 (accessed on 9th July 2025).

Ma, R., Yu, S., Tian, Y., Wang, K., Sun, C., Li, X., & Fang, J. (2016). Effect of non-thermal plasma-activated water on fruit decay and quality in postharvest Chinese bayberries. *Food and Bioprocess Technology, 9*(11), 1825–1834. https://doi.org/10.1007/s11947-016-1761-7 (accessed on 9th July 2025).

Małajowicz, J., Khachatryan, K., & Kozłowska, M. (2022). Properties of water activated with low-temperature plasma in the context of microbial activity. *Beverages, 8*(4), 63. https://doi.org/10.3390/beverages8040063 (accessed on 9th July 2025).

Mandal, R., Singh, A., & Singh, A. P. (2018). Recent developments in cold plasma decontamination technology in the food industry. *Trends in Food Science & Technology, 80*, 93–103. https://doi.org/10.1016/j.tifs.2018.07.014 (accessed on 9th July 2025).

Mao, L., Mhaske, P., Zing, X., Kasapis, S., Majzoobi, M., & Farahnaky, A. (2021). Cold plasma: Microbial inactivation and effects on quality attributes of fresh and minimally processed fruits and ready-to-eat vegetables. *Trends in Food Science & Technology, 116*, 146–175. https://doi.org/10.1016/j.tifs.2021.07.002 (accessed on 9th July 2025).

Matrose, N. A., Obikeze, K., Belay, Z. A., & Caleb, O. J. (2021). Plant extracts as alternative sources for post-harvest management of fungal pathogens: A review. *Food Bioscience, 41*, 100840. https://doi.org/10.1016/j.fbio.2020.100840 (accessed on 9th July 2025).

Mir, S. A., Shah, M. A., & Mir, M. M. (2016). Understanding the role of plasma technology in food industry. *Food and Bioprocess Technology, 9*(5), 734–750. https://doi.org/10.1007/s11947-016-1699-9 (accessed on 9th July 2025).

Mir, S. A., Siddiqui, M. W., Dar, B. N., Shah, M. A., Wani, M. H., Roohinejad, S., & Ali, A. (2020). Promising applications of cold plasma for microbial safety, chemical decontamination, and quality enhancement in fruits. *Journal of Applied Microbiology, 129*(3), 474–485. https://doi.org/10.1111/jam.14541 (accessed on 9th July 2025).

Misra, N. N. (2015). The contribution of non-thermal and advanced oxidation technologies towards dissipation of pesticide residues. *Trends in Food Science & Technology, 45*(2), 229–244. https://doi.org/10.1016/j.tifs.2015.06.005 (accessed on 9th July 2025).

Misra, N. N., Kaur, S., Tiwari, B. K., Kaur, A., Singh, N., & Cullen, P. J. (2015a). Atmospheric pressure cold plasma (ACP) treatment of wheat flour. *Food Hydrocolloids, 44*, 115–121. https://doi.org/10.1016/j.foodhyd.2014.08.019 (accessed on 9th July 2025).

Misra, N. N., Keener, K. M., Bourke, P., Mosnier, J. P., & Cullen, P. J. (2014a). In-package atmospheric pressure cold plasma treatment of cherry tomatoes. *Journal of Bioscience and Bioengineering, 118*(2), 177–182. https://doi.org/10.1016/j.jbiosc.2014.02.005 (accessed on 9th July 2025).

Misra, N. N., Martynenko, A., Chemat, F., Paniwnyk, L., Barba, F. J., & Jambrak, A. R. (2018). Thermodynamics, transport phenomena, and electrochemistry of external field-assisted nonthermal food technologies. *Critical Reviews in Food Science and Nutrition, 58*(11), 1832–1863. https://doi.org/10.1080/10408398.2017.1287660 (accessed on 9th July 2025).

Misra, N. N., Moiseev, T., Patil, S., Pankaj, S. K., Bourke, P., Mosnier, J. P., & Cullen, P. J. (2014c). Cold plasma in modified atmospheres for post-harvest treatment of strawberries. *Food and Bioprocess Technology, 7*(10), 3045–3054. https://doi.org/10.1007/s11947-014-1356-0 (accessed on 9th July 2025).

Misra, N. N., Pankaj, S. K., Frias, J. M., Keener, K. M., & Cullen, P. J. (2015b). The effects of nonthermal plasma on chemical quality of strawberries. *Postharvest Biology and Technology, 110*, 197–202. https://doi.org/10.1016/j.postharvbio.2015.08.023 (accessed on 9th July 2025).

Misra, N. N., Pankaj, S. K., Segat, A., & Ishikawa, K. (2016). Cold plasma interactions with enzymes in foods and model systems. *Trends in Food Science & Technology, 55*, 39–47. https://doi.org/10.1016/j.tifs.2016.07.001 (accessed on 9th July 2025).

Misra, N. N., Patil, S., Moiseev, T., Bourke, P., Mosnier, J. P., Keener, K. M., & Cullen, P. J. (2014b). In-package atmospheric pressure cold plasma treatment of strawberries. *Journal of Food Engineering, 125*, 131–138. https://doi.org/10.1016/j.jfoodeng.2013.10.023 (accessed on 9th July 2025).

Misra, N. N., Tiwari, B. K., Raghavarao, K. S. M. S., & Cullen, P. J. (2011). Nonthermal plasma inactivation of food-borne pathogens. *Food Engineering Reviews, 3*(3, 4), 159–170. https://doi.org/10.1007/s12393-011-9041-9 (accessed on 9th July 2025).

Moosavi, M. H., Khani, M. R., Shokri, B., Hosseini, S. M., Shojaee-Alibadi, S., & Mirmoghtadie, L. (2020). Modifications of protein-based films using cold plasma.

International Journal of Biological Macromolecules, 142, 769–777. https://doi.org/10.1016/j.ijbiomac.2019.10.017 (accessed on 9th July 2025).

Muhammad, A. I., Xiang, Q., Liao, X., Liu, D., & Ding, T. (2018). Understanding the impact of nonthermal plasma on food constituents and microstructure—A review. *Food and Bioprocess Technology, 11*(3), 463–486. https://doi.org/10.1007/s11947-017-2042-9 (accessed on 9th July 2025).

Nastasa, V., Pasca, A. S., Malancus, R. N., Bostanaru, A. C., Ailincai, L. I., Ursu, E. L., Vasiliu, A. L., Minea, B., Hnatiuc, E., & Mares, M. (2021). Toxicity assessment of long-term exposure to non-thermal plasma activated water in mice. *International Journal of Molecular Sciences, 22*(21), 11534. https://doi.org/10.3390/ijms222111534 (accessed on 9th July 2025).

Nishime, T. M. C., Borges, A. C., Koga-Ito, C. Y., Machida, M., Hein, L. R. O., & Kostov, K. G. (2017). Non-thermal atmospheric pressure plasma jet applied to inactivation of different microorganisms. *Surface and Coatings Technology, 312*, 19–24. https://doi.org/10.1016/j.surfcoat.2016.07.076 (accessed on 9th July 2025).

Nyamende, N. E., Domtchouang, F. R., Belay, Z. A., Keyser, Z., Oyenihi, A., & Caleb, O. J. (2021). Alternative postharvest pre-treatment strategies for quality and microbial safety of 'Granny Smith' apple. *Heliyon, 7*(5), e07104. https://doi.org/10.1016/j.heliyon.2021.e07104 (accessed on 9th July 2025).

Okyere, A. Y., Bertoft, E., & Annor, G. A. (2019). Modification of cereal and tuber waxy starches with radio frequency cold plasma and its effects on waxy starch properties. *Carbohydrate Polymers, 223*(1), 115075. https://doi.org/10.1016/j.carbpol.2019.115075 (accessed on 9th July 2025).

Onal-Ulusoy, B., Sen, Y., & Mutlu, M. (2019). Quality changes of hazelnut kernels subjected to different cold plasmas and gamma irradiation treatments. *LWT–Food Science & Technology, 116*, 108549. https://doi.org/10.1016/j.lwt.2019.108549 (accessed on 9th July 2025).

Paixão, L. M., Fonteles, T. V., Oliveira, V. S., Fernandes, F. A., & Rodrigues, S. (2019). Cold plasma effects on functional compounds of siriguela juice. *Food and Bioprocess Technology, 12*(1), 110–121. https://doi.org/10.1007/s11947-018-2197-z (accessed on 9th July 2025).

Pan, Y. W., Cheng, J. H., & Sun, D. W. (2021). Inhibition of fruit softening by cold plasma treatments: Affecting factors and applications. *Critical Reviews in Food Science and Nutrition, 61*(12), 1935–1946. https://doi.org/10.1080/10408398.2020.1776210 (accessed on 9th July 2025).

Pankaj, S. K., Bueno-Ferrer, C., Misra, N. N., Milosavljević, V., O'Donnell, C. P., Bourke, P., & Cullen, P. J. (2014). Applications of cold plasma technology in food packaging. *Trends in Food Science & Technology, 35*(1), 5–17. https://doi.org/10.1016/j.tifs.2013.10.009 (accessed on 9th July 2025).

Pankaj, S. K., Misra, N. N., & Cullen, P. J. (2013). Kinetics of tomato peroxidase inactivation by atmospheric pressure cold plasma based on dielectric barrier discharge. *Innovative Food Science & Emerging Technologies, 19*, 153–157. https://doi.org/10.1016/j.ifset.2013.03.001 (accessed on 9th July 2025).

Pankaj, S. K., Wan, Z., & Keener, K. M. (2018). Effects of cold plasma on food quality: A review. *Foods, 7*(1), 4. https://doi.org/10.3390/foods7010004 (accessed on 9th July 2025).

Pankaj, S. K., Wan, Z., Colonna, W., & Keener, K. M. (2017). Effect of high voltage atmospheric cold plasma on white grape juice quality. *Journal of the Science of Food and Agriculture, 97*(12), 4016–4021. https://doi.org/10.1002/jsfa.8268 (accessed on 9th July 2025).

Pathak, N., Grossi Bovi, G., Limnaios, A., Fröhling, A., Brincat, J. P., Taoukis, P., & Schlüter, O. (2020). Impact of cold atmospheric pressure plasma processing on storage of blueberries. *Journal of Food Processing and Preservation, 44*(8), e14581. https://doi.org/10.1111/jfpp.14581 (accessed on 9th July 2025).

Pathare, P. B., Caleb, O. J., Prasath, V. R., & Garud, S. R. (2023). Application of cold plasma for fresh produce quality and shelf-life extension. In *Postharvest Management of Fresh Produce*. Elsevier Inc. https://doi.org/10.1016/B978-0-323-91132-0.00009-5 (accessed on 9th July 2025).

Perinban, S., Orsat, V., & Raghavan, V. (2019). Nonthermal plasma–liquid interactions in food processing: A review. *Comprehensive Reviews in Food Science and Food Safety, 18*, 1985–2008. https://doi.org/10.1111/1541-4337.12503 (accessed on 9th July 2025).

Phan, K. T. K., Phan, H. T., Boonyawan, D., Intipunya, P., Brennan, C. S., Regenstein, J. M., & Phimolsiripol, Y. (2018). Non-thermal plasma for elimination of pesticide residues in mango. *Innovative Food Science & Emerging Technologies, 48*, 164–171. https://doi.org/10.1016/j.ifset.2018.06.009 (accessed on 9th July 2025).

Phan, K. T. K., Phan, H. T., Brennan, C. S., Regenstein, J. M., Jantanasakulwong, K., Boonyawan, D., & Phimolsiripol, Y. (2019). Gliding arc discharge non-thermal plasma for retardation of mango anthracnose. *LWT–Food Science and Technology, 105*, 142–148. https://doi.org/10.1016/j.lwt.2019.02.012 (accessed on 9th July 2025).

Phan, K. T. K., Phan, H. T., Uthaichana, K., & Phimolsiripol, Y. (2017). Effect of non-thermal plasma on physicochemical properties of 'Nam Dok Mai' mango. *International Journal on Advanced Science, Engineering, and Information Technology, 7*(1), 263–268. https://doi.org/10.18517/ijaseit.7.1.1620 (accessed on 9th July 2025).

Podolak, R., David, W., & Black, D. G. (2020). Factors affecting microbial inactivation during high pressure processing in juices and beverages: A review. *Journal of Food Protection, 83*(9), 1561–1575. https://doi.org/10.4315/JFP-20-096 (accessed on 9th July 2025).

Pour, A. K., Khorram, S., Ehsani, A., Ostadrahimi, A., & Ghasempour, Z. (2022). Atmospheric cold plasma effect on quality attributes of banana slices: Its potential use in blanching process. *Innovative Food Science & Emerging Technologies, 76*, 102945. https://doi.org/10.1016/j.ifset.2022.102945 (accessed on 9th July 2025).

Puligundla, P., Lee, T., & Mok, C. (2018a). Effect of intermittent corona discharge plasma treatment for improving microbial quality and shelf life of kumquat (*Citrus japonica*) fruits. *LWT–Food Science and Technology, 91*, 8–13. https://doi.org/10.1016/j.lwt.2018.01.019 (accessed on 9th July 2025).

Puligundla, P., Pyun, Y. R., & Mok, C. (2018). Pulsed electric field (PEF) technology for microbial inactivation in low-alcohol red wine. *Food Science and Biotechnology, 27*(6), 1691–1696. https://doi.org/10.1007/s10068-018-0422-1 (accessed on 9th July 2025).

Ramazzina, I., Berardinelli, A., Rizzi, F., Tappi, S., Ragni, L., Sacchetti, G., & Rocculi, P. (2015). Effect of cold plasma treatment on physio-chemical parameters and antioxidant activity of minimally processed kiwifruit. *Postharvest Biology and Technology, 107*, 55–65. https://doi.org/10.1016/j.postharvbio.2015.04.008 (accessed on 9th July 2025).

Ramazzina, I., Tappi, S., Rocculi, P., Sacchetti, G., Berardinelli, A., Marseglia, A., & Rizzi, F. (2016). Effect of cold plasma treatment on the functional properties of fresh-cut apples. *Journal of Agricultural and Food Chemistry, 64*(42), 8010–8018. https://doi.org/10.1021/acs.jafc.6b02730 (accessed on 9th July 2025).

Rana, S., Mehta, D., Bansal, V., Shivhare, U. S., & Yadav, S. K. (2020). Atmospheric cold plasma (ACP) treatment improved in-package shelf-life of strawberry fruit. *Journal of Food Science and Technology, 57*(1), 102–112. https://doi.org/10.1007/s13197-019-04035-7 (accessed on 9th July 2025).

Rothwell, J. G., Hong, J., Morrison, S. J., Vyas, H. K., Xia, B., Mai-Prochnow, A., & Carter, D. A. (2023). An effective sanitizer for fresh produce production: *In situ* plasma activated water treatment inactivates pathogenic bacteria and maintains the quality of cucurbit fruit. *BioRxiv*. https://doi.org/10.1101/2023.01.03.522676 (accessed on 9th July 2025).

Sarangapani, C., Devi, Y., Thirundas, R., Annapure, U. S., & Deshmukh, R. R. (2015). Effect of low-pressure plasma on physico-chemical properties of parboiled rice. *LWT–Food Science and Technology, 63*(1), 452–460. https://doi.org/10.1016/j.lwt.2015.03.026 (accessed on 9th July 2025).

Sarangapani, C., O'Toole, G., Cullen, P. J., & Bourke, P. (2017). Atmospheric cold plasma dissipation efficiency of agrochemicals on blueberries. *Innovative Food Science & Emerging Technologies, 44*, 235–241. https://doi.org/10.1016/j.ifset.2017.02.012 (accessed on 9th July 2025).

Sarvikivi, E., Roivainen, M., Maunula, L., Niskanen, T., Korhonen, T., Lappalainen, M., & Kuusi, M. (2012). Multiple norovirus outbreaks linked to imported frozen raspberries. *Epidemiology & Infection, 140*(2), 260–267. https://doi.org/10.1017/S0950268811000379 (accessed on 9th July 2025).

Schnabel, U., Niquet, R., Schlüter, O., Gniffke, H., & Ehlbeck, J. (2015). Decontamination and sensory properties of microbiologically contaminated fresh fruits and vegetables by microwave plasma processed air (PPA). *Journal of Food Processing and Preservation, 39*(6), 653–662. https://doi.org/10.1111/jfpp.12273 (accessed on 9th July 2025).

Scholtz, V., Pazlarova, J., Souskova, H., Khun, J., & Julak, J. (2015). Nonthermal plasma–A tool for decontamination and disinfection. *Biotechnology Advances, 33*, 1108–1119. https://doi.org/10.1016/j.biotechadv.2015.01.002 (accessed on 9th July 2025).

Schottroff, F., Fröhling, A., Zunabovic-Pichler, M., Krottenthaler, A., Schlüter, O., & Jäger, H. (2018). Sublethal injury and viable but non-culturable (VBNC) state in microorganisms during preservation of food and biological materials by non-thermal processes. *Frontiers in Microbiology, 9*, 2773. https://doi.org/10.3389/fmicb.2018.02773 (accessed on 9th July 2025).

Segat, A., Misra, N., Fabbro, A., Buchini, F., Lippe, G., Cullen, P., & Innocente, N. (2014). Effects of ozone processing on chemical, structural and functional properties of whey protein isolate. *Food Research International, 66*, 365–372. https://doi.org/10.1016/j.foodres.2014.10.002 (accessed on 9th July 2025).

Sehrawat, R., Kaur, B. P., Nema, P. K., Tewari, S., & Kumar, L. (2020). Microbial inactivation by high pressure processing: Principle, mechanism, and factors responsible. *Food Science and Biotechnology, 30*(1), 19–35. https://doi.org/10.1007/s10068-020-00831-6 (accessed on 9th July 2025).

Siddique, S. S., Hardy, G. E. St. J., & Bayliss, K. L. (2019). Cold plasma as a novel treatment to reduce the *in vitro* growth and germination of *Colletotrichum* species. *Plant Pathology, 68*(7), 1361–1368. https://doi.org/10.1111/ppa.13059 (accessed on 9th July 2025).

Stoica, M., Alexe, P., & Mihalcea, L. (2014). Atmospheric cold plasma as new strategy for foods processing–An overview. *Innovative Romanian Food Biotechnology, 15*. (accessed on 9th July 2025).

Sudheesh, C., & Sunooj, K. V. (2020). Cold plasma processing of fresh-cut fruits and vegetables. In *Fresh-Cut Fruits and Vegetables* (pp. 339–356). Academic Press. https://doi.org/10.1016/B978-0-12-816184-5.00014-8 (accessed on 9th July 2025).

Surowsky, B., Fröhling, A., Gottschalk, N., Schlüter, O., & Knorr, D. (2014). Impact of cold plasma on *Citrobacter freundii* in apple juice: Inactivation kinetics and mechanisms. *International Journal of Food Microbiology, 174*, 63–71. https://doi.org/10.1016/j.ijfoodmicro.2013.12.031 (accessed on 9th July 2025).

Surowsky, B., Schlüter, O., & Knorr, D. (2015). Interactions of non-thermal atmospheric pressure plasma with solid and liquid food systems: A review. *Food Engineering Reviews, 7*(2), 82–108. https://doi.org/10.1007/s12393-014-9088-5 (accessed on 9th July 2025).

Tappi, S., Berardinelli, A., Ragni, L., Dalla Rosa, M., Guarnieri, A., & Rocculi, P. (2014). Atmospheric gas plasma treatment of fresh-cut apples. *Innovative Food Science & Emerging Technologies, 21*, 114–122. https://doi.org/10.1016/j.ifset.2013.09.012 (accessed on 9th July 2025).

Tappi, S., Gozzi, G., Vannini, L., Berardinelli, A., Romani, S., Ragni, L., & Rocculi, P. (2016). Cold plasma treatment for fresh-cut melon stabilization. *Innovative Food Science & Emerging Technologies, 33*, 225–233. https://doi.org/10.1016/j.ifset.2015.12.022 (accessed on 9th July 2025).

Terpiłowski, K., Tomczyńska-Mleko, M., Nishinari, K., & Mleko, S. (2017). Surface properties of ion-induced whey protein gels deposited on cold plasma treated support. *Food Hydrocolloids, 71*, 17–25. https://doi.org/10.1016/j.foodhyd.2017.04.032 (accessed on 9th July 2025).

Thirumdas, R., Kadam, D., & Annapure, U. S. (2017b). Cold plasma: An alternative technology for starch modification. *Food Biophysics, 12*, 129–139. https://doi.org/10.1007/s11483-017-9468-5 (accessed on 9th July 2025).

Thirumdas, R., Sarangapani, C., & Annapure, U. S. (2015). Cold plasma: A novel non-thermal technology for food processing. *Food Biophysics, 10*(1), 1–11. https://doi.org/10.1007/s11483-014-9382-z (accessed on 9th July 2025).

Thirumdas, R., Trimukhe, A., Deshmukh, R. R., & Annapure, U. S. (2017a). Functional and rheological properties of cold plasma treated rice starch. *Carbohydrate Polymers, 157*, 1723–1731. https://doi.org/10.1016/j.carbpol.2016.11.050 (accessed on 9th July 2025).

Wang, J., Zhuang, H., Hinton, A., Jr., & Zhang, J. (2016). Influence of in-package cold plasma treatment on microbiological shelf life and appearance of fresh chicken breast fillets. *Food Microbiology, 60*, 142–146. https://doi.org/10.1016/j.fm.2016.07.007 (accessed on 9th July 2025).

Wang, R. X., Nian, W. F., Wu, H. Y., Feng, H. Q., Zhang, K., Zhang, J., & Fang, J. (2012). Atmospheric-pressure cold plasma treatment of contaminated fresh fruit and vegetable slices: Inactivation and physiochemical properties evaluation. *The European Physical*

Journal D, 66(10), 276. https://doi.org/10.1140/epjd/e2012-30053-1 (accessed on 9th July 2025).

Won, M. Y., Lee, S. J., & Min, S. C. (2017). Mandarin preservation by microwave-powered cold plasma treatment. *Innovative Food Science & Emerging Technologies, 39*, 25–32. https://doi.org/10.1016/j.ifset.2016.10.021 (accessed on 9th July 2025).

Wu, X., Zhao, W., Zeng, X., Zhang, Q. A., Gao, G., & Song, S. (2020). Effects of cold plasma treatment on cherry quality during storage. *Food Science and Technology International, 27*(5), 441–455. https://doi.org/10.1177/1082013220957134 (accessed on 9th July 2025).

Wu, Y., Cheng, J. H., & Sun, D. W. (2022). Subcellular damage of *Colletotrichum asianum* and inhibition of mango anthracnose by dielectric barrier discharge plasma. *Food Chemistry, 381*, 132197. https://doi.org/10.1016/j.foodchem.2022.132197 (accessed on 9th July 2025).

Wu, Y., Cheng, J. H., Keener, K. M., & Sun, D. W. (2023). Inhibitory effects of dielectric barrier discharge cold plasma on pathogenic enzymes and anthracnose for mango postharvest preservation. *Postharvest Biology and Technology, 196*, 112181. https://doi.org/10.1016/j.postharvbio.2022.112181 (accessed on 9th July 2025).

Yang, L., Wen, K. S., Ruan, X., Zhao, Y. X., Wei, F., & Wang, Q. (2018). Response of plant secondary metabolites to environmental factors. *Molecules, 23*(4), 762. https://doi.org/10.3390/molecules23040762 (accessed on 9th July 2025).

Yi, F., Wang, J., Xiang, Y., Yun, Z., Pan, Y., Jiang, Y., & Zhang, Z. (2022). Physiological and quality changes in fresh-cut mango fruit as influenced by cold plasma. *Postharvest Biology and Technology, 194*, 112105. https://doi.org/10.1016/j.postharvbio.2022.112105 (accessed on 9th July 2025).

Zhang, X. L., Zhong, C. S., Mujumdar, A. S., Yang, X. H., Deng, L. Z., Wang, J., & Xiao, H. W. (2019). Cold plasma pretreatment enhances drying kinetics and quality attributes of chili pepper (*Capsicum annuum* L.). *Journal of Food Engineering, 241*, 51–57. https://doi.org/10.1016/j.jfoodeng.2018.08.002 (accessed on 9th July 2025).

Zhou, D., Sun, R., Zhu, W., Shi, Y., Ni, S., Wu, C., & Li, T. (2023). Impact of dielectric barrier discharge cold plasma on the quality and phenolic metabolism in blueberries based on metabonomic analysis. *Postharvest Biology and Technology, 197*, 112208. https://doi.org/10.1016/j.postharvbio.2022.112208 (accessed on 9th July 2025).

Zhou, R., Zhou, R., Yu, F., Xi, D., Wang, P., Li, J., & Ostrikov, K. K. (2018). Removal of organophosphorus pesticide residues from *Lycium barbarum* by gas phase surface discharge plasma. *Chemical Engineering Journal, 342*, 401–409. https://doi.org/10.1016/j.cej.2018.02.107 (accessed on 9th July 2025).

Zhou, Y. H., Vidyarthi, S. K., Zhong, C. S., Zheng, Z. A., An, Y., Wang, J., & Xiao, H. W. (2020). Cold plasma enhances drying and color, rehydration ratio and polyphenols of wolfberry via microstructure and ultrastructure alteration. *LWT–Food Science and Technology*, 110173. https://doi.org/10.1016/j.lwt.2020.110173 (accessed on 9th July 2025).

Zimmermann, J. L., Shimizu, T., Schmidt, H., Li, Y., Morfill, G. E., & Isbary, G. (2012). Test for bacterial resistance build-up against plasma treatment. *New Journal of Physics, 14*(7), 073037. https://doi.org/10.1088/1367-2630/14/7/073037 (accessed on 9th July 2025).

CHAPTER 5

Ozone for Fresh Produce Quality and Safety

LAXMI KANT RAWAT and AMIT BARAN DAS*

Department of Food Engineering and Technology, Tezpur University, Napaam, Sonitpur, Assam, India

*Corresponding author

ABSTRACT

Strong oxidant ozone has become a viable technological tool for enhancing fresh product safety and quality. This chapter elaborately explains the most recent research on the use of ozone for handling fruits and vegetables after harvest. It encompasses the efficacy of ozone in reducing microbial contamination, extending shelf life, and preserving sensory attributes. This chapter critically assesses ozone's effects on various fresh produce varieties, taking into account variables including ozone concentration, length of treatment, and storage circumstances. It also addresses the drawbacks and safety issues of ozone, as well as its possible advantages over traditional sanitizers. This chapter intends to support the best possible application of ozone technology in fresh produce processing, enhancing food safety and quality, by offering a thorough summary of the existing studies.

5.1 INTRODUCTION

It is commonly recognized that greater food production is necessary to feed the world's population, which is developing quickly. The primary

Sustainable Approaches in Postharvest Handling and Management: Pankaj B. Pathare (Ed.)

DOI: 10.1201/9781779641076-5

sources of calories, proteins, and nutrients include cereals, pulses, fruits, and vegetables. Several nations' economies also depend heavily on spices and plantation crops. In terms of domestic and international commerce, wheat and rice are more significant due to their political and social ramifications. Increased production and decreased postharvest losses can improve the availability of grains and other food crops. The adoption of recently created high-yielding crops and effective research and development activities have enabled this. The phrase "Green Revolution" is used to characterize the influence of high-yielding cultivars on the world of agriculture. The unequal distribution, losses, and degradation of available food resources can result in hunger and malnutrition; thus, it's critical to maximize use and reduce postharvest food losses (Chakraverty, 2001).

During harvest, a crop is taken from the ground or divided from its parent plant during the postharvest handling phase of agricultural cultivation. Whether a crop is sold for fresh consumption or used as a component in a processed food product impacts the ultimate quality. Following harvest, a crop is taken from the ground or split off from its parent plant during the postharvest handling phase of agricultural cultivation. Whether a crop is sold for fresh consumption or utilized as a component in a processed food product impacts the ultimate quality. To delay deterioration, post-harvest management should concentrate on keeping the food cold, preventing moisture loss and chemical changes, and minimizing physical damage. To lessen the likelihood that fresh vegetables can harbor infections, sanitation is also significant.

Most of the post-harvest processing is done in a packing house, which can range from a small, basic structure with running water and some shelter to a huge, high-tech complex with conveyor belts, automated sorting and packing stations, walk-in refrigerators, and other equipment. Processing can start during the actual harvest process in mechanized harvesting when the harvesting equipment does the first cleaning and sorting (Gajanana et al., 2011). There is no need to emphasize the value of horticulture products, particularly fruits, and vegetables, in boosting the economic and nutritional status. India has a wide range of agro-climatic conditions that are favorable for the year-round production of fruits and vegetables at various stages.

The National Horticultural Board (NHB), APEDA, the creation of a separate Ministry of Food Processing (MFPI), and the implementation of a liberalized seed import policy are just a few of the actions the Indian government has taken to support the horticulture industry. A budgetary investment of Rs. 10,000 million was made under the VIII Plan, coinciding with the GOI's liberalization initiatives, and this provided a significant boost to horticulture development. Several measures were implemented during the liberalization phase. APEDA has created the idea of agri-export zones to raise the degree of processing, decrease waste, promote marketability, and assist farmers in realizing higher value (AEZ). Under the IX plan and the 10th FYP, the plan allocation was further raised to Rs. 1200 crores and Rs. 5580 crores, respectively, and the projected budget allocation for the 11th FYP was Rs. 49,640 crores (Singh, Shahi, and Singh, 2016).

Due to its effectiveness and use in the treatment of water and food, ozone applications are gaining interest in the fruit and vegetable business. Throughout time, it has been demonstrated (Greene and Seydim, 2004; Guzel-Seydim et al., 2001). An Expert Panel of Food Scientists assembled by the Electric Power Research Institute (EPRI) in 1997 backed the categorization of ozone as a food disinfectant as generally recognized as safe (GRAS). The EPRI submitted a Food Additive Petition to the FDA in 2000, asking for permission to use ozone in direct contact with food. The FDA authorized the use of ozone in 2001 for the treatment, preservation, and processing of foods in gaseous and aqueous phases (FDA, 2001).

Studies have been conducted to evaluate the effectiveness of ozone in various fruits and vegetables. It can be added continuously or intermittently to the atmosphere or washed or dipped in water containing ozone. Fruits and vegetables can be protected from bacteria, fungi, viruses, protozoa, and spores by using ozone, a potent antibacterial agent (Miller, Silva, and Brandao, 2013). This research aims to integrate and synthesize all studies and findings related to ozone-treated fruits and vegetables. It also examines how ozone affects the product's safety and quality attributes. If major advancements in the technology's quality and safety characteristics, as well as its economic and competitive benefits, are made, the industrial use of ozone may be standardized (Khadre, Yousef, and Kim, 2001).

5.2 FACTORS AFFECTING POST-HARVEST LOSS

Postharvest food losses depend on the crop variety, the year, the pest, the length of storage, and the threshing, drying, handling, storage, processing, transportation, and distribution techniques used. The precise size of losses is difficult to estimate, although postharvest technology-related research, development, and teaching initiatives are expanding. While postharvest losses for fruits and vegetables can range from 20% to 50%, they are often considered to be in the range of 5–20% for grains. Many nations might achieve food security if these losses could be reduced to a minimum (Abdullahi and Dandago, 2021). While it may also be produced synthetically, ozone is a naturally occurring molecule that can be found in our environment. Freshly produced ozone is what gives off the air's typical fresh, clean fragrance after a rainstorm, whereas electrical discharge might give off a little garlicky scent when electronic equipment is located (Mahapatra, Muthukumarappan, and Julson, 2005).

5.3 OZONE

In 1840, Christian Schonbein discovered ozone by recognizing an unpleasant gas created by water electrolysis (Rubin, 2001). Ozone has a boiling and melting point of –112°C and –193°C (Manley and Niegowski, 1967). The density of ozone is 2.14g/L at 0°C and atmospheric pressure; gaseous ozone is denser than air (Horvath, Bilitzky, and Huttner, 1985). Methane is created both above and below ground by UV light and photochemical processes (Graham, 1997). Only three substances—fluorine, fluorine dioxide, and the oxygen radical—have a higher oxidation potential, and they are not employed in culinary applications (Gurley, 1985).

Ozone is a potential decontamination method for fresh fruit that has uses in the food sector (Guzel-Seydim, Greene, and Seydim, 2004). Triatomic oxygen, or ozone, is created in the atmosphere by lightning and ultraviolet (UV) rays (Mahapatra, Muthukumarappan, and Julson, 2005). With a larger oxidation potential than other sanitizers used in the fresh produce business, ozone is a strong, highly reactive oxidant (Fan, 2021). There aren't many disinfection by-products produced when ozone breaks down into O_2 (Richardson et al., 1999). Ozone is created on-site from air or oxygen in two ways: corona discharge and UV. Both of these processes can result in the development of additional active substances such as hydrogen peroxide, nitrous oxide, and nitric acid (Peyrous, 1990). Strategies to limit microbiological contamination and post-harvest shelf life sometimes rely on chemical substances that are hazardous to both human health and the environment. To guarantee quality and safety, a workable replacement for conventional technologies must be found (Tzortzakis and Chrysargyris, 2017). Ozone is created by splitting a diatomic oxygen molecule (O_2) and combining it with two oxygen radicals to generate a triatomic ozone molecule (O_3) and (O) (Mustafa, 1990). It takes a lot of energy to rearrange the atoms into the ozone molecule, which energy is often produced by UV light, electrochemical reactions, or electrical discharges. Due to their high prices and poor returns, these procedures are rarely employed (Khadre, Yousef, and Kim, 2001). A non-thermal form of food preservation called ozone technology increases food safety without sacrificing quality or damaging the environment. It is impossible to collect, store, or transport ozone since it is an unstable molecule that self-decomposes at ambient temperature. It needs to be produced on-site (Guzel-Seydim, Greene, and Seydim, 2004) (Figure 5.1).

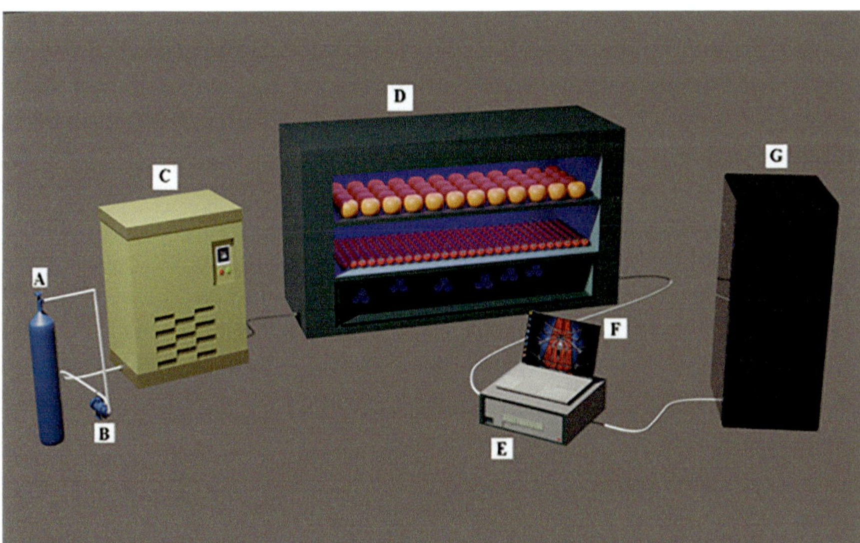

FIGURE 5.1 Gaseous ozone treatment setting. It includes an oxygen tank (A); oxygen supply pump (B); an ozone generator (C); Oxygen Treatment Chamber (D); Ozone Analyzer (E); Output Display (F); and Ozone destructor (G).

5.3.1 OZONE PRODUCTION

Ozone is a highly reactive gas that must be produced on-site as needed. Depending on the concentration, there are many ways to produce ozone (Oner and Demirci, 2016). The air might generate low levels of UV radiation by being exposed to UV lamps with a 185 nm wavelength (O'Donnell et al., 2012). During the passage of electrode feed gas through a dielectric medium, oxygen molecules are broken up into radical atoms and combined with molecular oxygen to generate ozone. Many variables, including voltage, current frequency, discharge gap, dielectric material, and thickness, affect the concentration of ozone (Horvath, Bilitzky, and Huttner, 1985).

Ozone concentrations in gas mixtures are expressed in milligrams per liter (mg/L) or parts per million (ppm). If air is used as the oxygen source, it needs to be dried to stop nitric acid from forming. Instead, it is possible to raise the ozone level in the gas mixture and sparge water by using oxygen or an oxygen concentrator (Kim, Yousef, and Chism, 1999; Kim, Yousef, and Dave, 1999).

Ozone is a versatile antibacterial agent that may be applied as a gas or dissolved in clean water. Although it has a lower partial pressure than oxygen and is 12 times more soluble in water, getting significant concentrations of it can be challenging. Lower temperatures and greater pressures can be used to boost the concentration of ozone in aqueous solutions. Although ozone is 12 times more soluble in water than oxygen, it is more difficult to achieve significant concentrations due to its lower partial pressure. Conditions that maximize transmission across the gas-water interface must be established to get the maximal oxidative impact. Alternative techniques involve permitting a lot of tiny ozone-filled bubbles to ascend through a water column while adjusting their volume and pace of ascent to maximize absorption. You may also create ozonation by aggressively combining ozone and water in emulsion turbines or injecting ozone into the water through a series of water jets (O'Donnell et al., 2012).

5.3.2 OZONE MEASUREMENT

Ozone's quick breakdown and high oxidation-reduction potential (ORP), which allow for little ozone losses, make it challenging to quantify ozone concentrations. Ozone concentration in aqueous and/or gaseous phases may be determined using several techniques (Oner and Demirci, 2016).

1. **Iodometric Method:** The iodometric approach relies on the release of free iodine from the oxidation of KI by ozone (Gottschalk, Libra, and Saupe, 2010).

$$KI + O_3 + H_2O \rightarrow I_2 + O_2 + KOH$$

Both the gaseous and aqueous phases of ozone may be measured using this approach, although the gaseous form requires bubbling the ozone gas through the KI solution. Due to the oxidation of iodide by any agent with an electrochemical potential higher than 0.54 eV, it is inexpensive but time-consuming and does not possess selectivity (Gottschalk, Libra, and Saupe, 2010).

2. **Indigo Trisulfonate Method:** The indigo trisulfonate reagent interacts with ozone, breaking the carbon-carbon double bond, which causes the indigo color of the reagent to be bleached (Bader and Hoigne, 1981). The indigo technique is straightforward, quick to use, and accurate to within 2% for determining the ozone content in the aqueous phase. It is the suggested approach (Grunwell et al., 1983).

3. **UV Absorption Method:** With the use of UV systems and the Beer-Lambert equation, it is possible to calculate the amount of ozone present in gas samples. The reduction in transmitted UV intensity and the level of ozone are correlated using this photometric approach (Oner and Demirci, 2016; Sharma et al., 2002). The formula used is as follows:

$$c = A * b / \varepsilon$$

Where b is the length of the light path, which is equal to the width of the quartz cuvette (cm), and is the molar absorptivity, which is equal to 2900/M cm. c is the concentration of ozone in water (ppm, mg/L), A is the absorbance value at UV 258 nm, and A is the absorbance value at IR 260 nm. The units are balanced by substituting values and conversion factors (48,000), which balance the units to yield:

$$c = A \times 1 \times 48{,}000 \text{ ppm } 2900$$

4. **Chemiluminescence Method:** When ozone performs a chemical reaction, light intensity is measured using the chemiluminescence technique (Gottschalk, Libra, and Saupe, 2010). In a reaction vessel, pure NO and air combine to form NO_2 and O_3, which are detected by red photomultiplier tubes. Continuous, sensitive, and quick describe it (Rice et al., 1981).

5.3.3 OZONE PROPERTIES

A high energy input separates the molecular oxygen (O_2) into two O molecules, forming the very unstable triatomic oxygen molecule (O_3) known as ozone. Generally, electrochemical processes, UV light, or electrical (corona) discharge are the sources of this high energy. Nevertheless, the first two processes are not widely used because of their high prices and subpar yields (Khadre, Yousef, and Kim, 2001). To produce aqueous ozone for washing and rising uses, ozone can be breathed in or ground up into water (Perry and Yousef, 2011). In water, ozone breaks down swiftly to oxygen, although the rate at which it does so depends on pressure, temperature, pH, the size of the ozone bubbles, the flow rate, the contact duration, the quality of the water, and the technology used for gas/liquid exchange. Ozone solubility is 580 mg/L at 27°C. Ozone becomes less stable at higher temperatures and higher pH levels in the solution. When water purity rises and smaller bubbles develop because of a larger contact surface area, ozone solubility rises (Miller, Silva, and Brandao, 2013). Proteins, lipids, carbohydrates, and nucleic acids may all react with ozone, a potent oxidant, to form new biomolecules (Mustafa, 1990).

5.3.4 APPLICATION OF OZONE

Although ozone is a powerful agent for preserving and ensuring the safety of food, its industrial uses are still not at the level needed. Ozone was used by a small cheese-making facility to reduce the levels of Enterobacteriaceae and the number of heterotrophic aerobic plate counts on surfaces that came into contact with food and the environment. Using 2 ppm ozone nightly for two months decreased the levels of Enterobacteriaceae and the heterotrophic aerobic plate count on surfaces that came into contact with food as well as non-food surfaces. It is essential to employ ozonation as a last disinfection step; it can't take the place of cleaning or excellent hygiene habits. When ozone usage was stopped, heterotrophic plate counts and levels of Enterobacteriaceae rose, although these drops were only noticed after cleaning (Oner and Demirci, 2016). Biofilm cells are more resilient to antimicrobial substances like cleaning agents (Lewis, 2001). Cells are shielded from the effects of cleaning chemicals by the biofilm structure, allowing them to carry on with normal growth after cleaning (Holah et al., 1994; Lewis, 2001).

We compared the efficiency of ozonated water with that of a conventional chemical beer line cleaner in removing biofilm from beer lines. According to the study, both ozone and chemical systems were successful in lowering biofilm from starting levels by 99.98% and 99.85%, respectively. This implies that it would be advantageous to use cleaning procedures that eliminate germs and remove the biofilm. For tube samples in a model beer line system, ozone delivered a much lower microbial population than chemical cleaners. According to epifluorescent microscopy, the chemical cleaner only destroyed a percentage of the cells, whereas the ozone eliminated a large portion of the biofilm from the glass slide (Oner and Demirci, 2016).

Microorganisms that can have a major adverse effect on wellness and decrease shelf life can be found in fruits and vegetables. Ozone has been used as an alternate sanitizer since washing them with water or chlorine solutions may not be sufficient to get rid of dangerous germs. Ozone may be employed in several stages of the preparation of products and is eco-friendly (Miller, Silva, and Brandao, 2013). When used industrially for fruit and vegetable preservation, ozone has been demonstrated to improve tomato yield when sprayed by drip irrigation (Rice, 2005). Industrially processed goods like apples and salad mix are treated with ozone to extend their shelf lives and minimize maintenance and wastewater disposal expenses. To stop the spread of fungal diseases, it is also sprayed on onions and potatoes (Botondi, Barone, and Grasso, 2021).

The kind and physiology of the treated product, reactor design, water quality, temperature, pH, and ozone demand of the medium all affect how well ozone inactivates microorganisms (Karaca and Velioglu, 2007; Kim, Yousef, and Chism, 1999). Ozone reacts with impurities in water or organic matter, lessening its sanitizing effect (Block, 1982). The amount used and the residual ozone concentration in the treatment medium after the gas has been administered to the food product determine how effective it is (Karaca and Velioglu, 2007).

5.3.4.1 FRUITS

Before considering treating fruit with ozone, it is important to keep in mind that a fruit's susceptibility to ozone differs based on its kind and species. The ideal application circumstances for each product must be chosen to prevent harm (Table 5.1).

5.3.4.1.1 Berries

Early research indicates that adding 2–3 ppm of gaseous ozone may be able to increase the shelf life of certain berries, although no time frame is specified (Ewell, 1950). The duration of intermittent treatments has not been specified. Other writers have not discovered any advantageous benefits of an O_3 treatment on a variety of berries. This could be brought on by variations in temperature, gas distribution systems, and O_3 concentration accuracy in storage rooms, among other factors. In the sections that follow, the findings of several berry studies will be compiled (Norton, Charig, and Demoranville, 1968; Spalding, 1966, 1968).

1. **Blackberries:** A continuous supply of 0.3 ppm gaseous O_3 resulted in an extension of the market quality of "Chester" blackberries. This treatment was effective in preventing fungal decay and maintaining the red color for up to 12 days of storage at 2°C. Additionally, the anthocyanins' content and the fruit quality were not affected by exposure to the gas, while the peroxidase (POD) enzyme activity was lower in the O_3-stored fruit than in the control ones (Barth et al., 1995).

2. **Blueberries:** Due to variations in storage conditions following the O_3 treatment, studies using blueberries produced inconsistent findings. Higher temperatures had the opposite impact on O_3, whereas low temperatures and controlled atmospheres (CA) boosted O_3's beneficial effects on blueberry quality. This could be accounted for by variations in storage circumstances (Horvitz and Cantalejo, 2014).

   The shelf life of blueberries with comparable percentages of rotting fruits as the control group was unaffected by O_3 treatment for two days at low temperatures, followed by four days at 21°C or six days at 15°C (Spalding, 1968). Compared to the control group, blueberries held for four weeks in CA with 700 ppb of O_3 exhibited greater marketability, indicating that O_3 application might slow deterioration (Fan et al., 2001).

   Blueberries infected with *P. fluorescens* and *E. agglomerans* had lower microbial counts after being sprayed with water containing 1 ppm O_3. For treatments lasting 60 and 120 seconds, the *P.*

fluorescens population fell by 2.57 and 2.80 log units, respectively. The decreases seen in *E. agglomerans* following O_3 treatment were >2.3 log, and no improvement in the antibacterial efficacy was seen. The reductions for both pathogens attained with the O_3 treatment (about 1 log) were noticeably greater than those attained with chlorine and water (Crowe et al., 2007).

The four-day exposure of blueberries to 700 ppb of O_3 did not affect their physicochemical properties (Fan et al., 2001). However, the synthesis of methanol, ethanol, and 2-nonanone was stimulated, whereas limonene production was decreased. However, treatment with $_{O3}$ did not significantly boost antioxidant capacity, anthocyanins, or phenolic substances.

3. **Cranberries:** The investigators studied how applying gaseous O_3 affected the quality of "Early Black" and "Howes" cranberries. During eight weeks of storage at 4.4°C, the treatment with 0.27 ppm O_3 increased weight loss but had no effect on the proportion of rotten cranberries. Fruit damage and weight loss increased with an increase in O_3 concentration and storage temperature to 0.60 ppm and 15°C, respectively (Norton, Charig, and Demoranville, 1968). Fruit that had been exposed to O_3 had cuticles that were degraded and contained 25% fewer lipids than the control group, which might have increased berry weight loss and fungal rot. However, it should be remembered that the temperature employed was significantly greater than that advised for tiny fruit preservation, leading to a synergistic impact with the loss of the O_3 in the cranberries.

4. **Raspberries:** The treatment with both gaseous and aqueous ozone (5% wt/wt in a flow air rate of 0.34 m^3/h) administered for 64 minutes was successful in lowering the populations of *Salmonella* and *E. coli* O157:H7 on inoculated raspberries without affecting the color of the fruit. For gaseous and aqueous ozone, respectively, bacteria counts may be reduced by 1.6 and 4.5 log CFU/g for *Salmonella*. O_3 administered in air and water decreased the counts of *E. coli* O157:H7 by 2.6 and 5.6 log CFU/g, respectively. The highest reductions in the populations of the examined pathogens after washing the fruit with tap water were 1.3 log CFU/g for *Salmonella* and *E. coli* O157:H7, respectively. With decreases

of 3.56 and 3.8 log units for *Salmonella* and *E. coli* O157:H7, respectively, the combination of 64 minutes of continuous exposure to O_3 and 64 minutes of exposure to pressurized ozone was more effective. It is crucial to look at other quality metrics like firmness and juice leakage because the length of this treatment is too long and might be harmful to the fruit's quality (Bialka and Demirci, 2007a, b).

5. **Strawberries:** The percentage of Botrytis or Rhizopus rot did not decrease after seven days of storage in an environment with 0.5 ppm O_3. Storage of strawberries in an environment with 0.5 ppm O_3 over air did not extend their shelf life, and the caps were harmed. Vitamin C content was similarly paradoxical, with fruits treated with $_{O3}$ having greater, lower, or identical quantities as controls (Spalding, 1968). The counts of mesophilic and psychrophilic bacteria, molds, and yeasts between control samples and those treated with 5000 mg O_3/L gas carriers for up to 12 days did not differ significantly (Allende et al., 2007). When strawberries were exposed to 0.35 ppm of O_3 for three days at 2°C, several pathogens were successfully eradicated from the strawberries. There was 15% less fungal decay than the control after two days at 20°C, but after four days at room temperature, the incidence of rot was identical. In contrast to the control, fruits held for three days in an environment with 0.35 ppm O_3 had lower amounts of fructose and glucose. However, the vitamin C content of the fruits was three times greater. This resulted from the antioxidative mechanism being activated, which encouraged the manufacture of vitamin C from carbohydrate reserves (Perez et al., 1999). The prevalence of Botrytis cinerea degradation was decreased when naturally infected "Camarosa" strawberries were stored cold for three days in air supplemented with 1.5 L O_3/L. Additionally, O_3 is beneficial against several infections (Nadas, Olmo, and Garcia, 2003).

Strawberry washing with 3 ppm O_3 eliminated the presence of *E. coli* O157:H7 and L. monocytogenes. While mesophilic bacteria, yeasts, and molds rose during storage rather than immediately declining following O_3 exposure, their end counts for both yeasts and molds were much larger than their beginning populations (Rodgers et al., 2004).

After 12 days, the fruit's total phenolic and ellagitannin concentrations were comparable in O_3-treated and untreated samples. Procyanidins and anthocyanins were impacted by O_3 after cold storage, and their levels decreased as a result of being exposed to the gas.

5.3.4.1.2 Table grapes

O_3 has been discovered to be efficient against native surface microflora but useless against microbes that have been injected into or are already present on fruits. According to this, when the fruits are artificially inoculated, there is less of a competitive microflora present and a larger microbial load of the target diseases, which may affect how successful the sanitizing treatment (Horvitz and Cantalejo, 2014).

After seven days of storage at 15.6°C, it was discovered that 0.5 ppm ozone inhibited the formation of surface mold but did not stop the rot induced by B. cinerea on infected "Thompson Seedless" and "Tokay" table grapes. By being exposed to 0.3 ppm O_3 over seven weeks of cold storage, gray mold incidence was not decreased (Palou et al., 2002; Spalding, 1968). After 20 and 40 minutes of exposure, it was discovered that a supply of 8 mg O_3/min completely eliminated the natural populations of molds, yeasts, and bacteria in "Alphonse Lavallee" and "Thompson Seedless" grapes. The microbiota on cv. "Zeiny" was also less impacted by the therapy. O_3 also caused the synthesis of resveratrol and pterostilbene, which, when paired with the gas's direct fungicidal impact, increased O_3's ability to prevent deterioration (Sarig et al., 1996).

They concluded that short-term postharvest exposure to O_3 might be an economically acceptable substitute for SO_2 during cold storage, since it was successful in preventing decay and preserving quality and freshness for up to nine weeks at 0°C.

After 72 days of cold storage at 5°C, three varieties of table grapes had considerably lower decay percentages when 2 ppm O_3 was added to the storage environment than when fruits were stored in the air (Cayuela et al., 2009). After 7 days of storage at 15°C ("Thompson Seedless") or after 28 days at 0.5°C ("Redglobe"), the combination of short-term fumigations

(60 minutes) and high concentrations of O_3 during pre-cooling of table grapes was shown to be similarly efficient in eliminating gray mold by around 50%. The frequency of gray mold decreased by around 50% among "Autumn Seedless" and "Black Seedless" grapes and by 65% among "Redglobe" grapes over six weeks of storage at 0.5°C after fumigation with 5000 L/L O_3 for 60 minutes in a commercial O_3 chamber. The scientists linked variations in cultivars' inherent resistance to gray mold as the cause of the variation in ozone's efficacy (Gabler et al., 2010).

O_3 therapy was unable to prevent infections brought on by *B. cinerea* that had already taken hold in tissues, as well as degradation brought on by *Alternaria* and *Penicillium* species (Gabler et al., 2010). The ineffective suppression of postharvest gray mold with low ozone dosages may be due to grapes' high ozone demand (Artés-Hernández, Artés, and Tomás-Barberán, 2003; Artés-Hernández et al., 2007; Palou et al., 2002).

In both ozonated and control rooms, "Flame Seedless" grapes treated with 0.3 ppm O_3 lost weight similarly and exhibited no outward signs of harm (Sarig et al., 1996). The most crucial information in this book is that grapes from three cultivars treated with either continuous or intermittent 2 ppm O_3 during 30 days of storage at 5°C resulted in a significantly higher weight loss than the control group stored in the air. In exposures lasting up to 40 minutes, ozone provided at a rate of 8 mg/min in an airflow of 500 mL/min did not cause phytotoxicity on berries, stems, or pedicels of either green or red cultivars, but prolonged exposures harmed some cultivars. Even after 80 minutes of exposure, O_3 treatments had no negative effects on certain cultivars' firmness or even had a beneficial impact on others. Intermittently O_3-treated fruits exhibited the lowest firmness losses during storage (Cayuela et al., 2009; Sarig et al., 1996).

5.3.4.1.3 Pome fruits

Studies on physicochemical, sensory, and nutritional factors will help us better understand the overall impacts of O_3 on these fruits. Research on O_3 application to pome fruit focuses on microbiological quality and superficial scald management.

1. **Apples:** It has been shown that O_3 can affect apple storage in both good and bad ways. Positive effects include a decrease in weight loss and spoilage after four daily hours of exposure to 5–6 mg/m^3 of ozone gas, while apples can keep for several weeks when

exposed to 2–3 cm^3/m^3 of ozone. Negative effects include apple damage from a rise in O_3 concentration to 10 cm^3/m^3 (Bazarova, 1982; Kuprianoff, 1953). In apple storage rooms, O_3 spraying reduced spore counts and managed surface molds (Schomer and McColloch, 1948; Smock and Watson, 1941). Ozone inhibited the fungus' aerial growth and spore production, but it had no effect on the deterioration and rot of infected or damaged fruit. With 3.25 ppm O_3, the gas damaged the fruit and changed its flavor. Some of the varieties' cuticles also became sticky and varnish-like. However, when the gas concentration was lowered to 1.95 ppm, none of these negative effects were observed (Schomer and McColloch, 1948).

Washing the fruit in water that was ozonated, or dipping the apples for one, three, or five minutes in ozonated water, was used to investigate the effectiveness of O_3 to decrease *E. coli* O157:H7 on infected apples. In comparison to unwashed control samples, the greatest pathogen population reductions on the fruit surface were 3.7 and 2.6 log CFU/g for the washing treatment and dipping treatment, respectively. For the bubbling ozone wash and dip methods, the counts in the stem-calyx region only decreased by 0.6 and 0.5 log CFU/g, respectively. This was attributed to the injected bacteria adhering to the rough stem-calyx area surfaces or to the microorganisms in this area being resistant to the sanitizer's activity (And and Yousef, 2001).

2. **Pears:** Although the lesion diameters in the ozone-treated fruit were significantly smaller than those in the control fruit, the effectiveness of a line spray of ozonated water (3.1 g O_3/mL) against *P. expansum* inoculated on 'd'Anjou' pears was ineffective in controlling decay (Spotts and Cervantes, 1992).

   Regardless of exposure duration, 81–100% of wounds were infected at ozone concentrations of 4.2–5.5 g/mL. The treatment of spores of *B. cinerea, M. piriformis*, and *P. expansum* in ozonated water (0.1–4 g O_3/mL) nevertheless prevented the germination of those spores. By reducing the concentration of viable fungal propagules, this might be employed as an indirect form of decay control (Spotts and Cervantes, 1992).

Fruit floated for five minutes in chlorinated (55 g/mL) and ozonated (0.31 g O_3/mL) dump solutions at the packing house showed no changes in decay levels, according to the scientists. Based on the LD99–100 of chlorine (about 50 g/mL) and oxygen (roughly 20 g/mL) for spores of *B. cinerea, M. piriformis, and P. expansum*, the scientists concluded that the latter's lack of impact was due to the gas's low concentration.

5.3.4.1.4 Stone fruits

1. **Peaches:** Continuous ozone exposure inhibited aerial mycelial growth and sporulation on peaches with *Monilinia fructicola, Botrytis cinerea, Mucor piriformis,* or *Penicillium expansum* which causes brown rot. Aerial growth and sporulation, however, resumed afterward in ambient atmospheres. Ozone exposure did not significantly reduce the incidence and severity of decay caused by these fungi with the exception of brown rot. Gray mold nesting among 'Thompson Seedless' table grapes were completely inhibited for ozone treatment when fruit were stored for 7 weeks at 5°C. Continuous ozone exposure at 0.3 ppm increased water loss after 5 weeks of storage at 5°C and 90% RH in 'Zee Lady' peaches but not after 4 weeks of storage in 'Flame Seedless' grapes. Respiration and ethylene production rates of 'O'Henry' peaches were not affected by exposure to 0.3 ppm ozone (Palou et al. 2002).
2. **Sweet Cherries:** Using ozonated water to precool sweet cherries of the variety "0900 Zirat" for 16 minutes had no effect on the fruit's color, firmness, SSC, TA, or outward appearance. But over a seven-day storage period, the treated cherries kept their stems greener and were more marketable than the control samples. A 1–2 log drop for yeasts and molds was seen starting on the fifth day, even though O_3 did not lower the bacterial populations (Koyuncu et al., 2005).

5.3.4.1.5 Citrus

1. **Clementines:** The "Nules" clementines that had been sporulated with B. cinerea were kept for eight days at 13°C and 95% RH in an ozone-enriched environment. When compared to fruit that was

air-stored, lesion development and spore production were significantly decreased by the O_3 treatment. This is surprising because a high temperature and low O_3 concentration would promote quicker O_3 breakdown into O_2 (Tzortzakis, Singleton, and Barnes, 2007).

2. **Lemons:** In three weeks of storage at 4.5°C, the authors found that adding 0.3 ppm O_3 to Eureka" lemons delayed the occurrence of blue mold but did not prevent it. Both the control and ozonated samples had 100% incidence after seven weeks, sporulation had significantly decreased, and none of the fruit had shown signs of damage (Palou et al., 2001).

3. **Oranges:** To inoculate "Valencia" oranges, exposure to continuous 0.3 ppm O_3 pushed back the appearance of green and blue mold by one week. Additionally, infections progressed more slowly, and the treatment prevented or inhibited *P. italicum* and *P. digitatum* external mycelial growth and conidia development. Oranges of the "Ovale" and "Valencia" varieties that were kept for eight weeks at 5°C and 90–95% RH had similar outcomes (Palou et al., 2001). According to the researchers, ozone reduced the number of spores in the storage area and prevented mold from growing on packages, walls, and floors. However, in the first case, after four weeks of storage at 5°C, gaseous O_3 was ineffective in lowering the final incidence and severity of the molds, nor was it successful in lowering the incidence of Penicillium in unwashed fruits in the combined treatment (Di Renzo et al., 2004).

4. **Tangerines:** Tangerines from the variety "Sai Nam Pung" were infected with *Penicillium digitatum*, cleaned with electrolyzed water (EW) for 4, 8, and 16 minutes, and then kept for 28 days at 5°C while being continuously exposed to 200 mg of ozone/L for two hours each day (Whangchai et al., 2010). While the disease incidence of the control and fruit washed for four minutes gradually increased after 14 days of storage, it was suppressed during 28 days of storage when EW for 8 and 16 minutes was combined with O_3. The combination therapy had no negative effects on weight loss, TSS, titratable acidity, or fruit peel color, and it was more successful at reducing illness symptoms than washing with EW alone.

5.3.4.1.6 Tropical fruit

1. **Bananas:** Recent studies have disregarded microbiological or sensory quality in favor of physiological factors like respiration rate and ripening. The effects of O_3 on bananas have not been recently studied. O_3 levels between 1.5 and 7 cm^3/m^3 of air produced physiological harm to the bananas but did not affect the ripening process or respiratory rate (Gane, 1937). A greater respiration rate was noticed with the blackening of the banana skin and a delay in the ripening phase due to the destruction of ethylene when the O_3 dose was raised to 25 to 90 cm^3/m^3 after eight days (Kuprianoff, 1953). When bananas were exposed to ozone at levels between 70 and 90 parts per million, the pace of ripening was delayed, but the fruits suffered physiological harm if not consumed soon after the climacteric stage (Gane, 1937).
2. **Kiwi:** To store "Hayard" kiwi fruit for seven months at 0°C and 90–95% RH, an environment enhanced with 4 mg/h of gaseous O_3 was utilized in place of air. B. cinerea was suppressed with exposure to O_3, but rot brought on by this fungus began to appear in fruits stored in the air as early as week 21. However, there was no mention of the equilibrium O_3 concentration that was attained in the treatment chambers (Barboni, Cannac, and Chiaramonti, 2010).

   The most significant information in this text is that treatment with O_3 lowered illness incidence by 56% and hindered fungal sporulation after a four-month storage period. Additionally, disease incidence was decreased, and a buildup of phenolic compounds was seen when the kiwis were exposed to O_3 for up to 144 hours prior to inoculation. This shows that O_3 could have caused the kiwis to establish a defense against Botrytis assaults (Minas et al., 2010).
3. **Longan:** The effectiveness of controlling *Lasiodiplodia* sp. and *Cladosporium* sp. inoculated on longan fruits for periods of 0, 15, 30, 60, and 120 minutes when exposed to 20 ppm gaseous ozone was investigated by the authors. They came to the conclusion that 60 minutes of exposure to the gas produced the best outcomes, whereas 120 minutes of exposure produced only marginal reductions in illness incidence (Whangchai, Saengnil, and Uthaibutra, 2004). The findings of this study suggest that prolonged fruit

cuticle treatments and high storage temperatures may promote fungus development. However, no mention is made of the temperature at which the O_3 treatment was conducted, which is crucial to take into account because ozone deteriorates more quickly at higher temperatures.

4. **Persimmon:** They investigated the duration that "Rojo Brillante," harvested at two separate times, would last in air or air that has been continuously enhanced with 0.15 ppm of oxygen for 30 days at 15°C and 90% relative humidity plus 7 days at 20°C and 90% RH. They discovered that O_3 did not alter the fruit's softening after the shelf-life simulation, keeping its firmness above the acceptable commercial limits. However, after shelf life, O_3-treated persimmons displayed greater weight loss and electrolyte leakage than the control fruits. On the other hand, the O_3 treatment had little to no impact on the formation of ethanol and acetaldehyde, TSS, pH, or color index. Additionally, the ozone-treated fruits showed no signs of phytotoxicity (Salvador et al., 2006).
5. **Watermelon:** The study looked at the physicochemical, microbiological, and sensory quality of the product after a nonaqueous treatment with UV light and washing with tap, ozonated (0.4 L/L, 3 minutes), and chlorinated water. The researchers came to the conclusion that O_3 was ineffective in reducing microbial populations and that, as compared to UV-irradiated or unwashed controls, the quality of the treated cubes was poorer overall. The mechanical harm caused by the centrifugation process was thought to be the cause of the discrepancies between the aqueous and non-aqueous treatments (Fonseca and Rushing, 2006).

5.3.4.1.7 Dried fruits and nuts

Due to the low water activity of the dried fruits and the requirement for O_3 to inactivate moisture in the cells, dried figs and pistachios performed better with higher gaseous O_3 concentrations.

1. **Figs:** *E. coli* was not found in any of the samples examined. Microbial counts of the three groups decreased with increasing O_3 concentration, while no effects of the exposure time were found

TABLE 5.1 Ozone Treatment Studies on Fruits

Fruit	O3 Treatment	Parameters Studied	References
Blackberries	0.3 ppm gaseous O_3	Color retention, anthocyanins Fungal decay	Barth et al. (1995)
Blueberries	0.5 ppm O_3 gas—2 d at low T 700 ppb gaseous O_3 + CA Spraying water with 1 ppm O_3	Rotting Anthocyanins and phenolic compounds Antioxidant capacity Decay incidence Esters and volatiles Ethylene production Respiration quotient *P. fluorescens* and *E. agglomerans* inhibition	Spalding (1968) Song et al. (2003a) Crowe et al. (2007)
Cranberries	0.27 ppm gaseous O_3—4.4°C 0.60 ppm gaseous O_3—15°C	Weight loss Rotting	Norton et al. (1968)
Raspberries	Aqueous and gaseous O_3 Flow air rate of 0.34 m^3/h with 5% O_3—64 min	Color Inoculated *Salmonella* and *E. coli* O157:H7 inhibition	Bialka and Demirci, (2007a, b)
Strawberries	0.5 ppm gaseous O_3 –7 days 5000 mg gaseous O_3/L—12 d 0.35 ppm O_3 gas—3 d at 2°C 1.5 µL/L gaseous O_3—3 d 0.3 and 0.7 ppm O_3 gas—7 days Aqueous and Gaseous O3 Flow air rate of 0.34 m^3/h with 5% O_3—64 min Aqueous O_3: 3 ppm O_3—5 min Aqueous O_3: 1.66 ppm—5 min	Botrytis and Rhizopus rot Effects on shelf-life Microbial growth Phenolic compounds Ellagitanin contents Sensory analysis Vitamin C content Aroma – Volatiles Fungal decay Phenolic compounds Vitamin C and sugar content Aroma Botrytis cinerea incidence Color, firmness, weight loss Sensory analysis Vitamin C, SSC Fruit surface color Inoculated *Salmonella* and *E. coli* O157:H7 inhibition Microbial inhibition Sensory analysis Color, firmness, TA	Spalding (1968(Allende et al. (2007) Perez et al. (1999) Nadas et al. (2003) Kute et al. (1995(Bialka and Demirci, (2007a, b) Rodgers et al. (2004) Rocculi et al. (2005)

TABLE 5.1 *(Continued)*

Fruit	O3 Treatment	Parameters Studied	References
Table grapes	Gaseous O_3 0.5 ppm O_3—7 days 0.3 ppm O_3—7 weeks of cold storage 8 mg O_3/min in an air flow of 500 mL/min—20 to 40 min 2 ppm—continuous or intermittent (12 h/d) 2500 and 5000 μL/Lxh—60 min 0.1 ppm O_3—continuous 8 ppm—30 min every 2.5 h 1.67 and 3.88 g/h O_3—1, 3, 5 h	Botrytis cinerea incidence Grey mold incidence Weight loss, physiological damage Microbial growth Phenolic compounds Phytotoxicity symptoms Decay Sensory analysis Resveratrol content Weight loss Grey mold, Alternaria and *Penicillium* spp incidence Anthocyanin and flavonol contents Botrytis cinerea incidence Physicochemical quality Weight loss Sensory evaluation Sugars and organic acids Phenolic compounds Sensory quality	Spalding (1968) Palou et al. (2002) Sarig et al. (1996) Cayuela et al. (2009) Mlikota-Gabler et al. (2010) Artes-Hern et al. (2003, 2004, 2007) Gonzalez-Barrio et al. (2006)
Apples	0.006 ppm O_3 gas—4 h/d 2 to 10 cm^3 gaseous O_3/m^3 of air "some few hours" 1.95 ppm gaseous O_3—1 to 2 h daily—5 months 3.25 ppm gaseous O_3—8 h/d—7 months 0.4 to 4 ppm gaseous O_3—continuous or intermittent 3 ppm aqueous O_3—5 min 25 mg/L aqueous O_3 – 4, 22 and 45°C—1-, 3-, and 5-min treatment	Spoilage, weight loss a Shelf-life extension Fruit decay and rotting Fungal spore counts Physiological damage Scald incidence Surface molds on packages and walls of apple storage rooms Off-odors elimination Ripening delay Spore counts and germination Scald incidence *E. coli* O157:H7 and L. monocytogenes inhibition Spoilage microflora growth Sensory quality *E. coli* O157:H7 growth on inoculated apples	Bazarova (1982) Kuprianoff (1953) Schomer and McColloch (1948) Smock and Watson (1941) Rodgers et al. (2004) Achen and Yousef (2001)

TABLE 5.1 *(Continued)*

Fruit	O3 Treatment	Parameters Studied	References
Pears	0.4 µL/L O_3 gas in the storage room Line spray of ozonated water—3.1 µg O_3/mL, about 5 sec or immersion in water with 4.2 or 5.5 µg/mL O_3—0.5 to 5 min Ozonated water—0.1 to 4 µg O_3/mL—1, 3, and 5 min 0.31 µg/mL aqueous O_3 – 5 min	Ethylene production Physicochemical parameters Scald index *P. expansum* incidence and severity on inoculated d'Anjou pears *B. cinerea*, *M. piriformis* and *P. expansum* spore germination Fungal propagules concentration in dump water Pear decay during 5-month storage	Skog and Chu (2001) Spotts and Cervantes (1992)
Clementines	Enrichment of the atmosphere with 0.1 µmol/mol O_3 gas—8 d	*B. cinerea* growth and spore production	Tzortzakis et al. (2007b)
Lemons	Intermittent 0.3 ppm O_3 gas—3 weeks of storage at 4.5°C	Blue mold incidence and spore production	Palou et al. (2001)
Oranges	Continuous 0.3 ppm gaseous O_3 0.72 ppm O_3 gas (v/v)—14 d Up to 40 ppm gaseous O_3 in the storage atmosphere Ozonated water (0.6 mg O_3/L) + 0.25 ppm gaseous O_3 in the storage room	Green and blue mold incidence Rate of ethylene destruction O_3 penetration and effectiveness when applied in different type of packages to control *P. digitatum* and *P. italicum* spores growth Ethylene reduction Physiological damage Ripening delay Fungal growth Spores load and surface growth of mold on packages, walls and floor	Palou et al. (2001) Palou et al. (2003) Kuprianoff (1953) Di Renzo et al. (2005)
Tangerines	Continuous exposure to 200 mg gaseous O_3/L for 2 h/day—28 d	*Penicillium digitatum* incidence Weight loss, TSS, TA, peel color	Whangchai et al. (2010)
Banana	Gaseous O_3 1.5 to 90 cm^3 O_3/m^3 air	Ethylene destruction Physiological damage Respiratory rate Ripening process	Gane (1937)
Kiwi	4 mg/h—7 months 0.3 µL/L—4 months	Botrytis cinerea rot Weight loss, firmness, °Brix, TA, pH, sugars and vitamin C Stem end rot incidence Phenolic compounds accumulation	Barboni et al. (2010) Minas et al. (2010)
Longan	20 ppm—15 to 120 min	*Lasiodiplodia* sp. and *Cladosporium* sp. incidence Mold, yeast and bacteria inhibition Browning	Whangchai et al. (2005) Whangchai et al. (2006)
Persimmon	Continuous 0.15 ppm—30 d	Color index, TSS, pH Ethanol and acetaldehyde Softening Weight loss, electrolyte leakage	Salvador et al. (2006)

TABLE 5.1 *(Continued)*

Fruit	O3 Treatment	Parameters Studied	References
Watermelon	Aqueous O_3: 0.4 µL/L—3 min	Microbiological, physicochemical and sensory analysis	Fonseca and Rushing (2006)
Fig	1, 5, and 10 ppm of gaseous O_3 for three or five hours at 20°C Eradicated with ozone treatment at 5 ppm	Reduce the total aerobic mesophilic, coliform, yeast, and mould counts *E. coli* and *B. cereus* Aerobic mesophilic, yeast, and mould counts can be reduced by 38–72% and coliform colonies	Oztekin, et al. (2006)
Pistachios	<1 ppm periods (0 to 360 minutes) at 20°C and 70% RH 9 mg/L of gaseous ozone for 420 minutes	*B. cereus* populations reduction Aflatoxin degradation	Akbas and Ozdemir (2008) Akbas and Ozdemir (2006)

other than for the total aerobic mesophilic microorganisms. Dried figs were treated with 1, 5, and 10 ppm of gaseous O_3 to reduce the total aerobic mesophilic, coliform, yeast, and mold counts on the fruits treated for three or five hours at 200°C (Oztekin, Zorlugenç, and Zorlugenç, 2006). Aerobic mesophilic, yeast, and mold counts can be reduced by 38–72%, and coliform colonies can be completely eradicated with ozone treatment at 5 ppm.

O_3 has been tested for its ability to lower populations of harmful *E. coli*, *B. cereus*, and *B. cereus* spores. For 360 minutes at 20°C and 70% RH (Akbas and Ozdemir, 2008), inoculated dried figs were exposed to 0.1, 0.5, and 1 ppm of gaseous O_3. The results revealed that with 0.1 and 0.5 ppm of the gas, *E. coli* and *B. cereus* counts decreased by 0.9–1.4 and 2.7–2.9 log units, respectively. It was feasible to get 3.5 log reductions for both bacteria at 1 ppm of O_3.

2. **Pistachios:** Whole and shelled kernels, as well as powdered pistachios infected with *E. coli* and B. cereus, were exposed to ozone for a range of periods (0 to 360 minutes) at 20°C and 70% RH. Ozone's ability to kill both bacteria became more effective with longer exposure times and higher ozone concentrations. *E. coli* populations were reduced by 2–3 log units in whole and shelled

kernels when O_3 doses were <1 ppm, but B. cereus populations were decreased by 1.5–2 log units in whole and shelled kernels (Akbas and Ozdemir, 2008).

There were several no differences between whole and shelled pistachios in the decrease of *E. coli* and *B. cereus* when the O_3 concentration was increased to 1 ppm. When ground, results with 1.5 and 2 log unit reductions were comparable (Horvitz and Cantalejo, 2014).

Aflatoxin degradation was facilitated by exposure to 9 mg/L of gaseous ozone for 420 minutes, with whole kernels responding more favorably than crushed nuts. The surface area of the pistachio samples was crucial to how well the ozone treatment worked (Akbas and Ozdemir, 2006).

5.3.4.2 ROOT VEGETABLES

5.3.4.2.1 Bulbs, tubers, and roots

The most crucial information in this book is that beneficial outcomes for potatoes and onions were shown with exposures to physiologically safe levels of gaseous O_3. However, because they lack protective skin and because O_3 has an oxidizing effect on the carotenoids found in these roots, carrots are more likely to experience physiological harm (Horvitz and Cantalejo, 2014). This could be partially explained by the fact that potatoes and onions lack protective skin and by the oxidative effects of O_3 on the carotenoids found in these roots.

1. **Onions:** After four weeks of cold storage and an additional two weeks of shelf life, weight loss and the occurrence of mold decreased in onion bulbs exposed to 50 ppb O_3 during the day and 250 ppb at night (Faitel'berg-Blank et al., 1979). Oxygen absorption, chemiluminescence, catalase, and peroxidase activity were all decreased in onions treated with 0.2 g O_3/L for eight hours each day, five days a week. Without altering internal decay, firmness, sprouting, or roots, O_3 was also efficient in lowering the airborne spore concentration in the storage rooms and the surface discoloration. As a result of the corona treatment, onions also showed no symptoms of phytotoxicity (Song et al., 2000).

2. **Potatoes:** Similar effects were shown in potatoes maintained for six months at 6–14°C and 93–97% RH, where they were inhibited, and the surface pathogenic microorganisms were eliminated in atmospheres containing 10–20 mg/m^3 of ozone (Baranovskaya et al., 1979; Kolodyaznaya and Suponina, 1975). During the storage of potatoes, exposure to 0.2 g O_3/L for eight hours a day, five days a week, decreased losses due to rotting from 6.7% in the controls to 0.8% in the treated tubers. Onions and sugar beets both had results like this (Akbas and Ozdemir, 2006). We investigated the effects of aqueous O_3 on infected potatoes. The microbial population was reduced by 1.6 log units after 30 seconds of exposure to ozonated water (5 ppm O_3), whereas counts of mesophilic and psychrotrophic bacteria, coliforms, and *L. monocytogenes* were reduced by 1.1, 0.7, 1.5, and 0.8 log units after a minute-long wash, respectively. When the exposure period was increased from one to seven minutes, the decreases in the microbial groups were not made worse (Selma et al., 2006).

3. **Carrots:** The effects of gaseous O_3 on *B. cinerea* and *S. sclerotiorum* during storage were investigated, and depending on the dosage and length of the treatment, both favorable and unfavorable outcomes were seen.

   Whole carrots that had been infected with *B. cinerea* and *S. sclerotiorum* were kept at 2, 8, and 16°C (Liew and Prange, 1994) while being exposed to O_3 concentrations varying from 0 to 60 L/L for eight hours each day for 28 days. With increasing O_3 concentration, both fungi's growth rates slowed down, with the maximum dose producing a 50% drop-in growth rate.

   When examining the effects of the gas on saprophytic mold growth (Song et al., 2002) and resistance to *B. cinerea* and *S. sclerotiorum*, whole carrots were exposed to 300 and 1000 nL/L of O_3 for one, two, and four days before storage at 10°C and high RH (Forney et al., 2007).

5.3.4.3 *LEAFY VEGETABLES*

1. **Spinach:** The most crucial information is that throughout the vacuum chilling process, fresh baby spinach leaves were treated

with O_3 and injected with *E. coli* O157:H7. 935 ppm, 10 psig of holding pressure, 30 minutes of holding duration, and continuous 10 ppm O_3 for up to three days of simulated transportation were the exposure parameters employed (Vurma et al., 2009). Vacuum chilling decreased *E. coli* levels by 1.8 log CFU/g, and the combination therapy had no negative effects on the treated lettuce's quality.

5.3.4.4 FLOWER BUDS

5.3.4.4.1 Broccoli

During 12 days of storage at 12°C, O_3 was effective in reducing or eliminating mold growth on broccoli flower buds and postponing the florets' yellowing (Forney et al., 2003). In comparison to control samples, broccoli kept with 40 nL/L O_3 at either 3 or 10°C exhibited decreased browning, yellowing, and opening (Skog and Chu, 2001).

The damage-causing maximum O_3 concentration (700 nL/L) resulted in the browning of the stem ends, desiccation of the sepals, a decrease in chlorophyll fluorescence, a change in volatile content, and accelerated weight loss. Despite increases in CO_2 and ethylene production for two and five days, respectively, the final results were comparable to the control group. None of these symptoms were brought on by 200 nL/L of O_3 (Forney et al., 2007).

5.3.4.4.2 Baby leaf brassica leaves

The total mesophilic and naturally occurring *Listeria* spp. counts of four *Brassica* leaves were decreased by ozonated water (10 mg/L) for one minute with or without UV-C activation without adversely influencing the respiration rate over eight days of cold storage (Martinez-Sánchez et al., 2008). While these microbial populations were unaffected by either O_3 alone, water wash, or heat-shock treatment, O_3 alone reduced the counts of yeasts and mold on mizuna, watercress, salad, and wild rocket leaves.

5.3.4.4.3 Cabbage

According to the authors, the PPO activity and total bacteria, *E. coli*, yeast, and mold counts of minimally processed cabbage dipped in a solution of 3 ppm O_3 were found to be reduced. This impact was noticed right away following the procedure and reportedly persisted for three days in cold storage. The scientists did find comparable numbers in the control and O_3-treated samples starting on day 4, though (Youm et al., 2004).

5.3.4.4.4 Cilantro

It was investigated if aqueous O_3 might effectively increase the shelf life of freshly cut cilantro. Initially, and during the four days of 0°C storage, the five-minute ozonated water wash and the five-minute ozonated water wash followed by the five-minute acidic electrolyzed water wash (AEW) reduced the total aerobic and Enterobacteriaceae counts in comparison to the control samples. Only the sequential washing (O_3 + AEW) method, nevertheless, produced fewer counts than the control group throughout the course of a 14-day storage period. On the other hand, O_3 alone was the most successful method for preserving the usual scent and general quality of freshly cut cilantro leaves, keeping them looking green and fresh (Wang, Feng, and Luo, 2004).

5.3.4.4.5 Rocket leaves

The effects of aqueous O_3 on rocket leaves (*D. tenuifolia* (L.) DC) were investigated in this study. Mesophilic and psychrophilic bacterial counts were decreased by around 1 log unit after washing for one minute in ozonated water (10 mg/L). The findings demonstrated that for 8 and 12 days, respectively, for samples held in MA and air, O_3-treated samples retained lower mesophilic counts than the control over the shelf-life period. The microbial counts on O_3-washed leaves for psychrophilic bacteria remained lower than the control for 15 and 12 days in the samples held in MA and air, respectively (Martinez-Sánchez et al., 2006). Only samples that were air-stored were able to successfully manage yeasts and molds, and O_3 was ineffective in lowering initial coliform counts by more than 0.5 log units. The treatment did not affect the rocket leaves' polyphenol and glucosinolate concentrations, visual quality, color, weight reduction, texture, chlorophyll content, or freshness. However, the treatment significantly decreased the samples' overall vitamin C content after eight days of storage, particularly in the leaves stored in MAP.

5.3.4.4.6 Spinach

After being submerged for three minutes at room temperature in ozonated water (5 ppm), freshly cut spinach leaves were compared to unwashed samples. The overall number of bacteria, yeasts, molds, *E. coli* O157:H7, and L. monocytogenes counts were all dramatically decreased after exposure to O_3. *E. coli* O157:H7 and L. monocytogenes populations were likewise decreased by this treatment by 1.22 and 1.4 log units, respectively (Rodgers et al., 2004). With a maximum reduction of 3–5 log CFU/leaf after 24 hours, ozone treatment of packaged spinach leaves inoculated with *E. coli* O157:H7 was successful in reducing the pathogen populations. However, the color of the O_3-treated leaves deteriorated after this time in storage (Klockow and Keener, 2009).

5.3.4.4.7 Lettuce

O_3 applications have been investigated for their impact on the microbiological, physicochemical, nutritional, and sensory aspects of fresh-cut lettuce, primarily iceberg type. These studies focus on the physicochemical, nutritional, sensory, pathogenic, and spoilage microflora impacts of O_3. Regardless of the exposure period, washing lettuce with 3 and 5 mg/L ozonated water decreased *E. coli* O157:H7 counts by 1 log unit. After a 10-minute wash, increasing the dosage to 9.7 or 16.5 mg/L resulted in a 1.4 log unit decrease (Singh et al., 2002; Yuk et al., 2006).

According to the scientists, the high ozone requirement of the organic material in the medium caused ozonated water to perform less effectively at low O_3 concentrations. However, after 10 days of storage at 15°C, no lingering antimicrobial effects were found despite a one-minute exposure to 3 ppm O_3 and 1% citric acid, which reduced *E. coli* O157:H7 counts by 2.31 units (Zhuang et al., 1996).

5.3.4.4.8 Broccoli

After four days of storage at 5°C, broccoli florets treated with water containing 1 ppm O_3 for 10 or 50 minutes decreased microbial development; nevertheless, after eight days, microbial counts were comparable to those seen in the control (Das and Kim, 2010). In comparison to tap, chlorinated, or electrolyzed water, broccoli exposed for three minutes to water containing 2 L/L of O_3 produced the lowest counts of total aerobic and coliform bacteria over the course of nine days of storage (Sothornvit, 2008). By the end of the storage period, it was discovered that O_3 accelerated surface discoloration and ascorbic acid loss in the treated florets (Das and Kim, 2010). However, the authors found no appreciable changes in the buds' overall carotenoid, protein, or lipid peroxidation contents. The O_3 had no effect on the composition or color of the gas, and no odors were noticed over the nine-day storage period. The varying lengths of O_3 exposure in the two tests may be the cause of these conflicting outcomes. For broccoli florets, an immersion time of 10 to 50 minutes seems excessive and too long to be of commercial relevance (Sothornvit, 2008).

5.3.4.4.9 Cauliflower

Freshly cut cauliflower that had *E. coli* counts of 1.88 log units and plate counts of 1.8 log units was treated with ozonated water. These reductions persisted after 18 days of cold storage and were greater than those made with tap or chlorinated water. The O_3-washed cauliflowers also kept their white look while being stored, receiving the highest color rating. Consumer acceptance was 18 days as opposed to 15 days for samples washed with tap water or left unwashed, and no off-flavors emerged during this time (Sothornvit, 2008).

5.3.4.5 FRUIT VEGETABLES

Both aqueous and gaseous O_3 treatments were successful in lowering the bacteria load while preserving sensory and nutritional quality. It took longer exposures to the gas and greater O_3 concentrations to totally inactivate the bacteria (Figure 5.2).

5.3.4.5.1 Cantaloupes

They investigated the outcomes of washing unwaxed cantaloupes (Eastern) with water containing 3 ppm of O_3 for five minutes after they had been exposed to *E. coli* O157:H7 and *L. monocytogenes*. They discovered that

E. coli O157:H7 and *L. monocytogenes* were no longer detected on the melons immediately following the treatment and remained undetectable for nine days of storage at 4°C. The pathogen populations were nevertheless decreased by around 1 log after washing the melons with tap water, and further growth over the next nine days of storage did not go over 1 log (Klockow and Keener, 2009).

At 4 to 5, 1, and 2.5 log units, respectively, mesophilic bacterial, yeast, and mold populations were decreased after exposure to O_3. Using tap water for cleaning did not work against yeasts. All microbial groups saw population growth during storage, with final counts exceeding the starting numbers. Sensory evaluations revealed no discernible changes between the control and O_3-treated melons.

5.3.4.5.2 Cucumbers

Compared to the control group stored in air, cucumbers exposed to 0.04 L/L of O_3 for 17 days at 3°C maintained their firmness, had a better look, and had lower microbial counts. However, there were no visible differences in the yellowing between the ozonated and control samples (Skog and Chu, 2001).

5.3.4.5.3 Tomatoes

B. cinerea spores on healthy tomato fruits were rendered inactive after 10 minutes of exposure to 3.8 g/mL ozone solutions. In comparison to control fruit stored in air, the scientists discovered that *B. cinerea*, *A. alternata*, and *C. coccodes* spore production was reduced by 94–99, 55–80, and 13–74% in wound-inoculated "Mareta" tomatoes preserved in ozone-enriched atmospheres for 2–312 hours (Tzortzakis, Singleton, and Barnes, 2007, 2008).

They discovered that tomatoes exposed to O_3 saw much less lesion formation, with bigger reductions seen at higher concentrations and over longer exposure durations. Even at the highest ozone concentration, no obvious signs of damage were seen.

The effectiveness of O_3 in reducing bacterial contamination was assessed. After being exposed to O_3 gas at a concentration of 10 mg/L for five minutes for low-dose inoculum, *S. enteritidis* cells inoculated on cherry tomatoes fully perished. For one- and four-hour attachment times for high-dose inoculum, 15 and 20 minutes, respectively, were required. While 20 mg/L completely reduced the pathogen population after 15 minutes for a four-hour attachment time, 5 mg/L produced no noticeable results.

TABLE 5.2 Ozone Treatment Studies on Vegetables

Vegetable	O3 Treatment	Parameters Studied	References
Onions	50 and 250 ppb O_3 gas (day and night, respectively) 0.2 µg gaseous O_3/L for 8 h/d, 5 d/week 50 and 250 ppb O_3 gas (day and night, respectively)	Firmness Mold incidence Sprouting Surface discoloration Weight loss Catalase and peroxidase activities Chemiluminescence Oxygen uptake Spoilage Airborne mold sampling Ethylene and volatile analysis Firmness Internal decay Roots and sprouts formation Surface discoloration Weight loss	Fan et al. (2001) Faitel'berg-Blank et al. (1979) Song et al. (2000)
Potatoes	10 to 20 mg/m³ of gaseous O_3 6 months at 6–14°C, 93–97% RH in an atmosphere with 3 mg gaseous O_3/L 0.2 µg gaseous O_3/L for 8 h/d, 5 d/week Aqueous O_3: 5 ppm—1–7 min 5 ppm −30 s to 5 min	Microbial growth Respiration rate Starch, sugars and vitamin C Superficial pathogenic microflora Chemical composition of the tubers Microbial growth Sensory quality Shelf-life extension Catalase and peroxidase activities Chemiluminescence Oxygen uptake Spoilage Mesophilic, psychrotrophic, coliforms, and *L. monocytogenes* counts *Y. enterocolitica* inactivation	Kolodyaznaya and Suponina, (1975) Baranovskaya et al. (1979) Faitel'berg-Blank et al. (1979) Selma et al. (2006)
Carrots	Gaseous O_3: 0 to 60 µL/L for 8 h/d—28 days 300 and 1000 nL/L of O_3 gas at 10°C for 1, 2, and 4 days before storage at 0°C for 24 weeks Continuous O_3 gas: 115, 208, and 530 ppb	*B. cinerea* and *S. sclerotiorum* growth rate Color changes Electrolyte leakage Respiration rate, weight loss	Liew and Prange (1994) Song et al. (2003b)

TABLE 5.2 *(Continued)*

Vegetable	O3 Treatment	Parameters Studied	References
	Continuous O_3 gas: 115, 208, and 530 ppb Continuous 50 nL/L O_3 gas—6 months of storage at 0.5°C and > 95% RH Aqueous O_3: 4 ppm—2–10 min	Decay and mold incidence Electrolyte leakage Surface discoloration, 6-methyoxymellein content Aroma and stress volatiles Firmness, weight loss Physiological damage Resistance to *B. cinerea* and *S. sclerotiorum* Respiration rate and ethylene production Sugar content Resistance to *B. cinerea* and *S. sclerotiorum* Resistance to *B. cinerea* and *S. sclerotiorum* Saprophytic molds growth Sprouting Sugar concentration, 6-MM accumulation Weight loss *P. carotovorum* control Respiration rate Tuber conductance Vitamin C content	Forney et al. (2007) Hildebrand et al. (2001) Hildebrand et al. (2008) Hassenberg et al. (2008)
Cantaloupes	Aqueous O_3: 3 ppm—5 min	*E. coli* O157:H7 and L monocytogenes inhibition Microbial growth Sensory analysis	Rodgers et al. (2004)
Cucumbers	0.04 μL/L of O_3 gas—17 d of storage at 3°C appearance	Firmness Microbial counts Yellowing	Skog and Chu (2001)
Tomatoes	Gaseous O_3: 0.05 to 5 μmol/mol for 2 to 312 h Gaseous O_3: 5–20 mg/L; 5 to 20 min	*B. cinerea*, *A. alternata* and *C. coccodes* spore production *S. enteritidis* inhibition Softening Color, weight loss Respiration rate Ethylene emission TA, SSC, organic acids Vitamin C content Sensory evaluation Antioxidant status β-carotene, lutein, and lycopene contents	Tzortzakis et al. (2007b, 2008) Das¸ et al. (2006)

TABLE 5.2 *(Continued)*

Vegetable	O3 Treatment	Parameters Studied	References
	Gaseous O_3: 4 ± 0.5 μL/L, 30 min every 3 h	Color, firmness Phenolic compounds	Aguayo et al. (2006)
	Gaseous O_3: 0.05 to 1 μmol/mol for 1 to 6 d	Respiration rate Ethylene emission	Tzortzakis et al. (2007a)
	Gaseous O_3: 10 μL/L—10 min Aqueous O_3: 3.8 μg/mL—10 min	Sensory analysis TA, SSC, organic acids Vitamin C content Weight loss β-Gal, PG, and PME activities Color Pectin solubilization and depolymerization Respiration rate Ethylene emission TA, SSC, organic acids Vitamin C content Total cell wall composition Hemicellulose content Weight loss *B. cinerea* spores inactivation	Ogawa et al. (1990)
Baby leaf	Aqueous O_3: 10 mg/L, 1 min with or without activation with UV-C light	*Listeria* spp. inhibition Mesophilic bacteria, yeasts, and molds growth	Martinez-Sanchez et al. (2008)
Brassica	Aqueous O_3: 3 ppm	*E. coli* inhibition Microbial counts PPO activity	Youm et al. (2004)
Cabbage	Aqueous O_3: 5 min (a) (a) + 5 min acidic electrolyzed water	Appearance, aroma Aerobic and Enterobacterias inactivation Yellowing, dehydration	Wang et al. (2004)
Cilantro	Aqueous O_3: 10 mg/L^{-1} min	Chlorophyll content Microbial analysis, O_2/CO_2 concentration Sensory analysis Vitamin C, polyphenol, and glucosinolates contents	Martinez-Sanchez et al. (2006)
Rocket leaves	In packaging gaseous O_3: 1.6 and 4.3 mg/L—5 min	*E. coli* O157:H7 inhibition Discoloration	Klockow and Keener (2009)

TABLE 5.2 *(Continued)*

Vegetable	O3 Treatment	Parameters Studied	References
Spinach	Aqueous O_3: 5 ppm—3 min	*E. coli* O157:H7 and L. monocytogenes inhibition Total bacteria and yeasts and molds inhibition	Rahman et al. (2010)
Broccoli	200 and 700 nL/L of O_3 –12 days of storage at 12°C 40 nL/L O_3, at either 3 or 10°C O_3 concentration (700 nL/L of O_3)	Effective in reducing or eliminating mold growth desiccation of the sepals browning of the stem ends reduction in chlorophyll fluorescence altered volatile composition, and enhanced weight loss	Zhuang et al. (1996) Das et al. (2010)
Lettuce	O_3 doses to 9.7 or 16.5 mg/L 3 ppm O_3 plus 1% citric acid for 1 min. O_3 was applied in gaseous phase (2.1, 5.2, and 7.6 mg/L for 5, 10, and 15 minutes)	Reducing pathogen populations of about 1.4 log units after 10-minutes *E. coli* O157:H7 counts in 2.31 units *E. coli* O157:H7 inactivated by 0.79 to 1.79 log cfu/g, with improved bactericidal effects with increased concentration and length of exposure	Singh et al. (2002) Yuk et al. (2006) Singh et al. (2002)
Cauliflower	ozonated water (0.31–0.35 ppm O_3, 15 minutes)	reduction in the total plate and *E. coli* counts of 1.8 and 1.88 log units No off flavor	Sothornvit (2010)

5.4 EFFECT OF OZONE ON PRODUCT SAFETY

Fresh food is frequently contaminated with pesticides and microorganisms, such as bacteria, viruses, parasites, fungi, and molds, which are problematic since they can degrade the produce and create mycotoxins (Miller, Silva, and Brandao, 2013).

Fruits and vegetables can get contaminated due to inappropriate handling, processing, distribution, or storage, as well as the inherent microbial load of the raw material. Proper hygiene procedures must be followed, and irrigation water must be properly treated, in order to disinfect these items. Before eating, an effective disinfection process is required (Miller, Silva, and Brandao, 2013).

Several microbes, including bacterial spores, viruses, yeasts, and molds, have been examined in relation to ozone. Ozone's microbicidal activity has a complicated mechanism since it targets a variety of biological components, such as proteins, unsaturated lipids, respiratory enzymes, peptidoglycans, enzymes, nucleic acids, and proteins and peptidoglycans in spore coatings and virus capsids (Khadre, Yousef, and Kim, 2001).

5.5 SAFETY AND SANITIZATION PRACTICES

Freshly cut vegetables have been connected to outbreaks of foodborne disease, while other items are safe to consume since heat kills dangerous germs (EUR-Lex, 2021). The HACCP system's important control points are identified by controls carried out in line with GMP and SQA (Callejón et al., 2015).

Due to their high-water activity (AW) and pH levels, cut fruit and vegetables are categorized as potentially hazardous foods. In addition to *Listeria monocytogenes*, *Escherichia coli*, *Enterococcus faecalis*, *Salmonella* enterica, *Pseudomonas* spp., and *Erwinia* spp., other microbial spoilage species found in fruits and vegetables include fungi and bacteria (Abadias et al., 2012; Wadamori, Gooneratne, and Hussain, 2017).

Norovirus and hepatitis are the two most common viruses detected in fresh produce that are known to cause foodborne illnesses. According to viral research done in the USA between 1998 and 2007, fresh produce contamination was the source of 18% of all foodborne diseases, and between 2004 and 2013, it was responsible for 24% of all foodborne illnesses. It is crucial to minimize the microbial burden of fresh vegetables in order to prevent foodborne diseases (Wadamori, Gooneratne, and Hussain, 2017). Raw materials are damaged mechanically and physiologically during preliminary processing, which causes chemical and enzymatic stress responses brought on by oxidative processes. In exposed wound sites, these processes lead to unfavorable phenomena such as tissue firmness loss, enzymatic browning, and microbial infection (Finnegan and O'Beirne, 2015).

5.6 CONCLUSION AND FUTURE TRENDS

Ozone has been shown to be a powerful antibacterial in a variety of situations, but it is not a panacea and has serious health and safety risks. Due to a variety of parameters, including the amount of organic material present, the intended impact, and the operating circumstances of the system, it is challenging to recommend the precise concentration of ozone needed for a given application. However, if individuals can be kept out of the application and degrading processes, it has the potential to be employed as a terminal sanitizer for environments and equipment that come into contact with food. Ozone concentrations of 2 ppm have been demonstrated to be effective in the laboratory and industry against a variety of bacteria. Ozonated water can be used in cleaning-in-place systems as well as for decontaminating surfaces and equipment. Compared to ozone gas, it has fewer health and safety concerns, but any usage must be preceded by a comprehensive examination. Ozone has been employed in many industrialized nations and is relatively cost-effective for long-term purposes, but further study is required in order to utilize the special properties of ozone in novel applications.

KEYWORDS

- **ozone treatment**
- **fresh produce**
- **postharvest decontamination**
- **shelf life extension**
- **food safety**
- **ozonated water**

REFERENCES

Abadias, M., Alegre, I., Oliveira, M., Altisent, R., & Viñas, I. (2012). Growth potential of *Escherichia coli* O157:H7 on fresh-cut fruits (melon and pineapple) and vegetables (carrot and escarole) stored under different conditions. *Food Control, 27*(1), 37–44.

Abdullahi Nura, & Dandago, M. A. (2021). Postharvest losses in food grains–A review. *Turkish Journal of Food and Agriculture Sciences, 3*(2), 25–36.

Akbas, M. Y., & Ozdemir, M. (2006). Effect of different ozone treatments on aflatoxin degradation and physicochemical properties of pistachios. *Journal of the Science of Food and Agriculture, 86*(13), 2099–2104.

Akbas, M. Y., & Ozdemir, M. (2008). Application of gaseous ozone to control populations of *Escherichia coli*, *Bacillus cereus* and *Bacillus cereus* spores in dried figs. *Food Microbiology, 25*(2), 386–391.

Allende, A., Marín, A., Buendía, B., Tomás-Barberán, F., & Gil, M. I. (2007). Impact of combined postharvest treatments (UV-C light, gaseous O_3, superatmospheric O_2 and high CO_2) on health promoting compounds and shelf-life of strawberries. *Postharvest Biology and Technology, 46*(3), 201–211.

And, M. A., & Yousef, A. E. (2001). Efficacy of ozone against *Escherichia coli* O157:H7 on apples. *Journal of Food Science, 66*(9), 1380–1384.

Artés-Hernández, F., Aguayo, E., Artés, F., & Tomás-Barberán, F. A. (2007). Enriched ozone atmosphere enhances bioactive phenolics in seedless table grapes after prolonged shelf life. *Journal of the Science of Food and Agriculture, 87*(5), 824–831.

Artés-Hernández, F., Artés, F., & Tomás-Barberán, F. A. (2003). Quality and enhancement of bioactive phenolics in cv. Napoleon table grapes exposed to different postharvest gaseous treatments. *Journal of Agricultural and Food Chemistry, 51*(18), 5290–5295.

Bader, H., & Hoigne, J. (1981). Determination of ozone in water by the indigo method. *Water Research, 15*(4), 449–456.

Baranovskaya, V. A., Zapolskii, O. B., Ovrutskaya, I. Y., Obodovskaya, N. N., Pschenichnaya, E. E., & Yushkevich, O. I. (1979). Use of ozone gas sterilization during storage of potatoes and vegetables. *Konservnaja i Ovoshecesushil'naya Promyshlennost, 4*, 10–12.

Barboni, T., Cannac, M., & Chiaramonti, N. (2010). Effect of cold storage and ozone treatment on physicochemical parameters, soluble sugars and organic acids in *Actinidia deliciosa*. *Food Chemistry, 121*(4), 946–951.

Barth, M. M., Zhou, C. E. N., Mercier, J., & Payne, F. A. (1995). Ozone storage effects on anthocyanin content and fungal growth in blackberries. *Journal of Food Science, 60*(6), 1286–1288.

Bazarova, V. I. (1982). Use of ozone in storage of apples. In *Food Science and Technology Abstracts, 14*(11), J1653.

Bialka, K. L., & Demirci, A. (2007a). Utilization of gaseous ozone for the decontamination of *Escherichia coli* O157:H7 and *Salmonella* on raspberries and strawberries. *Journal of Food Protection, 70*(5), 1093–1098.

Bialka, K. L., & Demirci, A. (2007b). Efficacy of aqueous ozone for the decontamination of *Escherichia coli* O157:H7 and *Salmonella* on raspberries and strawberries. *Journal of Food Protection, 70*(5), 1088–1092.

Block, J. C. (1982). Removal of bacteria and viruses by ozonation. In *Ozonation Manual for Water and Wastewater Treatment* (pp. 66–68). John Wiley & Sons, New York, New York.

Botondi, R., Barone, M., & Grasso, C. (2021). A review into the effectiveness of ozone technology for improving the safety and preserving the quality of fresh-cut fruits and vegetables. *Foods, 10*(4), 748.

Callejón, R. M., Rodríguez-Naranjo, M. I., Ubeda, C., Hornedo-Ortega, R., García-Parrilla, M. C., & Troncoso, A. M. (2015). Reported foodborne outbreaks due to fresh produce in the United States and European Union: trends and causes. *Foodborne Pathogens and Disease, 12*(1), 32–38.

Cayuela, J. A., Vázquez, A., Pérez, A. G., & García, J. M. (2009). Control of table grapes postharvest decay by ozone treatment and resveratrol induction. *Food Science and Technology International, 15*(5), 495–502.

Chakraverty, A. (2001). *Postharvest Technology*. Enfield, NH: Science Publishers.

Crowe, K. M., Bushway, A. A., Bushway, R. J., Davis-Dentici, K., & Hazen, R. A. (2007). A comparison of single oxidants versus advanced oxidation processes as chlorine-alternatives for wild blueberry processing (*Vaccinium angustifolium*). *International Journal of Food Microbiology, 116*(1), 25–31.

Das, B. K., & Kim, J. G. (2010). Microbial quality and safety of fresh-cut broccoli with different sanitizers and contact times. *Journal of Microbiology and Biotechnology, 20*(2), 363–369.

Di Renzo, G. C., Altieri, G., D'Erchia, L., Lanza, G., & Strano, M. C. (2004). Effects of gaseous ozone exposure on cold stored orange fruit. In *V International Postharvest Symposium, 682*, 1605–1610.

EUR-Lex. (2021). EUR-Lex—32016R0679—EN. https://eur-lex.europa.eu/eli/reg/2016/679/oj (accessed on 9th July 2025).

Ewell, A. W. (1950). Ozone and its application in food preservation. *Refrigerating Engineering*. URL (accessed on 9th July 2025).

Faitel'berg-Blank, V. R., Bykove, E. V., Orlova, A. V., Ostapenko, L. G., & Stepanenko, V. A. (1979). Improvement of keeping quality of potatoes and onions by means of ionized air. *Vestnik Selskokhoziaistvennoi Nauki, 4*, 110–112.

Fan, L., Forney, C. F., Jordan, M. A., Hildebrand, P. D., Kalt, W., Ryan, D. A. J., & Song, J. (2001). Effect of ozone treatment and controlled atmosphere storage on quality and phytochemicals in highbush blueberries. In *VIII International Controlled Atmosphere Research Conference, 600*, 417–423.

Fan, X. (2021). Gaseous ozone to preserve quality and enhance microbial safety of fresh produce: Recent developments and research needs. *Comprehensive Reviews in Food Science and Food Safety, 20*(5), 4993–5014.

FDA, U. (2001). Secondary direct food additives permitted in food for human consumption. *Federal Register, 66*(123), 33829–33830.

Finnegan, E., & O'Beirne, D. (2015). Characterizing deterioration patterns in fresh-cut fruit using principal component analysis. II: Effects of ripeness stage, seasonality, processing and packaging. *Postharvest Biology and Technology, 100*, 91–98.

Fonseca, J. M., & Rushing, J. W. (2006). Effect of ultraviolet-C light on quality and microbial population of fresh-cut watermelon. *Postharvest Biology and Technology, 40*(3), 256–261.

Forney, C. F., Song, J., Fan, L., Hildebrand, P. D., & Jordan, M. A. (2003). Ozone and 1-methylcyclopropene alter the postharvest quality of broccoli. *Journal of the American Society for Horticultural Science, 128*(3), 403–408.

Forney, C. F., Song, J., Hildebrand, P. D., Fan, L., & McRae, K. B. (2007). Interactive effects of ozone and 1-methylcyclopropene on decay resistance and quality of stored carrots. *Postharvest Biology and Technology, 45*(3), 341–348.

Gabler, F. M., Smilanick, J. L., Mansour, M. F., & Karaca, H. (2010). Influence of fumigation with high concentrations of ozone gas on postharvest gray mold and fungicide residues on table grapes. *Postharvest Biology and Technology, 55*(2), 85–90.

Gajanana, T. M., Sreenivasa Murthy, D., & Sudha, M. (2011). Post-harvest losses in fruits and vegetables in South India–A review of concepts and quantification of losses. *Indian Food Packer, 65*(6), 178–187.

Gane, R. (1937). The respiration of bananas in presence of ethylene. *The New Phytologist, 36*(2), 170–178.

Gottschalk, C., Libra, J. A., & Saupe, A. (2010). *Ozonation of Water and Wastewater: A Practical Guide to Understanding Ozone and Its Applications*. John Wiley & Sons.

Graham, D. M. (1997). Use of ozone for food processing. *Food Technology (Chicago), 51*(6), 72–75.

Grunwell, J., Benga, J., Cohen, H., & Gordon, G. (1983). A detailed comparison of analytical methods for residual ozone measurement. *The Journal of the International Ozone Association 5,* 203–223.

Gurley, B. (1985). Ozone: Pharmaceutical sterilant of the future? *PDA Journal of Pharmaceutical Science and Technology, 39*(6), 256–261.

Guzel-Seydim, Z. B., Greene, A. K., & Seydim, A. C. (2004). Use of ozone in the food industry. *LWT–Food Science and Technology, 37*(4), 453–460.

Holah, J. T., Bloomfield, S. F., Walker, A. J., & Spenceley, H. (1994). Control of biofilms in the food industry. In *Bacterial Biofilms and Their Control in Medicine and Industry* (pp. 163–168).

Horvath, M., Bilitzky, L., & Huttner, J. (1985). *Ozone*. Akademiai Kiado.

Horvitz, S., & Cantalejo, M. J. (2014). Application of ozone for the postharvest treatment of fruits and vegetables. *Critical Reviews in Food Science and Nutrition, 54*(3), 312–339.

Karaca, H., & Velioglu, Y. S. (2007). Ozone applications in fruit and vegetable processing. *Food Reviews International, 23*(1), 91–106.

Khadre, M. A., Yousef, A. E., & Kim, J. G. (2001). Microbiological aspects of ozone applications in food: A review. *Journal of Food Science, 66*(9), 1242–1252.

Kim, J. G., Yousef, A. E., & Chism, G. W. (1999). Use of ozone to inactivate microorganisms on lettuce. *Journal of Food Safety, 19*(1), 17–34.

Kim, J. G., Yousef, A. E., & Dave, S. (1999). Application of ozone for enhancing the microbiological safety and quality of foods: A review. *Journal of Food Protection, 62*(9), 1071–1087.

Klockow, P. A., & Keener, K. M. (2009). Safety and quality assessment of packaged spinach treated with a novel ozone-generation system. *LWT–Food Science and Technology, 42*(6), 1047–1053.

Kolodyaznaya, V. S., & Suponina, T. A. (1975). Storage of foods using ozone. *Kholodil'naya Tekhnika, 6*, 39–41.

Koyuncu, M. A., Seydim, A. C., Dilmaçünal, T., Savran, H. E., & Taş, T. (2005). Effects of different precooling treatments with ozonated water on the quality of '0900 Ziraat' sweet cherry fruit. In *V International Cherry Symposium, 795*, 831–836.

Kuprianoff, J. (1953). The use of ozone for the cold storage of fruit. *Z. Kalentechnik, 10*, 1–4.

Lewis, K. (2001). Riddle of biofilm resistance. *Antimicrobial Agents and Chemotherapy, 45*, 999–1007.

Liew, C. L., & Prange, R. K. (1994). Effect of ozone and storage temperature on postharvest diseases and physiology of carrots (*Daucus carota* L.). *Journal of the American Society for Horticultural Science, 119*(3), 563–567.

Mahapatra, A. K., Muthukumarappan, K., & Julson, J. L. (2005). Applications of ozone, bacteriocins and irradiation in food processing: A review. *Critical Reviews in Food Science and Nutrition, 45*(6), 447–461.

Manley, T. C., & Niegowski, S. J. (1967). Ozone. In *Encyclopedia of Chemical Technology* (Vol. 14).

Martinez-Sánchez, A., Allende, A., Bennett, R. N., Ferreres, F., & Gil, M. I. (2006). Microbial, nutritional and sensory quality of rocket leaves as affected by different sanitizers. *Postharvest Biology and Technology, 42*(1), 86–97.

Martinez-Sánchez, A., Allende, A., Cortés-Galera, Y., & Gil, M. I. (2008). Respiration rate response of four baby leaf *Brassica* species to cutting at harvest and fresh-cut washing. *Postharvest Biology and Technology, 47*(3), 382–388.

Miller, F. A., Silva, C. L., & Brandao, T. R. (2013). A review on ozone-based treatments for fruit and vegetables preservation. *Food Engineering Reviews, 5*(2), 77–106.

Minas, I. S., Karaoglanidis, G. S., Manganaris, G. A., & Vasilakakis, M. (2010). Effect of ozone application during cold storage of kiwifruit on the development of stem-end rot caused by *Botrytis cinerea*. *Postharvest Biology and Technology, 58*(3), 203–210.

Mustafa, M. G. (1990). Biochemical basis of ozone toxicity. *Free Radical Biology and Medicine, 9*(3), 245–265.

Nadas, A., Olmo, M., & Garcia, J. M. (2003). Growth of *Botrytis cinerea* and strawberry quality in ozone-enriched atmospheres. *Journal of Food Science, 68*(5), 1798–1802.

Norton, J. S., Charig, A. J., & Demoranville, I. E. (1968). Effect of ozone on storage of cranberries. In *Proceedings of the American Society for Horticultural Science, 93*(DEC), 792–+. 113 S West St, Ste 200, Alexandria, VA 22314-2851 USA: Amer Soc Horticultural Science.

O'Donnell, C., Tiwari, B. K., Cullen, P. J., & Rice, R. G. (2012). *Ozone in Food Processing*. John Wiley & Sons.

Oner, M. E., & Demirci, A. (2016). Ozone for food decontamination: Theory and applications. In *Handbook of Hygiene Control in The Food Industry* (pp. 491–501). Woodhead Publishing.

Oztekin, S., Zorlugenç, B., & Zorlugenç, F. K. (2006). Effects of ozone treatment on microflora of dried figs. *Journal of Food Engineering, 75*(3), 396–399.

Palou, L., Crisosto, C. H., Smilanick, J. L., Adaskaveg, J. E., & Zoffoli, J. P. (2002). Effects of continuous 0.3 ppm ozone exposure on decay development and physiological responses of peaches and table grapes in cold storage. *Postharvest Biology and Technology, 24*, 39–48.

Palou, L., Smilanick, J. L., Crisosto, C. H., & Mansour, M. (2001). Effect of gaseous ozone exposure on the development of green and blue molds on cold stored citrus fruit. *Plant Disease, 85*(6), 632–638.

Perez, A. G., Sanz, C., Rios, J. J., Olias, R., & Olias, J. M. (1999). Effects of ozone treatment on postharvest strawberry quality. *Journal of Agricultural and Food Chemistry, 47*(4), 1652–1656.

Perry, J. J., & Yousef, A. E. (2011). Decontamination of raw foods using ozone-based sanitization techniques. *Annual Review of Food Science and Technology, 2*, 281–298.

Peyrous, R. (1990). The effect of relative humidity on ozone production by corona discharge in oxygen or air. A numerical simulation. I, Oxygen. *Ozone: Science & Engineering, 12*(1), 19–40.

Ponte, J. G., & Kulp, K. (2000). *Handbook of Cereal Science and Technology* (2nd ed., rev. and expanded). New York: Marcel Dekker.

Rice, R. G. (2005). IOA-PAG user success reports—commercial applications of ozone in agri-foods. In *International Ozone Association Pan American Group Conference*, Georgia, USA (pp. 9-1–9-12).

Rice, R. G., Robson, C. M., Miller, G. W., & Hill, A. G. (1981). Uses of ozone in drinking water treatment. *Journal-American Water Works Association, 73*(1), 44–57.

Richardson, S. D., Thruston, A. D., Caughran, T. V., Chen, P. H., Collette, T. W., Floyd, T. L., Schenck, K. M., Lykins, B. W., Sun, G., & Majetich, G. (1999). Identification of new ozone disinfection by-products in drinking water. *Environmental Science & Technology, 33*(19), 3368–3377.

Ridley, J. D., & Sims, E. T. (1966). *Preliminary Investigations on The Use of Ozone to Extend the Shelf-Life and Maintain the Market Quality of Peaches and Strawberries*. South Carolina Agricultural Experiment Station, Clemson University.

Ridley, J. D., & Sims, E. T. (1967). Response of peaches to ozone during storage. *Plant Disease*. URL (accessed on 9th July 2025).

Rodgers, S. L., Cash, J. N., Siddiq, M., & Ryser, E. T. (2004). A comparison of different chemical sanitizers for inactivating *Escherichia coli* O157:H7 and *Listeria monocytogenes* in solution and on apples, lettuce, strawberries, and cantaloupe. *Journal of Food Protection, 67*(4), 721–731.

Rubin, M. B. (2001). The history of ozone. The Schönbein period, 1839–1868. *Bulletin for the History of Chemistry, 26*(1), 40–56.

Salvador, A., Abad, I., Arnal, L., & Martínez-Jávega, J. M. (2006). Effect of ozone on postharvest quality of persimmon. *Journal of Food Science, 71*(6), S443–S446.

Sarig, P., Zahavi, T., Zutkhi, Y., Yannai, S., Lisker, N., & Ben-Arie, R. (1996). Ozone for control of post-harvest decay of table grapes caused by *Rhizopus stolonifer*. *Physiological and Molecular Plant Pathology, 48*(6), 403–415.

Schomer, H. A., & McColloch, L. P. (1948). *Ozone in Relation to Storage of Apples* (USDA Circular No. 765, 23 pp.).

Selma, M. V., Beltrán, D., Chacón-Vera, E., & Gil, M. I. (2006). Effect of ozone on the inactivation of *Yersinia enterocolitica* and the reduction of natural flora on potatoes. *Journal of Food Protection, 69*(10), 2357–2363.

Sharma, R. R., Demirci, A., Beuchat, L. R., & Fett, W. F. (2002). Inactivation of *Escherichia coli* O157:H7 on inoculated alfalfa seeds with ozonated water under pressure. *Journal of Food Safety, 22*(2), 107–119.

Singh, D., Shahi, B., & Singh, K. M. (2016). Trends of pulses production, consumption and import in India: Current scenario and strategies. In K. M. Singh & B. Shahi (Eds.), *Trends of Pulses Production, Consumption and Import in India: Current Scenario and Strategies* (May 15, 2016).

Singh, N., Singh, R. K., Bhunia, A. K., & Stroshine, R. L. (2002). Efficacy of chlorine dioxide, ozone, and thyme essential oil or a sequential washing in killing *Escherichia coli* O157:H7 on lettuce and baby carrots. *LWT–Food Science and Technology, 35*(8), 720–729.

Skog, L. J., & Chu, C. L. (2001). Effect of ozone on qualities of fruits and vegetables in cold storage. *Canadian Journal of Plant Science, 81*(4), 773–778.

Smock, R. M., & Watson, R. D. (1941). Ozone in apple storage. *Refrigerating Engineering, 42*.

Song, J., Fan, L., Forney, C. F., Hildebrand, P. D., Jordan, M. A., Renderos, W., & McRae, K. B. (2002). Ozone and 1-MCP treatments affect the quality and storage life of fresh carrots. In *XXVI International Horticultural Congress: Issues and Advances in Postharvest Horticulture, 628*, 295–301.

Song, J., Fan, L., Hildebrand, P. D., & Forney, C. F. (2000). Biological effects of corona discharge on onions in a commercial storage facility. *HortTechnology, 10*(3), 608–612.

Sothornvit, R. (2008). Effect of ozonated and chlorinated water on quality of fresh-cut cauliflower and basil. In *III International Conference Postharvest Unlimited 2008, 858*, 319–324.

Spalding, D. H. (1966). *Appearance and Decay of Strawberries, Peaches, And Lettuce Treated with Ozone* (No. 756). Agricultural Research Service, US Department of Agriculture.

Spalding, D. H. (1968). *Effects of Ozone Atmospheres on Spoilage of Fruits and Vegetables After Harvest* (No. 2393-2021-2460).

Spotts, R. A., & Cervantes, L. A. (1992). Effect of ozonated water on postharvest pathogens of pear in laboratory and packinghouse tests. *Plant Disease, 76*(3), 256–259.

Tzortzakis, N., & Chrysargyris, A. (2017). Postharvest ozone application for the preservation of fruits and vegetables. *Food Reviews International, 33*(3), 270–315.

Tzortzakis, N., Singleton, I., & Barnes, J. (2007). Deployment of low-level ozone-enrichment for the preservation of chilled fresh produce. *Postharvest Biology and Technology, 43*(2), 261–270.

Tzortzakis, N., Singleton, I., & Barnes, J. (2008). Impact of low-level atmospheric ozone-enrichment on black spot and anthracnose rot of tomato fruit. *Postharvest Biology and Technology, 47*(1), 1–9.

Vurma, M., Pandit, R. B., Sastry, S. K., & Yousef, A. E. (2009). Inactivation of *Escherichia coli* O157:H7 and natural microbiota on spinach leaves using gaseous ozone during vacuum cooling and simulated transportation. *Journal of Food Protection, 72*(7), 1538–1546.

Wadamori, Y., Gooneratne, R., & Hussain, M. A. (2017). Outbreaks and factors influencing microbiological contamination of fresh produce. *Journal of the Science of Food and Agriculture, 97*(5), 1396–1403.

Wang, H., Feng, H., & Luo, Y. (2004). Microbial reduction and storage quality of fresh-cut cilantro washed with acidic electrolyzed water and aqueous ozone. *Food Research International, 37*(10), 949–956.

Whangchai, K., Saengnil, K., & Uthaibutra, J. (2004). Control of postharvest diseases in longan fruit by ozone. In *V International Postharvest Symposium, 682*, 2121–2126.

Whangchai, K., Saengnil, K., Singkamanee, C., & Uthaibutra, J. (2010). Effect of electrolyzed oxidizing water and continuous ozone exposure on the control of *Penicillium digitatum* on tangerine cv. 'Sai Nam Pung' during storage. *Crop Protection, 29*(4), 386–389.

Yahaya, S. M., & Mardiyya, A. Y. (2019). Review of post-harvest losses of fruits and vegetables. *Biomedical Journal of Scientific & Technical Research, 13*(4), 10192–10200.

Youm, H. J., Jang, J. W., Kim, K. R., Kim, H. J., Jeon, E. H., Park, E. K., & Song, K. B. (2004). Effect of chemical treatment with citric acid or ozonated water on microbial growth and polyphenol oxidase activity in lettuce and cabbage. *Preventive Nutrition and Food Science, 9*(2), 121–125.

Yuk, H. G., Yoo, M. Y., Yoon, J. W., Moon, K. D., Marshall, D. L., & Oh, D. H. (2006). Effect of combined ozone and organic acid treatment for control of *Escherichia coli* O157:H7 and *Listeria monocytogenes* on lettuce. *Journal of Food Science, 71*(3), M83–M87.

Zhuang, H., Lewis, L., Michelangeli, C., Hildebrand, D. F., Payne, F. A., Bastin, S., & Marth, M. M. (1996). Ozone water treatments for preserving quality of packaged, fresh-cut broccoli under refrigeration. *Science et Technique du Froid* (France).

CHAPTER 6

Role of Electrolyzed Water in Preserving Postharvest Quality and Safety of Fresh Fruits and Vegetables

HAROLD K. MALAHLELA,[1,2] REBOGILE R. MPHAHLELE,[3,*] ZINASH A. BELAY,[4] PANKAJ B. PATHARE,[5] and OLUWAFEMI J. CALEB[1,2,*]

[1]*Department of Food Science, Faculty of AgriSciences, Stellenbosch University, Stellenbosch, South Africa*

[2]*Africa Institute for Postharvest Technology, Faculty of AgriSciences, Stellenbosch University, Stellenbosch, South Africa*

[3]*Department of Agriculture, Private Bag, Pretoria, South Africa*

[4]*Agri-Food Systems and Omics Laboratory, Postharvest and Agro-Processing Technologies (PHATs), Agricultural Research Council (ARC) – Infruitec-Nietvoorbij, Stellenbosch, South Africa*

[5]*Department of Soils, Water and Agricultural Engineering, College of Agricultural and Marine Sciences, Sultan Qaboos University, Muscat, Oman*

*Corresponding author

ABSTRACT

Fresh fruits and vegetables (FFVs) are susceptible to rapid quality deterioration and cross-contamination with pathogenic microorganisms that could lead to severe foodborne illnesses. In the fresh fruits and

Sustainable Approaches in Postharvest Handling and Management: Pankaj B. Pathare (Ed.)

DOI: 10.1201/9781779641076-6

vegetables industry, most foodborne illnesses are caused by *Listeria monocytogenes*, *Salmonella* (*nontyphoidal*), *Toxoplasma gondii*, *Norovirus,* and *Campylobacter spp*. Therefore, disinfection and sanitization are one of the most important steps to ensure food safety and maintain quality. The use of electrolyzed water (EW) has gained more attention as a safe decontaminant in the FFV industry. Electrolyzed water is considered a green, sustainable, and most promising technology due to its effective bactericidal and germicidal ability, onsite production, safety for humans as well as the environment, and low running cost. This technique showed greater efficacy in reducing microbes without compromising the physiochemical qualities of fresh produce. The aim of the book chapter is, therefore, to present recent developments on the application of EW on FFVs postharvest quality and microbial safety.

6.1 INTRODUCTION

Fresh fruits and vegetables (FFV) consumption is vital to human health since they contain bioactive compounds such as polyphenols, organic acids, vitamins, and dietary fiber (Rodriguez-Casado, 2016). However, their production and consumption can be affected and limited by microbial pathogens. Moreover, FFV are susceptible to rapid deterioration and decay during production, postharvest storage, and retail stages (Duan et al., 2020). In addition, susceptibility of FFV to pathogenic microorganism infections greatly increases the possibility of foodborne diseases outbreaks (Pan et al., 2019). Therefore, disinfection of FFV after harvest is essential to reduce the prevalence of fungal and bacterial pathogens during storage, transportation, and consumption.

Recently, electrolyzed water (EW) has been applied in the food science and technology field due to its environmental friendliness, low cost, and convenience (Rahman et al., 2016). In addition, recent studies have shown that EW can be used as a postharvest washing treatment to sanitize and disinfect FFV against fungi and bacteria (Hussien et al., 2018), maintain postharvest quality (Aday, 2016), alleviate chilling injury (Shi et al., 2020), and remove pesticide residues in FFV (Qi et al., 2018). EW is an electrochemically activated water generated through electrolysis of dilute salt, such as sodium chloride (NaCl), in an electrolysis chamber. Electrolyzed water has antimicrobial effects due to its free available chlorine (FAC) content, high oxidation-reduction potential (ORP), and pH (Rahman et al., 2016). Due to this, acidic EW has been the most utilized EW for its sanitizing efficacy on fresh produce.

The efficacy of EW has been reported to be affected by its pH, ORP (ORP), and the interactive effects of hypochlorous acid (HOCl), chlorine gas (Cl_2), hydrogen peroxide (H_2O_2), and hydroxide (OH^-). These parameters, however, can be affected by the EW generating unit, the electrodes, the electric current, as well as the salt concentration and production time (Aniyyah et al., 2022). This book chapter presents the general principle and classification of EW, physical and chemical parameters affecting EW efficiency. In addition, possible antimicrobial mechanisms involved and recent studies on the application of EW for FFV postharvest quality and safety were discussed.

6.2 GENERAL PRINCIPLES AND CLASSIFICATION OF ELECTROLYZED WATER

Electrolyzed water is generated by passing an electric current of approximately 9–10 V through a dilute saline solution. Sodium chloride (NaCl) is the common salt used in the process; however, potassium chloride (KCl) and magnesium chloride ($MgCl_2$) salt compounds are also used (Iram and Wang, 2021). Electrolyzed water can be generated in three forms: acidic, alkaline, and neutral EW. The acidic and alkaline EWs can be generated in the electrolysis cell that consists of the anode (+) and cathode (–) electrodes separated by a diaphragm (Figure 6.1). When electric current is passed through the saline solution, NaCl dissociates into positively charged sodium (Na^+) and negatively charged chlorine (Cl^-). Concurrently, hydrogen ions (H^+) and hydroxyl ions (OH^-) are generated. These negatively charged ions (Cl^- and OH^-) migrate to the anode to give up electrons to form oxygen gas (O_2), chlorine gas (Cl_2), hypochlorite ion (OCl^-), hypochlorous acid (HOCl), and hydrochloric acid (HCl), thus forming acidic electrolyzed water (AEW) with a low pH ranging from 2 to 2.7 and a high ORP of over 1000 mV (Chen and Wang, 2022).

On the other hand, positively charged ions (H^+ and Na^+) migrate to the cathode to take up electrons and form hydrogen gas (H_2) and sodium hydroxide (NaOH). The cathode side of the electrolytic cell generates alkaline electrolyzed water (AEW). Alkaline EW is characterized by a

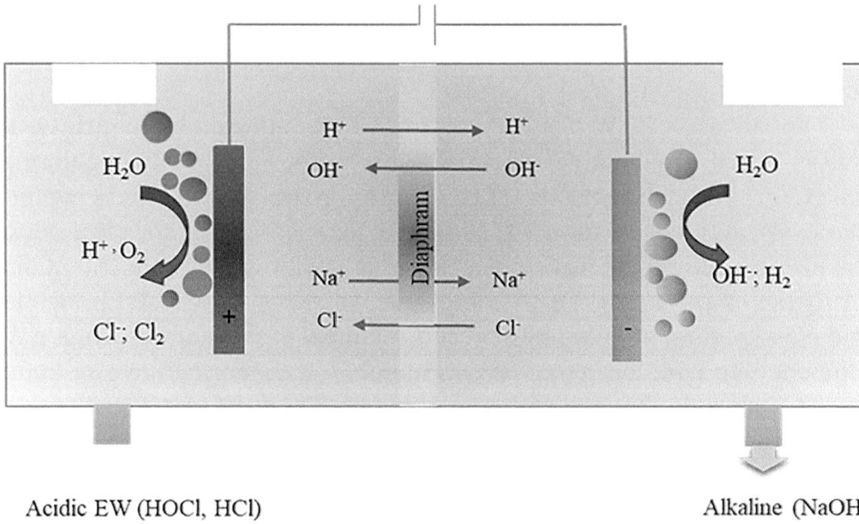

FIGURE 6.1 Electrolytic cell for the generation of acidic EW and alkaline EW.

high pH ranging from 10.0 to 13 and a low ORP ranging from –800 to –900 mV (Chen and Wang, 2022). Moreover, an electrolysis chamber without a membrane separating the cathode and anode produces neutral electrolyzed water (NEW). The positive and negative ions react to form a neutral solution (pH 7–8). In addition, NEW can be obtained by mixing the anode and cathode solutions. NEW is named after its characteristic close to neutral pH of 7–8, ORP of 750–900 mV with low free chlorine concentration (Hassan and Dann, 2019). Consequently, electrolyzed water is further classified as slightly acidic and slightly alkaline EWs mainly due to their pH ranges. Different types of EWs and their physical and chemical properties are shown in Table 6.1.

TABLE 6.1 Summary of Different EW Types and Their Properties

Type of Electrolyzed Water (EW)	pH	ORP (mV)	FAC (ppm)
Acidic EW	2–2.7	> 1000	20–60
Slightly acidic EW	5–6.5	850	10–30
Neutral EW	7–8	750–950	30–200
Alkaline EW	10–13	800–900	80–100
Slightly alkaline EW	11	800	100–300

6.3 MAJOR PARAMETERS THAT INFLUENCE EW EFFICIENCY

6.3.1 FREE AVAILABLE CHLORINE CONCENTRATION

The antimicrobial efficacy of electrolyzed water is attributed to free available chlorine concentration (FAC). Free available chlorine refers to the amount of chlorine in an aqueous solution (Hassan and Dann, 2019). Available chlorine can be found in different forms such as hypochlorite ion (OCl^-), chlorine gas (Cl_2), and hypochlorous acid (HOCl). Free available chlorine in the forms HOCl, Cl_2, and OCl^- are responsible for inactivation of pathogenic microorganisms (Akbulut and Eldeniz, 2019). The available forms and chlorine concentrations in the EW are influenced by pH as presented in Figure 6.2. Chlorine gas (Cl_2) and HOCl are found in lower pH, meanwhile, OCl^- is found in higher pH. However, HOCl is reported to be the most effective chlorine substance against growth of pathogens (Hiricova et al., 2008). From the food safety and decontamination of pathogens perspective, acidic EW has a strong sanitizing effect due to low pH. At low pH, the target membrane surface is more susceptible to HOCl attack, thus maximizing the effectiveness of HOCl. Therefore, EW presenting low pH and abundant HOCl is desirable for sanitization. The sanitization effects of chlorine compounds (Cl_2, HOCl, OCl^-) however, can be reduced during the reaction with organic matter that exists in the fresh produce. Thus, in recent advances on the EW generation techniques, a circulating electrolyzed water is therefore introduced in which 1 L of EW can be made in 8 minutes and the process can be repeated multiple times a day to increase the stability (Gil et al., 2015; Rahman et al., 2016).

Pre-harvest application of pesticides is an important practice to ensure high quality of FFV after harvesting. However, pesticide residues on FFV can be toxic to humans and cause serious health problems. Alkaline EW can be utilized as a detergent and for removing pesticide residues on FFV. Alkaline EW (100 mg L^{-1} FAC) washing for 20 minutes was effective in removing six pesticide residues ($\geq$ 95% pure; phorate, chlorpyrifos, lambdacyhalothrin, cyfluthrin, procymidone, and chlorothalonil) on color pepper vegetable when compared with tap water, sodium hypochloride (NaClO) and xinjinju detergent solution (Liu et al., 2021). Moreover, six pesticides ($\geq$ 95% pure; isoprocarb, chlorpyrifos, bifenthrin, beta-cypermethrin; difenoconazole and azoxystrobin) residues were also removed on cowpea with alkaline EW (Han et al., 2017). However, these authors

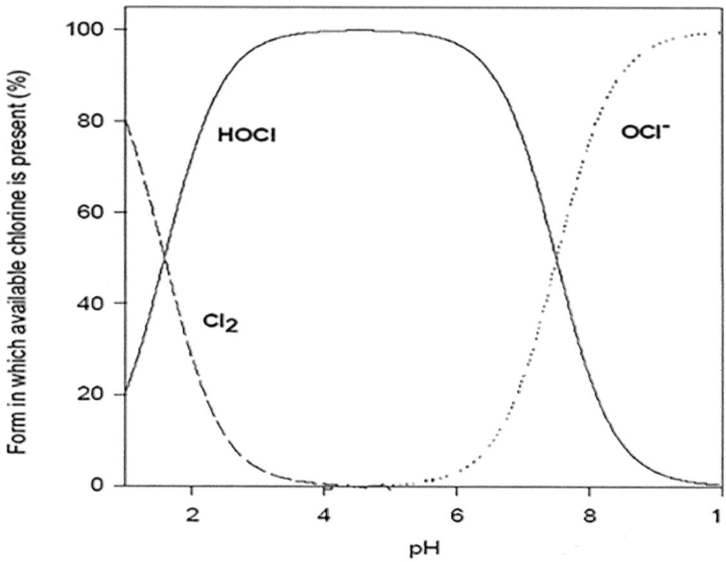

FIGURE 6.2 Effect of pH on chlorine species.

did not mention the FAC of the alkaline EW treatment. In another study by Yang et al. (2020), the effects of alkaline EWs with a pH value of 11.0 and 12.5 on the removal of pesticide residues from kumquats fruits were studied. The results showed that alkaline EW was better than tap water for removal of 10 pesticide residues from kumquats. Additionally, the pesticide reduction rate with pH 12.5 alkaline EW was higher than that of pH 11.0 EW. In the same study, the pesticide residue reduction rate gradually increased as the washing duration increased. These findings suggest that pH and washing duration influence the effectiveness of EW in removing pesticides on FFV (Zhang et al., 2021). Therefore, EW is an excellent postharvest washing treatment for removal of pesticides on FFV. Although EW has shown great degradation ability for pesticides, the mechanism and mode of action for pesticide degradation by EW is still unknown, which implies that further investigations should be conducted to facilitate the application of EW in removal of pesticide residues on FFV.

6.3.2 OXIDATION-REDUCTION POTENTIAL (ORP)

One of the intrinsic factors that influences pathogenic microorganisms' growth on FFV surfaces includes ORP, also known as redox potential.

Thermodynamically, ORP is defined as the sum of all the oxidizing and reducing agents in a chemical system (Turantas et al., 2018). ORP plays a significant role in determining the biocidal efficacy of EW. High ORP destabilizes microbial cell membranes and induces changes in metabolic flux and adenosine triphosphate (ATP) production (Chen and Wang, 2022). This is due to changes in electron flow in microorganisms' cells (Hricova et al., 2016).

The sterilization effects of ORP are mostly associated with the pH, where an upsurge in pH from acidic (2.5) to alkaline (9.0) results in a sharp decline in ORP and subsequent decline in sterilization efficacy (Rebezov et al., 2022). Some researchers have proposed that an increased ORP increases EW antimicrobial efficiency (Rahman et al., 2010). Quan et al. (2010) also reported that the antimicrobial efficiency of weak acidic EW against *Vibrio vulnificus* and *Vibrio parahaemolyticus* bacterial pathogens ceased at pH 9. In general, a high ORP facilitates the oxidation of sulfhydryl mixtures in the bacterial cell, destroys metabolic pathways, and inhibits bacterial growth (Rahman et al., 2010). Therefore, a high ORP and low pH result in the inactivation of microorganisms (Rebezov et al., 2022).

6.3.3 PH

pH value influences the formation of chlorine compounds in EW. When pH is less than 4, the solution is a mixture of Cl_2 and HOCl. At pH 5 to 7, the most predominant compound is HOCl; at this pH range, the concentration of HOCl is optimum and its stability is high. For pH higher than 7, OCl^- is the predominant chlorine compound. Furthermore, there is a correlation between pH value, ORP, and FAC of EW. A previous study showed that ORP and FAC decreased significantly when pH increased from 2.5 to 9 (Rahman et al., 2010). Electrolyzed water is a potent sanitizer at an acidic state. At a lower pH, pathogenic microorganism cell membranes are affected and prevents them from reproducing (Cheng et al., 2016; Ye et al., 2017). Moreover, low pH enables the cell to be susceptible to the effects of active chlorine that leads to cell membrane damages, destruction of enzymes, and alteration of the normal metabolic function (Aniyyah et al., 2022).

Kurahash et al. (2021) showed that slightly acidic EW spatial spraying with pH 5.9 was more effective in reducing *Bacillus cereus*, *B. subtilis*, *Escherichia coli* (O157:H7), *Pseudomonas aeruginosa*, *Salmonella enterica subsp. enterica*, *Staphylococcus aureus subsp. aureus*, *Cladosporium cladosporioides*, and *Staphylococcus epidermidis* when compared with distilled water (pH 7–8). Moreover, *Cronobacter sakazakii* biofilms were reduced by 5–6.5 pH of slightly acidic EW (Tao et al., 2022). Additionally, a 1-minute treatment of slightly acidic EW (pH=6.0) was efficient to kill 8–9 Log CFU/mL of *Escherichia coli*, *Salmonella enterica*, *Typhimurium*, *Staphylococcus aureus*, and *Bacillus cereus* spores (Kim et al., 2019). However, the presence of low pH in acidic EW could accelerate rapid valorization of dissolved Cl_2 that has an adverse effect on human health, thus promoting the use of EW with a neutral to alkaline pH.

6.4 ANTIMICROBIAL MECHANISM OF ELECTROLYZED WATER

Underlying antimicrobial mechanisms of EW have not been fully explained in the literature. The antimicrobial mechanisms of EW are due to FAC substances such as OCl^- and HOCl (Rahamn et al., 2016). Other researchers propose that the disinfectant effect of EW mainly depends on its low pH, high ORP, and the synergistic effect of HOCl, Cl_2, H_2O_2, and OH^- (Chen and Wang, 2022). This suggests that acidic EW offers the best disinfection efficiency due to its low pH, high ORP, and FAC species. A low pH disintegrates the pathogenic microorganism cellular membrane, allowing entry of HOCl by passive diffusion. Thereafter, cell surface morphology is altered from smooth to rough and shrunken. Following the entry of HOCl into the microbial cell, reactive oxygen species (ROS) such as O^-, Cl^-, and OH^- further damage the cell lipid membrane, denature proteins, ultimately destroying the pathogens' DNA (Figure 6.3). Subsequently, this causes substantial disordered intracellular components, normal cellular functions, and bacterial ultra-structures (Yan et al., 2021). In addition, high ORP disrupts metabolic compounds in bacterial cells and leads to apoptosis (Ye et al., 2017). Nevertheless, OCl^- disinfection potential is limited to oxidation action to inactivate functional proteins localized in the plasma membrane outside the cell due to the hydrophobic nature of the lipid bilayer of the cell membrane (Zhang et al., 2021). Therefore, OCl^- has a poor sterilization ability, and the mechanism of OCl^- is reflected in the breakdown of the microorganism cytoderm and membrane. However, HOCl has a stronger germicidal ability than OCl^- due to the neutrality and small molecules of HOCl that can freely enter the intracellular space of the microorganism and directly denature the nucleic acid and proteins.

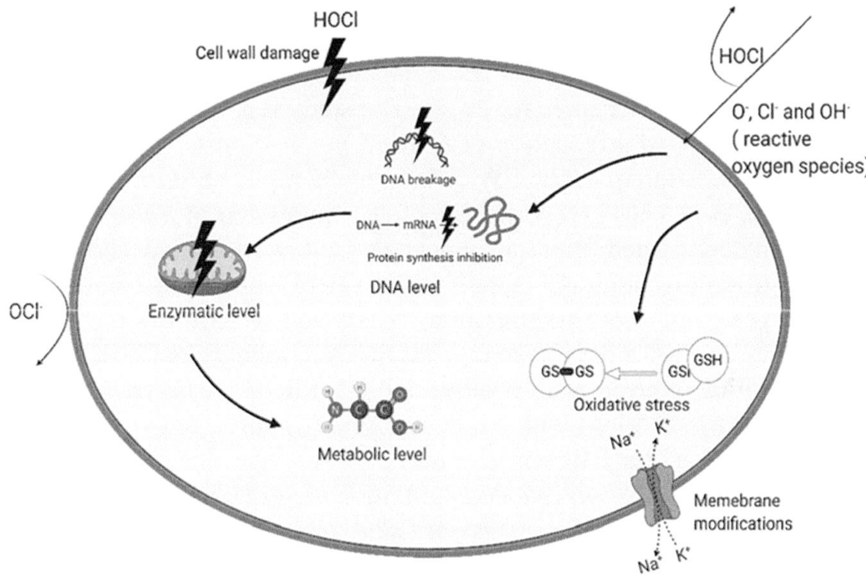

FIGURE 6.3 Schematic presentation of antimicrobial mechanism of electrolyzed water.

6.5 DIFFERENT TYPES OF ELECTROLYZED WATER AND THEIR IMPACT ON FRESH PRODUCE

6.5.1 *ACIDIC ELECTROLYZED WATER (AEW)*

Various studies reported the application of different EWs to disinfect or sanitize fresh produce, as presented in Table 6.2. Of the various EWs, acidic EW is the most utilized EW to inactivate the prevalence of pathogenic microorganisms in fresh produce. AEW (4 mg L^{-1} FAC, pH 3.84 ± 0.12, and 920.5 ± 30.5 mV ORP) showed positive results for sterilization of lettuce and reduced incidence of *E. coli* ATCC 25922 and *Listeria innocua* Seeliger ATCC 33090 during 7 days' storage at 7.0 ± 1.0°C (Zhao et al., 2019). The bactericidal effect could be attributed to the low pH (3.84) and high ORP (920.5 mV). These results were consistent with Huang et al. (2008), who reported that aerobic and anaerobic bacteria can grow optimally at ORP of 200–800 mV and -700–200 mV, respectively, therefore suggesting that the optimal ORP of EW for bacterial inactivation is above 800 mV. Similarly, acidic EW treatment containing 2.34 pH, 1170 mV ORP, and 51 mg L^{-1} FAC significantly inhibited the growth of pathogenic microorganisms on fresh-cut eggplant (Li et al., 2020). In addition, acidic

EWs (100 and 150 mg L^{-1} FAC) effectively inactivated aerobic bacteria, molds, and yeasts from red cabbage inoculated with *Salmonella enterica serovar Typhimurium* strain DT104 compared to 50 mg L^{-1} FAC of EW and distilled water (Chen et al., 2018). The study reported by Hopkins et al. (2021) indicated a reduction of *Listeria innocua* on fresh peaches by minimal application of acidic EW containing 22 mg L^{-1} FAC with pH 2.8. Whangchai et al. (2017) reported effective suppression of *Fusarium* spp. growth on de-crowned 'Phu Lae' pineapple fruit by acidic EW (FAC, 300 mg L^{-1}). In another study, Chiabrando et al. (2017) showed that acidic EW reduced yeast and mold proliferation, decay, and weight loss on 'Duke' blueberries during 15 days of storage at 0°C. Accordingly, acidic EW with 50 mg L^{-1} FAC reduced gram-positive and gram-negative bacteria populations by more than 5 logs with 1 min exposure (Chauret, 2014). Similarly, application of acidic EW with 50 mg L^{-1} FAC significantly decreased *Escherichia coli*, *Listeria innocua,* and *Salmonella choleraesuis* populations on minimally processed 'Royal Gala' apples when compared with distilled water treatment (Graca, 2011). Nevertheless, the FAC of acidic EW can decrease over time and lose its antimicrobial potential quickly (Block et al., 2020). On the other hand, the high ORP and FAC of acidic EW can cause metal corrosion (Yan et al., 2021).

6.5.2 SLIGHTLY ACIDIC ELECTROLYZED WATER

Slightly acidic EW with a proximate below neutral pH has been recognized as having decontamination effects for fresh produce. Bacterial counts on broccoli sprouts were reduced to acceptable levels of under 8 log CFU/g by 30–50 mg L^{-1} FAC and pH 5.47–5.59 of slightly acidic EW treatment (Li et al., 2018). Pre-wash treatment with slightly acidic EW (pH 6.6) also eliminated the prevalence of fungal spores and prolonged the shelf-life of 'Camarosa' strawberry fruits stored for 3 days at $\approx$ 25°C (Sierra et al., 2019). In a recent study, Tao et al. (2022) studied the bactericidal effect of slightly acidic EW (25, 50, and 100 mg L^{-1} FAC) on *Cronobacter sakazakii* cultures. Based on their findings, 25 mg L^{-1} slightly acidic EW significantly reduced *C. sakazakii* cultures from 8.98 to 5.34 log CFU/mL, with a further reduction to 3.11 log CFU/mL in the 100 mg L^{-1} slightly acidic EW treatment. The sensitivity of *C. sakazakii* to FAC could be attributed to its distinct thin cell wall. Additionally, slightly acidic EW with pH 6.40,

910 mV ORP, and 60 mg L^{-1} of FAC gave the most sterilization effect and apoptosis of *E. coli* (Ye et al., 2017). Furthermore, treatment with slightly acidic EW for 30 seconds also resulted in a 6.02 and 5.83 log reduction for *E. coli* and *S. aureus*, respectively (Liao et al., 2017). Rahman et al. (2010) results indicated that slightly acidic EW with 5 mg L^{-1} FAC was more effective than 50 mg L^{-1} FAC of acidic EW in reducing the prevalence of bacterial strains in cabbage stored at 50°C. In comparison with acidic EW, slightly acidic EW is colorless and odorless, thus not altering food taste and aroma. Therefore, slightly acidic EW shows more stable decontamination efficacy than acidic EW.

6.5.3 NEUTRAL ELECTROLYZED WATER

In recent years, neutral EW has been a novel disinfectant used for inactivation of food-borne pathogens (Machado et al., 2016; Zhang et al., 2016). Moreover, neutral EW is stable, more productive, convenient, and economic because the ion-selective septum membrane is not utilized during electrolysis (Chen and Wang, 2022). Numerous studies have reported the effectiveness of neutral EW against fresh produce pathogenic microorganisms (Table 6.2). For instance, 10 s exposure to neutral EW with pH 6.5–7.5 and 10.0 mg L^{-1} of FAC applied through an overhead irrigation was effective for killing *Colletotrichum fructicola* pathogen, which causes anthracnose in strawberry (Hirayama et al., 2016). Graca et al. (2020) reported a yeast reduction of 0.61 and 0.63 Log CFU/g, respectively, for acidic (pH of 2.87 ± 0.05, an ORP of 11132 mV and a FAC of 102 ± 3 mg L^{-1}) and neutral EW (pH of 7.95 ± 0.06, an ORP of 757 ± 4 mV and a FAC of 101 ± 2 mg L^{-1}) compared with the 0.22 Log CFU/g attained by the disinfection done with sodium hypochlorite (pH value of 6.8 ± 0.02, an ORP of 597 ± 2 mV and a FAC of 101 ± 2 mg L^{-1}) solution on 'Royal gala' apple pieces packed in bags of biaxially oriented polypropylene (BOPP) (0.030 mm thick) and kept at 4±0.5°C for 9 days. Hsu et al. (2019) showed that neutral EW with pH in the range of 7.0–7.2 and 50 mg L^{-1} FAC inactivated *Salmonella spp.* and *S. aureus* in a test suspension after 10 s of contact time. This treatment presented <10 and 9.0×106 CFU/mL survival rate for *S. aureus* and *Salmonella spp.*, respectively. In addition, Ogunniyi et al. (2020) study showed that neutral EW treatment could be used for sanitization for fresh vegetables. Neutral EW treatment (50 and 85 mg L^{-1} FAC) significantly reduced bacterial load on fresh spinach leaves by approximately 10-fold than control-tap water (Ogunniyi et al., 2020). In the same study, the investigators did not observe any negative effects on spinach leaves overall quality. Neutral EW can also be used to sterilize fruits. Sheng et al. (2020) observed that treatment with 100 mg L^{-1} neutral EW prevented *Listeria monocytogenes* cross-contamination between 'Granny Smith' and 'Fuji' apples and successfully reduced *L. monocytogenes* prevalence. Nonetheless, in contrast with acidic EW (pH $\approx$ 2.87, ORP $\approx$ 1113 mV and FAC $\approx$ 102 mg L^{-1}), neutral EW (pH $\approx$ 7.95, ORP $\approx$ 757 mV and FAC $\approx$ 101 mg L^{-1}) was found to be ineffective in reducing *E. coli* and *C. sakazakii* populations on 'Tommy Atkins' mangoes when held at temperatures of 4, 8 and 12°C for 10 days (Santo et al., 2018). The differences in decontamination efficacy of EW technologies depends on the initial microbial load on fresh produce surface and physicochemical characteristics of EW. This highlights the importance of preventing contamination during harvesting and processing stages and combining different disinfection methods to increase the safety of FFV.

6.5.4 ALKALINE ELECTROLYZED WATER

Alkaline EW is not an effective sterilizer and disinfectant when compared to acidic, slightly acidic, and neutral EW, and this has led to limited application in sterilizing FFV. Alkaline EW is mainly studied for its health promotion, such as inhibiting the growth of anaerobic bacteria in the oral cavity (Vasella et al., 2021). Furthermore, alkaline EW is widely used to remove pesticide residues from fresh produce. Nevertheless, alkaline EW contains high concentrations of sodium hydroxide (NaOH), which poses a detergent action of dissolving proteins, fats, and polymeric compounds outside the bacterial membrane. However, several studies have demonstrated the antimicrobial effects of alkaline EW. Alkaline EW treatment suppressed the growth and disease development of *Penicillium* on 'Valencia' oranges stored for three weeks at temperatures between 18 and 28°C and high relative humidity (Hussien et al., 2018). Nonetheless, in this study, alkaline EW was not as effective as acidic EW. Similar observations were found on *Euginia uniflora* fruit treated with alkaline EW containing pH 11.02 (Dilarri et al., 2016). Although alkaline EW showed inhibitory effects on fungi, its inhibitory effects are short-lived and could expose fresh produce that are susceptible to latent pathogenic microorganisms during storage. Nyamende et al. (2021) found that slightly alkaline EW treatments (50–500 mg L^{-1} FAC) resulted in a significant reduction in lesion zones of 'Granny

Smith' apples inoculated with *B. cinerea* compared to the untreated control fruit during 5 and 24°C storage for four weeks (Figure 6.4). Furthermore, curative efficacy was most effective at concentrations of 200–500 mg L^{-1} for 5°C and 300–500 mg L^{-1} for 24°C (Nyamende et al., 2021).

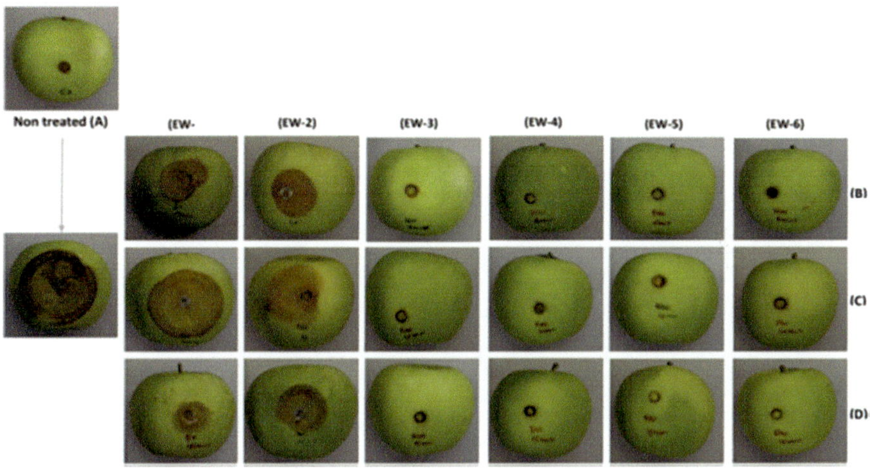

FIGURE 6.4 Differences in lesion area inoculated with *B. cinerea* on 'Granny Smith' apples: non treated (A); treated with different concentrations (EW-1=50 mg L^{-1}, EW-2=100 mg L^{-1}, EW-3=200 mg L^{-1}, EW-4=300 mg L^{-1}, EW-5=400 mg L^{-1} and EW-6=500 mg L^{-1} FAC) of electrolyte water treatment for 5 min (B); for 10 min (C); and for 15 min (D) after four weeks' storage at 24°C.

6.6 EFFECTS OF ELECTROLYZED WATER ON QUALITY OF FRESH FRUITS AND VEGETABLES

6.6.1 *INHIBITION OF BROWNING*

Fruits and vegetables' surface browning or darkening is one of the main physiological disorders that leads to substantial quality loss during storage and retail markets. Surface browning is due to oxidation of phenolic compounds in fresh produce catalyzed by polyphenol oxidase (PPO) and peroxidase (POD) enzyme activities (Zhang et al., 2021). Browning severity is dependent on the concentration of available PPO, phenolic substrates, antioxidant compounds in the produce, pH, temperature, and available oxygen (Fufa et al., 2021). During fresh produce ripening and senescence, PPO and POD enzymes react with the phenolic substrates, causing browning in the presence of oxygen (Zhang et al., 2021). Electrolyzed water has shown great efficiency in mitigating surface browning of FFV. Dipping in acidic-EW

TABLE 6.2 Recent Studies on the Application of EW on Fresh Produce Microbiological Quality

Fresh Produce	Pathogenic Microorganisms	Type of EW	Exp. Time (min)	FAC (ppm)	pH	ORP (mV)	References
Cauliflower	Total bacterial, mould and yeast	Slightly acidic	10	20–22	5.5–5.6	900–950	Akther et al. (2023)
Apple	AMB, yeast and moulds	Alkaline	10, 15	200 and 300	11–13	> −800	Nyamende et al. (2022)
Apple	*S. epidermidis*, *S. capitis*, *O. soli*, and *A. inuii*	Slightly alkaline	10, 15	200 and 300	10–11.5	> −800	Nyamende et al. (2022)
Potato	Total bacterial count, mould and yeast	EW	2, 5, 10	–	–	–	Procaccini et al. (2022)
Pea sprouts	*Escherichia coli*	EW	10	4	3.5 ± 0.1	1021.1 ± 9.9	Wang et al. (2022)
Fig	Mesophilic aerophilic bacteria	Neutral	1	71.4	7.65	855	Yamaner (2022)
Organic strawberry	*E. coli O157:H7 and Salmonella*	**Acidic	5	4	–	–	Zhao et al. (2022)
Apple	*Botrytis cinerea*	Slightly alkaline	5, 10, 15	50–500	≈11	> −800	Nyamende et al. (2021)
Fresh-cut bell peppers	*L. monocytogenes*	Slightly acidic	2	–	–	–	Saravanakumar et al. (2021)
Longan fruit	Mould and yeasts	Acidic	10	80	2.5	1490 ± 5	Tang et al. (2021)
Lettuce	*Salmonella*	Slightly acidic	0.75	50	6.38	872–885	Cap et al. (2020)
Fresh-cut apple	Yeasts	Acidic/Neutral	5	102/101	2.87/7.95	1113/757	Graça et al. (2020)
Coriander	*E. coli and Salmonella*	Slightly acidic	5	20, 40 & 60	5.0–6.0	–	Jiang et al. (2020)
Fresh-cut eggplant	Aerobic bacteria, yeast and mould	Acidic/Slightly acid	5	51/31	2.34/6.25	1170/861	Li et al. (2020)
Spinach leaves	*E. coli, S. Enteritidis* and *L. innocua*	Neutral	1	50	7.0	857	Ogunniyi et al. (2020)
Orange	*P. digitatum* and *P. italicum*	Acidic/ Alkaline	/	100/2.8	2.6/11.0	−240/ 420	Youssef and Hussien (2020)
Black olives	Aerobic bacteria, and yeast	Acidic	1	80	2.7	1100	Gok and Pazır (2019)
Apples, mandarins, cherry tomato	*E. coli* O157:H7, *L. monocytogenes*	Slightly acidic	3	30	5.42	818	Chen et al. (2019)
Carrot	*E. coli O157:H7, Salmonella*	Slightly acidic	3	4	4.02	956	Liu et al. (2019)

TABLE 6.2 *(Continued)*

Fresh Produce	Pathogenic Microorganisms	Type of EW	Exp. Time (min)	FAC (ppm)	pH	ORP (mV)	References
Spinach, beet leaf and iceberg lettuce	*Bacillus cereus*	Slightly acidic	15	80	5.74	832	Hussain et al. (2019)
Avocado	*Colletotrichum* spp.	Neutral	0.5	/8.2	906	832	Hassan and Dann (2019)
Lettuce	*E. coli* and *L. innocua*	**Acidic	7	4	3.84	920.5	Zhao et al. (2019)
Grapes	*Brettanomyces bruxellensis*	EW	6 and 12	400	–	–	Cravero et al. (2018)
Broccoli sprouts	Total bacterial	Slightly acidic	–	50.7 ± 1.10	5.48 ± 0.31	-	Li et al. (2018)
Wheat grains	*Fusarium graminearum*	Acidic and Alkaline	–	60	2.5–6.5 & 8.5–12.5	–	Lyu et al. (2018)
Broccoli sprouts	Aerobic bacteria, molds and yeasts	Acidic EW	0.33	230	3.66	–	Puligundla et al. (2018)
Fresh-cut Mangoes	*E. coli and Cronobacter sakazakii*	Acidic/Neutral	5	102/101	2.87/7.95	1113/757	Santo et al. (2018)
Fresh-Sliced Button Mushrooms	Total bacterium, yeast and mould	EW	3	16.86 ± 0.3	5.50 ± 0.02	514.67 ± 1.53	Wu et al. (2018)
Apple and tomato	*E coli* O157:H7 *and L. monocytogenes*	Slightly acidic	3	30	5.42	854	Tango et al. (2017)
Fresh-cut pears	*E. coli, S. enterica,* and *Listeria* spp.	Acidic/Neutral	3	99/102	2.9/8.2	1121/754	Graça et al. (2017)
Romaine and iceberg lettuces	*E. coli* O157:H7	Slightly acidic	5, 15, 30	50	6	–	Pang and Hung (2016)
Cherry tomato/ Strawberry	Aerobic bacteria, yeast and mould	Slightly acidic	10	34.33	6.49	853.7	Ding et al. (2015)
Fresh-cut kale	*E. coli* O157:H7, *L. monocytogenes*, TBC, Enterobacteriaceae, *Pseudomonas* spp., yeast and mould counts	Slightly acidic	5, 15, 30	–	5.51 ± 0.25, 5.93 ± 0.18 & 6.38 ± 0.2	898 ± 15, 915 ± 20 & 963 ± 15	Mansur and Oh (2015)

AMB = Aerobic mesophilic bacteria, total bacterial counts [TBC], **combined with other techniques, /=Not determined.

minimized browning in fresh-cut 'Florida' and 'Ionathan' apples packaged in plastic containers under atmospheric conditions for 14 days at 8°C (Plesoianu et al., 2022). The authors observed 70.7 and 72.0 *L* values for non-treated samples and 75.6 and 73.5 **L* values for AEW-treated samples for 'Florina' and 'Ionathan' cultivars, respectively. Furthermore, the effectiveness of acidic-EW as an anti-browning agent also became evident according to the results obtained in the **a*** values of both cultivars. Postharvest washing with EW for 90 and 180 seconds delayed surface browning incidence on fresh-cut iceberg lettuce when compared with 90 and 180 seconds washing with tap water during 9 days of 5°C storage (Das et al., 2011). Liu et al. (2021) results showed that 1 hour EW (pH 2 ± 3; 55.98 ± 2.27 mg L^{-1} FAC) treatment led to a lower surface browning degree than untreated samples on 'Jingan No. 9' sweet potato slices stored at 4°C for 8 days.

There are various reports about the application of EW to mitigate browning in postharvest fruits and vegetables. AEW containing 55.98 ± 2.27 mg L^{-1} FAC and pH 2.7 significantly reduced browning severity and activities of PPO and POD enzymes of sweet potato slices when compared with control during 8 days of storage at 4°C (Liu et al., 2021). The low acidic pH value of EW significantly influenced enzyme activities, since browning promoting enzymes are less active under acidic conditions. Similarly, PPO and POD activities of button mushrooms were inhibited by SAEW treatment during 8 days' storage at 5°C (Wu et al., 2018). In addition, suppression of browning in mushrooms by different concentrations (5–25 mg L^{-1}) of EW were reported by Aday (2016). Moreover, browning in apples is indicated by high *a* and low **L* colorimetric values. 'Florina' and 'Ionathan' apple cultivars treated with AEW had **L* values of 75.6 and 73.5, respectively, when compared with **L* values (70.7 and 72.0) of non-treated samples during 14 days of storage at 8°C (Plesoianu et al., 2021). Furthermore, browning inhibition by EW was also evaluated on fresh-cut vegetables (Li et al., 2017; Wu et al., 2018). Nonetheless, the anti-browning mechanism by EW in fresh produce is still unknown, but it could be due to HOCl and low pH since PPO is less reactive under acidic conditions (Zhang et al., 2021).

6.6.2 TEXTURE QUALITY CHANGES

Tissue softening of fresh produce during storage and in retail markets is associated with senescence and quality loss. Softening is due to structural changes in the primary cell walls initiated by degrading enzymes such as polygalacturonase (PG), and pectin methylesterase (PME) (Zhang et al., 2020). Maintenance of fresh produce firmness is an important aspect for prolonging the shelf-life of fresh produce. Furthermore, consumers associate firmness, crunchiness, and crispness and other texture parameters with freshness of fresh produce (Fufa, 2021). Therefore, application of EW to retain fresh produce firmness has been explored. Chen et al. (2017) evaluated the effect of acidic EW (48 mg L^{-1} FAC at pH 2.8) on extending the shelf-life of 'Brightwell' and 'Camellia' blueberries during postharvest storage. In the investigation, the postharvest wash treatment delayed softening of both cultivars, while a higher efficacy of delaying softening was observed on 'Camellia' blueberries than 'Brightwell' blueberries. The investigators suggested that these differences could be influenced by differences in thickness of the blueberries' skin and integrity of the edible portion (Chen et al., 2017). In the same study, acidic EW treatment inactivated cell wall degrading enzymes and inhibited degradation of cell wall components (Na_2CO_3–soluble pectin (NSP)), cellulose, and hemicellulose).

Effects of acidic EW treatment (pH = 2.5, FAC = 80 mg L^{-1}, 10 min) on pulp firmness, amounts of cell wall materials and cell wall polysaccharides, activities, and expression of relevant genes of cell wall degrading enzymes in pulp of 'Fuyan' longan during 5 days' storage at 25°C were evaluated (Sun et al., 2022). Based on the observations of the study, acidic EW-treated fruit retained a higher pulp firmness, prevented water soluble pectin formation, reduced the degradation of covalent soluble pectin, cellulose, and hemicellulose, and lowered cell wall degrading enzymes activities and their corresponding gene expression. When stored for 5 days, pulp firmness (113.6 g mm^{-1}), cell wall materials (13.9 g kg^{-1}), and covalent soluble pectin (1.4 g kg^{-1}) in acidic EW-treated fruit displayed clearly higher contents than those in control samples. These data suggest that acidic EW treatment can slow down the pulp softening and retain higher pulp cell wall particles levels in postharvest fresh longans, which was because acidic EW lowered activities of cell wall degrading enzymes and its gene expression levels and maintained the cell wall structure's integrity. In addition, slightly acidic EW significantly retarded the loss of 'Jiancui' jujube fruit firmness and maintained tissue structure (Li et al., 2020). Belay et al. (2021) found that alkaline EW (200 mg L^{-1} FAC, ORP of –800 mV and 11–13 pH) dipping for 10 minutes retained 'Crimson Blaze' nectarines firmness when compared with non-treated samples stored at –0.5°C, 95% RH for 21 days. In addition, alkaline EW treated fruits had the lowest decay incidence followed by chlorine-treated fruits after 31 days of storage (Figure 6.5). According to Zhang and Jiang (2019), invasion of pathogenic microorganisms on the produce surface may contribute to further production of ethylene, subsequent degradation of cell wall, and accelerate softening and firmness loss. Additionally, ethylene plays a role in metabolic processes related to maturation, softening, and senescence and directly influences activities of cell wall degrading enzymes. Thus, the ability of EW to suppress cell wall degrading enzymes activities may be linked with inhibition of ethylene biosynthesis and production and inactivating pathogenic microorganism on FFV surface. Furthermore, enhancement of antioxidant bioactive compounds of fresh produce by EW is reported to be responsible for maintaining the integrity of the cell membrane (Zhang et al., 2021).

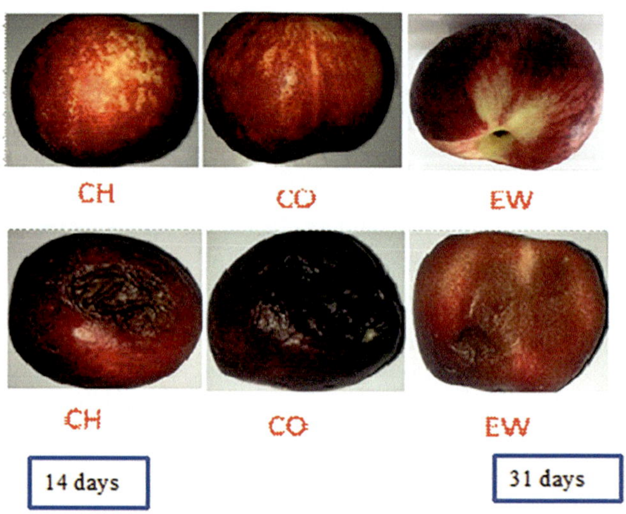

FIGURE 6.5 Effects of alkaline electrolyzed water (EW) and chlorine treatments on decay incident of fresh nectarine stored at –0.5°C and 95% RH for 31 days. EW; alkaline electrolyzed water treatments; CH, chlorine; CO, control.

6.6.3 *MITIGATING CHILLING INJURY*

Cold storage has been used extensively over the years for retarding fresh produce quality deterioration and extending shelf life. However, long-term cold storage may lead to physiological and metabolic disorders such as chilling injury, particularly in tropical and subtropical fruits.

General symptoms of chilling injury include surface and internal browning, skin pitting, and pulp flocculation, which are accompanied by the degradation of cell membrane integrity (Zhang et al., 2020). Thus, chilling injury damages produce texture and appearance and reduces consumer's acceptance. Chilling injury is another physiological disorder that has been reported to be alleviated by EW. Application of hot functional EW with pH 2.6–2.65, 1125 mV ORP, and 62 mg L^{-1} FAC physical properties showed the best results in the reduction of chilling injury of 'Satsuma' orange fruits when compared with hot water and untreated control (Shi et al., 2021). In addition, the treatment increased antioxidant enzyme activities such as superoxide dismutase (SOD) of 'Satsuma' orange fruit. Wei et al. (2015) reported that EW reduced chilling injury indexes of banana fruit and maintained higher firmness compared with control fruits during low 4 ± 1°C temperature storage and 85% relative humidity for 16 days. Treatment with EW enhances antioxidant systems of postharvest fresh produce (Zhang et al., 2021), and chilling injury alleviation may be related to the enhancement of antioxidant enzymes and regulation of ROS metabolism.

6.7 CONCLUSION AND FUTURE PROSPECTS

Electrolyzed water has shown efficiency as a potent cleaner and sanitizer for fresh produce. This chapter presented the general principle and application of EW for improvement of fruits and vegetables' safety and quality. With a foundation in acidic, neutral, and alkaline EW, recent advances in EW introduced slightly acidic and slightly alkaline EW. Acidic EW, produced at the anode side during electrolysis, has a very powerful effect as a disinfectant due to its low pH and high HOCl and FAC contents. On the other hand, alkaline EW, produced at the cathode side during electrolysis, is a novel cleaner with high pH and a high content of dilute NaOH and OCl^-. Neutral EW is considered the least effective EW in inhibiting microbial growth compared to AEW; however, NEW is stable, less corrosive, and can easily enter the microbial cytoderm. The decontamination effect of electrolyzed water is dependent on factors such as pH, ORP, and FAC. These factors are responsible for the inactivation of pathogenic microorganisms.

Previous research in the application of EW mainly focused on the sanitization of fresh produce; however, there is still limited research about the optimization of EW physical parameters (pH, ORP, and FAC) for washing FFV to attain the best sanitization protocol. Furthermore, the detailed antimicrobial mode of action of EW is not well elucidated. Additionally, there is little research on the effects of EW on nutritional compounds and the physiological response and metabolisms of FFV. Therefore, more research is necessary to (i) optimize EW physical parameters for achieving the best treatment for the preservation of produce and controlling pathogenic microorganisms; (ii) elucidate the germicidal mechanism of EW; and (iii) investigate the effects of EW on nutritional compounds and the physiological response of fresh produce. Considering this knowledge, EW can be utilized as an alternative to synthetic chemicals for postharvest sanitization and quality improvement of fresh produce.

FUNDING

This work is based upon research supported wholly or in part by the National Research Foundation (NRF), South Africa (Grant No.: 137990) awarded to Dr. O.J. Caleb.

CONFLICT OF INTEREST

All authors declare that there is no conflict of interest.

KEYWORDS

- **electrolyzed water**
- **food safety**
- **fresh fruits and vegetables**
- **microbial decontamination**
- **physiochemical quality**
- **postharvest sanitization**

REFERENCES

Aday, M. S. (2016). Application of electrolyzed water for improving postharvest quality of mushroom. *LWT–Food Science and Technology, 68*, 44–51.

Aghdam, M. S., Luo, Z., Jannatizadeh, A., Sheikh-Assadi, M., Sharafi, Y., Farmani, B., & Razavi, F. (2019). Employing exogenous melatonin applying confers chilling tolerance in tomato fruits by upregulating ZAT2/6/12 giving rise to promoting endogenous polyamines, proline, and nitric oxide accumulation by triggering arginine pathway activity. *Food Chemistry, 275*, 549–556.

Akbulut, M. B., & Eldeniz, A. Ü. (2019). *In vitro* antimicrobial activity of different electrochemically activated solutions on *Enterococcus faecalis*. *European Oral Research, 53*, 44–50.

Akther, S., Islam, Md. R., Alam, M., Alam, Md. J., & Ahmed, S. (2023). Impact of slightly acidic electrolyzed water in combination with ultrasound and mild heat on safety and quality of fresh-cut cauliflower. *Postharvest Biology and Technology, 197*.

Aniyyah, M. N., Idhamnulhadi, Z., Shah, A. A., Shakirah, H. L., Suhaila, A., Norazlina, H., & Najwa, M. H. (2022). Electrolysis study effect on electrolyzed water as disinfectant and sanitizer. In *Journal of Physics: Conference Series, 2266*, 012004. IOP Publishing.

Belay, Z. A., Botes, W. J., & Caleb, O. J. (2021). Effects of alkaline electrolyzed water pretreatment on the physicochemical quality attributes of fresh nectarine during storage. *Journal of Food Processing and Preservation, 45*, e15879. https://doi.org/10.1111/jfpp.15879 (accessed on 9th July 2025).

Block, Z., Eyles, A., Corkrey, R., Stanley, R., Ross, T., & Kocharunchitt, C. (2020). Effect of storage conditions on shelf stability of undiluted neutral electrolyzed water. *Journal of Food Protection, 83*, 1838–1843.

Cap, M., Rojas, D., Fernandez, M., Fulco, M., Rodriguez, A., Soteras, T., & Mozgovoj, M. (2020). Effectiveness of short exposure times to electrolyzed water in reducing *Salmonella* spp and imidacloprid in lettuce. *LWT*, 109496.

Chauret, C. P. (2014). Sanitization. In C. A. Batt & M. L. Tortorello (Eds.), *Encyclopedia of Food Microbiology* (2nd ed., pp. 360–364). Academic Press.

Chen, B., & Wang, C. (2022). Electrolyzed water and its pharmacological activities: A mini-review. *Molecules, 27*, 1222.

Chen, J., Xu, B., Deng, S. G., & Huang, Y. T. (2016). Effect of combined pretreatment with slightly acidic electrolyzed water and botanic bio preservative on quality and shelf life of Bombay duck (*Harpadon nehereus*). *Journal of Food Quality, 39*, 116–125.

Chen, X., Tango, C. N., Daliri, E. B. M., Oh, S. Y., & Oh, D. H. (2019). Disinfection efficacy of slightly acidic electrolyzed water combined with chemical treatments on fresh fruits at the industrial scale. *Foods, 8*, 497.

Chen, X., Xue, S. J., Shi, J., Kostrzynska, M., Tang, J., Guévremont, E., Villeneuve, S., & Mondor, M. (2018). Red cabbage washing with acidic electrolyzed water: Effects on microbial quality and physicochemical properties. *Food Quality and Safety, 2*, 229–237.

Chen, Y., Hung, Y. C., Chen, M., & Lin, H. (2017). Effects of acidic electrolyzed oxidizing water on retarding cell wall degradation and delaying softening of blueberries during postharvest storage. *LWT, 84*, 650–657.

Chiabrando, V., Peano, C., & Giacalone, G. (2017). The efficacy of different postharvest treatments on physico-chemical characteristics, bioactive components and microbiological quality of fresh blueberries during storage period. *Food Research, 6*, 240–248.

Cravero, F., Englezos, V., Rantsiou, K., Torchio, F., Giacosa, S., Segade, S. R., Gerbi, V., Rolle, L., & Cocolin, L. (2018). Control of *Brettanomyces bruxellensis* on wine grapes by post-harvest treatments with electrolyzed water, ozonated water and gaseous ozone. *Innovative Food Science and Emerging Technologies, 47*, 309–316.

Das, B. K., Kim, J. G., & Choi, J. W. (2011). Edge browning and microbial quality of fresh-cut iceberg lettuce with different sanitizers and contact times. *Bulgarian Journal of Agricultural Science, 17*, 55–62.

Dilarri, G., Silva, V. L., Pecora, H. B., Montagnolli, R. N., Corso, C. R., & Bidoia, E. D. (2016). Electrolytic treatment and biosurfactants applied to the conservation of *Eugenia uniflora* fruit. *Journal of Food Science and Technology, 36*, 456–460.

Ding, T., Ge, Z., Shi, J., Xu, Y. T., Jones, C. L., & Liu, D. H. (2015). Impact of slightly acidic electrolyzed water (SAEW) and ultrasound on microbial loads and quality of fresh fruits. *LWT–Food Science and Technology, 60*, 1195–1199.

Duan, Y., Wang, G. B., Fawole, O. A., Verboven, P., Zhang, X. R., Wu, D., & Chen, K. (2020). Postharvest precooling of fruit and vegetables: A review. *Trends in Food Science and Technology, 100*, 278–291.

Dziedzic, E., Błaszczyk, J., Bieniasz, M., Dziadek, K., & Kopeć, A. (2020). Effect of modified (MAP) and controlled atmosphere (CA) storage on the quality and bioactive compounds of blue honeysuckle fruits (*Lonicera caerulea* L.). *Scientia Horticultural, 265*, 109226.

Fufa, D. D. (2021). Novel approach to enhance the shelf life of fresh-cut fruits and vegetables: A review. *Journal of Food Processing Technology, 12*, 891.

Gil, M. I., Selma, M. V., Suslow, T., Jacxsens, L., Uyttendaele, M., & Allende, A. (2015). Pre and postharvest preventive measures and intervention strategies to control microbial food safety hazards of fresh leafy vegetables. *Critical Reviews in Food Science and Nutrition, 55*, 453–468. https://doi.org/10.1080/10408398.2012.657808 (accessed on 9th July 2025).

Gok, S. B., & Pazır, F. (2019). Effect of treatments with UV-C light and electrolyzed oxidizing water on decontamination and the quality of Gemlik black olives. *Journal of Consumer Protection and Food Safety*, 1–9.

Graça, A., Abadias, M., Salazar, M., & Nunes, C. (2011). The use of electrolyzed water as a disinfectant for minimally processed apples. *Postharvest Biology and Technology, 61*, 172–177.

Graça, A., Santo, D., Pires-Cabral, P., & Quintas, C. (2020). The effect of UV-C and electrolyzed water on yeasts on fresh-cut apple at 4 °C. *Journal of Food Engineering, 282*, 110034. https://doi.org/10.1016/j.jfoodeng.2020.110034 (accessed on 9th July 2025).

Graça, A., Santo, D., Quintas, C., & Nunes, C. (2017). Growth of *Escherichia coli*, *Salmonella enterica* and *Listeria* spp., and their inactivation using ultraviolet energy and electrolyzed water, on 'Rocha' fresh-cut pears. *Food Control, 77*, 41–49.

Han, Y., Song, L., An, Q., & Pan, C. (2017). Removal of six pesticide residues in cowpea with alkaline electrolyzed water. *Journal of the Science of Food and Agriculture, 97*, 2333–2338.

Hirayma, Y., Asano, S., Watanabe, K., Sakamoto, Y., Ozaki, M., & Ohki, S. T. (2016). Control of *Colletotrichum fructicola* on strawberry with a foliar spray of neutral electrolyzed water through an overhead irrigation system. *Journal of General Plant Pathology, 82*, 186–189.

Hopkins, D. Z., Parisi, M. A., Dawson, P. L., & Northcutt, J. K. (2021). Surface decontamination of fresh, whole peaches (*Prunus persica*) using sodium hypochlorite or acidified electrolyzed water solutions. *International Journal of Fruit Science, 21*, 1–11. https://doi.org/10.1080/15538362.2020.1822269 (accessed on 9th July 2025).

Hricova, D., Stephan, R., & Zweifel, C. (2008). Electrolyzed water and its application in the food industry. *Journal of Food Protection, 71*, 1934–1947. https://doi.org/10.4315/0362-028X-71.9.1934 (accessed on 9th July 2025).

Hsu, Y. F., Chuang, C. Y., Huang, H. C., & Yang, S. (2019). Applying membrane-less electrolyzed water for inactivating pathogenic microorganisms. *Applied Ecology and Environmental Research, 17*, 15019–15027.

Huang, Y., Hung, Y., Hsu, S., Huang, Y., & Hwang, D. (2008). Application of electrolyzed water in the food industry. *Food Control*, 329–345.

Hussien, A., Ahmed, Y., Al-Essawy, A. H., & Youssef, K. (2018). Evaluation of different salt-amended electrolyzed water to control postharvest molds of citrus. *Tropical Plant Pathology, 43*, 10–20.

Jiang, Y., Ai, C., Liao, X., Liu, D., & Ding, T. (2020). Effect of slightly acidic electrolyzed water (SAEW) and ultraviolet light illumination pretreatment on microflora inactivation of coriander. *LWT*, 109898.

Kim, H. J., Tango, C. N., & Chelliah, R. (2019). Sanitization efficacy of slightly acidic electrolyzed water against pure cultures of *Escherichia coli*, *Salmonella enterica* Typhimurium, *Staphylococcus aureus* and *Bacillus cereus* spores, in comparison with different water hardness. *Scientific Reports, 9*, 4348.

Kurahashi, M., Ito, T., & Naka, A. (2021). Spatial disinfection potential of slightly acidic electrolyzed water. *PLOS ONE, 16*, 1–10.

Li, H., Ren, Y., Hao, J., & Liu, H. (2017). Dual effects of acidic electrolyzed water treatments on the microbial reduction and control of enzymatic browning for fresh-cut lotus root. *Journal of Food Safety, 37*, 2333.

Li, L., Hao, J., Song, S., Nirasawa, S., Jiang, Z., & Liu, H. (2018). Effect of slightly acidic electrolyzed water on bioactive compounds and morphology of broccoli sprouts. *Food Research International, 105*, 102–109.

Li, X., Yue, H., Xu, S., Tian, J., Zhao, Y., & Xu, J. (2020). The effect of electrolyzed water on fresh-cut eggplant in storage period. *LWT, 123*, 109080.

Liao, X., Xuan, X., Li, J., Suo, Y., Liu, D., Ye, X., Chen, S., & Ding, T. (2017). Bactericidal action of slightly acidic electrolyzed water against *Escherichia coli* and *Staphylococcus aureus* via multiple cell targets. *Food Control, 79*, 380–385.

Liu, Q., Jin, X., Feng, X., Yang, H., & Fu, C. (2019). Inactivation kinetics of *Escherichia coli* O157:H7 and *Salmonella typhimurium* on organic carrot (*Daucus carota* L.) treated with low concentration electrolyzed water combined with short-time heat treatment. *Food Control, 106*, 106702.

Liu, R., Yu, Z., & Sun, Y., & Zhou, S. (2021). The enzymatic browning reaction inhibition effect of strong acidic electrolyzed water on different parts of sweet potato slices. *Food Bioscience, 43*, 101252. https://doi.org/10.1016/j.fbio.2021.101252 (accessed on 9th July 2025).

Liu, Y., Wang, J., Zhu, X., Liu, Y., Cheng, M., Xing, W., Wan, Y., Li, N., Yang, L., & Song, P. (2021). Effects of electrolyzed water treatment on pesticide removal and texture quality in fresh-cut cabbage, broccoli, and color pepper. *Food Chemistry, 353*, 129408.

Lyu, F., Gao, F., Zhou, X., Zhang, J., & Ding, Y. (2018). Using acid and alkaline electrolyzed water to reduce deoxynivalenol and mycological contaminations in wheat grains. *Food Control, 88*, 98–104.

Machado, I., Meireles, A., Fulgêncio, R., Mergulhão, F., Simões, M., & Melo, L. F. (2016). Disinfection with neutral electrolyzed oxidizing water to reduce microbial load and to prevent biofilm regrowth in the processing of fresh-cut vegetables. *Food and Bioproducts Processing, 98*, 333–340.

Mansur, A. R., & Oh, D. H. (2015). Combined effect of thermosonication and slightly acidic electrolyzed water to reduce foodborne pathogens and spoilage microorganisms on fresh-cut kale. *Journal of Food Science, 80*, M1277–M1284.

Nyamende, N. E., Belay, Z. A., Keyser, Z., Oyenihi, A. B., & Caleb, O. J. (2022). Impacts of alkaline-electrolyzed water treatment on physicochemical, phytochemical, antioxidant properties and natural microbial load on 'Granny Smith' apples during storage. *International Journal of Food Science and Technology, 57*, 447–456.

Nyamende, N. E., Domtchouang, F. R., Belay, Z. A., Keyser, Z., Oyenihi, A., & Caleb, O. J. (2021). Alternative postharvest pre-treatment strategies for quality and microbial safety of 'Granny Smith' apple. *Helion, 7*, e07104.

Nyamende, N. E., Hoff, J. W., & van Brede, V. (2022). Isolation and characterization of culturable microbes on the surface of 'Granny Smith' apples treated with electrolyzed water during cold storage. *Food Science and Biotechnology, 31*, 1603–1614.

Ogunniyi, A. D., Tenzin, S., Ferro, S., Venter, H., Pi, H., Amorico, T., & Trott, D. J. (2020). A pH-neutral electrolyzed oxidizing water significantly reduces microbial contamination of fresh spinach leaves. *Food Microbiology, 93*, 103614.

Pan, Y., Cheng, J. H., & Sun, D. W. (2019). Cold plasma-mediated treatments for shelf-life extension of fresh produce: A review of recent research developments. *Comprehensive Reviews in Food Science and Food Safety, 18*, 1312–1326.

Pang, Y. H., & Hung, Y. C. (2016). Efficacy of slightly acidic electrolyzed water and UV-ozonated water combination for inactivating *Escherichia coli* O157:H7 on romaine and iceberg lettuce during spray washing process. *Journal of Food Science, 81*, 1743–1748. https://doi.org/10.1111/17503841.13364 (accessed on 9th July 2025).

Plesoianu, A. M., Felicia, V. N., & Ionica, T. M. E. (2022). Quality of fresh-cut apples as affected by dip wash treatments with organic acids and acidic electrolyzed water. *Food Science and Technology Campinas, 42*, e62620.

Plesoianu, A. M., Nour, V., Tutulescu, F., & Ionica, M. E. (2021). Quality of fresh-cut apples as affected by dip wash treatments with organic acids and acidic electrolyzed water. *Food Science and Technology, 42*, 62620.

Ponce-Valadez, M., Escalona-Buendía, H. B., Villa-Hernández, J. M., de León-Sánchez, F. D., Rivera-Cabrera, F., & Alia-Tejacal, I. (2016). Effect of refrigerated storage (12.5 °C) on tomato (*Solanum lycopersicum*) fruit flavor: A biochemical and sensory analysis. *Postharvest Biology and Technology, 111*, 6–14.

Procaccini, L. M. G., Mu, T., & Sun, H. (2022). Effect of innovative food processing technologies on microbiological quality, color and texture of fresh-cut potato during storage. *International Journal of Food Science and Technology, 57*, 898–907.

Puligundla, P., Kim, J. W., & Mok, C. (2018). Broccoli sprout washing with electrolyzed water: Effects on microbiological and physicochemical characteristics. *LWT, 92*, 600–606.

Qi, H., Huang, Q., & Hung, Y. C. (2018). Effectiveness of electrolyzed oxidizing water treatment in removing pesticide residues and its effect on produce quality. *Food Chemistry, 239*, 561–568.

Quan, Y., Choi, K. D., Chung, D., & Shin, I. S. (2010). Evaluation of bactericidal activity of weakly acidic electrolyzed water (WAEW) against *Vibrio vulnificus* and *Vibrio parahaemolyticus*. *International Journal of Food Microbiology, 136*, 255–260.

Rahman, S. M. E., Jin, Y. G., & Oh, D. H. (2010). Combined effects of alkaline electrolyzed water and citric acid with mild heat to control microorganisms on cabbage. *Journal of Food Science, 75*, M111–M115.

Rahman, S. M. E., Khan, I., & Oh, D. H. (2016). Electrolyzed water as a novel sanitizer in the food industry: Current trends and future perspectives. *Comprehensive Reviews in Food Science and Food Safety, 15*, 471–490.

Rebezov, M., Saeed, K., Khaliq, A., Rahman, S. J. U., Sameed, N., Semenova, A., Khayrullin, M., Dydykin, A., Abramov, Y., & Thiruvengadam, M. (2022). Application of electrolyzed water in the food industry: A review. *Applied Sciences, 12*, 6639.

Rodriguez-Casado, A. (2016). The health potential of fruits and vegetables phytochemicals: Notable examples. *Critical Reviews in Food Science and Nutrition, 56*, 1097–1107.

Santo, D., Graça, A., Nunes, C., & Quintas, C. (2018). *Escherichia coli* and *Cronobacter sakazakii* in 'Tommy Atkins' minimally processed mangos: Survival, growth and effect of UV-C and electrolyzed water. *Food Microbiology, 70*, 49–54. https://doi.org/10.1016/j.fm.2017.09.008 (accessed on 9th July 2025).

Saravanakumar, K., Sathiyaseelan, A., Mariadoss, A. V. A., Chelliah, R., Shin, S., Park, S., & Wang, M. H. (2021). Slightly acidic electrolyzed water combination with antioxidants and fumaric acid treatment to maintain the quality of fresh-cut bell peppers. *LWT*, 111565.

Sheng, L., Shen, X., Ulloa, O., Suslow, T. V., Hanrahan, I., & Zhu, M. J. (2020). Evaluation of JC9450 and neutral electrolyzed water in controlling *Listeria monocytogenes* on fresh apples and preventing cross-contamination. *Frontiers in Microbiology, 10*, 3128.

Shi, F., Li, X., Meng, H., Wei, W., & Wang, Y. (2020). Reduction in chilling injury symptoms by hot electrolyzed functional water treatment may function by regulating ROS metabolism in Satsuma orange fruit. *LWT, 125*, 109218.

Sierra, B. E. G., Meza, A. X. S., & Sánchez, L. T. G. (2019). Antifungal activity of acidic electrolyzed water against strawberry postharvest molds (*Fragaria* × *ananassa* Duch cv. Camarosa). *Acta Agronómica, 68*, 126–133.

Singh, D., & Sharma, R. R. (2018). Postharvest diseases of fruits and vegetables and their management. In *Postharvest Disinfection of Fruits and Vegetables* (pp. 1–52). Academic Press: Elsevier.

Sun, J., Chen, H., Xie, H., Li, M., Chen, Y., Hung, Y. C., & Lin, H. (2022). Acidic electrolyzed water treatment retards softening and retains cell wall polysaccharides in pulp of postharvest fresh longans and its possible mechanism. *Food Chemistry, 23*, 100265.

Tang, J., Chen, H., Lin, H., Hung, Y. C., Xie, H., & Chen, Y. (2021). Acidic electrolyzed water treatment delayed fruit disease development of harvested longans through inducing the disease resistance and maintaining the ROS metabolism systems. *Postharvest Biology and Technology, 171*, 111349.

Tango, C. N., Khan, I., Kounkeu, P. F. N., Momna, R., Hussain, M. S., & Oh, D. H. (2017). Slightly acidic electrolyzed water combined with chemical and physical treatments to decontaminate bacteria on fresh fruits. *Food Microbiology, 67*, 97–105.

Tao, H., Liao, Q., Xu, Y., & Wang, H. (2022). Efficacy of slightly acidic electrolyzed water for inactivation of *Cronobacter sakazakii* and biofilm cells. *Journal of Food Protection, 85*, 511–517.

Turantaş, F., Ersus-Bilek, S., Sömek, Ö., & Kuşçu, A. (2018). Decontamination effect of electrolyzed water washing on fruits and vegetables. *Journal of Microbiology, Biotechnology and Food Sciences, 7*, 337–342.

Wang, Y., Wu, J., & Yang, H. (2022). Comparison of the metabolic responses of eight *Escherichia coli* strains including the "big six" in pea sprouts to low concentration electrolyzed water by NMR spectroscopy. *Food Control, 131*.

Wei, W., Hao, L., & Wang, Y. (2015). Effect of cold shock treatment of different ACC (available chlorine concentration) electrolyzed functional water on chilling tolerance in bananas. *Food Science and Technology, 77*.

Whangchai, K., Khayankarn, S., & Uthaibutra, J. (2017). Effect of acidic electrolyzed oxidizing water treatments on the control of postharvest disease and pathogenesis-related protein production in pineapple fruit. *Journal of Advanced Agricultural Technologies, 4*, 3.

Wu, S., Nie, Y., Zhao, J., Fan, B., Huang, X., Li, X., Sheng, J., Meng, D., Ding, Y., & Tang, X. (2018). The synergistic effects of low-concentration acidic electrolyzed water and ultrasound on the storage quality of fresh-sliced button mushrooms. *Food and Bioprocess Technology, 11*, 314–323.

Yamaner, Ç. (2022). The effect of neutral electrolyzed water on the microbial population and quality of dried figs (*Ficus carica* L.) during storage. *Journal of Agricultural Sciences, 28*, 232–238.

Yan, P., Chelliah, R., Jo, K. H., & Oh, D. H. (2021). Research trends on the application of electrolyzed water in food preservation and sanitation. *Processes, 9*, 2240.

Yan, P., Daliri, E. B., & Oh, D. H. (2021). New clinical applications of electrolyzed water: A review. *Microorganisms, 9*, 136. https://doi.org/10.3390/microorganisms9010136 (accessed on 9th July 2025).

Yang, J., Song, L., Pan, C., Han, Y., & Kang, L. (2020). Removal of ten pesticide residues on/in kumquat by washing with alkaline electrolyzed water. *International Journal of Environmental Analytical Chemistry, 102*, 3638–3651.

Ye, Z., Wang, S., Chen, T., Gao, W., Zhu, S., He, J., & Han, Z. (2017). Inactivation mechanism of *Escherichia coli* induced by slightly acidic electrolyzed water. *Scientific Reports, 7*, 6279.

Youssef, K., & Hussien, A. (2020). Electrolyzed water and salt solutions can reduce green and blue molds while maintaining the quality properties of 'Valencia' late oranges. *Postharvest Biology and Technology, 159*, 111025.
Zhang, C., Li, B., Jadeja, R., Fang, J., & Hung, Y. C. (2016). Effects of bacterial concentrations and centrifugations on susceptibility of *Bacillus subtilis* vegetative cells and *Escherichia coli* O157:H7 to various electrolyzed oxidizing water treatments. *Food Control, 60*, 440–446.
Zhang, C., Zhao, Z., Yang, G., Shi, Y., Zhang, Y., Shi, C., & Xia, X. (2021). Effect of slightly acidic electrolyzed water on natural *Enterobacteriaceae* reduction and seed germination in the production of alfalfa sprouts. *Food Microbiology, 97*, 103414.
Zhang, W., & Cao, J., & Jiang, W. (2021). Application of electrolyzed water in postharvest fruits and vegetables storage: A review. *Trends in Food Science and Technology, 114*, 599–607.
Zhang, W., & Jiang, W. (2019). UV treatment improved the quality of postharvest fruits and vegetables by inducing resistance. *Trends in Food Science and Technology, 92*, 71–80.
Zhang, W., Li, X., & Jiang, W. (2020). Development of antioxidant chitosan film with banana peels extract and its application as coating in maintaining the storage quality of apple. *International Journal of Biological Macromolecules, 154*, 1205–1214.
Zhang, W., Shu, C., Chen, Q., Cao, J., & Jiang, W. (2019). The multi-layer film system improved the release and retention properties of cinnamon essential oil and its application as coating in inhibition to *Penicillium* expansion of apple fruit. *Food Chemistry, 299*, 125109.
Zhang, W., Zhao, H., Zhang, J., Sheng, Z., Cao, J., & Jiang, W. (2019). Different molecular weights chitosan coatings delay the senescence of postharvest nectarine fruit in relation to changes of redox state and respiratory pathway metabolism. *Food Chemistry, 289*, 160–168.
Zhao, L., Li, H., Wang, K., Li, X., Guo, C., & Yang, H. (2022). Effects of electrolyzed water and levulinic acid combination on microbial safety and polysaccharide nanostructure of organic strawberry. *Food Chemistry, 394*.
Zhao, L., Zhao, M. Y., Phey, C. P., & Yang, H. S. (2019). Efficacy of low concentration acidic electrolyzed water and levulinic acid combination on fresh organic lettuce (*Lactuca sativa* var. *crispa* L.) and its antimicrobial mechanism. *Food Control, 101*, 241–250.

CHAPTER 7

Edible Coating for Fresh Produce Shelf-Life Extension

BERNARD MARINGGAL[1,*] and NORHASHILA HASHIM[2,3]

[1]*Faculty of Resource Science and Technology, Universiti Malaysia Sarawak, Sarawak, Malaysia*

[2]*Department of Biological and Agricultural Engineering, Faculty of Engineering, Universiti Putra Malaysia, Selangor, Malaysia*

[3]*SMART Farming Technology Research Centre (SFTRC), Faculty of Engineering, Universiti Putra Malaysia, Selangor, Malaysia*

*Corresponding author

ABSTRACT

A confirmed finding reveals that an edible coating serves as a protective barrier on the surface of fresh produce, influencing the internal gas environment, minimizing water losses, and delaying the ripening of the fruit. To maintain the safety and quality of fresh produce, attempts have been made to introduce novel natural coating materials. This chapter seeks to summarize recent studies on the application of edible coatings to various fresh produce. The basic idea underlying the edible coating treatment is highlighted, as is the effect on the physical and chemical properties, sensory, and antimicrobial aspects of fresh produce. Mechanisms of the action of edible coatings in extending the shelf life of fresh produce are also discussed. To enhance the longevity of fresh produce, an alternative method involving using edible coating can be utilized. The materials used in the edible coating have a significant impact on its effectiveness and consumer acceptance. The efficacy of the selected materials to extend the

Sustainable Approaches in Postharvest Handling and Management: Pankaj B. Pathare (Ed.)

DOI: 10.1201/9781779641076-7

shelf life of fresh produce without compromising sensory and nutritional properties is one of the primary issues in edible coating techniques that require additional research.

7.1 INTRODUCTION

Edible coatings refer to thin layers of food-grade substances that are applied to the surface of fresh produce, serving the purpose of prolonging its shelf life and preserving its overall quality (Armghan et al., 2022; Tavassoli-Kafrani et al., 2022). The use of edible coatings has become increasingly popular in the fresh produce industry as a means to address the challenges of preserving perishable products for longer periods. In addition, postharvest losses resulting from the decline in quantity and quality of fresh produce after harvest pose a formidable obstacle (Maringgal et al., 2020a). These postharvest losses are attributed to inadequate handling and storage, insufficient packaging, and the prevalence of microbial and fungal infections. With the growing demand for fresh produce, prolonging its shelf life using an edible coating is becoming increasingly important to reduce food waste and meet consumer expectations.

The utilization of edible coatings to prolong the shelf life of fresh produce is not new. According to Woods (1990), the earliest use of edible coatings was to inhibit the loss of moisture, which led to a reduction in the softening and shriveling of fresh produce, and to enhance the appearance by imparting shine. During ancient times, fruits and vegetables were coated with edible materials such as wax, honey, and tree sap to safeguard them from physical damage and environmental influences. Currently, the use of edible coatings has evolved and expanded, with advances in food science and technology providing new opportunities to enhance the performance and effectiveness of these coatings.

The primary mechanism of action of edible coatings is to form a barrier around the produce that protects it from physical damage and environmental factors, such as moisture, oxygen, and light (Hamzah et al., 2022; Sarker and Grift, 2021). Guimaraes et al. (2018) revealed that edible coatings are one of the modified atmosphere methods for preserving fresh produce that has demonstrated promising results. This is supported by Maringgal et al. (2021), who uncover that edible coatings can also help to maintain the fresh produce's quality by controlling the exchange of gases, such as carbon dioxide and oxygen, which can affect its taste, texture, and appearance.

Additionally, edible coatings use biological or edible chemical materials as a protective layer on the surface of fresh produce, which contains antimicrobial properties and inhibits gaseous exchange, thus halting the degradation and ripening processes. For instance, Yadav et al. (2022) found that edible coatings can decelerate the enzymatic and microbial processes that contribute to spoilage, further extending the shelf life of fresh produce. According to Sharma et al. (2019), a composite coating known as an edible coating has been commonly applied in fresh produce to create an effective barrier, as illustrated in Figure 7.1. Thus, in this chapter, we focus on types of edible coatings and their effect on physiological, physicochemical, sensory, and antimicrobial properties to prolong the shelf life of fresh produce after harvest, the mechanisms of action of edible coatings, regulations on edible coatings, and challenges facing edible coatings and their future trends.

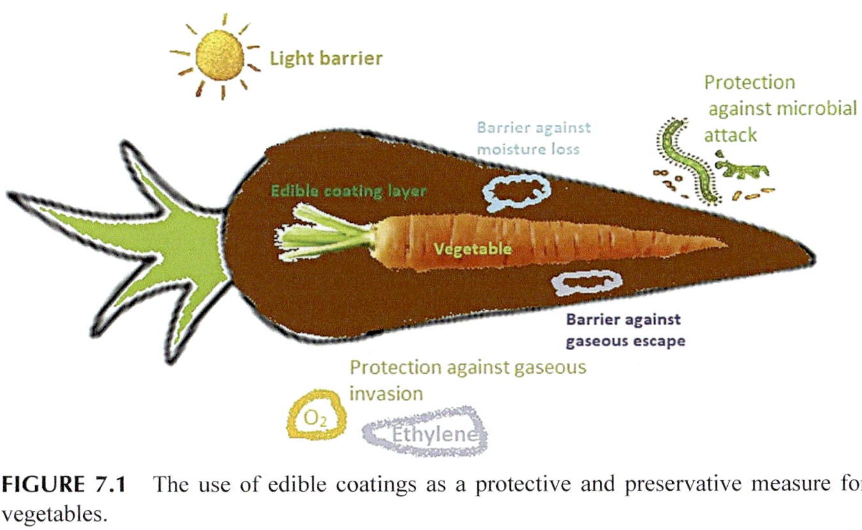

FIGURE 7.1 The use of edible coatings as a protective and preservative measure for vegetables.

Source: Modified from Sharma et al. (2019).

7.2 TYPE OF EDIBLE COATINGS

A wide range of natural and synthetic materials can be used to create edible coatings, including polysaccharides, proteins, lipids, and polyethene (Sharma et al., 2019). Among the frequently utilized base materials are chitosan, carrageenan, pectin, and lipids. The composition of the coating depends on the intended application and the type of fresh produce being treated. There are several types of edible coatings, as shown in Figure 7.2, each with its composition and properties. The types of edible coating are as follows:

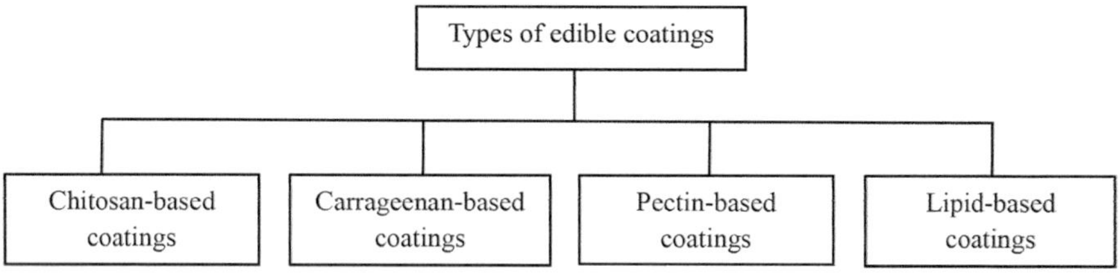

FIGURE 7.2 Type of edible coating for fresh produce.

7.2.1 CHITOSAN-BASED COATINGS

Chitosan, a natural polymer obtained from chitin, is sourced from the exoskeletons of crustaceans such as shrimp and crabs (Shapi'i et al., 2020). Chitosan has excellent antimicrobial properties and is an interesting biopolymer material. It is biodegradable and biocompatible and can be used to form non-toxic coatings for fresh produce (Arroyo et al., 2020). In addition, a chitosan-based edible coating may help to control the exchange of gases, such as carbon dioxide and oxygen, which can affect the fresh produce's quality (El-Sayed et al., 2021; Escamilla-Garcia et al., 2018). Table 7.1 comprises a summary of the recently reported effect of chitosan-based coating on fresh produce.

A study conducted recently by Chetia et al. (2023) discovered that the combination of chitosan and Assam lemon peel essential oil extraction can be utilized to maintain the quality of grapes and prolong their shelf life. The authors noted that coating grapes with 1% essential oil chitosan resulted in the highest quality retention for up to 15 days of storage at room temperature (25 ± 2°C). On the other hand, Zárate-Moreno et al. (2023) have designed and assessed chitosan-based food coatings for the preservation of exotic fruit, specifically feijoa. Their research revealed that the chitosan-based coating acted as a permeable membrane that facilitated suitable oxygen exchange to preserve fruit freshness and prevent natural weight loss, thereby slowing down oxidative degradation and extending the shelf life of the fruit.

TABLE 7.1 A summary of the Effect of Chitosan-Based Coating on Fresh Produce

Fresh Produce	Remarks	References
Grape	• Combination of chitosan and Assam lemon peel essential oil extraction. • Maintaining the quality of grapes and prolonging their shelf life up to 15 days of storage at room temperature (25 ± 2°C).	Chetia et al. (2023)
Feijoa	• Chitosan-based food coatings for the preservation of exotic fruit. • Significant effect on antimicrobial activity and act as a layer that can improve gas exchange and physiological properties of fruits during storage.	Zárate-Moreno et al. (2023)
Mandarin	• Chitosan-based layer-by-layer edible coating. • Hydroxypropyl methylcellulose is the inner layer and chitosan is the outer layer. • Markedly decrease the degradation of bioactive compounds and organic acids in mandarin fruit during 28 days of cold storage at 5°C.	Jurić et al. (2023)
Orange	• Alginate-Chitosan based coating enriched with Zinc Oxide (ZnO) nanoparticles. • Maintaining the physicochemical properties and increasing the shelf life of oranges up to 20 days at 4°C.	Dulta et al. (2022)
Bell pepper	• Combination of polyamine treatment (spermine) and chitosan coating. • Prevent the weight loss of bell pepper and extend the shelf life up to 28 days at 10°C.	Sharma et al. (2022)
Tomato	• Chitosan-Pullulan composite edible coating. • Improve the shelf life and postharvest quality of tomato over 18 days of storage at 23°C and 4°C.	Kumar et al. (2021)
Strawberry	• Chitosan-based coatings incorporated with apple peel polyphenols. • Improve the storage quality of strawberries in terms of firmness, weight loss, decay, total soluble solids, titratable acidity, and bioactive compounds.	Riaz et al. (2020)

Jurić et al. (2023) revealed that chitosan-based layer-by-layer edible coatings significantly reduce the degradation of bioactive compounds and organic acids in mandarin fruit over 28 days of cold storage at 5°C. Their study recommends a two-step dipping process, where fruits are first dipped in a primary coat, such as hydroxypropyl methylcellulose, followed by a second coat, such as chitosan, for effective coating.

Chitosan-based coatings have been proven effective in preserving tomatoes and bell peppers. For instance, Kumar et al. (2021) employed a chitosan-pullulan composite edible coating infused with pomegranate peel extract to treat tomatoes. The outcome was a significant extension in the tomatoes' shelf life to over 18 days, both at ambient temperatures of 23°C and under refrigeration at 4°C. The composite coating significantly improved postharvest quality by reducing weight loss, maintaining TSS, titratable acidity, color, and pH, as well as retaining higher levels of phenolic and flavonoid content and antioxidant activity during storage at both room and cold temperatures. Another significant finding by Sharma et al. (2022) explored the advantageous effects of a combined treatment utilizing polyamines, particularly 1.5 mM spermine, in conjunction with chitosan to prolong the shelf life of bell peppers. This treatment resulted in an extension of the bell pepper's storability by approximately 28 days, with the lowest observed weight loss, making it the most effective treatment for prolonging the bell pepper's shelf life.

According to Riaz et al. (2020), chitosan is a widely utilized biopolymer for applying edible coatings with various antioxidant agents. In their recent study, a composite coating comprising chitosan-based apple peel polyphenols was found to enhance the storage quality of strawberries at 20°C with relative humidity ranging between 35–40%. The results showed that the edible coatings had a significant effect on physicochemical quality, that is, firmness, weight loss, decay, TSS, titratable acidity, and bioactive compounds. These findings suggest that chitosan-based apple peel polyphenols edible coatings could be used to extend the shelf life of strawberries and to reduce food processing industrial waste by exploiting apple peel as an antioxidant ingredient.

7.2.2 CARRAGEENAN-BASED COATINGS

In recent years, there has been growing interest in carrageenan-based coatings as a promising alternative to synthetic coatings for preserving fresh produce. Carrageenan, derived from red seaweed, is a natural polysaccharide widely employed in the food industry as a thickener and stabilizer (Shafie et al., 2022). Carrageenan-based coatings are efficient in controlling moisture loss, which is a major contributor to spoilage in fresh produce (Tavassoli-Kafrani et al., 2016). They are also known for their good mechanical properties, making them ideal for use in fresh-cut fruits and vegetables (da Silva Bruni et al., 2023; Suryanto et al., 2023).

Table 7.2 provides a comprehensive summary of various research endeavors that have examined the potential of carrageenan-based coatings to preserve different varieties of fresh produce. Meindrawan et al. (2018) established a nanocomposite coating using carrageenan and ZnO nanoparticles to enhance the storage quality of mangoes by reducing the respiration rate and total acidity, maintaining firmness, and delaying discoloration and decay. The addition of ZnO nanoparticles also endowed the carrageenan coating with antimicrobial properties against *Escherichia coli*.

TABLE 7.2 A Summary of Carrageenan-Based Coating on the Fresh Produce

Fresh Produce	Remarks	References
Mango	• Carrageenan-based coatings incorporated with ZnO nanoparticles. • Improve the storage quality of mangoes by reducing their respiration rate and maintaining their physicochemical quality. • Enhance the antimicrobial properties.	Meindrawan et al. (2018)
Strawberry	• Carrageenan gum coating containing lemongrass essential oil. • Retain the physicochemical quality of strawberries for up to 12 days under refrigeration at 4°C.	Wani et al. (2021)
Mango (fresh-cut)	• Composite edible coating consisting of carrageenan, beeswax, and two plasticizers (glycerol and monosaccharide). • The physicochemical quality is preserved throughout a 6-day refrigerated storage period at 6°C. • Sensory evaluation of fresh-cut mangoes was not affected.	Afifah et al. (2019)

In a similar vein, Wani et al. (2021) exposed that strawberries coated with carrageenan gum coating added with 1% w/v lemon grass essential oil exhibited superior quality retention for 12 days when stored under refrigeration at 4°C. The experimental results demonstrated that the carrageenan-coated fruits delayed weight loss, decay percentage, retained ascorbic acid, antioxidant activity, firmness, and fruit color changes. Strawberries coated with carrageenan gum also demonstrated the lowest cellulase activity, pectin methylesterase activity, and β-galactosidase activity, while displaying the maximum reduction in polygalacturonase activity at the end of storage. In addition, during storage, the fruit coating formula, which includes lemon grass essential oil, demonstrated a significant reduction in psychrophilic bacteria, yeast, and mold count. Furthermore, the coating formulation containing lemongrass essential oil exhibited a significant reduction in psychrophilic bacteria, yeast, and mold counts on the fruits during storage.

Additionally, Afifah et al. (2019) applied an edible coating consisting of a composite of beeswax, carrageenan, glycerol, and monosaccharide to fresh-cut mangoes during refrigerated storage at 6°C for 6 days. Glycerol and monosaccharides act as plasticizers. The application of the edible coating resulted in reduced weight loss, maintenance of pH and total acidity, delayed increase of TSS, and inhibited the growth of microorganisms in fresh-cut mangoes. Moreover, there was no significant difference in sensory perception between the coated fruit and the uncoated fruit.

7.2.3 PECTIN-BASED COATINGS

Pectin is a naturally occurring polysaccharide present in various fruits and vegetables. It is a soluble component of plant fibers that can be extracted from the cell walls of different plants (Al-Tayyar et al., 2020). Due to its good gel-forming properties, pectin is a popular choice for edible coatings. Pectin-based coatings have been shown to slow down the enzymatic and microbial processes that contribute to spoilage, thus lengthening the shelf life of fresh produce (Nastasi et al., 2022; Panahirad et al., 2021). These coatings are frequently applied to fresh produces such as strawberries (Da Silva et al., 2019; Hernández-Carrillo et al., 2021; Muñoz-Almagro et al., 2021), raspberry (Abdi and Bakhshi, 2019; Guerreiro et al., 2015), blackberry (Tumbarski et al., 2020), tomato (Rodriguez-Garcia et al., 2016), and lime (Maftoonazad and Ramaswamy, 2019) to maintain their physicochemical quality during storage as listed in Table 7.3.

Hernández-Carrillo et al. (2021) discovered that dipping strawberries in a coating made from orange peel extract, lemon essential oil, and reuterin resulted in a reduction of color changes in the strawberries during the cold storage period of 31 days. The coating also exhibited antimicrobial effects, with the reuterin reducing *Penicillium conidia* by more than two logarithmic cycles. Moreover, the study demonstrates the great potential of using these coatings for strawberry preservation, as they are capable of preventing fungal spoilage without reducing the quality.

TABLE 7.3 A summary of Pectin-Based Coating on the Fresh Produce

Fresh Produce	Remarks	References
Strawberry	• Pectin edible coating (extracted from orange peels) incorporated with lemon essential oil and reuterin. • Decreases color changes in strawberries during 31 days of cold storage. • Antimicrobial effect.	Hernández-Carrillo et al. (2021)
	• Combination of sunflower pectin gel, elaborated with calcium and stevia/saccharin. • Prolong the shelf life of strawberries up to 12 days with storage temperature at 4°C by maintaining firmness, reducing weight loss, and keeping the microbial load constant. • Combining this edible coating with modified atmosphere packaging further prolonged the shelf life by up to 23 days with the same storage temperature.	Muñoz-Almagro et al. (2021)
	• Apple pectin suspension is incorporated with cellulose nanocrystals, glycerol, and lemongrass essential oil. • Reduced the weight loss and anthocyanin content during 8-day storage at 10°C ± 1°C.	Da Silva et al. (2019)
Raspberry	• Pectin edible coating enriched with essential oils of lemon and thyme. • Delayed the degradation of anthocyanin, and vitamin C, and reduced weight loss during storage at 5°C for up to 12 days.	Abdi and Bakhshi (2019)
	• Pectin-based coating incorporated with citral and eugenol. • While the coating proved effective in reducing microbial spoilage, its impact on physicochemical properties, such as fruit color and Trolox equivalent antioxidant capacity, was not statistically significant during the 14-day storage at 0.5°C.	Guerreiro et al. (2015)

TABLE 7.3 *(Continued)*

Fresh Produce	Remarks	References
Blackberry	• Pectin-based edible coating and incorporating the bacteriocin of *Bacillus methylotrophicus* BM47. • Prolong the shelf life of coated blackberries by maintaining the physicochemical properties during the 16 days of storage at 4°C with 75% relative humidity. • Decreased the percentage of decay and retained the antioxidant levels of the coated blackberries.	Tumbarski et al. (2020)
Tomato	• Pectin edible coating incorporated with oregano essential oil. • Antifungal effect against the growth of *Alternaria alternate*. • The total phenols and antioxidant activity of tomatoes increased throughout the 12-day storage period at 12.5°C, without adversely affecting their sensory acceptability.	Rodriguez-Garcia et al. (2016)
Lime	• Pectin edible coating incorporated with beeswax. • Prolonged the shelf life, slowed down the ripening process, and maintained the physicochemical properties of lime fruit during 32 days of storage at 10°C.	Maftoonazad and Ramaswamy (2019)

Strawberries are a fruit with high nutritional value. They are characterized by a short shelf-life and rapid deterioration (Riaz et al., 2020). Muñoz-Almagro et al. (2021) obtained that strawberries coated with a mixture of sunflower pectin gel, calcium, and stevia/saccharin coating maintained their firmness, reduced weight loss, and kept the microbial load constant throughout a 12-day storage period at 4°C. They further extended their research by combining this edible coating with modified atmosphere packaging (MAP), which increased the shelf life of strawberries to 23 days at the same storage temperature. The results emphasize the appropriateness of utilizing an edible pectin coating in combination with MAP to achieve a significant extension of shelf life while maintaining the high quality of the fresh produce.

Meanwhile, Da Silva et al. (2019) apply an apple pectin suspension incorporated with cellulose nanocrystals, glycerol, and lemongrass essential oil on strawberries. Their study indicated that the edible coating can reduce the weight loss and anthocyanin content during 8 days of storage at 10°C ± 1°C. Recently, in a study conducted by Piechowiak and Skóra

(2023), an edible coating was applied to strawberries, which were then combined with cinnamon oil. The study showed that the edible coating was able to prevent the growth of yeast and mold, minimize the loss of soluble solids and ascorbic acid, and decrease the level of oxidative stress during 72 hours of storage at room temperature. Overall, these findings offer valuable insights that can be used to develop sustainable and effective methods for preserving fresh produce.

Raspberries are an economically important soft fruit species (Davik et al., 2022). Due to their softness, post-harvest treatment is important to maintain their quality throughout the logistic and retail periods. Abdi and Bakhshi (2019) conducted research that demonstrated how pectin-based edible coatings infused with lemon and thyme essential oils can delay the degradation of anthocyanin and vitamin C and reduce weight loss during the storage of raspberries at 5°C for 12 days. Guerreiro et al. (2015) reported that a pectin-based coating incorporated with citral and eugenol was effective in lowering microbial spoilage in raspberries during storage, allowing for the fruit to be stored for at least 7 days at 0.5°C. However, during the 14-day storage period at 0.5°C, the application of this coating did not result in significant alterations in the physicochemical properties of the raspberries, including color and Trolox equivalent antioxidant capacity.

Blackberries are small fruits with significant antioxidant properties. However, preserving their quality and extending their storage capacity has become a significant challenge in the distribution of premium-quality berries (Maringgal et al., 2020a). This is because they are highly vulnerable to pathogen attack, over-ripening, and tremendous softening. Tumbarski et al. (2020) employed pectin-based edible coatings containing *Bacillus methylotrophicus* BM47 bacteriocin, which demonstrated the ability to extend the shelf life of blackberries. The physicochemical properties of the coated blackberries were maintained during 16 days of storage at 4°C with 75% relative humidity. Additionally, the coating reduced the percentage of decay and preserved the antioxidant levels of the blackberries during storage.

Tomatoes are climacteric fruits that experience gradual deterioration after harvest, leading to a reasonably short postharvest lifespan. Furthermore, tomato fruits are prone to postharvest diseases caused by various pathogenic fungi, which can result in significant financial losses. As a result, the application of an antifungal edible coating has been extensively utilized to alleviate these issues. Rodriguez-Garcia et al. (2016) discovered that an oregano essential oil incorporated pectin-based edible coating on tomatoes had an antifungal effect against *Alternaria alternata* growth. The coating also increased the total phenols and antioxidant activity of the coated tomatoes during the 12 days of storage at 12.5°C, without any negative impact on the sensory acceptability of the tomatoes. Meanwhile, Maftoonazad and Ramaswamy (2019) conducted a study on lime fruit, in which they found that a pectin-based edible coating incorporated with beeswax was able to prolong the shelf life, slow down the ripening process, and maintain the physicochemical properties during 32 days of storage at 10°C. It is worth noting that all the aforementioned studies concluded that a pectin-based edible coating can prolong the shelf life and maintain the physicochemical quality of fresh produce while activating its antimicrobial properties during storage.

7.2.4 LIPID-BASED COATINGS

Lipid-based coatings consist of fats and oils, such as beeswax, carnauba wax, and vegetable wax. These coatings form a barrier around the fresh produce, helping to control moisture loss and respiration rate, and maintain its quality. In addition, Al-Tayyar et al. (2020) described that lipids are effective moisture-resistance barriers. The authors added that the incorporation of lipids with polysaccharides and proteins will develop the edible coating with a greater moisture barrier and mechanical resistance. Thus, lipid-based coatings are often used on fruits and vegetables that are prone to physical damage, such as cucumber, tomato, lemon, guava, orange, and eggplant, to protect them from physical damage during storage.

Rux et al. (2023) recently tested a commercial lipid-based coating called Liquidseal, which is formulated from a mixture of neutral glycerides such as esters of glycerol and fatty acids. This product was observed to prolong the shelf life of fresh cucumbers by mitigating water loss and fruit respiration during retail storage. Additionally, the authors reported that Liquidseal can also reduce tissue stiffness in fresh cucumbers, which is important to enhance the appearance of the product during retail.

Furthermore, Zewdie et al. (2022) researched to explore the potential of coating tomatoes with a combination of beeswax and the extraction of neem leaf. The authors found that tomatoes treated with 9% beeswax coating and 25% neem leaf extract exhibited reduced weight loss and changes in titratable acidity, TSS, and pH during storage at ambient conditions (15.2°C–20.4°C) with relative humidity ranging from 55.53% to 69.46%. The developed edible coating has the potential to extend the shelf life of tomato fruits up to 36 days and maintain their quality, making it a feasible option for farmers, retailers, and wholesalers.

Nazrin et al. (2020) have developed an integration of coconut oil-beeswax coating to maintain lemon quality for up to 18 days under ambient conditions with a temperature of 21 ± 2°C and relative humidity of 50 ± 5%. According to the researchers, coating lemons with a 90:10 or 80:20 mixture of coconut oil-beeswax increases shelf life and preserves the fruit's quality. This is accomplished by retaining the fruit's green color, cutting down respiration and production of ethylene, preventing shriveling and weight loss, and preserving the moisture content and firmness of the lemon throughout the storage period. Other lipid-based coating materials that have been used for fresh produce include vegetable wax on guava (Venu et al., 2020), carnauba wax incorporated with montmorillonite nanoclay on blood orange (Nasirifar et al., 2018), carnauba wax incorporated with nanoclay emulsions on 'Valencia' orange (Motamedi et al., 2018), and carnauba wax emulsion dip coating on eggplant (Singh et al., 2016). All of the above-mentioned materials have demonstrated remarkable efficacy in conserving the condition of the fruits and extending their shelf life, as presented in Table 7.4.

TABLE 7.4 A summary of Lipid-Based Coating on the Fresh Produce

Fresh Produce	Remarks	References
Cucumber	• Commercial lipid-based coatings, namely LiquidSeal, are used in this study. The main ingredients are neutral glycerides, i.e., esters of glycerol and fatty acids. • Reduce the water loss (54–68%) and fruit respiration (approximately 33%) of fresh cucumber under simulated retail conditions at 20°C and 65% relative humidity for a duration of up to 8 days. • Reduce the tissue stiffness of fresh cucumbers, thus extending their shelf life.	Rux et al. (2023)
Tomato	• Combination of beeswax coating (9%) and neem leaf extract (25%). • Increased the shelf life of tomato fruits during the 36-day storage period. • Efficiently cut down weight loss by 55–68%, the revision in titratable acidity by 20–66.7%, pH by 6.3–14.1%, and total soluble solids by 2.8–6.9%.	Zewdie at al. (2022)

TABLE 7.4 *(Continued)*

Fresh Produce	Remarks	References
Lemon	• Integration of coconut oil-beeswax coating (90:10/ 80:20). • Increase the shelf life and maintain the quality of the lemon in terms of reducing respiration and ethylene production, retaining its green color, preventing weight loss and shriveling, and preserving the moisture content and firmness of the lemon throughout the 18 days of storage.	Nasrin et al. (2020)
Guava	• Guava fruits were coated with vegetable wax (1:4 v/v). • Reduce the physiological losses in weight, pectin methyl esterase activity, and malondialdehyde content. • Effective in delaying the fruit's skin yellowing. • Throughout the 12-day storage period at 10°C, the treated samples exhibited higher firmness, total phenolic and ascorbic contents, as well as enhanced total antioxidant activity.	Venu et al. (2020)
Blood orange	• Carnauba wax coatings incorporated with montmorillonite nanoclay are used in this study. • Resulting in the highest acidity and antioxidant activity. • Show the lowest level of deformation and dissolved solids. • Fruits coating showed better brightness, which was reflected in the maximum changes in components "*L*" and "*a*."	Nasirifar et al. (2018)
'Valencia' orange	• 'Valencia' orange was coated with carnauba wax incorporated with 1 w % of nanoclay emulsions. • Effectively slowed down the respiration rates and weight loss of fruits, while also preserving their sensory and nutritional quality over a period of 8 weeks, under storage conditions of 4°C and 80% relative humidity.	Motamedi et al. (2018)
Eggplant	• Carnauba wax emulsion dip coating. • Reduced physiological weight loss, glossiness effect, and improved moisture retention. • Enhancing the storage life under ambient temperature.	Singh et al. (2016)

7.3 MECHANISMS OF ACTION OF EDIBLE COATINGS IN EXTENDING SHELF LIFE OF FRESH PRODUCE

Miteluț et al. (2021) emphasized that edible coatings play a crucial role in prolonging the shelf life of fresh produce by safeguarding it against physical, chemical, and biological factors that lead to spoilage.

According to Maringgal et al. (2020a), an edible coating refers to a thin layer applied to the surface of a fruit, serving as a protective barrier that separates the fruit and its surrounding environment. The mechanisms of action of edible coatings can vary depending on the type of coating and the fresh produce being treated, but some of the most common mechanisms include:

7.3.1 CONTROLLING MOISTURE LOSS AND FRESH WEIGHT LOSS

Fresh produce can lose moisture through transpiration, a process where water vapor is released from the surface of the product (Mahajan and Lee, 2023). The moisture content decreased as the storage period increased, suggesting that the fresh weight loss percentage of the fruit was impacted by the loss of water from the fruit. Moreover, moisture loss is a crucial factor that significantly contributes to the decline in the quality of fresh produce, potentially leading to reduced nutritional value, limp texture, flaccidity, withering, and shriveling (Al-Tayyar et al., 2020).

Edible coatings can help to slow down this process by forming a barrier around the produce, minimizing the exchange of moisture between the produce and its surrounding environment. This can help to maintain the quality and texture of the fresh produce after harvest. Parven et al. (2020) supported this claim with their finding that aloe vera gel coating facilitated retaining moisture content in fruit, thus reducing weight loss of papaya during storage at ambient temperature. This might be due to the ability of edible coatings to slow down the transpiration loss of fresh produce, which may be attributed to their capacity to limit changes in the internal gas atmosphere within the intercellular spaces of the fruit (Maringgal et al., 2020a). The results of this investigation also show that an aloe vera gel coating could be a promising solution to mitigate storage, transportation, and marketing issues with papaya.

Another finding by Maringgal et al. (2020b) revealed that fresh weight loss is linked to the firmness of papayas, both coated and uncoated, with Malaysian stingless bee honey. Their results also showed that weight loss from fruit increased with the decrease in firmness, indicating a proportional relationship. The observed low correlation between firmness and fresh weight loss also resulted in textural loss and changes in cellular composition in papayas. The research has also demonstrated that edible coating acts as an ideal barrier that partially reduces water movement and minimizes moisture loss from the surface of fresh produce (Maringgal et al., 2020a).

7.3.2 CONTROLLING GAS EXCHANGE

Fresh produce continues to release and absorb gases such as carbon dioxide and oxygen even after harvest, which can affect its quality and shelf life (Jafarzadeh et al., 2021; Maringgal et al., 2021). However, edible coatings can help to regulate the exchange of gases, maintaining an optimal balance that supports the produce's respiration and prevents the growth of microorganisms. In addition, this preservation method entails applying a layer of biological or chemical material onto the surface of the product, creating a barrier that restricts gaseous exchange and ultimately delays the ripening process. Ma et al. (2021) demonstrated through their research that edible coatings can decelerate the respiration rate of mango fruit by limiting alterations in the internal gas atmosphere within the intercellular spaces of fruits. As a result, the metabolism rate of fruits decreased by reducing the internal ethylene concentration and increasing the carbon dioxide concentration.

The use of edible coatings as a modified atmosphere technique has demonstrated effective results in preserving fruits (Saleem et al., 2020; Tabassum and Khan, 2020). The method employs biological or chemical materials as a coating layer on the product's surface in order to halt gaseous exchange, thereby slowing down the ripening process. Sousa et al. (2021) assessed the influence of synergic edible coatings of hydroxypropyl methylcellulose and beeswax in concentrations of 10, 20, and 40% on 'Palmer' mangoes retained at 21°C for 15 days. The results of the study indicate that edible coating can offer remarkable advantages for preserving the quality of 'Palmer' mango postharvest by slowing down the ripening process and preserving the texture and color of both the peel and pulp. The authors highlighted that the application of the edible coating preserves the titratable acidity and soluble solids, reduces weight loss and disease incidence, and minimizes the synthesis of sugars by inhibiting the activities of alcohol dehydrogenase and fruit fermentation.

7.3.3 PROVIDING A PHYSICAL BARRIER

Edible coatings can help to protect fresh produce from physical damage, such as bruising, that can lead to spoilage. Physical damage to the fruit's tissue may result in microbial contamination (Zhao et al., 2022). The coatings can also reduce the exposure of the produce to contaminants, such as dust and bacteria, that can cause spoilage (Armghan et al., 2022).

According to Chaudhary et al. (2020), edible coatings serve as protective coverings for fresh produce and also act as carriers for antimicrobial agents and various functional compounds. Furthermore, it was reported that an edible coating, namely Decco Shield, made from micronized calcium carbonate, can maintain firmness retention, weight loss retention, act as a physical barrier to pathogens, delay the development of scald, and maintain the natural appearance of apples (Decco, 2023).

Taher et al. (2020) and Pirozzi et al. (2020) added that the edible coating acts as a physical barrier on tomatoes that helps in maintaining firmness during storage and thus reduces weight loss. Similarly, Kumar et al. (2021) demonstrated that a composite coating synergizing chitosan-pullulan with pomegranate peel extract was beneficial for preserving the firmness and minimizing the weight loss of tomatoes throughout the 18-day storage at room temperature and cold storage at 4°C. This might be due to the fact that the edible coating has decreased the process of respiration, which has aided in inhibiting the actions of enzymes that break down cell walls and promote weight loss. Some researchers also believed that by providing a protective covering over the stem scars of tomatoes, they could reduce moisture loss during storage (Yadav et al., 2022).

7.3.4 INHIBITING ENZYMATIC ACTIVITY

Fruits and vegetables contain enzymes that can break down the product and cause spoilage that leads to economic losses (Kaczmarek et al., 2019). Edible coatings can help to slow down the activity of these enzymes, extending the shelf life of the fresh produce (Miteluţ et al., 2021). For instance, the combination of gum Arabic and roselle extract as edible coating materials has been shown to have a strong inhibitory effect on the activity of the enzymes polyphenol oxidase (PPO) and guaiacol peroxidase (POD), which contribute to the physicochemical quality of the stored blueberry (Yang et al., 2019). According to Zhao et al. (2019), inhibiting the PPO enzyme activity will maintain the cellular membrane of the coated fresh produce, thus slowing down the firmness deterioration process. Meanwhile, inhibiting the POD enzyme activity will reduce the degradation of total anthocyanin content in fresh produce, where it is associated with antioxidant activities (Yang et al., 2019).

A seminal study in this area is the work of Saleem et al. (2021), where they incorporated chitosan with an ascorbic acid-based edible coating to enhance the postharvest quality and storage stability of strawberry fruits. The edible coating was found to be effective in improving the fruit's firmness by reducing the activities of cell wall-degrading enzymes, that is, polygalacturonase, cellulase, and pectin methyl esterase. Additionally, the incorporation of ascorbic acid into chitosan coating has been shown to stimulate the activities of reactive oxygen species (ROS) scavenging enzymes, such as ascorbate peroxidase, catalase, peroxidase, and superoxide dismutase (SOD). Thus, the role of edible coating is undeniable in maintaining the postharvest quality of fresh produce during storage, especially by inhibiting enzymatic activities.

7.3.5 PREVENTING MICROBIAL GROWTH

The development of microorganisms such as bacteria and fungi can lead to the spoilage of fresh produce (Alegbeleye et al., 2022). Edible coatings can help to prevent the growth of these microorganisms by creating an inhospitable environment, reducing the exchange of gases, and providing a physical barrier. Chitosan-based coatings have been shown to have strong antimicrobial properties, making them effective in preventing the growth of a range of microorganisms. Arroyo et al. (2020) have created an antimicrobial active edible coating made from alginate and chitosan added with ZnO nanoparticles for guava (*Psidium guajava* L.) fruits. The results of their study indicate that coatings have the ability to prevent the appearance of rot in all guava fruits, which is associated with the antibacterial activity of nanoZnO. These results further support the idea of Esparza-González et al. (2016), who stated that the metallic oxide exhibited antimicrobial properties and inhibits the growth of pathogenic microorganisms very effectively.

Prakash et al. (2020) investigated the impact of a sodium alginate-based edible coating that contained 0.5% and 1% concentrations of citral nanoemulsion on the physical and chemical properties, microbial activity, and sensory analysis of fresh-cut pineapples preserved at 4°C with relative humidity at 90% for 12 days. The researchers discovered that by applying a citral nanoemulsion coating, the fresh-cut pineapples had excellent color retention (with higher *L* and **b* values), reduced microbial growth, and a lower respiration rate during storage. Additionally, the application of citral nanoemulsion coating at 0.5% concentration led to a reduction of 2.52 and 2.23 log CFU/g of artificially inoculated **Salmonella* enterica and Listeria monocytogenes, respectively, in coated fresh cut pineapples. Surprisingly, higher concentrations of citral coating (1%) were found to reduce texture and sensory tolerance.

7.3.6 IMPROVING NUTRITIONAL VALUE

In some cases, edible coatings can be formulated to provide additional nutritional benefits. For example, coatings can be enriched with antioxidants, vitamins, and minerals that are beneficial to human health (Zehiroglu et al., 2019). This can help enhance the nutritional value of fresh produce and make it more appealing to consumers.

The study by Huang et al. (2019) offers favorable effects for the quality maintenance of mushrooms (*Lentinus edodes*) during 16 days of postharvest storage (4 ± 1°C) by using a chitosan and guar gum-based composite edible coating. The authors added that the edible coating slowed the rate of declines in soluble protein and ascorbic acid and had a significant effect on the mushroom's firmness during the storage period, especially on the concentration of 1% chitosan and 15% guar gum. Research findings by Sathiyaseelan et al. (2021) also point towards the fact that the shelf life and quality of fresh-cut red bell pepper coated with chitosan-tea tree oil nanoemulsion and calcium chloride were increased when stored at 4°C. Furthermore, the high nutritional value and distinct flavor profile of whole or fresh-cut bell peppers have been identified to extend the shelf-life and enhance the quality of fresh-cut red bell peppers for up to 18 days at 4°C, thereby emphasizing their industrial significance.

A longitudinal study of edible coating on fresh produce by Farina et al. (2020) reports that freshly sliced 'Fuji' apples coated with an aloe vera gel-based edible coating combined with natural anti-browning and antioxidant compounds enhanced post-harvest quality. The results of the proximate analysis of this study, including minerals, essential elements, nutrients, and vitamin content, indicated that the coating did not modify the innate properties of the coated fresh-cut apples and maintained constant values throughout the low-temperature storage (4 ± 1°C) and 90% ± 5% relative humidity (RH) for 9 days. The evidence from this study suggests that edible coating did not alter the nutritional value of the fresh produce while maintaining the other physicochemical qualities.

7.4 REGULATION ON EDIBLE COATINGS FOR FRESH PRODUCE

Edible coatings are becoming a popular postharvest processing method due to their eco-friendly nature, and they are typically made from animal and vegetable products (Al-Tayyar et al., 2020; Chavan et al., 2023). The main ingredients of edible coatings are proteins, polysaccharides, and lipids, along with minor components like plasticizers, emulsifiers, and active ingredients such as antimicrobials and antioxidants. However, the amount of each component needs to be carefully balanced to achieve the desired effect, and the composition of the coating must adhere to specific regulations for each food product. This agrees with Galus et al. (2020), who emphasize that edible coatings must adhere to all food additive regulations in the applicable jurisdiction.

In the United States, the constituents used in edible coatings must be classified as generally recognized as safe (GRAS) and listed in the Code of Federal Regulations. Similarly, the European Directive (1995) permits the use of Arabic gum, karaya gum, pectins, shellac, beeswax, candelilla wax, and carnauba wax in edible coatings, with an expansion in 1998 to include lecithin, polysorbates, fatty acids, and fatty acid salts. Furthermore, the US Food and Drug Administration (FDA, 2006) has granted approval for additional additives to be used in protective coatings for fresh fruits and vegetables (FFVs), such as polydextrose, sorbitan monostearate, sucrose fatty acid esters, cocoa butter, and castor oil.

Several edible coating materials have been developed, including chitosan, aloe vera, cellulose, and protein-based materials, which can be combined with active ingredients to provide superior barrier properties and antimicrobial activity while maintaining taste and texture (Dhall, 2013). As Chhikara and Kumar (2022) suggested, ideal edible coatings should be transparent, tasteless, and odorless, while also allowing for sufficient water vapor and solutes to pass through, as well as selectively permitting the exchange of gases and volatile compounds.

7.5 CHALLENGES AND FUTURE TRENDS

Edible coatings have emerged as a promising technology to prolong the shelf life and maintain the physicochemical quality of fresh produce. However, despite their advantages, there are still certain challenges and future trends that must be addressed to fully harness the potential of this technology.

One of the main challenges of edible coatings is to achieve a balance between the functional properties of the coatings and their sensory characteristics. Consumers demand high-quality products with desirable appearance, texture, and flavor. However, some edible coatings may affect the organoleptic properties of the treated products, leading to decreased consumer acceptance. Therefore, it is essential to develop coatings that can provide adequate protection to fresh produce and are non-toxic while maintaining their sensory attributes.

Another challenge is related to the scalability and cost-effectiveness of the technology. The development of edible coatings requires specialized equipment, materials, and processes that may increase production costs. Hence, it is crucial to optimize the formulation and application processes to make them more affordable and feasible for large-scale applications. Moreover, the use of natural and sustainable materials is becoming increasingly important to meet the demand for eco-friendly products.

In addition, the efficacy of edible coatings can vary depending on the type of fresh produce, the storage conditions, and the pathogens present. Consequently, it is essential to conduct extensive research to evaluate the effectiveness of the coatings under different scenarios and optimize their performance accordingly. Besides, the combination of edible coatings with other preservation methods, such as controlled atmosphere (CA) and (MAP, can enhance their effectiveness and provide better preservation results. The effectiveness of edible coatings can be further amplified through the use of advanced disinfection methods, active packaging, and hurdle technologies to counteract the various forms of spoilage.

Future trends in edible coatings for fresh produce include the development of multi-functional coatings that can provide multiple benefits simultaneously, such as antimicrobial activity, antioxidant activity, and sensory improvement. The use of nanotechnology in edible coatings is also a promising area for future research, as it can enhance the performance of the coatings by providing better control over the release of active compounds and improving their mechanical properties. The reason for this is that the nanomaterial has a larger surface area, which enables it to have better contact with the cell membrane and allows for improved absorption and migration of the nanomaterial into the fresh produce. Additionally, the development of intelligent coatings that can respond to external stimuli, such as temperature, humidity, or light, can provide better protection to fresh produce and increase its shelf life.

7.6 CONCLUSION

In this chapter, edible coatings have shown great potential for preserving the quality and prolonging the shelf life of fresh produce. The most recent advancements in this area involve the widespread application of chitosan, carrageenan, pectin, and lipids as the primary components for creating edible coatings. These bases are combined with various functional additives, such as essential oils, plant extracts, antioxidant extracts, and nanoparticles in their nanoforms. The functional ingredients added to the main bases of edible coatings play a crucial role beyond providing a protective barrier for the fresh produce. These ingredients not only extend the shelf life and maintain the physicochemical quality during storage but also enhance the nutritional and antimicrobial values of the produce. It is crucial to understand the mechanisms of action of edible coatings in extending the shelf life of fresh produce to achieve maximum benefits. Nevertheless, some challenges, such as maintaining sensory attributes, toxicity, scalability, and efficacy, need to be addressed to fully exploit the potential of this technology. Future trends include the development of multi-functional coatings, nanotechnology-based coatings, and intelligent coatings, which can provide better protection and enhance the performance of the coatings. The continuous development of this technology can significantly benefit the fresh produce industry, reduce food waste, and meet the growing demand for high-quality and sustainable products.

KEYWORDS

- **edible coatings**
- **fresh produce preservation**
- **functional additives**
- **nanotechnology-based coatings**
- **physicochemical quality**
- **shelf life extension**

REFERENCES

Abdi, S., & Bakhshi, D. (2019). Pectin edible coatings enriched with essential oils of lemon and thyme to improve storage of black raspberry. *Journal of Postharvest Technology, 7*(3), 18–29.

Afifah, N., Ratnawati, L., & Darmajana, D. A. (2019). Evaluation of plasticizer addition in composite edible coating on quality of fresh-cut mangoes during storage. In *IOP Conference Series: Earth and Environmental Science, 251*(1), 012029. IOP Publishing.

Alegbeleye, O., Odeyemi, O. A., Strateva, M., & Stratev, D. (2022). Microbial spoilage of vegetables, fruits and cereals. *Applied Food Research, 2*(1), 100122.

Al-Tayyar, N. A., Youssef, A. M., & Al-Hindi, R. R. (2020). Edible coatings and antimicrobial nano emulsions for enhancing shelf life and reducing foodborne pathogens of fruits and vegetables: A review. *Sustainable Materials and Technologies, 26*, e00215.

Armghan Khalid, M., Niaz, B., Saeed, F., Afzaal, M., Islam, F., Hussain, M., & Al-Farga, A. (2022). Edible coatings for enhancing safety and quality attributes of fresh produce: A comprehensive review. *International Journal of Food Properties, 25*(1), 1817–1847.

Arroyo, B. J., Bezerra, A. C., Oliveira, L. L., Arroyo, S. J., de Melo, E. A., & Santos, A. M. P. (2020). Antimicrobial active edible coating of alginate and chitosan add ZnO nanoparticles applied in guavas (*Psidium guajava* L.). *Food Chemistry, 309*, 125566.

Chavan, P., Lata, K., Kaur, T., Jambrak, A. R., Sharma, S., Roy, S., & Rout, A. (2023). Recent advances in the preservation of postharvest fruits using edible films and coatings: A comprehensive review. *Food Chemistry, 418*, 135916.

Chetia, J., Adhikary, P., Devi, L. M., & Badwaik, L. S. (2023). Extraction of essential oil from Assam lemon peels and its incorporation in chitosan-based coating for maintaining grape quality. *Sustainable Chemistry and Pharmacy, 32*, 101034.

Chhikara, S., & Kumar, D. (2022). Edible coating and edible film as food packaging material: A review. *Journal of Packaging Technology and Research, 6*, 1–10.

da Silva Bruni, A. R., Friedrichsen, J. D. S. A., de Jesus, G. A. M., da Silva Alves, E., da Costa, J. C. M., Souza, P. R., & Bonafe, E. G. (2023). Characterization and application of active films based on commercial polysaccharides incorporating ZnONPs. *International Journal of Biological Macromolecules, 224*, 1322–1336.

Da Silva, I. S. V., Prado, N. S., De Melo, P. G., Arantes, D. C., Andrade, M. Z., Otaguro, H., & Pasquini, D. (2019). Edible coatings based on apple pectin, cellulose nanocrystals, and essential oil of lemongrass: Improving the quality and shelf life of strawberries (*Fragaria ananassa*). *Journal of Renewable Materials, 7*(1), 73.

Davik, J., Røen, D., Lysøe, E., Buti, M., Rossman, S., Alsheikh, M., & Sargent, D. J. (2022). A chromosome-level genome sequence assembly of the red raspberry (*Rubus idaeus* L.). *PLOS ONE, 17*(3), e0265096.

Decco Postharvest. (2023). http://www.decopostharvest.com/ (accessed on 9th July 2025).

Dhall, R. K. (2013). Advances in edible coatings for fresh fruits and vegetables: A review. *Critical Reviews in Food Science and Nutrition, 53*, 435–450.

Dulta, K., Koşarsoy Ağçeli, G., Thakur, A., Singh, S., Chauhan, P., & Chauhan, P. K. (2022). Development of alginate-chitosan based coating enriched with ZnO nanoparticles for increasing the shelf life of orange fruits (*Citrus sinensis* L.). *Journal of Polymers and the Environment, 30*(8), 3293–3306.

ED-European Parliament and Council Directive N 98/72/EC. (1998). On food additive other than colors and sweeteners. http://ec.europa.eu/food/fs/sfp/addit_flavor/flav11_en.pdf (accessed on 9th July 2025).

El-Sayed, H. S., El-Sayed, S. M., Mabrouk, A. M., Nawwar, G. A., & Youssef, A. M. (2021). Development of eco-friendly probiotic edible coatings based on chitosan, alginate and carboxymethyl cellulose for improving the shelf life of UF soft cheese. *Journal of Polymers and the Environment, 29*, 1941–1953.

Escamilla-García, M., Rodríguez-Hernández, M. J., Hernández-Hernández, H. M., Delgado-Sánchez, L. F., García-Almendárez, B. E., Amaro-Reyes, A., & Regalado-González, C. (2018). Effect of an edible coating based on chitosan and oxidized starch on shelf life of *Carica papaya* L., and its physicochemical and antimicrobial properties. *Coatings, 8*(9), 318.

Esparza-González, S. C., Sánchez-Valdés, S., Ramírez-Barrón, S. N., Loera-Arias, M. J., Bernal, J., Meléndez-Ortiz, H. I., & Betancourt-Galindo, R. (2016). Effects of different surface modifying agents on the cytotoxic and antimicrobial properties of ZnO nanoparticles. *Toxicology in Vitro, 37*, 134–141.

Farina, V., Passafiume, R., Tinebra, I., Palazzolo, E., & Sortino, G. (2020). Use of *Aloe vera* gel-based edible coating with natural anti-browning and anti-oxidant additives to improve post-harvest quality of fresh-cut 'Fuji' apple. *Agronomy, 10*(4), 515.

FDA 21CFR172. (2006). Food additives permitted for direct addition to food for human consumption, Subpart C. Coatings, films and related substances. *Coatings*. http://www.ecfr.gov (accessed on 9th July 2025).

Galus, S., Arik Kibar, E. A., Gniewosz, M., & Kraśniewska, K. (2020). Novel materials in the preparation of edible films and coatings—A review. *Coatings, 10*(7), 674.

Guerreiro, A. C., Gago, C. M., Faleiro, M. L., Miguel, M. G., & Antunes, M. D. (2015). Raspberry fresh fruit quality as affected by pectin- and alginate-based edible coatings enriched with essential oils. *Scientia Horticultural, 194*, 138–146.

Guimaraes, A., Abrunhosa, L., Pastrana, L. M., & Cerqueira, M. A. (2018). Edible films and coatings as carriers of living microorganisms: A new strategy towards bio preservation and healthier foods. *Comprehensive Reviews in Food Science and Food Safety, 17*, 594–614.

Hamzah, M. H., Rahim, A. Z. M., Maringgal, B., Basri, M. S. M., & Ibrahim, S. (2022). Optimization of silk fibroin coating during storage using response surface methodology and its effect on the physicochemical properties of *Solanum ferox* (*S. ferox*). *Journal of Food Measurement and Characterization, 16*(5), 3385–3401.

Hernández-Carrillo, J. G., Orta-Zavalza, E., González-Rodríguez, S. E., Montoya-Torres, C., Sepúlveda-Ahumada, D. R., & Ortiz-Rivera, Y. (2021). Evaluation of the effectivity of reuterin in pectin edible coatings to extend the shelf-life of strawberries during cold storage. *Food Packaging and Shelf Life, 30*, 100760.

Huang, Q., Qian, X., Jiang, T., & Zheng, X. (2019). Effect of chitosan and guar gum-based composite edible coating on quality of mushroom (*Lentinus edodes*) during postharvest storage. *Scientia Horticultural, 253*, 382–389.

Jafarzadeh, S., Nafchi, A. M., Salehabadi, A., Oladzad-Abbasabadi, N., & Jafari, S. M. (2021). Application of bio-nanocomposite films and edible coatings for extending the shelf life of fresh fruits and vegetables. *Advances in Colloid and Interface Science, 291*, 102405.

Jurić, S., Bureš, M. S., Vlahoviček-Kahlina, K., Stracenski, K. S., Fruk, G., Jalšenjak, N., & Bandić, L. M. (2023). Chitosan-based layer-by-layer edible coatings application for the preservation of mandarin fruit bioactive compounds and organic acids. *Food Chemistry: X, 17*, 100575.

Kaczmarek, M., Avery, S. V., & Singleton, I. (2019). Microbes associated with fresh produce: Sources, types and methods to reduce spoilage and contamination. In *Advances in Applied Microbiology* (Vol. 107, pp. 29–82). Academic Press.

Kumar, N., Neeraj, P., & TrajkovskaPetkoska, A. (2021). Improved shelf life and quality of tomato (*Solanum lycopersicum* L.) by using chitosan-pullulan composite edible coating enriched with pomegranate peel extract. *ACS Food Science & Technology, 1*(4), 500–510.

Ma, J., Zhou, Z., Li, K., Li, K., Liu, L., Zhang, W., & Zhang, H. (2021). Novel edible coating based on shellac and tannic acid for prolonging postharvest shelf life and improving overall quality of mango. *Food Chemistry, 354*, 129510.

Maftoonazad, N., & Ramaswamy, H. S. (2019). Application and evaluation of a pectin-based edible coating process for quality change kinetics and shelf-life extension of lime fruit (*Citrus aurantifolium*). *Coatings, 9*(5), 285.

Mahajan, P. V., & Lee, D. S. (2023). Modified atmosphere and moisture condensation in packaged fresh produce: Scientific efforts and commercial success. *Postharvest Biology and Technology, 198*, 112235.

Maringgal, B., Hashim, N., Mohamed Amin Tawakkal, I. S., Mohamed, M. T. M., Hamzah, M. H., & Mohd Ali, M. (2021). Effect of Kelulut honey nanoparticles coating on the changes of respiration rate, ascorbic acid, and total phenolic content of papaya (*Carica papaya* L.) during cold storage. *Foods, 10*(2), 432.

Maringgal, B., Hashim, N., Tawakkal, I. S. M. A., & Mohamed, M. T. M. (2020a). Recent advance in edible coating and its effect on fresh/fresh-cut fruits quality. *Trends in Food Science & Technology, 96*, 253–267.

Maringgal, B., Hashim, N., Tawakkal, I. S. M. A., Mohamed, M. T. M., Hamzah, M. H., Ali, M. M., & Abd Razak, M. F. H. (2020b). Kinetics of quality changes in papayas (*Carica papaya* L.) coated with Malaysian stingless bee honey. *Scientia Horticulturae, 267*, 109321.

Meindrawan, B., Suyatma, N. E., Wardana, A. A., & Pamela, V. Y. (2018). Nanocomposite coating based on carrageenan and ZnO nanoparticles to maintain the storage quality of mango. *Food Packaging and Shelf Life, 18*, 140–146.

Miteluț, A. C., Popa, E. E., Drăghici, M. C., Popescu, P. A., Popa, V. I., Bujor, O. C., & Popa, M. E. (2021). Latest developments in edible coatings on minimally processed fruits and vegetables: A review. *Foods, 10*(11), 2821.

Motamedi, E., Nasiri, J., Malidarreh, T. R., Kalantari, S., Naghavi, M. R., & Safari, M. (2018). Performance of carnauba wax-nano clay emulsion coatings on postharvest quality of 'Valencia' orange fruit. *Scientia Horticultural, 240*, 170–178.

Muñoz-Almagro, N., Herrero-Herranz, M., Guri, S., Corzo, N., Montilla, A., & Villamiel, M. (2021). Application of sunflower pectin gels with low glycemic index in the coating of fresh strawberries stored in modified atmospheres. *Journal of the Science of Food and Agriculture, 101*(14), 5775–5783.

Nasirifar, S. Z., Maghsoudlou, Y., & Oliyaei, N. (2018). Effect of active lipid-based coating incorporated with nano clay and orange peel essential oil on physicochemical properties of *Citrus sinensis*. *Food Science & Nutrition, 6*(6), 1508–1518.

Nasrin, T. A. A., Rahman, M. A., Arfin, M. S., Islam, M. N., & Ullah, M. A. (2020). Effect of novel coconut oil and beeswax edible coating on postharvest quality of lemon at ambient storage. *Journal of Agriculture and Food Research, 2*, 100019.

Nastasi, J. R., Kontogiorgos, V., Daygon, V. D., & Fitzgerald, M. A. (2022). Pectin-based films and coatings with plant extracts as natural preservatives: A systematic review. *Trends in Food Science & Technology, 120*, 192–211.

Panahirad, S., Dadpour, M., Peighambardoust, S. H., Soltanzadeh, M., Gullón, B., Alirezalu, K., & Lorenzo, J. M. (2021). Applications of carboxymethyl cellulose- and pectin-based active edible coatings in preservation of fruits and vegetables: A review. *Trends in Food Science & Technology, 110*, 663–673.

Parven, A., Sarker, M. R., Megharaj, M., & Meftaul, I. M. (2020). Prolonging the shelf life of papaya (*Carica papaya* L.) using *Aloe vera* gel at ambient temperature. *Scientia Horticultural, 265*, 109228.

Piechowiak, T., & Skóra, B. (2023). Edible coating enriched with cinnamon oil reduces the oxidative stress and improves the quality of strawberry fruit stored at room temperature. *Journal of the Science of Food and Agriculture, 103*(5), 2389–2400.

Pirozzi, A., Del Grosso, V., Ferrari, G., & Donsì, F. (2020). Edible coatings containing oregano essential oil nano emulsion for improving postharvest quality and shelf life of tomatoes. *Foods, 9*(11), 1605.

Prakash, A., Baskaran, R., & Vadivel, V. (2020). Citral nanoemulsion incorporated edible coating to extend the shelf life of fresh cut pineapples. *LWT, 118*, 108851.

Riaz, A., Aadil, R. M., Amoussa, A. M. O., Bashari, M., Abid, M., & Hashim, M. M. (2020). Application of chitosan-based apple peel polyphenols edible coating on the preservation of strawberry (*Fragaria ananassa* cv. Hongyan) fruit. *Journal of Food Processing and Preservation, 45*(1), e15018.

Rodriguez-Garcia, I., Cruz-Valenzuela, M. R., Silva-Espinoza, B. A., Gonzalez-Aguilar, G. A., Moctezuma, E., Gutierrez-Pacheco, M. M., & Ayala-Zavala, J. F. (2016). Oregano (*Lippia graveolens*) essential oil added within pectin edible coatings prevents fungal decay and increases the antioxidant capacity of treated tomatoes. *Journal of the Science of Food and Agriculture, 96*(11), 3772–3778.

Rux, G., Labude, C., Herppich, W. B., & Geyer, M. (2023). Investigation on the potential of applying bio-based edible coatings for horticultural products exemplified with cucumbers. *Current Research in Food Science, 6*, 100407.

Saleem, M. S., Anjum, M. A., Naz, S., Ali, S., Hussain, S., Azam, M., & Ejaz, S. (2021). Incorporation of ascorbic acid in chitosan-based edible coating improves postharvest quality and storability of strawberry fruits. *International Journal of Biological Macromolecules, 189*, 160–169.

Saleem, M. S., Ejaz, S., Anjum, M. A., Nawaz, A., Naz, S., Hussain, S., & Canan, İ. (2020). Postharvest application of gum Arabic edible coating delays ripening and maintains quality of persimmon fruits during storage. *Journal of Food Processing and Preservation, 44*(8), e14583.

Sarker, A., & Grift, T. E. (2021). Bioactive properties and potential applications of *Aloe vera* gel edible coating on fresh and minimally processed fruits and vegetables: A review. *Journal of Food Measurement and Characterization, 15*, 2119–2134.

Sathiyaseelan, A., Saravanakumar, K., Mariadoss, A. V. A., Ramachandran, C., Hu, X., Oh, D. H., & Wang, M. H. (2021). Chitosan–tea tree oil nano emulsion and calcium chloride tailored edible coating increase the shelf life of fresh cut red bell pepper. *Progress in Organic Coatings, 151*, 106010.

Shafie, M. H., Kamal, M. L., Zulkiflee, F. F., Hasan, S., Uyop, N. H., Abdullah, S., & Zafarina, Z. (2022). Application of carrageenan extract from red seaweed (*Rhodophyta*) in cosmetic products: A review. *Journal of the Indian Chemical Society, 99*(9), 100613.

Shapi'i, R. A., Othman, S. H., Nordin, N., Basha, R. K., & Naim, M. N. (2020). Antimicrobial properties of starch films incorporated with chitosan nanoparticles: *In vitro* and *in vivo* evaluation. *Carbohydrate Polymers, 230*, 115602.

Sharma, P., Shehin, V. P., Kaur, N., & Vyas, P. (2019). Application of edible coatings on fresh and minimally processed vegetables: A review. *International Journal of Vegetable Science, 25*(3), 295–314.

Sharma, S., Krishna, H., Barman, K., Kole, B., Singh, S. K., & Behera, T. K. (2022). Synergistic effect of polyamine treatment and chitosan coating on postharvest senescence and enzyme activity of bell pepper (*Capsicum annuum* L.) fruit. *South African Journal of Botany, 151*, 175–184.

Singh, S., Khemariya, P., Rai, A., Rai, A. C., Koley, T. K., & Singh, B. (2016). Carnauba wax-based edible coating enhances shelf-life and retain quality of eggplant (*Solanum melongena*) fruits. *LWT, 74*, 420–426.

Sousa, F. F., Junior, J. S. P., Oliveira, K. T., Rodrigues, E. C., Andrade, J. P., & Mattiuz, B. H. (2021). Conservation of 'Palmer' mango with an edible coating of hydroxypropyl methylcellulose and beeswax. *Food Chemistry, 346*, 128925.

Suryanto, H., Yanuhar, U., Pradana, Y. R. A., & Bintara, R. D. (2023). Starch/carrageenan blend-based bio composites as packaging materials. In *Composites from the Aquatic Environment* (pp. 139–161). Springer, Singapore.

Tabassum, N., & Khan, M. A. (2020). Modified atmosphere packaging of fresh-cut papaya using alginate-based edible coating: Quality evaluation and shelf-life study. *Scientia Horticultural, 259*, 108853.

Taher, M. A., MennatAllah, E. A., Tadros, L. K., & Sanad, M. I. (2020). The effects of new formulations based on gum Arabic on antioxidant capacity of tomato

(*Solanum lycopersicum* L.) fruit during storage. *Journal of Food Measurement and Characterization, 14*, 2489–2502.

Tavassoli-Kafrani, E., Gamage, M. V., Dumée, L. F., Kong, L., & Zhao, S. (2022). Edible films and coatings for shelf-life extension of mango: A review. *Critical Reviews in Food Science and Nutrition, 62*(9), 2432–2459.

Tavassoli-Kafrani, E., Shekarchizadeh, H., & Masoudpour-Behabadi, M. (2016). Development of edible films and coatings from alginates and carrageenans. *Carbohydrate Polymers, 137*, 360–374.

Tumbarski, Y., Petkova, N., Todorova, M., Ivanov, I., Deseva, I., Mihaylova, D., & Ibrahim, S. A. (2020). Effects of pectin-based edible coatings containing a bacteriocin of *Bacillus methylotrophicus* BM47 on the quality and storage life of fresh blackberries. *Italian Journal of Food Science, 32*(2).

Wani, S. M., Gull, A., Ahad, T., Malik, A. R., Ganaie, T. A., Masoodi, F. A., & Gani, A. (2021). Effect of gum Arabic, xanthan and carrageenan coatings containing antimicrobial agent on postharvest quality of strawberry: Assessing the physicochemical, enzyme activity and bioactive properties. *International Journal of Biological Macromolecules, 183*, 2100–2108.

Woods, J. L. (1990). Moisture loss from fruits and vegetables. *Postharvest News and Information, 1*, 195.

Yadav, A., Kumar, N., Upadhyay, A., Sethi, S., & Singh, A. (2022). Edible coating as postharvest management strategy for shelf-life extension of fresh tomato (*Solanum lycopersicum* L.): An overview. *Journal of Food Science, 87*(6), 2256–2290.

Yang, Z., Zou, X., Li, Z., Huang, X., Zhai, X., Zhang, W., & Tahir, H. E. (2019). Improved postharvest quality of cold stored blueberry by edible coating based on composite gum Arabic/roselle extract. *Food and Bioprocess Technology, 12*, 1537–1547.

Zárate-Moreno, J. C., Escobar-Sierra, D. M., & Ríos-Estepa, R. (2023). Development and evaluation of chitosan-based food coatings for exotic fruit preservation. *BioTech, 12*(1), 20.

Zehiroglu, C., & Ozturk Sarikaya, S. B. (2019). The importance of antioxidants and place in today's scientific and technological studies. *Journal of Food Science and Technology, 56*, 4757–4774.

Zewdie, B., Shonte, T. T., & Woldetsadik, K. (2022). Shelf life and quality of tomato (*Lycopersicon esculentum* Mill.) fruits as affected by neem leaf extract dipping and beeswax coating. *International Journal of Food Properties, 25*(1), 570–592.

Zhao, H., Liu, B., Zhang, W., Cao, J., & Jiang, W. (2019). Enhancement of quality and antioxidant metabolism of sweet cherry fruit by near-freezing temperature storage. *Postharvest Biology and Technology, 147*, 113–122.

Zhao, P., Ndayambaje, J. P., Liu, X., & Xia, X. (2022). Microbial spoilage of fruits: A review on causes and prevention methods. *Food Reviews International, 38*(sup1), 225–246

CHAPTER 8

Distribution Packaging of Fresh Produce and Its Sustainability Trends

SAOWAPA CHAIWONG,[1,2,*] RAVINUN SAENGWONG-NGAM,[2] RATTAPON SAENGRAYAP,[1,2] JUTARAT RATTANAKARAN,[2] CHUREERAT PRAHSARN,[3] and TATIYA TRONGSATITKUL[4]

[1]*School of Agro-Industry, Mae Fah Luang University, Chiang Rai, Thailand*

[2]*Integrated Agri-Tech Ecosystem Research Group, Mae Fah Luang University, Chiang Rai, Thailand*

[3]*National Metal and Materials Technology Center, National Science and Technology Development Agency, Pathum Thani, Thailand*

[4]*School of Polymer Engineering, Institute of Engineering, Suranaree University of Technology, Nakhon Ratchasima, Thailand*

*Corresponding author

ABSTRACT

Fruit cushioning material serves as a primary packaging to provide mechanical damage protection from major impact and vibration forces. Nowadays, cushioning materials, either synthetic or natural based, are available in various forms, and their effectiveness in protection relies on many factors, including design, product shape, size, and weight, as well as choice of use. In this chapter, example cases have shown that impact force depends on various factors such as drop height, number of drops, and surface material, while vibration force level varies on acceleration, frequency, and time journey. Expanded polyethylene (EPE) with foam

Sustainable Approaches in Postharvest Handling and Management: Pankaj B. Pathare (Ed.)

DOI: 10.1201/9781779641076-8

net design has been widely used for an individual fruit cover to protect fruit bruising. An eco-friendly cushion material for distribution packaging systems has been developed from natural materials such as paper, natural fibers, and natural rubber latex. Nevertheless, little academic research has been conducted on the development of cushioning materials from natural resources in terms of their designs and functions. In addition, this chapter also discusses distribution packaging of fresh produce, serving as a secondary packaging during transportation and distribution, such as corrugated fiberboard boxes, foam boxes, and plastic crates. Packaging systems with thermal insulation are currently focused on cold chain management of fresh produce to maintain temperature fluctuation and freshness during transportation. Foam boxes are still commercially used to keep cold temperatures of food products and fresh produce for shipment. Other multilayer thermal insulation materials applied in covers and boxes are mainly synthetic materials such as aluminum foil, polystyrene, polyurethane, nonwoven, and EPE. Recently, natural fiber has been considered as an alternative material for developing sustainable packaging systems. Utilization of natural materials as distribution packaging systems has gained interest both in companies and consumers who seek sustainable alternatives to conventional plastic packaging. With success in development, these alternative packaging systems from natural resources offer effective solutions for protecting fresh produce during transportation as well as minimizing environmental impact.

8.1 INTRODUCTION

Distribution packaging of fresh produce prevents damage during physical handling and transportation. Sustainable packaging has recently been adopted in fresh produce applications to satisfy consumer demands and environmental concerns. Taxes on nondegradable packaging and environmental improvement fees have also been implemented (Sohn et al., 2019). Cushioning, as a primary packaging, plays an important role in controlling mechanical damage to fruits, reducing postharvest losses of fresh produce (Kitazawa, 2018) as well as improving visual appearance and consumer acceptance. Conventional plastic foams are commercially applied as cushioning materials to protect against mechanical damage of fruits during transportation (Dubey and Mishra, 2019). Until recently, scant research has addressed the design of natural packaging cushioning for fruit protection. Most natural cushioning materials are conventionally based on paper, such as trays and partition designs. Cold chain management of fresh produce is another important issue to reduce postharvest losses by controlling temperature throughout the supply chain (Centobelli et al., 2020). Thermal insulation materials are used to maintain fruit freshness under ambient temperature in small-scale businesses (Kitinoja, 2013). Foam sheets/boxes have been widely used for commercial packing of food products due to their excellent thermal insulation properties. Aluminum foil (ALF) is also frequently used to improve thermal insulation efficiency (Singh et al., 2008; Wang et al., 2020; Zeng et al., 2022). Research studies now concentrate on biodegradable packaging to reduce the adverse effects of environmental pollution.

This chapter describes primary packaging cushioning materials, which include corrugated fiberboard boxes and foam boxes, as well as pallet covers as secondary or tertiary packaging. Impact or drop tests in laboratories illustrate different primary factors such as drop height and surface material. Simulated vibration tests focus on acceleration, frequency, and time for vibration conditions. Cushioning designs of both natural and synthetic materials offer protection against mechanical fruit damage under impact, drop, and vibration tests. Corrugated fiberboard boxes impact ventilation and compressive strength. Thermal insulation materials, employed as either pallet covers or placed inside corrugated fiberboard boxes, help maintain cold temperature during fresh produce storage and transportation, thus improving cold chain management.

8.2 PACKAGING SYSTEM, FUNCTION AND FORMAT FOR FRESH PRODUCE

8.2.1 PACKAGING SYSTEM FOR FRESH PRODUCE

Packaging is an extremely complicated and interconnected system, which can be defined as a series of operations that serve the purpose of producing product sales units (Pongrácz, 2007). Three types of packing are generally considered as primary, secondary, and tertiary. Primary packaging involves the basic product and is carried home by the end consumer from the store (Figure 8.1). Secondary packages, also known as transport packages, are used to house multiple principal shipments. A secondary package could be carried home by the end user or may be utilized by retailers as product support when stocking shelves in the store. Tertiary packaging is used when a group of primary or secondary packages is assembled, for example, stretch films for covering a pallet, tension nets, or ties for strapping the unit load are examples of tertiary packaging. Table 8.1 defines some commonly used terms, as well as the correlation between them and the three packaging types (Gustafsson et al., 2009).

Common primary packaging includes punnets, bags, plastic trays, and net bags, which are used to display berry fruits, bananas, cabbage, cauliflower, broccoli, and oranges in supermarkets (Figure 8.2). Common footprint packaging (secondary packaging) is used to pack various vegetables and fruits for international shipping, as well as in US and EU countries (Figure 8.3A), while regular slotted carton (RSC) and full telescope design (FTD) boxes are commonly used for tropical fruits exported from Thailand (Figure 8.3B and 8.3C). Palletization as tertiary packaging by column stacking is shown for exported Jaffa tangerines in Israel and Cavendish bananas at Dole plc, UK (Figure 8.4).

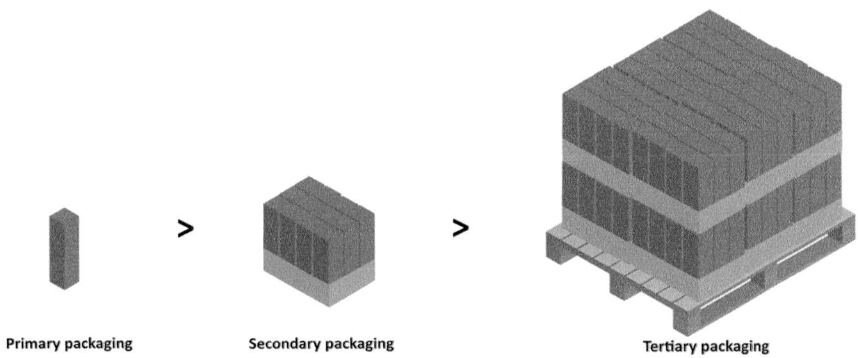

FIGURE 8.1 Packaging types as primary, secondary and tertiary.
Source: Adapted from Gustafsson et al. (2009).

TABLE 8.1 Definitions of Different Packaging Types

Packaging Type	Definition
Primary packaging	Can contact food and is usually taken home.
Secondary packaging	Designed to contain and support multiple primary packaging.
Tertiary packaging	Designed to be easier to move, display, handle and/or protect various primary or transport packages.
Consumer packaging	Primary packaging.
Sales packaging	Primary packaging.

TABLE 8.1 *(Continued)*

Packaging Type	Definition
Transport packaging	Designed to make it easier to use primary packages for efficient production and distribution together with preventing physical handling and transport damage.
Box	Secondary packaging for transport.
Bulk packaging	Similar to transport packaging with size larger than 1 cubic meter.
Distribution packaging	Properties are the same as transport packaging.
Display packaging	Grouping packaging that focuses on displaying the features of the product.
Retail packaging	Focuses on the design to fit the product shelf.

Source: Gustafsson et al. (2009).

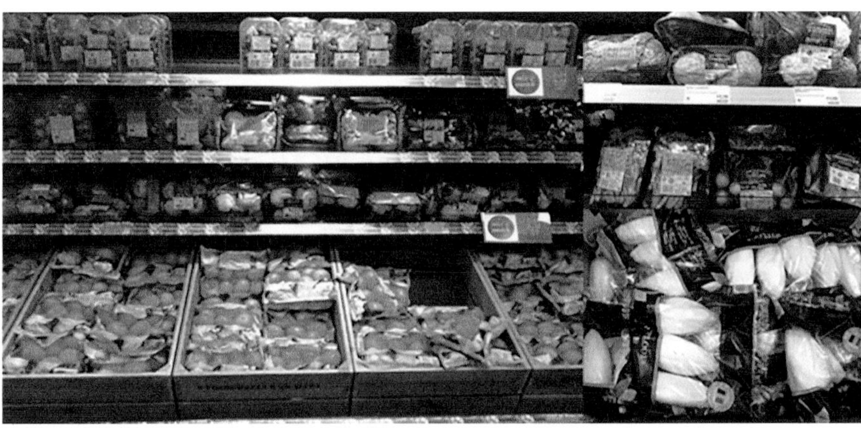

FIGURE 8.2 Primary packaging of fresh produce on display at retail stores.

Source: Authors.

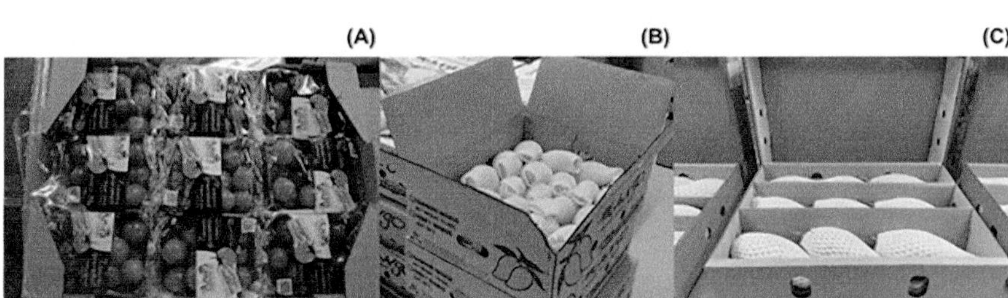

FIGURE 8.3 Secondary packaging as a common footprint package of fresh produce in the UK (A); RSC (B); and FTD design box of 'Nam Dok Mai See Thong' mangoes (C).

Source: Authors.

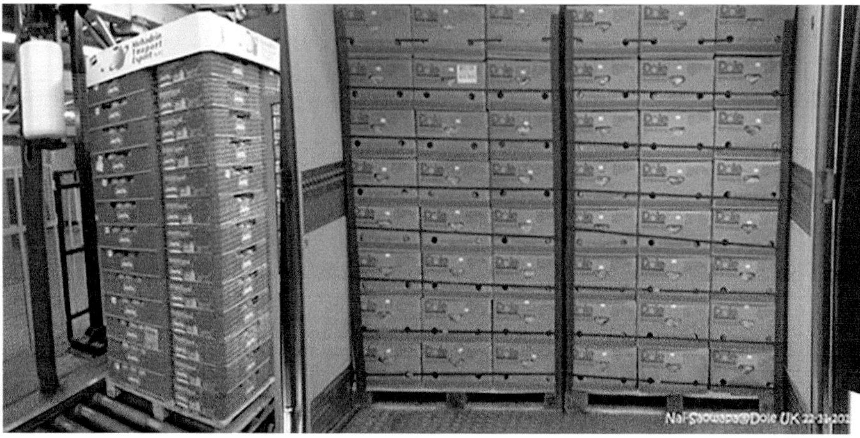

FIGURE 8.4 Tertiary packaging of Jaffa tangerine in Israel and column stacking of cavendish banana at Dole plc, UK.

Source: Authors.

8.2.2 PACKAGING FORMATS FOR AGRICULTURAL PRODUCE

Fresh produce can be provided in either bulk or retail packing options. Bulk packaging is used to transport large amounts of fresh fruit through a supply chain and protect products from physical damage while streamlining delivery and handling. It is utilized for harvesting, storing, wholesaling, and even selling fresh products for different supply chain functions. Structural qualities of bulk packaging include strength, stackability, usability, and efficient use of available space (Figure 8.5) (FAO, 2011).

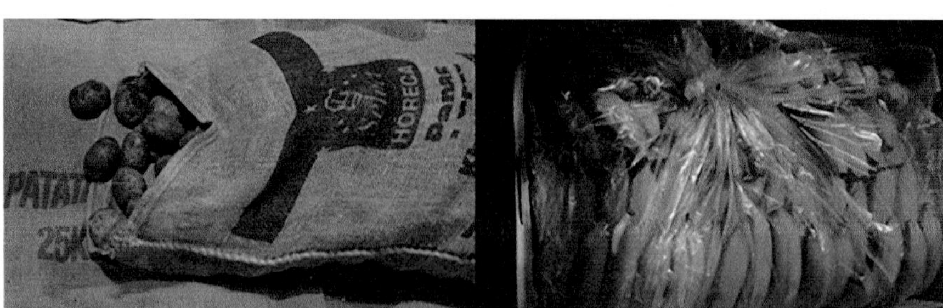

FIGURE 8.5 Bulk packaging of potato at High Tree Packers, Ltd. and Cavendish banana at Dole plc, UK.

Source: Authors.

A retail produce package is ready to sell, such as a packed bunch of bananas or salad, a punnet or tray of strawberries or tomatoes or peaches, or an individually shrink-wrapped zucchini (Figure 8.6). The primary benefits of fruit and vegetable packaging for retail are as follows: (i) the package protects the produce from physical damage; (ii) the package ensures food safety by keeping the produce clean and free of dust, dirt, and microorganism contamination; (iii) the package enables the display of printed information, such as product identification and storage guidelines; and (iv) the package extends shelf life by creating modified atmosphere packaging (MAP) (Porat et al., 2018).

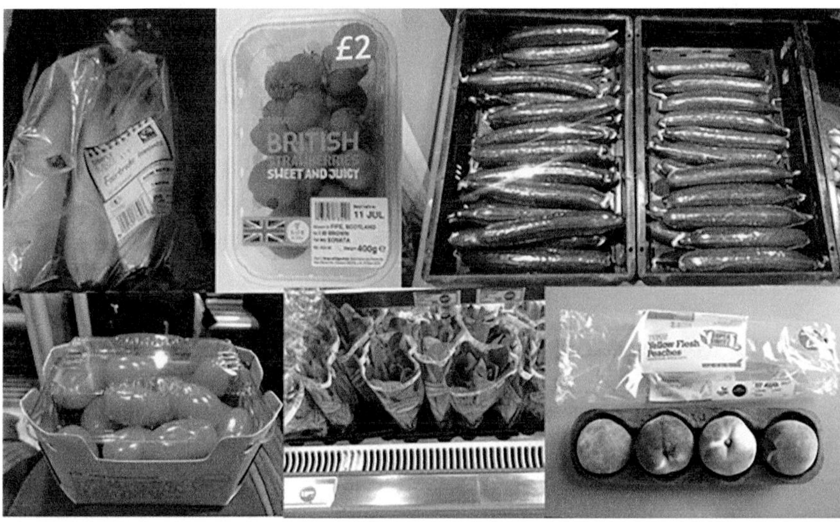

FIGURE 8.6 Retail packages of fruit and vegetables.

Source: Authors.

8.3 EFFECTS OF CUSHIONING ON IMPACT AND VIBRATION FRUIT DAMAGES

8.3.2 FACTORS AFFECTING IMPACT AND VIBRATION FRUIT DAMAGES

8.3.2.1 FACTORS AFFECTING IMPACT FRUIT DAMAGE

Several impact tests, including drop tests, pendulum impactor tests, and spherical impactor tests, are used to examine fruit susceptibility to damage (Lin et al., 2022). The impact energy (E) of the impact test is computed using the equation *E=mgh*, where "*m*" indicates the mass of the fruit or sample, "*g*" denotes the acceleration of gravity (9.81 m/s^2), and "*h*" specifies the height of the drop (m) (Ruiz-Altisent and Moreda, 2011). As the pendulum swings from various heights, the fruit is impacted by the hard surface (Opara and Pathare, 2014). Impact bruising of fruit is reported as internal and external factors. To study internal factors, the radius of curvature was varied on apples (Van Zeebroeck et al., 2007; Zarifneshat et al., 2010), peaches (Ahmadi et al., 2010), kiwifruits (Ahmadi, 2012), and pomegranates (Shafie et al., 2015). A small radius of curvature caused greater damage, area, or volume than a large radius of curvature because more energy was absorbed at a small radius of curvature, increasing the chances of bruising injury (Ahmadi, 2012).

External factors of impact bruising, such as drop height, impact surface, and number of drops, which produce different impact energy levels, are reviewed in this section. Copious research on fruit bruising drop tests has been conducted (Table 8.2). Apples were dropped from 0.05 to 1.4 m (Lu et al., 2010a, b, 2012; Unuigbe and Onuoha, 2013). In an apple postharvest handling study, possible drop heights ranged from 0.6 m in an orchard and 0.05 to 0.3 m at the retail display (Lewis et al., 2008). The range of drop heights in the berry test was 0.05 to 1.2 m, similar to that for apples (Kitazawa et al., 2014; Yu et al., 2014). Individual or packaged strawberries were dropped from 0.05 to 0.38 mm (Ferriera et al., 2008; Kitazawa et al., 2014). The minimum drop height of peach, tangerine, and tomato was 0.5 m (Idah et al., 2007; Montero et al., 2009; Reza, 2013; Vergano et al., 1991), while various drop heights were investigated, such as 0.05 to 0.60 m (pomegranate) (Hussein et al., 2019, 2020; Shafie et al., 2015), 0.20 to 0.60 m (pear) (Pathare, 2021; Pathare et al., 2021), 0.05 to 0.15 m (peach) (Tabatabaekoloor, 2013), and 0.2 to 0.6 m (guava) (Htike et al., 2021).

Paper (cardboard and corrugated fiberboard), metal or steel, rubber, wood, foam, hard plastic, and firm ceramic were all used to compare impact bruising (Idah et al., 2007; Lu et al., 2010a, b, 2012; Montero et al., 2009; Reza, 2013; Unuigbe and Onuoha, 2013). Hard surface material (steel or wood) produced the most impact bruising in apples (Lu et al., 2010a; Unuigbe and Onuoha, 2013), peaches (Reza, 2013), tomatoes (Idah et al., 2007), kiwifruits (Mencarelli et al., 1996), and table olive fruits (Saracoglu et al., 2011). While cardboard or corrugated fiberboard produced less bruise area or volume of impact bruising than on metal,

TABLE 8.2 Impact Test Conditions as Drop Tests from Various Heights Using Different Impact Surfaces

Commodity	Drop Height (m)	Impact Surface	References
Apple	0.05–0.3	• Rubber	Lu et al. (2012)
	0.05–0.5	• Double-wall corrugated fiberboard • Rubber • Wood*	Lu et al. (2010a)
	0.2–0.5 (5 times)	• Double-wall and single-wall corrugated fiberboard	Lu et al. (2010b)
	0.5–1.4	• Foam • Cardboard • Metal • Wood*	Unuigbe and Onuoha (2013)
Peach	0.5–1.5	• Steel* • Rubber	Reza (2013)
	0.31–0.91	• Steel (0.31 m was a critical drop height)	Vergano et al. (1991)
Guava	0.2–0.6	• Steel ball	Hitke et al. (2021)
Pomegranate	0.1–0.2	• Rigid flat ceramic	Hussein et al. (2019)
Strawberry	0.25–1.0	• Mild steel	Chaiwong (2016)
	0.05–0.3	• Corrugated fiberboard • Silicon rubber*	Kitazawa et al. (2014)
	0.13–0.38	• Solid aluminum	Ferreira et al. (2008)
Blueberry	0.6–1.2	• Hard plastic	Yu et al. (2014)
Tomato	0.2–0.5	• Plastic box • Paper box	Cui et al. (2018)
	0.5–1.4	• Foam • Cardboard • Plastic • Metal* • Wood	Idah et al. (2007)
Kiwifruit	300	• Steel* • Wood	Mencarelli et al. (1996)
Tangerine	400–1000 (2 times)	• Rigid ceramic	Montero et al. (2009)

* The impact surface gave the greatest impact bruise of fruits.

Source: Chaiwong (2016).

wood, plastic, and rubber (Idah et al., 2007; Kitazawa et al., 2014; Lu et al., 2010a) (Table 8.2).

Fewer drop test studies were conducted on a number of drops for impact fruit bruising (Aboud, 2006; Hussein et al., 2019; Lu et al., 201; Pathare, 2021; Tabatabaekoloor, 2013). A number of drops (1 to 3 times) was investigated in some fruit studies such as apple, pomegranate, peach, and pear (Aboud, 2006; Hussein et al., 2019; Lu et al., 2011; Pathare, 2021; Tabatabaekoloor, 2013). Most studies conducted a fixed number of drops from different height levels under diverse storage temperatures (Celik et al., 2021; Hussein et al., 2019; Pathare, 2021; Shafie et al., 2015). However, these experiments could not clearly determine the significant factors in impact bruising of fruit. Htike et al. (2021) examined three factors (drop height, number of drops, and storage temperature) and used response surface methodology (RSM) to analyze guava impact bruising. Minimal impact bruising resulted from a drop height of 0.53 m for five drops under storage temperature at 30°C.

8.3.2.2 FACTORS AFFECTING VIBRATION FRUIT DAMAGE

Vibration research on fresh fruit can be classified into three areas: in-transit experiments, simulation experiments, and transit-simulation (Trans-Sim) type experiments that combine these two methodologies. Studies of the interactions of various transport variables and their effects on damage or changes in fresh produce quality are the focus of in-transit studies, while in Trans-Sim studies on vibration damage, frequency, acceleration, and duration are the major independent simulation variables. These values are obtained from field data as actual transport, while for simulation tests, various vibration treatments have been used as the input variables to assess the effect on fresh produce (Fernando et al., 2018).

For in-transit study, a power density (PD) plot monitors the actual transport condition and is a crucial tool for laboratory simulation of vibration conditions. High or low PD level indicates frequency, and each traveling vehicle has a strong or weak point (Singh et al., 2006). A high PD level at a particular frequency can indicate vehicle trouble; consequently, PD represents the road and/or vehicle quality (Marcondes, 2009). Tire vibration produces a frequency of 15–20 Hz (Singh et al., 2006). Several studies of actual transport vibration levels have been conducted in Asian countries (Chonhenchob et al., 2009, 2010, 2012; Ishikawa et al., 2009; Park et al., 2020; Zhou et al., 2007). During actual transportation in Thailand, 10–20 Hz vibration frequency levels were commonly observed (Chonhenchob et al., 2010) and connected to ASTM D4169 (2008) and ISTA PROJECT 4AB (2009). Also, frequency peaks in truck transportation trials in Japan and Taiwan were 15 Hz and 2–3 Hz, respectively (Ishikawa et al., 2009), while China and Korea reported peak frequencies of 2.5–4 and 1.5–3 Hz, respectively (Park et al., 2020; Zhou et al., 2007).

Many actual transportation studies have examined factors influencing varied vibration levels. In truck transport, vehicle characteristics were most significant, such as: 1) position of the vehicle and the package along the stack (Barchi et al., 2002; Berardinelli et al., 2005; Hinsch et al., 1993; Ranathunga et al., 2010; Zhou et al., 2007); 2) payload and vehicle size (Garcia-Romeu-Martinez et al., 2008); 3) vehicle suspension (Garcia-Romeu-Martinez et al., 2008; Timm et al., 1996; Singh et al., 2006) while; and 4) speed and road surface condition also affected vibration levels in transit (Çakmak et al., 2010; Lu et al., 2010a).

Positions were commonly compared at two or three locations, such as the front, middle, and rear. The top, center, and bottom packages along the stack also had different vibrating levels, especially the top package. The rear position provided higher acceleration and PD value compared to the middle or front position (Barchi et al., 2002; Berardinelli et al., 2005; Hinsch et al., 1993; Soleimani and Ahmadi, 2014; Zhou et al., 2007). The top package had the highest vibration level, followed by the center and bottom levels (Barchi et al., 2002; Berardinelli et al., 2005; Hinsch et al., 1993; Ranathunga et al., 2010; Slaughter et al., 1993; Soleimani and Ahmadi, 2014).

In simulation laboratory experiments, a shaker is driven by a known vibration intensity given by a small number of interesting frequencies or a standard vibration profile (Fernando et al., 2018). Chaiwong (2021) examined three vibration variables (acceleration, frequency, and vibration duration) for simulated vibration transportation. Acceleration exhibited the most significant influence on guava bruising under simulated transportation compared to frequency and vibration duration. Table 8.3 summarizes vibration damage at different vibration frequency, acceleration, and vibration duration for fresh produce during truck transportation.

TABLE 8.3 Simulated Conditions for Vibration Damage of Fresh Produce During Road Transport

Commodity	Frequency (Hz)	Acceleration (ms^{-2})	Time (min)	References
Apple	8 to 9	6.18	20	Vursavuş and Özgüven (2004)
	4.17	n/a	10	Acıcan et al. (2007)
Pear	5 to 200	3.92	5	Berardinelli et al. (2005)
Peach	6	9.22	5	Vergano et al. (1991)
Tomato	3	n/a	60	Sharan et al. (2009)
	24	n/a	n/a	Bello et al. (2013)
Figs	16	2.45	30	Çakmak et al. (2010)
Kiwifruit	13	6.86	n/a	Tabatabaekoloor et al. (2013)
Watermelon	7.5	6.86	60	Shahbazi et al. (2010)
Strawberry	5–10	5.88	10	Fischer et al. (1992)
	5	15.69	0.6	Jiang et al. (2001)
	7	9.81	60	Nakamura et al. (2007b)
	7 to 35	5.88	n/a	Nakamura et al. (2008)
	3–5	3.92–10.79	150	Chaiwong and Bishop (2015)
	3 and 5	3.92 and 10.79	150	Chaiwong and Bishop (2020)
Guava	7, 13.5 and 20	2.94, 5.88 and 8.83	15, 30 and 45	Chaiwong et al. (2021)

n/a is not available.

Source: Adapted from Chaiwong (2016).

8.3.3 CUSHIONING MATERIALS AND FUNCTIONS

The packaging system is convenient for merchants and agriculturists to ensure good quality delivery of postharvest products to customers. Nowadays, the use of cushioning materials contributes to excellent packaging efficiency. Cushioning material's functions are 1) to keep produce fresh after harvesting; 2) to store the harvested product; and 3) to prevent bruising during transportation to a destination (Dubey and Mishra, 2018). Cushioning material contained within a package decreases degradation of fruits and vegetables, blocks and fills gaps to reduce vibration and other mechanical stresses, including drops, shocks, and constant movement. The cushioning materials also absorb kinetic energy from package vibrations (Gao, 2018; Deshwal et al., 2019; Nechita and Năstac, 2022). The product must not be adversely affected by contact with the cushioning material.

Adjusting the cushioning material depending on product type will ensure that the product arrives undamaged (Jarimopas et al., 2007). The cushioning material can be selected or modified according to the product type for high-quality transportation (Chen et al., 2020; Chitranshi et al., 2020).

Many types of cushioning materials are now available, including plastic or natural fibers, with appropriate choice relying on the design, application, product shape, size, weight, and transportation vehicle. This review classifies the types of natural cushioning and synthetic material for functional use, as shown in Table 8.4. Cushioning materials have high compressive strength (compressive strength increases with increasing density), reduced water absorption, grease resistance, easy molding, and low cost. Da Costa Castro et al. (2012) reviewed the development of both natural and synthetic cushioning materials. Natural materials include plant fibers or wool. Plant fibers such as coconut fiber and wood straw are ready to use immediately as cushioning in papaya and mango (da Costa et al., 2014) and can be combined with other materials (da Costa et al., 2012). Bamboo fibers and water lettuce roots were used to produce cushioning materials to reduce banana bruising during actual transportation (Saengwong-ngam et al., 2022). Molded paper from recycled paperboard and/or newsprint can be used for wrapping and cushioning items (Semple et al., 2022), with paper wraps and wrapping tissue made from the synthesis of cellulose (Deshwal et al., 2019). Paperboard carton packaging is used for interior packaging and shows more function as a cushioning material for partitioning or external packaging in corrugated fiberboard box form (CFB) (Pathare and Opara, 2014). Recently, natural rubber latex (NRL) without bamboo leaf fiber as a foam net prototype successfully reduced vibration mechanical damage of guava fruits due to a lower cushion coefficient value as compared to EPE foam net (Chaiwong et al., 2022). Cushioning performance was shown through the cushion coefficient, which measured the material's ability to absorb energy under stress (Song et al., 2018).

Synthetic plastic foam or elastic film cushioning materials are made from polystyrene (PS), polyurethane (PU), and polyethylene (PE) (Farrelly and Shaw, 2017), while plastic trays are derived from fossil fuel-based chemicals like natural gas or petroleum (Maga et al., 2019). Plastic is also made into bubble wrap, which is an elastic film inflated with air (Bwambok et al., 2014; Tuval et al., 2018), while loose fill or foam peanuts made from expanded PS are commonly used as interior packaging during transportation (El-Sonbati, 2012). Most cushioning research has addressed interior packaging that provides a more effective cushioning performance than external packaging and can further slow or prevent external mechanical forces from being transmitted to the fruit. Therefore, interior packaging is commonly considered, in the fruit supply chain, to effectively protect against fruit damage. Paper-based materials and foam materials employed as interior packaging are widely used for fruit protection (Lin et al., 2022). Interior packaging is classified by the two main origins as natural cushioning material and synthetic cushioning material (Siddiqui et al., 2009).

TABLE 8.4 Cushioning Materials for Distribution Packaging

Materials	Structure	Figure	References
	Natural		
Rubberized fiber cushioning	Fiber coated with rubber and vulcanized to form solid bonded sheets.	7	da Costa Castro et al. (2012)
• Corn straw • Coconut fiber • Bamboo fiber	Bamboo fiber and water lettuce root used as a cushioning material to protect bananas from mechanical damage.		Saengwong-ngam et al. (2022)
	Molded Paper		
Pulp tray	Typically made from recycled paperboard and/or newsprint.	11	Semple et al. (2022)
Paper wrap	Creped cellulose wadding		Deshwal et al. (2019)
Wrapping tissue	derived from the synthesis of cellulose, or translucent thin tissue paper used for wrapping and cushioning items.	10 (A) (B)	Deshwal et al. (2019)
Paperboard carton packaging - CFB	A corrugated cardboard flute with one or two flat linerboards as a paperboard partition.	3 (C)	Pathare and Opara (2014)
Natural rubber latex (NRL)	Formed as a foam net prototype to reduce mechanical damage of guava fruits.	12	Chaiwong et al. (2022)
	Synthetic		
Plastic foam cushioning materials • PS • PU • PE	An elastic film/foam	8	Farrelly and Shaw, (2017)
Plastic tray	Derived from fossil fuel-based chemicals like natural gas or petroleum.	9	Maga et al. (2019)

TABLE 8.4 *(Continued)*

Materials	Structure	Figure	References
Bubble wrap	An elastic film inflated with air.	10 (A)	Tuval et al. (2018)
			Bwambok et al. (2014)
Airbags	An elastic film inflated with air. Used only rarely in trucks.	–	Nayak et al. (2013)
Loose fill/ foam peanut	Made of expanded PS as similar sized pieces with a starch base.	–	El-Sonbati (2012)

8.3.3.1 NATURAL CUSHIONING MATERIALS

Natural cushioning materials are usually produced from agricultural products or biowaste, frequently using bamboo and coconut fiber (da Costa et al., 2014). Natural fibers provide a number of benefits over synthetic fibers, including low density, low cost, high strength-to-weight ratio, ease of processing, outstanding specific strength, high specific modulus, and especially their recyclability (Lu et al., 2014; Ying-Chen et al., 2010). Most current research has focused on natural cushioning materials, including foam nets, molded trays, crates, and liners (Dubey and Mishra, 2018). The generalizability of much-published research on this issue is problematic, and novel cushioning materials combining natural and synthetic material features are of interest, with increased biodegradability, recyclability, high resilience, low compression, low moisture absorption, and sensitivity to microbes.

Coconut fiber pad cushioning material was tested for shock absorption by assessing the interaction between mass (g), thickness (m), and static pressure (kPa). The fiber cushion reduced impact acceleration when static loads increased. Low thickness gave low absorption (da Costa et al., 2012) and did not protect the contents from shocks (Marcondes et al., 2003). Coconut fiber and wood straw packaging reduced serious injuries in papaya and mango with no significant differences in weight loss, skin color, and respiration rate (da Costa Castro et al., 2014), while coconut fiber combined with rubber improved tensile strength, modulus hardness, and abrasion resistance to form strongly bonded sheets (da Costa et al., 2012).

Bamboo baskets can be reused and are resistant to weight load during the transportation of mango and carambola (*Averrhoa carambola*)

(Chonhenchob and Singh, 2004; Phukon and Barua, 2015). Bamboo fiber and water lettuce root have been used as a natural cushioning material to improve banana qualities and reduce bruising area during actual transportation compared to air bubble bags. Figure 8.7 shows a cushioning design made from bamboo fiber and water lettuce root (Saengwong-Ngam et al., 2022). This study first compared NRL foam net to expanded polyethylene (EPE) foam net to reduce vibration bruising of guava as cushioning material to protect against mechanical damage (Figure 8.12).

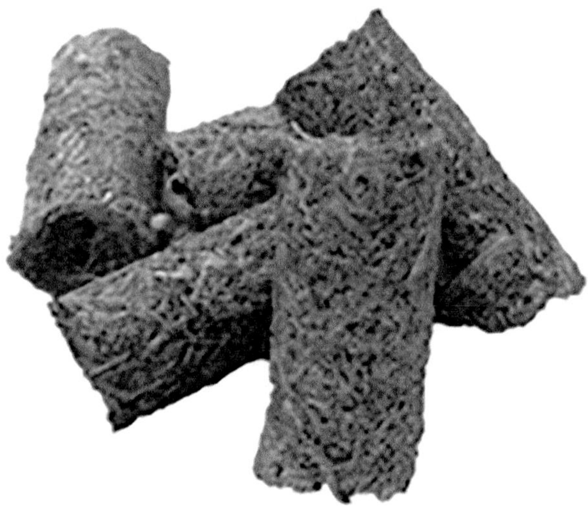

FIGURE 8.7 Cushioning natural material from bamboo fiber and water lettuce root reduced banana bruising.

Source: Authors.

Recent trends have led to widespread use of natural molded paper cushioning material as the most economical and eco-friendly packaging to transport products over long distances. Molded paper is available in various designs and a wide range of colors and sizes. Molded pulp trays are used to pack melon and apple as corrugated common footprint (CCF) trays designed appropriately for the shape and size of fruits (Figure 8.11). Pulp trays are made from recycled paperboard and/or newsprint (Semple et al., 2022). Wrapping tissue or paper sheet cushioning materials are derived from the synthesis of cellulose, and translucent thin tissue paper is used to underlie or wrap mango in a box (Deshwal et al., 2019) (Figure 8.10C).

Paperboard carton packaging is also popular as CFB (Figure 8.3C). It is applied to underlie a plastic tray, used as a paperboard partition to separate individual fruit and liner, and made from a corrugated cardboard flute with one or two flat linerboards (Pathare and Opara, 2014).

8.3.3.2 SYNTHETIC CUSHIONING MATERIALS

Foam cushioning materials made from PS, PU, and PE are flexible, semi-rigid, or rigid. These types of cushions have different characteristics depending on the specific weight of the product and the structure of the foam cushioning materials. Foam is used worldwide and demonstrates many advantages such as: (1) PS is non-hygroscopic, closed-cell, soft elastic, and has limited recovery; (2) PU is soft, semi-hard, and hard, open-cell, has better cushioning with increasing hardness but with reduced recovery and elasticity; and (3) PE has excellent cushioning properties, is closed-cell, but is not weather resistant (Farrelly and Shaw, 2017). Foam net is used to cover mango and guava fruits to protect against mechanical damage during domestic transportation in Thailand (Figure 8.8). Other commercial fruits such as apple, pear, and pineapple also use foam net to reduce mechanical damage from vibration (Chonhenchob et al., 2008; Eissa et al., 2012, 2013; Zhou et al., 2008).

Plastic trays have a good cushioning effect, immobilize the produce within the pack (Siddiqui et al., 2009), and are derived from fossil fuel-based chemicals like natural gas or petroleum (Maga et al., 2019). Plastic trays in Figure 8.9 were used as a cushioning material for kiwifruit and tomato inside CCF. Bubble cushioning material provides outstanding protection from damage caused by shock, vibration, or abrasion (Siddiqui et al., 2009). An air bubble sheet was placed under ‘Elsanta’ strawberry punnets and laid between the banana layer in the CCF tray (Figure 8.10A).

The use of cushioning materials has increased, but they are typically constructed of non-biodegradable materials. Foam materials, in particular, are often used for commercial packaging, although they are neither environmentally friendly nor biodegradable (Nechita and Năstac, 2022). Nowadays, environmental problems and consumer demand for eco-friendly materials are increasing as environmental laws, such as disposal fees for non-degradable packaging materials and environmental improvement fees, become more stringent. As a result, biomass-based material research and development are being aggressively pursued globally (Sohn et al., 2019).

Composite materials made from biomass are now frequently employed in technology and packaging materials as eco-friendly, lightweight substitutes to prevent damage and prolong the shelf life of fruit (Karimah et al., 2021; Li et al., 2014).

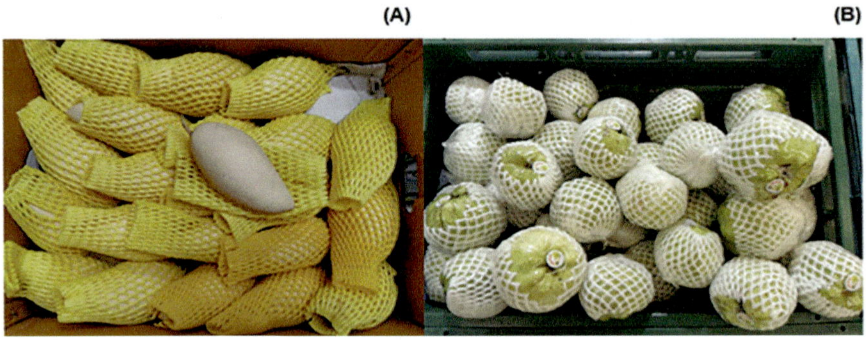

FIGURE 8.8 Foam net covering on 'Nam Dok Mai See Thong' mango (A); and guava (B) fruits for protection from mechanical damage during domestic transportation in Thailand.

Source: Authors.

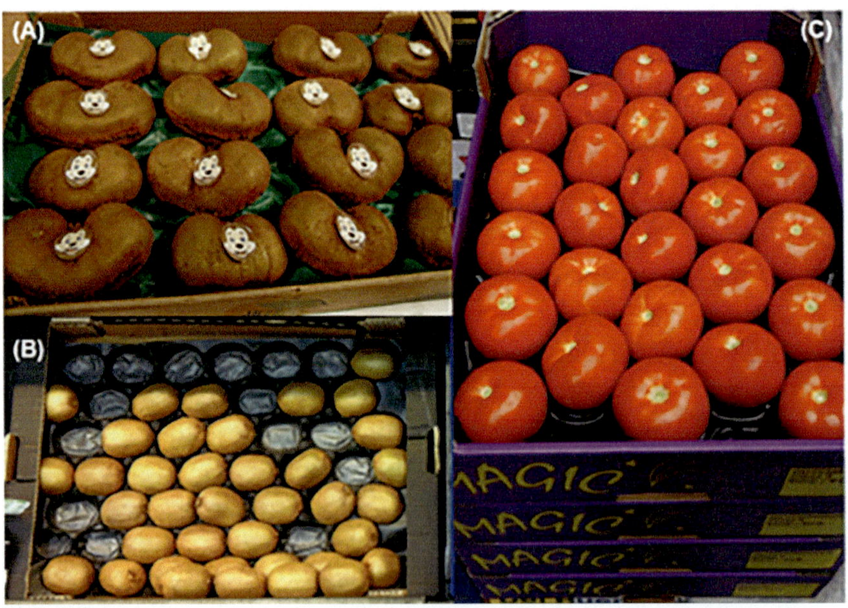

FIGURE 8.9 Plastic tray for kiwifruit (A, B); and tomato (C) fruits inside CCF.

Source: Authors.

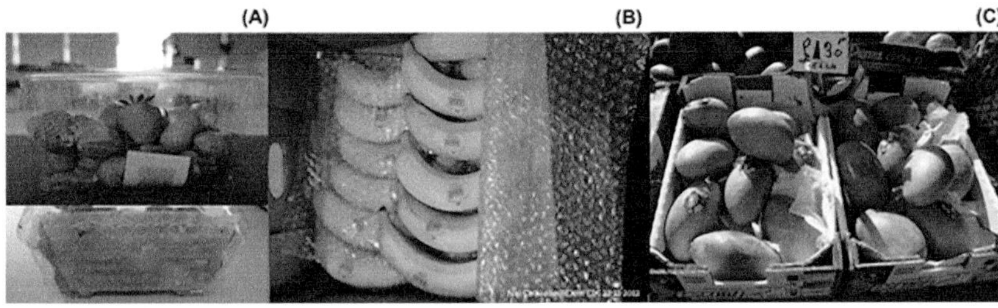

FIGURE 8.10 Air bubble sheet under 'Elsanta' strawberry punnet (A); laid between banana layer in CCF tray (B); and paper sheet for mango (C).
Source: Authors.

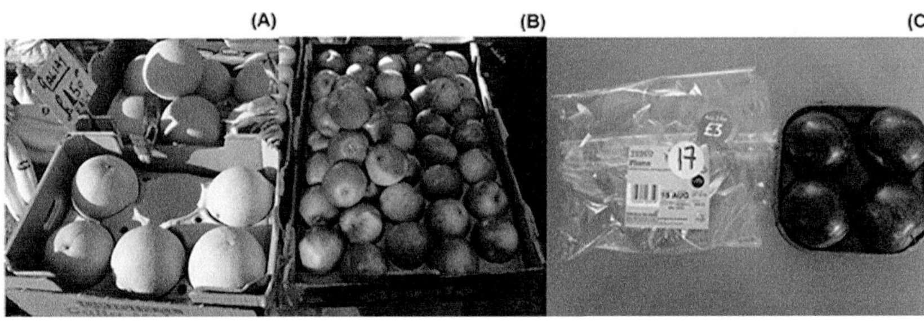

FIGURE 8.11 Molded pulp tray for packing melon and apple in CCF tray (A, B) and plums as a retail package.
Source: Authors.

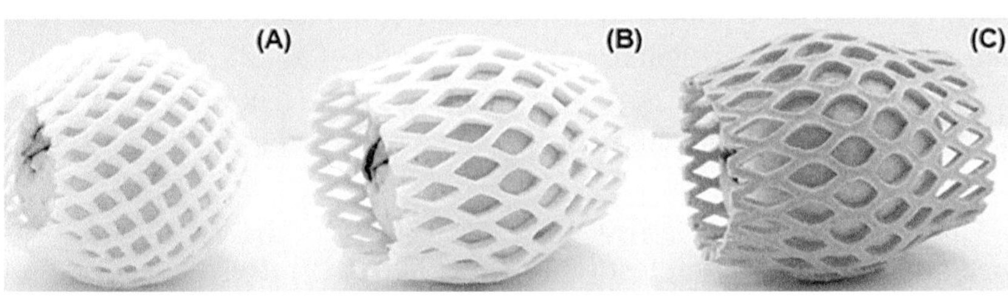

FIGURE 8.12 EPE foam net (A) was investigated and compared for cushioning performance with NRL foam net either with bamboo leaf fiber (BLF) or without BLF.
Source: Authors.

8.3.4 CUSHIONING MATERIALS TO PROTECT AGAINST SHOCK AND VIBRATION DAMAGES

Cushioning materials with various qualities and structures are now often used inside packaging, such as boxes and bags, to prevent the product from shaking or vibrating in the packaging, thereby preventing damage (Zhou et al., 2008), depending on the kind of goods, substance, vibration level, and transportation vehicle (Jarimopas et al., 2007). Research has focused on many kinds of commercial fruit that require different cushioning materials for safe and undamaged transport (Chen et al., 2020).

Table 8.5 lists studies focusing on various cushioning materials and vibration effects from drop (Dunno et al., 2021; Kitazawa et al., 2015) or impact effects (Dunno et al., 2021). Most of the cushioning materials are foam nets used to wrap fruits and prevent vibration damage during transportation (Chonhenchob et al., 2008; Eissa et al., 2012, 2013; Hussein et al., 2020; Ríos-Mesa et al., 2020; Zhou et al., 2008). Foam nets are generally applied to climacteric fruits such as apples (Eissa et al., 2012, 2013; Jarimopas et al., 2007; Kitzawa et al., 2018), pears (Zhou et al., 2008), and avocados (Ríos-Mesa et al., 2020), as well as a non-climacteric fruit such as pineapples (Chonhenchob et al., 2008). Cushioning designs as tray styles in CFB were used for apples (Dunno et al., 2021; Kitazawa et al., 2018), pears (Thompson et al., 2008; Wang et al., 2022), avocados (Thompson et al., 2008), and cantaloupes (Azam et al., 2022). Foam nets and tray styles in CFB are often used for reducing vibration damage to fruit during transportation. Most cushioning materials have been investigated as foam nets (Chonhenchob et al., 2008; Eissa et al., 2012, 2013; Jarimopas et al., 2007; Kitazawa et al., 2018; Ríos-Mesa et al., 2020; Zhou et al., 2008), foam trays (Dunno et al., 2021; Lin et al., 2020; Tao et al., 2021; Wang et al., 2022), corrugated board (Fernando et al., 2020; Jarimopas et al., 2007; Wang et al., 2022), plastic boards or trays (Kitazawa et al., 2015; Thompson et al., 2008), and paper trays (Azam et al., 2022; Kitazawa et al., 2018).

The key design focus is to wrap the fruit to protect it from damage, especially in the vibration test (Hussein et al., 2019). Results suggest that the development of cushioning material still lacks the function of maintaining and preserving fruit during transportation, and stopping or slowing down changes in product quality during and after transportation (Cherono and Workneh, 2018). Future challenges remain to prolong the ripening life, preserve color, and prevent deterioration by microorganisms (Yadav et al., 2022). Environmentally friendly cushioning materials reduce waste contamination (Zhang et al., 2021), with low cost of production, and are becoming an increasing marketing trend (Singh et al., 2022).

TABLE 8.5 Cushioning Materials for Protecting Mechanical Fruit Damages Under Impact, drop and Vibration Tests

Fruits	Experiment Approach	Cushioning Materials and Packing	Notable Results	References
Strawberry	• Drop test	• Foamed plastic board (FPB) • Corrugated plastic board (CPB) • Foamed rubber sheet (FRS) • CFB	• The drop could be controlled individually between the stackable packaging. • The board or sheet-like cushioning materials were laid between each layer or outside the bottom layer.	Kitazawa et al. (2015)
Apple	• Drop test	• Expanded polystyrene (EPS) trays • CFB	• EPS trays reduced bruise susceptibility. • ESP tray demonstrated a 70% decrease in impact acceleration.	Dunno et al. (2021)
	• Shock test	• A two-ply pulp molded tray • Foam net • Crushed paper • CFB	• The reduction of fruit bruising was made possible by the space between the fruit and the inner surface of the hollow of the top layer by using a two-ply pulp molded tray.	Kitazawa et al. (2018)
	• Impact test • Compression test	• Corrugated board • Foam net	• The single face corrugated board with flutes on the outside provided shock protection and reduced bruises on the apple.	Jarimopas et al. (2007)
	• Vibration test	• Foam net	• Foam net was more efficient at reducing damage to apples and maintaining firmness.	Eissa et al. (2013)
	• Vibration test	• Foam net • CFB	• The use of foam-net reduced the amount of fruit damaged by 50–63%.	Eissa et al. (2012)
Banana	• Vibration test (shaking)	• Plant cushioning material • CFB	• Cushioning material reduced the bruised area, inhibited mold and extended banana quality after transportation.	Saengwong-ngam, Matan, and Matan (2022)
	• Vibration test	–	–	Fernando et al. (2020)

TABLE 8.5 *(Continued)*

Fruits	Experiment Approach	Cushioning Materials and Packing	Notable Results	References
		• One-piece corrugated paperboard cartons • Plastic bag (low-density polyethylene)	• Corrugated paperboard containers reduced damage caused by the vibration effect. • he combination of plastic bags and vacuum tightening demonstrated that banana damage levels were reduced.	–
Pear	• Vibration test	• EPS tray • EPE net cover • Corrugated board • Paper wrapping • FB	• Mechanical damage of pears decreased to the lowest level at 9% by using EPS tray + EPE net cover.	Wang et al. (2022)
	• Vibration test	• Foam net • Paper-wrap packages • A reusable plastic container	• Foam net reduced vibration effect during transportation. • ear presented decent quality during transportation and distribution.	Zhou et al. (2008)
Pear and avocado	• Vibration test	• Suspended tray	• The suspended tray demonstrated reduced transit vibration damage levels.	Thompson et al. (2008)
Avocado	• Vibration test	• PE foam mesh (Foam net) • Plastic basket	• Mechanical damage generated for vibration levels were low in avocado with foam net.	Ríos-Mesa et al. (2020)
Cantaloupe	• Vibration test	• Paper pulp tray packaging • CFB	• ruit packed in a paper pulp tray had smaller resonant vibration and less bruising.	Azam et al. (2022)
Mango	• Vibration test	• Cardboard boxes	• Quality and shelf life of mango were affected by each vibration frequency during simulated transport.	Costa et al. (2021)

TABLE 8.5 *(Continued)*

Fruits	Experiment Approach	Cushioning Materials and Packing	Notable Results	References
Peach	• Vibration test	• PU cushion material tray • EPE sheet • CFB	• Cushion material reduced susceptibility to vibration damage. • The bruised area and slow degradation rate reduced mechanical harm. • Ripe peaches were less susceptible to mechanical damage because of the PU+CFB and vibration at a low temperature of 10°C.	Lin et al. (2020)
Tomato	• Vibration test	• Wooden box	• Increase in transportation distance and storage temperature caused greater changes in the physical qualities of tomatoes.	Al-Dairi et al. (2021)
Shiitake mushroom	• Vibration test	• Foam cushion material tray • CFB	• Foam cushion material reduced essential effects as respiration rate, weight loss, weight reduction, degree of browning and lipid oxidation.	Tao et al. (2021)
Papaya	• Vibration test	• Newspaper filler • Dried banana leaves • Dried rice straw • Plastic basket	• Newspaper filler reduced the degradation effect (weight loss and mechanical damage) and maintained the freshness of fruit as high hardness in papaya.	Sigalingging et al. (2019)
Pineapple	• Vibration test	• Foam net • CFB • Reusable plastic container • Foam box	• Lowest damage levels were produced by CFB with paperboard partitions. • Foam net reduced bruise damage of pineapples in all containers (reusable plastic container, corrugated fiberboard box and foam box).	Chonhenchob et al. (2008)

8.4 CORRUGATED FIBERBOARD BOX AND VENTILATION

8.4.1 CORRUGATED FIBERBOARD OF FRESH PRODUCE

Corrugated fiberboard (often mistakenly called cardboard or pasteboard) consists of a central corrugating (called the corrugating medium or the medium) and the outer and inner liners of kraft (Smith et al., 2004). Corrugated fiberboard is commonly divided into nine flute types that vary in pitch (the distance between the two flute tips) and number of flutes per meter (Table 8.6) (Poustis, 2005). Kraft paper is made from unbleached pulp with brown color and strong characteristics. The grade of paperboard depends on weight and thickness (Boyette et al., 1996). Constructions of corrugated fiberboard are typically single wall, double wall, and triple wall (Figure 8.13) (FEFCO, 2021). The B flute for double wall configuration is usually used in horticultural crops (Boyette et al., 1996; Thompson and Mitchell, 2002). The most common flutes used for fresh produce in Thailand are the C and BC flutes for single wall and double wall corrugated fiberboard, respectively (Chonhenchob et al., 2011).

TABLE 8.6 Characteristics of the Nine Flute Sizes

Type of Flute	Pitch (mm)	Average Flutes/m	Average Thickness
D	14.96	75	8.0
K	11.70	95	6.5
A	8.66	110	4.8
C	7.95	129	4.2
B	6.50	154	2.8
E	3.50	295	1.7
F	2.40	310	1.2
G	1.80	350	1.0
O	1.25	360	0.7

Source: Poustis (2005).

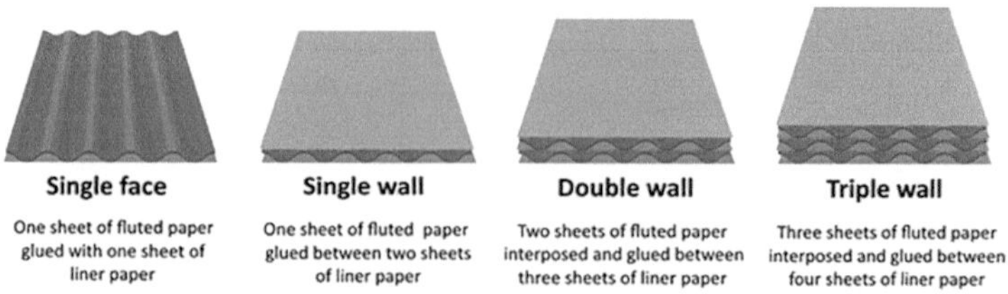

FIGURE 8.13 Various structures of corrugated fiberboard.
Source: Adapted from FEFCO (2021).

8.4.2 DISTRIBUTION PACKAGING FOR FRESH PRODUCE

The most commonly used corrugated fiberboard package is known as a regular slotted container (RSC) (Figure 8.14) (Poustis, 2005). Singh et al. (2009) reported that the three most used styles of corrugated boxes for fresh produce were slotted boxes, telescoping boxes, and rigid/bliss boxes with three codes FEFCO 0201, FEFCO 0320, and FEFCO 0606, respectively (Figure 8.14). A survey of fresh produce packaging in Southeast Asia found that RSC, full telescope design (FTD), and full telescope Hak slotted (FTHS) boxes were the most popular shipping carton to pack various tropical fruits, particularly in the Philippines, Thailand, and Vietnam (Bihn, 2011; Chonhenchob et al., 2011; Villahermosa et al., 2011).

CCFs first appeared in 2000 and have been developed in the United States by the Fiberboard Box Association and the European Federation of Corrugated Board Manufacturers (FEFCO) (Figure 8.15). The standardized CCFs are compatible with a global standard (FEFCO) to provide uniform dimensions and tab and receptacle system. The CCFs are stacked efficiently and safely to protect fresh produce located in the bottom layers of a pallet (Chonhenchob et al., 2011). These versatile packages provide lightweight configuration of vent design, colorful graphic design, and printing to attract customer attention. CCFs increased space efficiency by 7.8–22% by loading more products per truckload and can be displayed at retail stores (Singh and Singh, 2007). When comparing CCFs and returnable plastic containers (RPCs) of strawberries, CCFs had an 11% greater payload of berries with significantly less bruising with the same cooling rate. In a case study of system cost analysis of packages in California table grapes, overall system costs (cash cost) of RPCs increased by 12% when compared to CCFs. Retailer's system costs also increased significantly by about 15% because of higher RPCs transportation and handling cost (American Forest and Paper Association, 2021).

Corrugated fiberboard loses strength over time. Thompson et al. (2002) reported that fiberboard in moisture equilibrium with air at 90% RH retained only 40% of initial stacking strength. However, wax-coated corrugated fiberboard containers delay reduction of their strength and rate of moisture absorption. Waxed corrugated containers are noticeably higher in price than packages that are appropriate for dry conditions. These containers are recycled only in specific processes and not mixed with regular corrugated containers (Thompson and Mitchell, 2002).

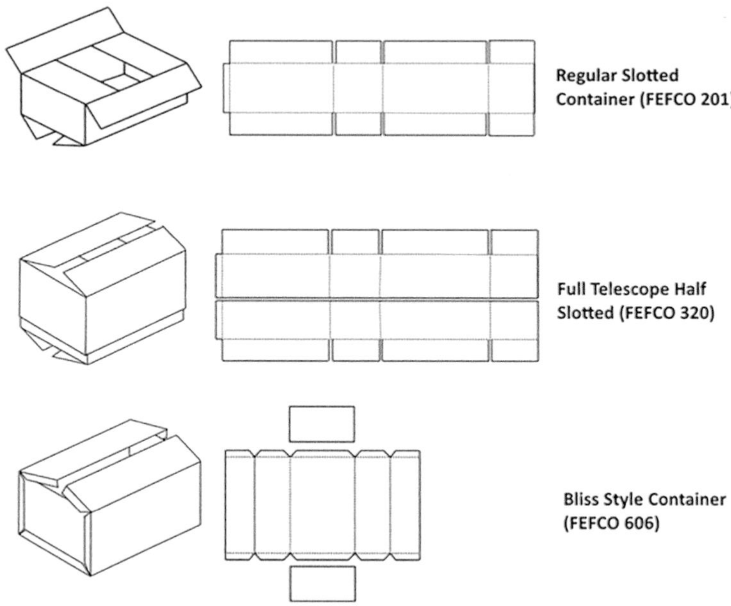

FIGURE 8.14 Common styles of boxes used for fresh produce.

Source: Adapted from Singh et al. (2009).

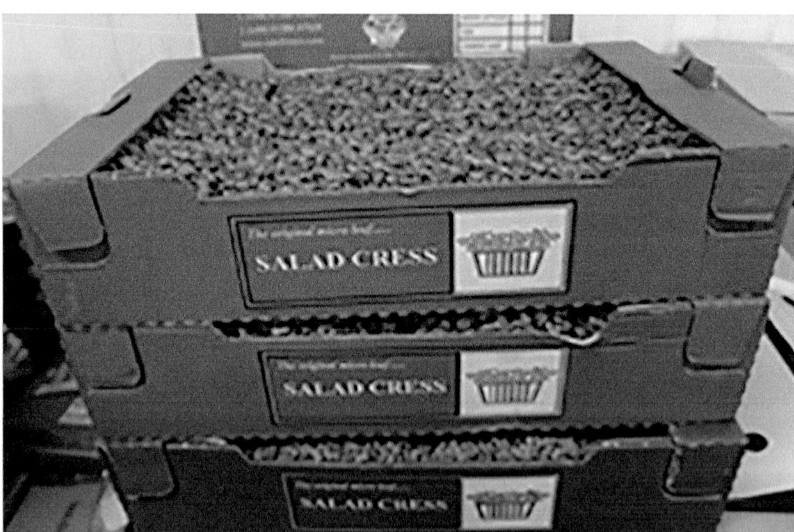

FIGURE 8.15 A corrugated common footprint.

Source: Authors.

Plastic crates, such as trapezoid-shaped crates, rectangular crates, and round plastic crates, are commonly manufactured from high-density polyethylene (HDPE) and polypropylene (PP) (Chonhenchob et al., 2011; Rapusas and Rolle, 2009). In Southeast Asia, most styles of plastic crates differ from those in the United States and European markets. Rectangular plastic crates reduce losses with more space efficiency for storage and distribution in comparison to trapezoid-shaped crates. Rectangular plastic crates provide variable depths with fixed length dimensions for standardization, giving a higher payload with less packing. Plastic crates are resistant to water and moisture and can be cleaned and sanitized before packing fresh produce (Chonhenchob et al., 2011).

In the United States and Europe, reusable/returnable plastic containers for the distribution of fresh produce have significantly increased for bulk packaging because RPCs are durable, high-quality containers and have good pooling systems for supply chain management (Chonhenchob et al., 2011; Vigneault et al., 2009). A key role of RPCs is as an environmentally friendly package due to 39% less total energy, 95% less total solid waste, and 29% less total greenhouse emission (Franklin Associates, 2004). RPCs have the efficiency to replace corrugated fiberboard with reduction of waste and safe energy. Innovative foldable RPCs designed by IFCO (Figure 8.16) were introduced to the U.S. market in 1995 and are now the world's largest RPC pool. The major efficiency of IFCO RPCs is to reduce cooling times and product damage, eliminate disposal waste, remove the volatility of CFB market pricing, and decrease workman's compensation claims at the distribution center and the retail store. Chonhenchob et al. (2011) investigated the cooling rate between RPCs and corrugated boxes in other tropical fruits (mangoes, papayas). RPCs also provided a significantly faster cooling rate than corrugated boxes; however, faster air movement for heat removal could enhance water loss.

8.4.3 VENTILATION DESIGN FOR DISTRIBUTION PACKAGING OF PRODUCE

Forced-air precooling is one of the most widely used techniques for maintaining fresh produce quality, with high efficiency and low operating cost. Cold air circulating inside the cooling chamber permeates through the fresh produce packaging by ventilation holes. Ventilation design of

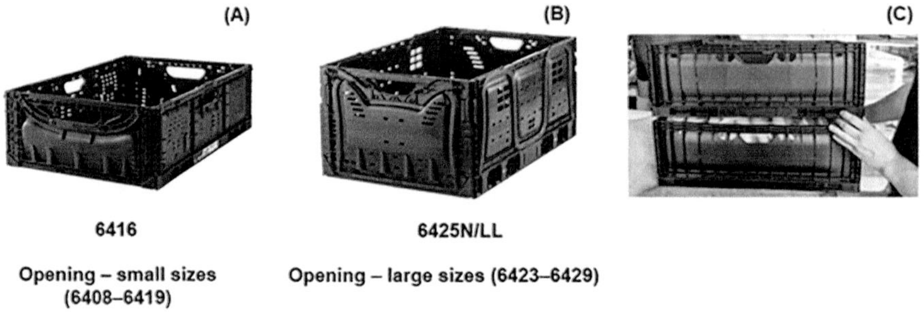

FIGURE 8.16 Foldable FICO RPCs for fresh produce.

Source: https://www.ifco.com/explore-our-products/?solution=fruit-vegetables (A, B). https://www.ifco.com/how-to-make-your-banana-supply-chain-sustainable/ (C) Selvatica bananas traveled from Ecuador to Paris-Rungis International Market, where they were ripened before being sent to customers across Europe.

distribution packaging must be considered to maximize cooling performance and mechanical strength of the packages.

Internal airflow and temperature distribution inside the packages are critical to maintain fresh produce quality. Heterogeneous distribution of cooling air due to poor package ventilation design causes overcooling, chilling injury, and higher mass loss (Han et al., 2017, 2018). A previous study indicated that the area around the vent provided higher convective heat transfer coefficients (Berry et al., 2017), while the area near the vent showed high air velocity and turbulence intensity (Delele et al., 2013). Conversely, at the blind spot, field heat of fresh produce is not efficiently removed. Berry et al. (2017) designed a multi-vent hole aligned on the package wall. Results showed that cooling uniformity significantly improved and reduced energy consumption by 58% compared to the standard vent design. The vent area is another factor related to the optimization of ventilation design. Increasing the vent area accelerates the cooling rate of produce (Berry et al., 2017; Ferrua and Singh, 2009), while increasing the vent area beyond the optimal point either increases the cooling rate or cooling uniformity (De Castro et al., 2004; Delele et al., 2013; Tutar et al., 2009; Wang et al., 2019). Another concern in ventilation design is package integrity; the strength of packages decreases with increase in vent area (Berry et al., 2017). Compressive strength reduced by 2–20% with increased number of vent areas. Flute number, size of liner, and geometry of vent hole are also additional factors that influenced the strength of the package (Berry et al., 2017; Fadiji et al., 2016; Singh et al., 2008). Berry et al. (2022) suggested various approaches to find the optimal ventilation design by simultaneously assessing performance, mechanical strength, logistics, cost, environmental impact, and fresh produce condition.

8.4.4 STACKING AND COMPRESSIVE STRENGTH OF FRESH PRODUCE PACKAGING

Corrugated fiberboard cartons (CFC) are commonly used for fresh produce distribution because of their lightweight, recyclable, and cost-effective characteristics (Pathre and Opera, 2014). CFCs are also superior to reusable plastic containers (RPCs) in terms of lower mechanical damage from impacts and vibrations. Package integrity is important, and CFCs also face various mechanical damage along the distribution chain. The load on the bottom layer of the pallet must withstand the maximum compression force, and the package must have sufficient strength to avoid bulking (Mukama et al., 2020).

The box compression test (BCT) is usually used to evaluate empty CFC strength, which is related to flute size, the perimeter of the box, and properties of corrugated board such as bending stiffness and edge crush test (ECT) value that are calculated by McKee's formula (Fadiji et al., 2018). ASTM D642 (ASTM, 2010) is the standard method for determining CFC compressive strength. Higher stress is usually found at the corners of packages as well as at the vent holes (Figure 8.17) (Fadiji et al., 2019). The design of CFC vent holes allows better cooling performance; however, the area and number of vent holes, orientation, and shape affect CFC strength (Fadiji et al., 2016). On a large scale, pallet stacking, internal packaging, bearing, and transport conditions also affect the performance of CFCs (Berry et al., 2022). Singh et al. (2011) reported that box stacking configuration, that is, interlock stacking, column stacking, and overhang, affect the compressive strength of a palletized load of the box. Storage and transport conditions also affect the structural strength of CFCs. Low temperature and high humidity in cold storage/transportation also weaken the bonds of the cellulose structure of the fiberboard, resulting in deformation under mechanical loads (Berry et al., 2019). Proper ventilation design reduces moisture accumulation in CFCs and prevents deformation during storage/transport.

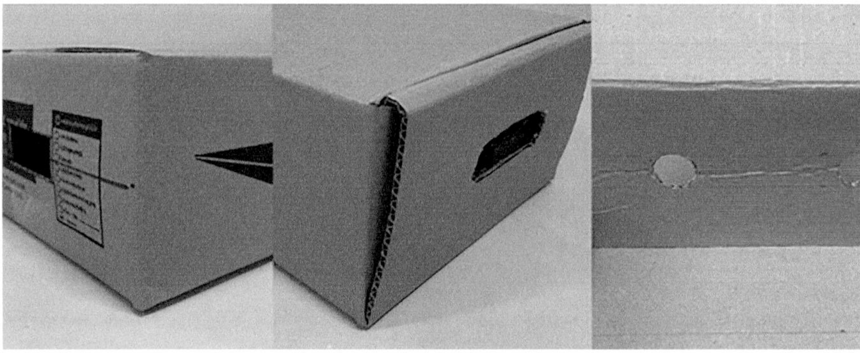

FIGURE 8.17 Box failure on corners, handholes and vent holes after compression test.
Source: Author.

8.5 PLASTIC AND THERMAL INSULATION COVERS

Plastic and thermal insulation covers are classified as tertiary packaging during the distribution and transportation of fresh produce. Plastic covers are mainly used as active packaging by flushing gas to reduce fruit deterioration, particularly for soft fruits. Only a few studies have addressed the efficiency of thermal insulation covers to maintain the cold temperature of fresh produce throughout the supply chain. This section compares thermal insulation cover packaging performance of foam sheet and other alternative thermal insulation materials combined with ALF material to improve thermal insulation properties. These alternative materials reduce foam sheet application and increase the use of sustainable materials.

8.5.1 POLYETHYLENE PLASTIC COVERS

Pallet covers are used to ameliorate the effects of rapid changes in temperature and humidity and protect fresh produce from spoiling (Melis, 2016; Wheeler et al., 2015). A few studies have described the use of pallet covers for fresh produce. Polyethylene plastic and thermal insulation covers are mainly used. Polyethylene (PE) plastic covers create active MAP by flushing mixed gases or high CO_2 to remove ethylene and promote anti-fog properties using a porous and breathable membrane (Table 8.7). Commercial covers require proper cooling before placing on containers. PEAK*fresh* is a polyethylene bag impregnated with minerals that extracts ethylene gas. It has excellent permeability and good deodorizing properties (Figure 8.18) (PEAK*fresh*, 2021).

TransFresh Corporation (2011) studied consumer acceptance of California fresh strawberries by visiting 114 retail stores in 39 cities. 'Tectrol' covers were prepared by flushing high CO_2 (10% CO_2) into the strawberries. The quality attributes of fresh strawberries in Tectrol covers were compared to fruit with no sealing covers. Tectrol covers resulted in a significantly higher percentage of purchase decisions with low product mold and decay. Macnish et al. (2012) examined how four commercial pallet covers (CO_2 west, PEAK*fresh*, PrimePro, and Tectrol) maintained strawberry quality during refrigerated transport (0–3.8°C) for 2.3–4.7 days. The sealed Tectrol covers had the highest CO_2 concentration (11–16%) compared to CO_2 west, PEAK*fresh*, and PrimePro covers (0.06–0.3% CO_2). Tectrol covers exhibited significantly less decay (36%) than the non-covered pallet (control) (41%) and other pallet covers (39–43%) after a 2-day shelf life at 20°C. Development in pallet cover design has improved the storage of perishable products damaged by ethylene production. Boxes are separated from other boxes by a plastic film between each layer. Each layer of boxes contains its own separate atmosphere to reduce cross-contamination of harmful gasses or diseases (Figure 8.19) (Lehn and Herrmann, 2013).

TABLE 8.7 Commercial Polyethylene Plastic Covers for Fresh Produce

Commodities	Properties	References
Strawberry, Berry, Cherry, Avocado, Stone fruit, Asparagus, Tomato, Cucumber	• Breathable PE impregnated with C_2H_4 absorber • Unsealed pallet covers • Active MAP by C_2H_4 flushing for long-distance shipping to induce ripening	PEAK*fresh* (2021)
Strawberry, Raspberry, Blackberry, Blueberry	• 'Tectrol' cover • Active MAP by gas flushing with high CO_2 (10%CO_2) • Inhibition of mold and decay	TransFresh Corporation (2011)
Strawberry	• 'Tectrol' cover (11–16%CO_2) with less decay (36%) than non-covered pallet (control) (41%) and three other pallet covers (39–43%)	Macnish et al. (2012)

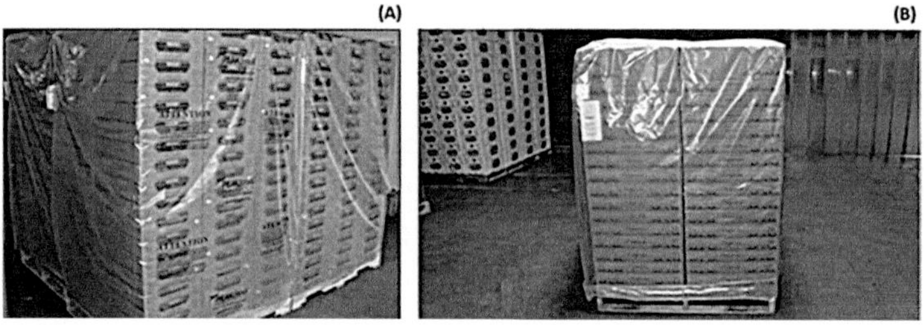

FIGURE 8.18 PEAK*fresh* cover for active MAP strawberry transportation.

Source: https://www.peakfreshusa.com/pallet-covers.

8.5.2 THERMAL INSULATION MATERIALS

To guarantee product integrity, many commercial businesses concentrate on product transportation at the batch (pallet) level, as it is the most timely and economically feasible option (Melis, 2016). Pallet cover materials are used in commercial practices to maintain humidity within the pallets by attenuating rapid temperature fluctuations. Pallet covers are placed on the container of fresh produce when the optimal temperature and humidity have been reached, to maintain these ideal conditions as long as possible (Pelletier et al., 2011).

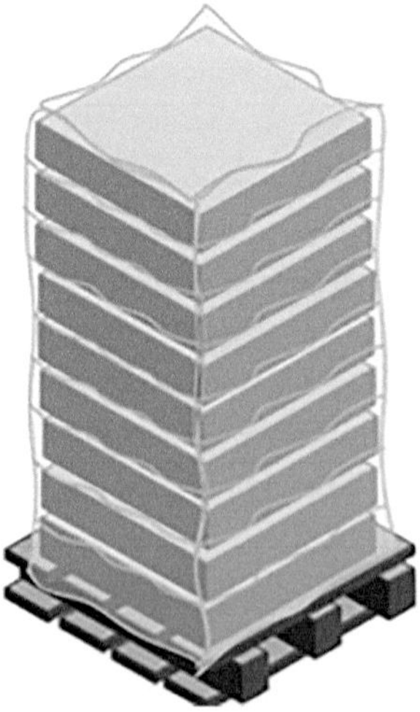

FIGURE 8.19 Innovative design of plastic cover film illustrating the location of film layers between boxes.

Source: Adapted from Lehn and Herrmann (2013).

Insulating materials have low thermal conductivity to limit heat transmission, while radiation and convection also play roles (Singh et al., 2008). Thermal conductivity of most materials decreases with increasing temperature. By replacing gas inside the cellular structure, the absorbed moisture could reduce the thermal performance of cellular polymers to a degree that depends on the temperature of each side of the insulation material. Latent heat transfer may also occur as a consequence of evaporation and condensation (Desjarlais and Zarr, 2002). The most common materials used for pallet cover applications are thermal-insulated materials such as ALF, polyurethane (PU), and nonwovens. As shown in Table 8.8, thermal conductivity differs depending on the material type. Thermal-insulated materials, including PU foam and aerogel blanket, possess low thermal conductivity and constrain heat transfer. ALF is a reflective material that has high thermal conductivity and reflects heat to effectively reduce heat radiation (Wang and Guan, 2017).

TABLE 8.8 Thermal Conductivity at 20°C of Different Materials

Materials	**Thermal Conductivity (MW m^{-1} K^{-1})**
Polyisocyanurate	24.6
Aerogel blanket	16.2
Polyethylene	61.0
Expanded polystyrene	42.5
Cardboard box	43.9

Source: Wang et al. (2020).

Thermal insulation material, employed as a single substance or a combination of different materials, retards thermal flow and is adaptable to any shape, structure, or surface (Shukla, 2011). Insulating materials are used to thermally isolate a system and significantly decrease the heat transfer rate between the system and surrounding area or environment (Deshmukh et al., 2017). Insulation materials decrease thermal flow by reducing convection, radiation, and conduction while performing one or more of the following functions: energy conservation by reducing thermal loss or gain, regulating the surface for individual safety and convenience, and enabling vapor flow and water condensation (Khandelwal, 2010). Fibrous insulation is made up of small diameter fibers that delicately partition the material's air space. Small individual cells are isolated from one another in cellular insulations.

Glass or foamed plastics such as polystyrene (PS) (closed cell), polyurethane (PU), polyisocyanurate (PIR), polyolefin (PO), or elastomer may be used as the cellular material. Small nodules in granular insulations contain voids or hollows. However, gas may pass between the separate gaps, and these materials are not regarded as genuine cellular materials. It may be made into a loose or pourable substance or as rigid insulation with the addition of a binder and fibers (TIASA, 2001). PS is normally used as pallet cover material, in combination with other materials such as ALF or coated with PU, to cover fresh produce during transportation (Figure 8.20A).

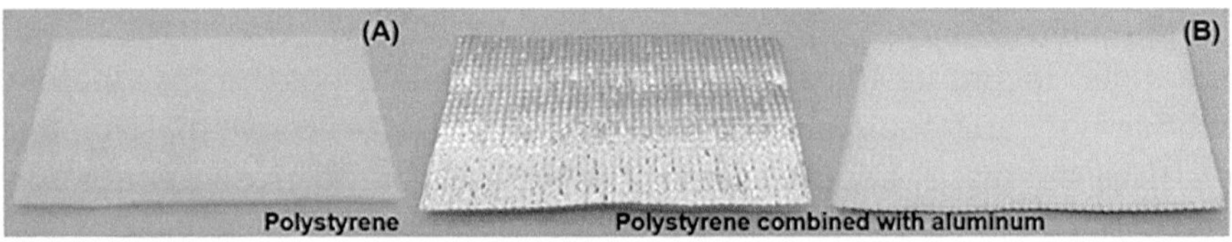

FIGURE 8.20 PS (A); and combined with ALF (B, C) to increase thermal insulation material performance.

Source: Authors.

ALF is a reflective insulation material, which consists of one or more low-emittance surfaces and can reflect heat back out, thus effectively reducing heat radiation (Wang and Guan, 2017). ALF has a low radiation coefficient and good anti-radiation ability that effectively reduce thermal radiation (Tong and Tien, 1983). Since the 1950s, ALF has shown excellent performance in many countries in Europe and America. It is also used in the building industry as a thermal insulation material (Juan, 2011). For pallet covers, ALF is often used in combination with other materials such as white foam to cover fresh produce during shipping delays (Wheeler et al., 2015) (Figures 8.20 and 8.21).

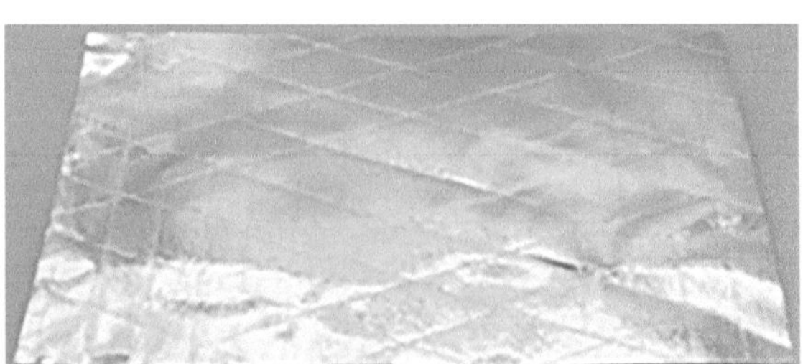

FIGURE 8.21 Aluminum foil (ALF).

Source: Authors.

Spun-bond nonwovens are made by combined processes of fiber spinning, fiber depositing, web binding, and winding to create rolls (Bhat and Malkan, 2007). Nonwovens can be produced from horizontal or transverse webs or randomly bound together using heated adhesive or thermoplastic fibers (Patel and Bhrambhatt, 2011) (Figure 8.22). Nonwovens are useful in a variety of applications including transportation, construction management, manufacturing, and, more recently, agriculture (Tausif, 2016). In agricultural areas, nonwovens are developed for various applications including crop cover, frost protection, landscape fabric, greenhouse shading, insect protection, and also to reduce extreme temperature differences (Gupta, 1987).

FIGURE 8.22 Nonwoven.

Source: Authors.

8.5.3 THERMAL INSULATION COVER FOR BOXES OF FRESH PRODUCE

In cold chain management, evaporatively cooled insulated transport boxes or trailers are recommended for small-scale businesses, while passive cooling (insulated pallet covers) is recommended for large-scale businesses (Kitinoja, 2013). Recently, interest in thermal insulation covers for fresh produce, instead of highly valuable products such as pharmaceutical or medical products, has increased. However, few academic publications have addressed the efficiency of thermal covers in retaining cooled temperatures for fresh produce.

Pallet covers are applied as a technological packaging to reduce waste from food spoilage by reducing temperature and humidity changes during transportation (Melis, 2016). Insulated pallet covers decrease temperature fluctuations during transportation either in a refrigerated vehicle or in a shaded area with no refrigerated dock (Sharp and Irving, 1981). Bycroft et al. (1996) investigated combinations of an insulated pallet covering and a supplemental coolant using asparagus pallets. Insulated pallet wraps were the most beneficial to reduce temperature fluctuation.

Various commercial thermal covers used to isolate perishables and prevent cross-contamination in refrigerated transport are shown in Table 8.9. These innovative cover materials based on ALF, polyester fiberfill, nylon, PU, and nonwovens can provide control of temperature fluctuation as well as thermal protection from solar radiation. ICE-BRIX®, Reflectix™, WEICO®, TempShield, Kodiakooler®, and ISO KIT are new commercial pallet cover brands. Nonwovens manufactured by Dupont under the brand name Tyvek® are used as cargo cover material for perishable goods such as fruits, vegetables, and cut flowers during air transportation. Pallet cover materials come in various forms depending on the manufacturing process. The Raindall® brand for flower, food, and beverage transportation uses a combination of nylon, PU coated, and polyester fiberfill as thermal insulation cover. Figure 8.23 illustrates several styles of pallet covers used in commercial operations. On a limited scale, insulated containers are employed for main packing (individual package), while Chill buddy™ is used for various applications including retail pods, pallet shrouds, and insulated bags for transporting fresh produce.

Few published studies have described the beneficial effects of pallet covers on reducing postharvest losses of fresh produce (Table 8.10). Pallet covering on sides and bottom by Reflectix™ reduced weight loss and wilting of amaranth and preserved the desirable dark green color. Using a pallet cover gave a higher score in overall quality than the uncovered product (Wheeler et al., 2015). Chaiwong and Bishop (2015) studied lightweight insulated bags as effective cool temperature management that reduced cool chain strawberry breakdown from supermarket to domestic refrigerator. Double-bubble foil insulation cover kept pre-chilled lettuce at low temperature and was also suitable for low-temperature phosphine fumigation to control western flower thrips on harvested lettuce (Liu, 2011). Melis (2016) reported that insulated pallet covers gave better temperature preservation than no covers, and temperature changes occurred slower

TABLE 8.9 Pallet Covers for Fresh Produce in Commercial Practices

Commodities	Properties	Branding	References
Perishable crops and cut flowers	Nonwoven with white color. Breathable cover with good O_2 transmission and high-water vapor permeability.	Tyvek®, DuPont	https://www.dupont.com/brands/tyvek.html
Fresh fruits and vegetables	Polyester fiberfill and PU coating	Randall Manufacturing	https://www.randallmanufacturing.com/
Fresh produce	Seven layers; Alu /PE/Aerogel/woven fabric/PA/Alu/PET	WEICO®	https://www.made-in-china.com/showroom/weicopackaging/product-detailrCFmhiHbbGVp/China-Thermal-Pallet-Cover-and-Waterproof-Pallet-Covers.html
Food and fresh produce	Alu exterior and 4 mm white foam interior	ICE-BRIX®	https://www.polar-tech.com/shop/category/containers-science-transport-pallet-covers/filter:/
Fresh produce	Aluwith white foam	Reflectix™	https://www.reflectixinc.com/applications/shipping-products/pallet-cover/

Remarks: Alu: Aluminum, PA: Polyamide, PET: Polyethylene terephthalate.

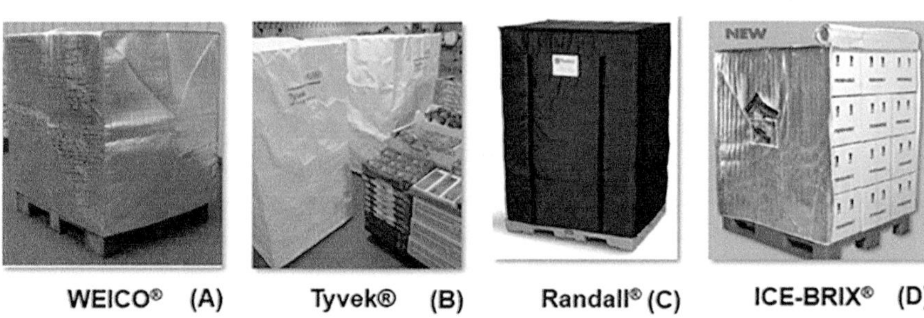

FIGURE 8.23 Pallet covers used in commercial practices including WEICO® (A); Tyvek® (B); Randall® (C); and ICE-BRIX® (D).

Source: https://www.made-in-china.com/showroom/weicopackaging/product-detailrCFmhiHbbGVp/China-Thermal-Pallet-Cover-and-Waterproof-Pallet-Covers.html (A); http://www.dupont.com/products-and-services/fabrics-fibers-nonwovens/protective-fabrics/brands/tyvek.html (B); https://tempcontrol.sftruckandtrailer.net/insulated-bags-insulated-pallet-covers-insulated-containers/randall-temp-control-insulated-covers (C); https://www.polar-tech.com/shop/category/containers-science-transport-pallet-covers/filter:/ (D).

than with no covers in chard, cucumber, and carrot. A combination of room cooling and two layers of heat-reflective sheet with thin nonwoven (HRS+TNNW) showed the highest efficiency in maintaining cool temperature and retarding the deterioration of okra during simulated storage and transportation (Rattanakaran et al., 2021b). HRS+TNNW also exhibited high potential as a thermal insulation cover to reduce postharvest loss in okra (5%) compared to typical handling (11–18%) and effectively reduced the use of foam sheets in cool chain management distribution packaging of okra under ambient environment conditions (Rattanakaran et al., 2021a).

TABLE 8.10 Pallet Covers for Fresh Produce in Academic Research

Commodities	Materials	Results	References
Lettuce	Double-bubble foil insulation cover	Cover reduced the effect of changes in ambient temperature on lettuce temperature profiles during phosphine fumigation treatments.	Liu (2011)
Amaranth	Reflectix™ insulation material (ALF/0.8 cm polyethylene/bubble pack) for pallet cover compared with no cover	Improved overall quality and reduced weight loss.	Wheeler et al. (2015)
Strawberry	Lightweight insulated bags; nonwoven material made from HDPE	Kept strawberry cool and delayed increase of air and pulp temperatures.	Chaiwong and Bishop (2015)
Chard, cucumber, carrot	Tyvek®, Metalized PET, Metalized PET bubbles and no cover as control	Insulated pallet covers showed better temperature preservation than no cover. Temperature fluctuations were slower than when using no cover.	Melis (2016)
Okra	P-LLDPE, HRS+TNNW, and MFS	Room cooling with HRS+TNNW was more efficient for temperature control of okra by slowing deterioration during simulated storage and transport.	Rattanakaran et al. (2021b)
Okra	P-LLDPE, HRS+TNNW, HRS+TKNW, MTyvek, MFS and no cover as control.	Thermal insulation covering maintained a better cool temperature than no cover. HRS + TNNW showed potential as thermal insulation cover for okra.	Rattanakaran et al. (2021a)

Remarks: PET: Polyethylene terephthalate, P-LLDPE: Perforated linear low-density polyethylene, HRS+TKNW: Heat-reflective sheet with thick nonwoven, MFS: Metalized foam sheet, MTyvek: Metalized Tyvek®.

PS with excellent thermal insulation and physical protection is commonly used to make foam boxes for packing fresh produce (Figure 8.24). Many shippers and distributors in Thailand use foam boxes to transport fresh produce. Foam boxes, as excellent insulators, are packed with gel ice to maintain fresh produce cool on long-distance flights (Chonhenchob, 2011). As shown in Table 8.11, copious research exists on chilled food products such as fish (Navaranjan et al., 2013), beer (Paternoster et al., 2017), dairy and food industry (Deshmukh et al., 2017), and cooked rice (Lee and Yoo, 2020). Most studies focused only on thermal insulation box performance for controlling cold temperature without determining fresh produce quality. ALF was highlighted as an important material to improve efficiency of thermal insulation boxes (Singh et al., 2008; Wang et al., 2020; Zeng et al., 2022). Some research has been conducted on thermal insulation packaging for food products such as frozen cooked rice, beer, and chilled fish (Lee and Yoo, 2020; Navaranjan et al., 2013; Paternoster et al., 2017;), with a single study that investigated thermal insulation boxes (thermal insulation material inside corrugated fiberboard) of fresh produce (Paquette et al., 2017). Most commercial thermal insulation boxes for fresh produce are presented on websites (Figure 8.25).

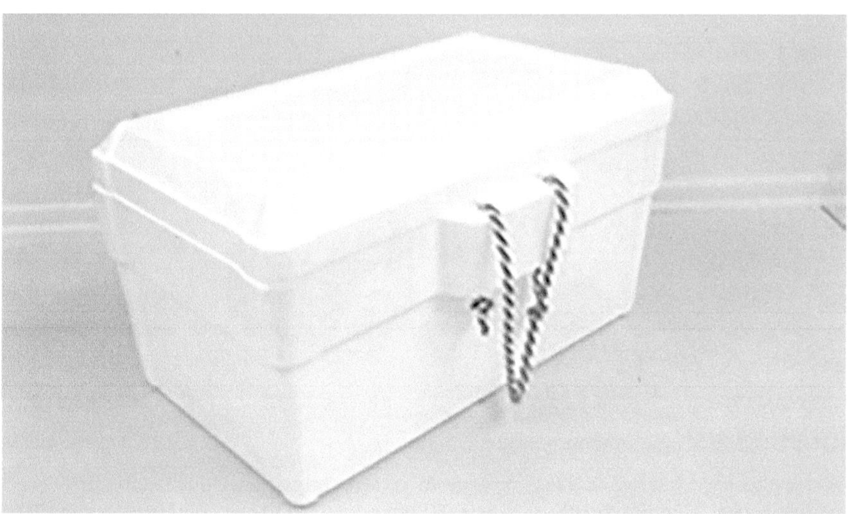

FIGURE 8.24 Commercial foam box made from PS.

Source: Authors.

TABLE 8.11 Thermal Insulation Boxes for Food Products and Their Performance

Box/Food Product	Materials	Results	References
		Box Testing	
Thermal insulation material of foam box	Addition of ALF on the inner and outside surfaces.	Thermal insulation performance improved.	Zeng et al. (2022)
Standard cardboard box	Addition of ALF on the internal liner surface.	Insulative performance increased together with maximum insulation time (MIT).	Wang et al. (2020)
Gel pack	ThermalCor® laminated with ALF.	Lamination of foil on ThermalCor® improved the R-value of the package.	Singh et al. (2008)
		Food Products	
Frozen cooked rice	Aluminum pouch and PE foam	Performance of the box improved and successfully suppressed quality deterioration of frozen cooked rice.	Lee and Yoo (2020)
Food can, meat pack, vegetable pack and fresh-cut lettuce pack	Addition of ALF on the inner surface.	Use of ALF led to 13% and 10% lower meat and lettuce temperatures, respectively.	Paquette et al. (2017)
Dairy and food industry	Glass wool, polystyrene and polyurethane foam	These poor conductors with low thermal conductivity prevented heat loss or heat gain of the product.	Deshmukh et al. (2017)
Beer	Cardboard combined with plastic foil (Bp-B)	The foil improved thermal insulation properties, reduced air movement and maintained the quality of beer.	Paternoster et al. (2017)
Chilled fish	Cardboard combined with EPS foam	The EPS foam improved the R value of the package and maintained the quality of the fish.	Navaranjan et al. (2013)

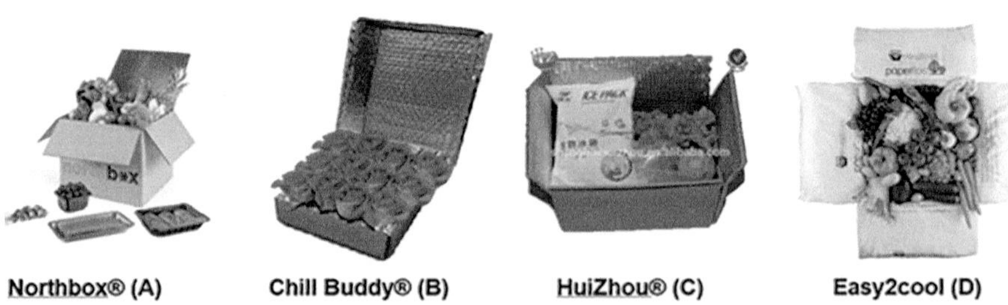

FIGURE 8.25 Commercial thermal insulation boxes.

Source: https://packaging.cascades.com/northbox/ (A) https://www.havi.com/sites/default/files/chill_buddy_brochure_3.pdf (B) https://www.alibaba.com/product-detail/Aluminum-Foil-Pizza-Box-Thermal-Food_60410872924. l?fbclid=IwAR2nGBpH byIrTVhKNPZX34Okv4pmAjqx5OedS3YXvdExzkAxnvke_UIixr (C) https://www.easy2cool.de/versandk%C3%BChlung_en.htmlv (D).

KEYWORDS

- **cold chain management**
- **distribution packaging**
- **fruit cushioning materials**
- **mechanical damage protection**
- **natural fiber materials**
- **sustainable packaging**

REFERENCES

Aboud, A. J. (2006). Study on factors affecting apple bruises under drop loading. *New Trends in Agricultural Engineering, 876–887.*

Acıcan, T., Alibaş, K., & Özelkök, I. S. (2007). Mechanical damage to apples during transport in wooden crates. *Biosystems Engineering, 96*(2), 239–248.

Ahmadi, E. (2012). Bruise susceptibilities of kiwifruits as affected by impact and fruit properties. *Research in Agricultural Engineering, 58*(3), 107–113.

Ahmadi, E., Ghassemzadeh, H. R., Sadeghi, M., & Moghaddam, M. (2010). The effect of impact and fruit properties on the bruising of peach. *Journal of Food Engineering, 97*, 110–117.

Al-Dairi, M., Pathare, P. B., & Al-Yahyai, R. (2021). Effect of postharvest transport and storage on color and firmness quality of tomato. *Horticultural, 7*(7), 163.

American Forest and Paper Association. (2021). *California Table Grapes: A Packaging and Distribution System Case Scenario* [www.document]. https://www.fibrebox.org/upload/CaseStudy_CaliforniaGrapes.pdf (accessed on 9th July 2025).

ASTM D4169–08. (2008). *Standard Practice for Performance Testing of Shipping Containers and Systems*. American Society of Testing and Materials, West Conshohocken, PA.

ASTM D642. (2010). *Standard Test Method for Determining Compressive Resistance of Shipping Containers, Components, and Unit Loads*. American Society of Testing and Materials International.

Azam, M. M., Saad, A., & Amer, B. M. (2022). Assessment of the quality losses of cantaloupe fruit during transportation. *Processes, 10*(6), 1187.

Barchi, G. L., Berardinelli, A., Guarnieri, L., Ragni, C., & Fila, C. T. (2002). Damage to loquats by vibration-simulating intra-state transport. *Biosystems Engineering, 83*(3), 305–312.

Bello, K., Idah, P. A., & Fadeyibi, A. (2013). Damage of tomatoes in traditional palm baskets of different shape subjected to force vibration. *Swiss Journal of Applied Sciences, 2*(8), 1–8.

Berardinelli, A., Donati, V., Giunchi, A., Guarnieri, A., & Ragni, L. (2005). Damage to pears caused by simulated transport. *Journal of Food Engineering, 66*, 219–226.

Berry, T. M., Ambaw, A., Defraeye, T., Coetzee, C., & Opara, U. L. (2019). Moisture adsorption in palletized corrugated fiberboard cartons under shipping conditions: A CFD modelling approach. *Food and Bioproducts Processing, 114*, 43–59.

Berry, T. M., Defraeye, T., Shrivastava, C., Ambaw, A., Coetzee, C., & Opara, U. L. (2022). Designing ventilated packaging for the fresh produce cold chain. *Food and Bioproducts Processing, 134*, 121–149.

Berry, T. M., Fadiji, T. S., Defraeye, T., & Opara, U. L. (2017). The role of horticultural carton vent hole design on cooling efficiency and compression strength: A multi-parameter approach. *Postharvest Biology and Technology, 124*, 62–74.

Bhat, G. S., & Malkan, S. R. (2007). Polymer-laid web formation. In S. J. Russell (Ed.), *Handbook of Nonwovens* (pp. 143–195). Cambridge: Woodhead Publishing Limited.

Binh, L. N. (2011). Packaging in fresh produce supply chains in Viet Nam. In A. A. S. Villahermosa, L. N. Binh, R. S. Rolle, & V. Chonhenchob, *Packaging in Fresh Produce Supply Chain in Southeast Asia* (pp. 101–119). Bangkok: Food and Agriculture Organization of the United Nations.

Boyette, M. D., Sanders, D. C., & Rutledge, G. A. (1996). *Package Requirements for Fresh Fruits and Vegetables*. The North Carolina Agricultural Extension Service. North Carolina State University, Raleigh, NC, USA. Publication, (9/96).

Bwambok, D. K., Christodouleas, D. C., Morin, S. A., Lange, H., Phillips, S. T., & Whitesides, G. M. (2014). Adaptive use of bubble wrap for storing liquid samples and performing analytical assays. *Analytical Chemistry, 86*(15), 7478–7485.

Bycroft, B. L., Brash, D. W., & Bollen, F. (1996). Using insulation and cooling to improve the asparagus cool chain. *Acta Horticultural, 415*, 323–332.

Çakmak, B., Alayunt, F. N., Akdeniz, R. C., Aksoy, U., & Can, H. Z. (2010). Assessment of the quality losses of fresh fig fruits during transport. *Journal of Agricultural Sciences, 16*, 183–193.

Celik, H. K., Ustun, H., Erkan, M., Rennie, A. E. W., & Akinci, I. (2021). Effects of bruising of 'Pink Lady' apple under impact loading in drop test on firmness, colour and gas exchange of fruit during long term storage. *Postharvest Biology and Technology, 179*, 111561.

Centobelli, P., Cerchione, R., & Ertz, M. (2020). Food cold chain management: What we know and what we deserve. *Supply Chain Management: An International Journal*.

Chaiwong, S. (2016). *Effect of Impact and Vibration on Quality and Damage in The British Strawberries* (Doctoral dissertation, University of Essex).

Chaiwong, S., & Bishop, C. F. H. (2015). Effect of vibration damage on the storage quality of 'Elsanta' strawberry. *Australian Journal of Crop Science, 9*(9), 859–864.

Chaiwong, S., & Bishop, C. F. H. (2015). Use of an insulated bag from the supermarket to maintain 'Elsanta' strawberry temperature to households. *Acta Horticultural, 1079*, 187–192.

Chaiwong, S., & Bishop, C. F. H. (2020). The changes of physical properties in 'Elsanta' strawberries from the winter and summer cultivations after vibration tests. *Australian Journal of Crop Science, 14*(4), 697–704.

Chaiwong, S., Saengrayap, R., Rattanakaran, J., Chaithanarueang, A., Arwatchananukul, S., Aunsri, N., Tontiwattanakul, K., Jitkokkruad, K., Kitazawa, H., & Trongsatitkul, T.

(2022). Eco-friendly cushioning performance for reducing vibration damage in guava during simulated transportation. *Manuscript Submitted for Publication.*

Chaiwong, S., Yoythaisong, P., Arwatchananukul, S., Aunsri, N., Tontiwattanakul, K., Trongsatitkul, T., Kitazawa, H., & Saengrayap, R. (2021). Vibration damage in guava during simulated transportation assessed by digital image analysis using response surface methodology. *Postharvest Biology and Technology, 181*, 111641.

Chen, R., Sui, L., Liu, Q., & Qiu, Q. (2020). Research on the cushioning effect of protective materials under high impact. In *Journal of Physics: Conference Series* (*Vol. 1635, No. 1*, p. 012091). IOP Publishing. https://doi.org/10.1088/1742-6596/1635/1/012091 (accessed on 9th July 2025).

Cherono, K., & Workneh, T. S. (2018). A review of the role of transportation on the quality changes of fresh tomatoes and their management in South Africa and other emerging markets. *International Food Research Journal, 25*(6), 2211–2228.

Chitranshi, S., Dubey, N., & Sajjad, M. (2020). Sustainable botanical products for safe post-harvest management of perishable produce: A review. *Journal of Horticulture and Postharvest Research, 3*(1), 125–140.

Chonhenchob, V., & Singh, S. P. (2004). Testing and comparison of various packages for mango distribution. *Journal of Testing and Evaluation, 32*(1), 1–4.

Chonhenchob, V., Chriyachotilert, S., & Singh, S. P. (2011). Packaging in fresh produce supply chains in Thailand. In A. A. S. Villahermosa, L. N. Bihn, R. S. Rolle, & V. Chonhenchob (Eds.), *Packaging in Fresh Produce Supply Chain in Southeast Asia* (pp. 43–99). Bangkok: Food and Agriculture Organization of the United Nations.

Chonhenchob, V., Kamhangwong, D., & Singh, S. P. (2008). Comparison of reusable and single-use plastic and paper shipping containers for distribution of fresh pineapples. *Packaging Technology and Science: An International Journal, 21*(2), 73–83.

Chonhenchob, V., Singh, S. P., Singh, J. J., Sittipod, S., Swasdee, D., & Pratheepthinthong, S. (2010). Measurement and analysis of truck and rail vibration levels in Thailand. *Packaging Technology and Science, 23*(3), 91–100.

Chonhenchob, V., Singh, S. P., Singh, J. J., Stallings, J., & Grawal, G. (2012). Measurement and analysis of vehicle vibration for delivering packages in small-sized and medium-sized trucks and automobiles. *Packaging Technology and Science, 25*, 31–38.

Chonhenchob, V., Sittipod, S., Swasdee, P., Rachtanapun, S., Singh, S. P., & Singh, J. (2009). Effect of truck vibration during transport on damage to fresh produce shipments in Thailand. *Journal of Applied Packaging Research, 3*(1), 27–38.

Costa, J. D. D. S., Figueiredo Neto, A., Olivier, N. C., Irmão, M. A. D. S., Costa, M. D. S., & Gomes, J. P. (2021). Road transport vibration stress impact on 'Palmer' mangoes quality and shelf life. *Revita Brasileira de Fruticulture, 43.*

Cui, J., Yang, M., Son, D., Park, S., & Cho, S. I. (2018). Estimation of tomato bruising by mechanical impact force using multivariate analysis. *Hort Science, 53*(9), 1352–1359.

Da Costa Castro, C. D. P., de Assis Fonseca Faria, J., & Dantas, T. B. H. (2014). Evaluating the performance of coconut fiber and wood straw as cushioning materials to reduce injuries of papaya and mango during transportation. *International Journal of Advanced Packaging Technology, 2*(1), 84–95.

Da Costa Castro, C. D. P., Faria, J. D. A. F., & Dantas, T. B. H. (2012). Testing the use of coconut fiber as a cushioning material for transport packaging. *Materials Sciences and Applications, 3*, 151–156.

De Castro, L. R., Vigneault, C., & Cortez, L. A. B. (2004). Container opening design for horticultural produce cooling efficiency. *Food, Agriculture & Environment, 1*, 135–140.
Delele, M. A., Ngcobo, M. E. K., Getahun, S. T., Chen, L., Mellmann, J., & Opara, U. L. (2013). Studying airflow and heat transfer characteristics of a horticultural produce packaging system using a 3-D CFD model. Part I: Model development and validation. *Postharvest Biology and Technology, 86*, 536–545.
Deshmukh, G., Birwal, P., Datir, R., & Patel, S. (2017). Thermal insulation materials: A tool for energy conservation. *Journal of Food Processing & Technology, 8*(4), 1–5.
Deshwal, G. Kr., Panjagari, N. R., & Alam, T. (2019). An overview of paper and paper-based food packaging materials: Health safety and environmental concerns. *Journal of Food Science and Technology, 56*(10), 4391–4403.
Desjarlais, A. O., & Zarr, R. R. (2002). *Insulation Materials, Testing and Applications* (*Vol. 1426*). Pennsylvania: ASTM International.
Dubey, N., & Mishra, V. (2018). Cushioning materials for fruits, vegetables and flowers. In M. W. Siddiqui, M. S. Rahman, & A. A. Wani (Eds.), *Innovative Packaging Fruits and Vegetable Strategies for Safety and Quality Maintenance* (pp. 275–313). Apple Academic Press.
Dunno, K., Stoeckley, I., & Hofmeister, M. (2021). Susceptibility of impact damage to whole apples packaged inside molded fiber and expanded polystyrene trays. *Foods, 10*(9), 1980.
Eissa, A. H. A., Albaloushi, N. S., & Azam, M. M. (2013). Vibration analysis influence during crisis transport of the quality of fresh fruit on food security. *Agricultural Engineering International: CIGR Journal, 15*(3), 181–190.
Eissa, A., Gamaa, G. R., Gomaa, F. R., & Azam, M. M. (2012). Comparison of package cushioning materials to protect vibration damage to golden delicious apples. *International Journal of Latest Trends in Agriculture and Food Sciences, 2*(1), 36–57.
El-Sonbati, A. (2012). Thermoplastic elastomers; starch protective loose-fill foams. In *Thermoplastic Elastomers* (Chapter 15). Tech Europe.
Fadiji, T., Coetzee, C. J., Berry, T. M., & Opara, U. L. (2019). Investigating the role of geometrical configurations of ventilated fresh produce packaging to improve the mechanical strength–Experimental and numerical approaches. *Food Packaging and Shelf Life, 20*, 100312.
Fadiji, T., Coetzee, C. J., Berry, T. M., Ambaw, A., & Opara, U. L. (2018). The efficacy of finite element analysis (FEA) as a design tool for food packaging: A review. *Biosystems Engineering, 174*, 20–40.
Fadiji, T., Coetzee, C., & Opara, U. L. (2016). Compression strength of ventilated corrugated paperboard packages: Numerical modelling, experimental validation and effects of vent geometric design. *Biosystems Engineering, 151*, 231–247.
Farrelly, T. A., & Shaw, I. C. (2017). Polystyrene as hazardous household waste. In *Household Hazardous Waste Management* (p. 45).
FEFCO. (2021). Corrugated board production. https://www.fefco.org/lca/dscription-of-production-system/corrugated-board-production (accessed on 9th July 2025).
Fernando, I., Fei, J., Stanley, R., & Enshaei, H. (2018). Measurement and evaluation of the effect of vibration on fruits in transit—Review. *Packaging Technology and Science, 31*(11), 723–738.

Fernando, I., Fei, J., Stanley, R., & Rouillard, V. (2020). Evaluating packaging performance for bananas under simulated vibration. *Food Packaging and Shelf Life, 23*, 100428.

Ferreira, M. D., Sargent, S. A., Brecht, J. K., & Chandler, C. K. (2008). Strawberry fruit resistance to simulated handling. *Scientia Agricola (Piracicaba, Braz.), 65*(5), 490–495.

Ferrua, M. J., & Singh, R. P. (2009). Design guidelines for the forced-air cooling process of strawberries. *International Journal of Refrigeration, 32*, 1932–1943.

Fischer, D., Craig, W. L., Watada, A. E., Douglas, W., & Ashby, B. H. (1992). Simulated in transit vibration damage to packaged fresh market grapes and strawberries. *Applied Engineering in Agriculture, 8*(3), 363–366.

Food and Agriculture Organization of the United Nations (FAO). (2011). Basic principles of fresh produce packaging. In A. A. S. Villahermosa, L. N. Bihn, R. S. Rolle, & V. Chonhenchob (Eds.), *Packaging in Fresh Produce Supply Chain in Southeast Asia* (pp. 1–7). Bangkok: Food and Agriculture Organization of the United Nations.

Franklin Associates. (2004). Life cycle inventory of reusable plastic container and display-ready corrugated containers used for fresh produce application. Retrieved from http://usereusables.org/sites/all/themes/usereusables/images/LCI_Preface_and_Executive_Summary.pdf (accessed on 9th July 2025).

Freeston Jr, W. D., & Platt, M. M. (1965). Mechanics of elastic performance of textile materials: Part XVI: Bending rigidity of nonwoven fabrics. *Textile Research Journal, 35*(1), 48–57.

Gao, Y. (2018). *Research on Properties and Design Methods of Cushion Packaging Materials for Consumer Electronic* (Master's thesis, Lappeenranta University of Technology LUT School of Energy Systems LUT Mechanical, Lappeenranta, Finland).

Garcia-Romeu-Martinez, M. A., Singh, S. P., & Cloquell-Ballester, V. A. (2008). Measurement and analysis of vibration levels for truck transport in Spain as a function of payload, suspension and speed. *Packaging Technology and Science, 21*, 439–451.

Gupta, N. P. (1987). Influence of medullated fiber on mechanical properties and product performance. *Indian Journal of Textile Research, 12*, 46–52.

Gustafsson, K., Jönson, G., Smith, D., & Sparks, L. (2009). *Retailing Logistics & Fresh Food Packaging: Managing Change in the Supply Chain*. London: Kogan Page Limited.

Han, J. W., Qian, J. P., Zhao, C. J., Yang, X. T., & Fan, B. L. (2017). Mathematical modelling of cooling efficiency of ventilated packaging: Integral performance evaluation. *International Journal of Heat and Mass Transfer, 111*, 386–397.

Han, J. W., Zhao, C. J., Qian, J. P., Ruiz-Garcia, L., & Zhang, X. (2018). Numerical modeling of forced-air cooling of palletized apple: Integral evaluation of cooling efficiency. *International Journal of Refrigeration, 89*, 131–141.

Hinsch, R. T., Slaughter, D. C., Craig, W. L., & Thompson, J. F. (1993). Vibration of fresh fruits and vegetables during refrigerated truck transport. *Transactions of the ASAE (American Society of Agriculture Engineers), 36*(4), 1039–1042.

Htike, T., Saengrayap, R., Aunsri, N., Tontiwattanakul, K., & Chaiwong, S. (2021). Investigation and evaluation of impact bruising in guava using image processing and response surface methodology. *Horticultural, 7*(10), 411.

Hussein, Z., Fawole, O. A., & Opara, U. L. (2019). Determination of physical, biochemical and microstructural changes in impact-bruise damaged pomegranate fruit. *Journal of Food Measurement and Characterization, 13*, 2177–2189.

Hussein, Z., Fawole, O. A., & Opara, U. L. (2020). Effects of bruising and storage duration on physiological response and quality attributes of pomegranate fruit. *Scientia Horticultural, 267*, 109306.

Hussein, Z., Fawole, O. A., & Opara, U. L. (2020). Harvest and postharvest factors affecting bruise damage of fresh fruits. *Horticultural Plant Journal, 6*(1), 1–13.

Idah, P. A., Ajisegiri, E. S. A., & Yisa, M. G. (2007). An assessment of impact damage to fresh tomato fruits. *Assumption University Journal of Technology, 10*(4), 271–275.

Ishikawa, Y., Kitazawa, H., & Shina, T. (2009). Vibration and shock analysis of fruit and vegetables transport–Cherry transport from Yamagata to Taipei. *Japan Agricultural Research Quarterly, 43*(2), 129–135.

ISTA PROJECT 4AB. (2009). *Packaged-Products for Shipment in Known Distribution Channels*.

Jarimopas, B., Singh, S. P., Sayasoonthorn, S., & Singh, J. (2007). Comparison of package cushioning materials to protect post-harvest impact damage to apples. *Packaging Technology and Science: An International Journal, 20*(5), 315–324.

Jiang, Y., Shina, T., Nakamura, N., & Nakahara, A. (2001). Electrical conductivity evaluation of postharvest strawberry damage. *Journal of Food Science, 66*(9), 1392–1395.

Juan, L. (2011). Characteristics and fabrication technology of polyurethane aluminum foil composite air duct. *Installation, 03*, 32–34.

Karimah, A., Ridho, M. R., Munawar, S. S., Adi, D. S., Damayanti, I. R., Subiyanto, B., Fatriasari, W., & Fudholi, A. (2021). A review on natural fibers for development of eco-friendly bio-composite: Characteristics, and utilizations. *Journal of Materials Research and Technology, 13*, 2442–2458.

Khandelwal, M. (2010). *Basics About Insulations*. Gujarat: Nirma Industries.

Kitazawa, H. (2018). Cushioning packaging for fresh produce. *Reference Module in Food Science*, 1–8.

Kitazawa, H., Li, L., Hasegawa, N., Rattanakaran, J., & Saengrayap, R. (2018). Evaluation of shock-proof performance of new cushioning system for portable packaging of apples. *Environmental Control in Biology, 56*(4), 167–172.

Kitazawa, H., Saito, K., & Ishikawa, Y. (2014). Effect of difference in acceleration and velocity change on product damage due to repetitive shock. *Packaging Technology and Science, 27*, 221–230.

Kitazawa, H., Saito, K., & Ishikawa, Y. (2015). Method for controlling damage to products subjected to cumulative fatigue considering damage degree at each layer in stacked packaging. *Journal of Packaging Science and Technology, Japan, 24*(2), 69–78.

Kitinoja, L. Use of cold chains for reducing food losses in developing countries. http://www.postharvest.org/Cold_chains_PEF_White_Paper_13_03.pdf (accessed on 9th July 2025).

Lee, H. G., & Yoo, S. (2020). Changes in the physical properties of frozen cooked rice depending on thermal insulation levels of packaging during freeze-thaw. *Journal of Food Science, 85*(12), 4342–4350.

Lehn, I. M., & Herrmann, M. L. (2013). Compartment pallet packaging system for perishable products. *United States Patent Application Publication, US 2013/0026061 A1*, 31 January 2013.

Lewis, R., Yoxall, A., Marshall, M. B., & Canty, L. A. (2008). Characterizing pressure and bruising in apple fruit. *Wear, 264*, 37–46.

Li, F., Guan, K., Liu, P., Li, G., & Li, J. (2014). Ingredient of biomass packaging material and compare study on cushion properties. *International Journal of Polymer Science*, 1–7.

Lin, M., Chen, J., Chen, F., Zhu, C., Wu, D., Wang, J., & Chen, K. (2020). Effects of cushioning materials and temperature on quality damage of ripe peaches according to the vibration test. *Food Packaging and Shelf Life, 25*, 100518.

Lin, M., Fawole, O. A., Saeys, W., Wu, D., Wang, J., Opara, U. L., Nicolai, B., & Chen, K. (2022). Mechanical damages and packaging methods along the fresh fruit supply chain: A review. *Critical Reviews in Food Science and Nutrition.*

Liu, Y. B. (2011). Low-temperature phosphine fumigation of chilled lettuce under insulated cover for postharvest control of western flower thrips, *Frankliniella occidentalis* (Pergande) (Thysanoptera: Thripidae). *Journal of Asia-Pacific Entomology, 14*(3), 323–325.

Lu, F., Ishikawa, Y., Kitazawa, H., & Satake, T. (2010a). Effect of vehicle speed on shock and vibration levels in truck transport. *Packaging Technology and Science, 23*, 101–109.

Lu, F., Ishikawa, Y., Kitazawa, H., & Satake, T. (2010b). Measurement of impact pressure and bruising of apple fruit using pressure-sensitive film technique. *Journal of Food Engineering, 96*, 614–620.

Lu, F., Ishikawa, Y., Kitazawa, H., & Satake, T. (2012). Assessment and prediction of repetitive impact damage to apple fruit using pressure-sensitive film technique. *Journal of Food Agriculture and Environment, 10*(2), 156–160.

Lu, H., Zheng, H., Hu, Y., Lou, H., & Kong, X. (2011). Bruise detection on red bayberry (*Myrica rubra* Sieb. & Zucc.) using fractal analysis and support vector machine. *Journal of Food Engineering, 104*, 149–153.

Lu, T., Liu, S., Jiang, M., Xu, X., Wang, Y., Wang, Z., Gou, J., Hui, D., & Zhou, Z. (2014). Effects of modifications of bamboo cellulose fibers on the improved mechanical properties of cellulose reinforced poly (lactic acid) composites. *Composites Part B: Engineering, 62*, 191–197.

Macnish, A. J., Padda, M. S., Pupin, F., Tsouvaltzis, P. I., Deltsidis, A. I., Sims, C. A., Brecht, J. K., & Mitcham, E. J. (2012). Comparison of pallet cover systems to maintain strawberry fruit quality during transport. *Hort Technology, 22*(4), 493–501.

Maga, D., Hiebel, M., & Aryan, V. (2019). A comparative life cycle assessment of meat trays made of various packaging materials. *Sustainability, 11*(19), 5324.

Marcondes, J. (2009). Vibration. In K. L. Yam (Ed.), *The Wiley Encyclopedia of Packaging Technology* (pp. 1266–1270). New York: John Wiley & Sons Inc.

Marcondes, J., Hatton, K., Graham, J., & Schueneman, H. (2003). Effect of temperature on the cushioning properties of some foamed plastic materials. *Packaging Technology and Science, 16*(2), 69–76.

Melis, R. B. (2016). *New Techniques and Methods for Cold Chain Monitoring and Tracking in Perishable Products* (Doctoral dissertation). Universidad Politécnica de Madrid, Madrid.

Mencarelli, F., Massantini, R., & Botondi, R. (1996). Influence of impact surface and temperature on the ripening response of kiwifruit. *Postharvest Biology and Technology, 8*, 165–177.

Montero, C. R. S., Schwarz, L. L., Santos, L. C., Andreazza, C. S., Kechinski, C. P., & Bender, R. J. (2009). Postharvest mechanical damage affects fruit quality of 'Montenegrina' and 'Rainha' tangerines. *Pesquisa Agropecuária Brasileira, 44*(12), 1639–1640.

Mukama, M., Ambaw, A., & Opara, U. L. (2020). Advances in design and performance evaluation of fresh fruit ventilated distribution packaging: A review. *Food Packaging and Shelf Life, 24*, 100472.

Nakamura, N., Umehara, H., Nei, D., Okadome, H., Ishikawa, Y., Nakano, K., Maezawa, S., & Shina, T. (2008). Effect of package conditions on the damage of strawberries. *Journal of the Society of Agricultural Structures, Japan, 39*(1), 1–8.

Nakamura, N., Umehara, H., Okadome, H., Nakano, K., Maezawa, S., & Shina, T. (2007b). Effect of vibration frequency and direction on damage of strawberries. *Journal of the Society of Agricultural Structures, Japan, 38*(2), 101–108.

Navaranjan, N., Fletcher, G. C., Summers, G., Parr, R., & Anderson, R. (2013). Thermal insulation requirements and new cardboard packaging for chilled seafood exports. *Journal of Food Engineering, 119*(3), 395–403.

Nayak, R., Padhye, R., Sinnappoo, K., Arnold, L., & Behera, B. K. (2013). Airbags. *Textile Progress, 45*(4), 209–301.

Nechita, P., & Năstac, S. M. (2022). Overview on foam forming cellulose materials for cushioning packaging applications. *Polymers, 14*(10), 1963.

Opara, U. L., & Pathare, P. B. (2014). Bruise damage measurement and analysis of fresh horticultural produce–A review. *Postharvest Biology and Technology, 91*, 9–24.

Paquette, J. C., Mercier, S., Marcos, B., & Morasse, S. (2017). Modeling the thermal performance of a multilayer box for the transportation of perishable food. *Food and Bioproducts Processing, 105*, 77–85.

Park, J., Choi, S., & Jung, H. M. (2020). Measurement and analysis of vibration levels for truck transport environment in Korea. *Applied Sciences (Basel), 10*(19), 6754.

Patel, M., & Bhrambhatt, D. (2011). Nonwoven technology. https://textlnfo.files.wordpress.com/2011/10/nonwoven-fabrics1.pdf (accessed on 9th July 2025).

Paternoster, A., Van Camp, J., Vanlanduit, S., Weeren, A., Springael, J., & Braet, J. (2017). The performance of beer packaging: Vibration damping and thermal insulation. *Food Packaging and Shelf Life, 11*, 91–97.

Pathare, P. B. (2021). Bruise susceptibility and impact on quality parameters of pears during storage. *Frontiers in Sustainable Food Systems, 5*, 658132.

Pathare, P. B., & Opara, U. L. (2014). Structural design of corrugated boxes for horticultural produce: A review. *Biosystems Engineering, 125*, 128–140.

Pathare, P. B., Al-Dairi, M., & Al-Mahdouri, A. (2021). Bruise damage susceptibility and fruit quality assessment of pear. *The Open Agriculture Journal, 15*, 82–90.

PEAKfresh. (2021). Pallet cover. https://www.peakfreshusa.com/about-pallet-covers (accessed on 9th July 2025).

Pelletier, W., Brecht, J. K., do Nascimento Nunes, M. C., & Émond, J. P. (2011). Quality of strawberries shipped by truck from California to Florida as influenced by postharvest temperature management practices. *Hort Technology, 21*, 482–493.

Phukon, R. M., & Barua, P. (2015). Effect of different packing systems and transportation on physio-chemical qualities of carambola (*Averrhoa carambola*). *Scientists Joined as Life Member of Society of Krishi Vigyan, 3*(2), 39–42.

Pongrácz, E. (2007). The environmental impacts of packaging. In M. Kutz (Ed.), *Environmentally Conscious Materials and Chemicals Processing* (pp. 237–278). NJ, USA: John Wiley & Sons, Inc.

Porat, R., Lichter, A., Terry, L. A., Harker, R., & Buzby, J. (2018). Postharvest losses of fruit and vegetables during retail and in consumers' homes: Quantifications, causes, and means of prevention. *Postharvest Biology and Technology, 139*, 135–149.

Poustis, J. (2005). Corrugated fiberboard packaging. In M. J. Kirwan (Ed.), *Paper and Paperboard Packaging Technology* (pp. 317–372). Oxford: Blackwell Publishing Ltd.

Ranathunga, C. L., Jayaweera, H. H. E., Suraweera, S. K. K., Wattage, S. C., Ruvinda, K. K. D. L., & Ariyaratne, T. R. (2010). Vibration effects in vehicular road transportation. *Proceedings of the 26th Technical Sessions, Institute of Physics*, Colombo, Sri Lanka, March 2010, 9–16.

Rapusas, R., & Rolle, R. S. (2009). *Management of Reusable Plastic Crates in Fresh Produce Supply Chains*. Bangkok: Food and Agriculture Organization of the United Nations.

Rattanakaran, J., Saengrayap, R., Aunsri, N., Padee, S., Prahsarn, C., Kitazawa, H., Bishop, C. F. H., & Chaiwong, S. (2021a). Performance of thermal insulation covering materials to reduce postharvest losses in okra. *Horticultural, 7*(10), 392.

Rattanakaran, J., Saengrayap, R., Prahsarn, C., Kitazawa, H., & Chaiwong, S. (2021b). Application of room cooling and thermal insulation materials to maintain quality of okra during storage and transportation. *Horticultural, 7*(7), 188.

Reza, T. (2013). Engineering properties and bruise susceptibility of peach fruits. *Agricultural Engineering International: CIGR Journal, 15*(4), 244–252.

Ríos-Mesa, A. F., Zuluaga Gallego, R., Osorio, M., Ciro-Velásquez, H. J., & Márquez Cardozo, C. J. (2020). Effect of vehicle vibration on the mechanical and sensory properties of avocado (*Persea americana* Mill. cv. Hass) during road transportation. *International Journal of Fruit Science, 20*(sup3), S1904–S1919.

Ruiz-Altisent, M., & Moreda, G. P. (2011). Fruits, mechanical properties and bruise susceptibility. In J. Gliński, J. Horabik, & J. Lipiec (Eds.), *Encyclopedia of Agrophysics* (pp. 318–321). Dordrecht: Springer.

Saracoglu, T., Ucer, N., & Ozarslan, C. (2011). Engineering properties and susceptibility to bruising damage of table olive (*Olea europaea*) fruit. *International Journal of Agriculture and Biology, 13*, 801–805.

Semple, K. E., Zhou, C., Rojas, O. J., Nkeuwa, W. N., & Dai, C. (2022). Moulded pulp fibers for disposable food packaging: A state-of-the-art review. *Food Packaging and Shelf Life, 33*, 100908.

Shafie, M., Rajabipour, A., Castro-Garcia, S., Jiménez-Jiménez, F., & Mobli, H. (2015). Effect of fruit properties on pomegranate bruising. *International Journal of Food Properties, 18*, 1837–1846.

Shahbazi, F., Rajabipour, A., Mohtasebi, S., & Rafie, Sh. (2010). Simulated in-transit vibration damage to watermelons. *Journal of Agricultural Science and Technology, 12*, 23–24.

Sharan, G., Srivastav, S., Rawale, K. P., & Dave, U. (2009). Development of corrugated fiber board cartons for long distance transport of tomatoes in India. *International Journal of Service Learning in Engineering, 4*(1), 31–43.

Sharp, A. K., & Irving, A. R. (1981). *Insulating Covers for Pallets of Food*. Scotland: AK, Sharp.

Siddiqui, M. W., Rahman, S., & Wani, A. A. (2009). *Innovative Packaging of Fruits and Vegetables: Strategies for Safety and Quality Maintenance* (Vol. 38, pp. 2434–2446).

Sigalingging, R., Nasution, H. A., Rindang, A., & Ayu, P. C. (2019). Effect of packaging fillers materials on the quality of papaya fruit (*Carica papaya* L.). In *IOP Conference Series: Earth and Environmental Science, 260*(1), 012036. IOP Publishing.

Singh, A. K., Itkor, P., Lee, M., Shin, J., & Lee, Y. S. (2022). Promoting sustainable packaging applications in the circular economy by exploring and advancing molded pulp materials for food products: A review. *Critical Reviews in Food Science and Nutrition*, 1–16.

Singh, J., & Singh, S. P. (2007). Damage reduction to food products during transportation and handling. In M. Kutz (Ed.), *Handbook of Farm, Dairy, And Food Machinery* (pp. 655–693). New York: William Andrew, Inc.

Singh, J., Kisch, R., Chhun, J., & Olsen, E. (2009). Design—An opportunity in reducing corrugated fiberboard carbon footprint. *Journal of Applied Packaging Research, 3*(2), 105–118.

Singh, J., Olsen, E., Singh, S. P., Manley, J., & Wallace, F. (2008). The effect of ventilation and hand holes on loss of compression strength in corrugated boxes. *Journal of Applied Packaging Research, 2*(4), 227–238.

Singh, J., Singh, S. P., & Joneson, E. (2006). Measurement and analysis of US truck vibration for leaf spring and air ride suspensions, and development of tests to simulate these conditions. *Packaging Technology and Science, 19*, 309–323.

Singh, R. P., Singh, J., & Saha, K. (2011). Effect of palletized box offset on compression strength of unitized and stacked empty corrugated fiberboard boxes. *Journal of Applied Packaging Research, 5*(3), 157–168.

Singh, S. P., Burgess, G., & Singh, J. (2008). Performance comparison of thermal insulated packaging boxes, bags and refrigerants for single-parcel shipments. *Packaging Technology and Science: An International Journal, 21*(1), 25–35.

Slaughter, D. C., Hinsch, R. T., & Thompson, J. F. (1993). Assessment of vibration injury to Bartlett pears. *Transactions of the ASAE (American Society of Agricultural Engineers), 36*(4), 1043–1047.

Smith, J. P., Zagory, D., & Ramaswamy, H. S. (2004). Packaging of fruits and vegetables. In D. M. Barrett, L. Somogyi, & H. Ramaswamy (Eds.), *Processing Fruits: Science and Technology* (2nd ed., pp. 355–395). New York: CRC Press.

Sohn, J. S., Kim, H. K., Kim, S. W., Ryu, Y., & Cha, S. W. (2019). Biodegradable foam cushions as ecofriendly packaging materials. *Sustainability, 11*(6), 1731.

Soleimani, B., & Ahmadi, E. (2014). Measurement and analysis of truck vibration levels as a function of packages locations in truck bed and suspension. *Computers and Electronics in Agriculture, 109*, 141–147.

Song, X., Zhang, G., Lu, J., Zhang, L., & Zhang, S. (2018). Study on the cushion performance of the cushion material composed of EPE and corrugated paperboard. In *Applied Sciences in Graphic Communication and Packaging* (pp. 467–474). Singapore: Springer.

Tabatabaekoloor, R. (2013). Engineering properties and bruise susceptibility of peach fruits (*Prunus persica*). *Agricultural Engineering International: CIGR Journal, 15*, 244–252.

Tao, F., Chen, W., & Jia, Z. (2021). Effect of simulated transport vibration on the quality of shiitake mushroom (*Lentinus edodes*) during storage. *Food Science & Nutrition, 9*(2), 1152–1159.

Tausif, M. (2016). Application based approach of nonwoven industry. https://www.technicaltextile.net/articles/application-based-approach-of-nonwoven-industry-7523 (accessed on 9th July 2025).

The Thermal Insulation Association of Southern Africa (TIASA). (2001). *Thermal Insulation Handbook.* https://www.aaamsa.co.za/docs_new/TIASA/Handbook_Chapter1.pdf (accessed on 9th July 2025).

Thompson, J. F., & Mitchell, F. G. (2002). Strawberries and cane berries. In A. A. Kader (Ed.), *Postharvest Technology of Horticultural Crops* (3rd ed., pp. 85–95). Oakland: University of California, Division of Agriculture and Natural Resources.

Thompson, J. F., Brecht, P. E., & Hinsh, T. (2002). Refrigerated trailer transport of perishable products. California: Agriculture and Natural Resources, University of California, Davis.

Thompson, J. F., Slaughter, D. C., & Arpaia, M. L. (2008). Suspended tray package for protecting soft fruit from mechanical damage. *Applied Engineering in Agriculture, 24*(1), 71–75.

Timm, E. J., Brown, G. K., & Armstrong, P. R. (1996). Apple damage in bulk bins during semitrailer transport. *Applied Engineering in Agriculture, 12*(3), 369–377.

Tong, T. W., & Tien, C. L. (1983). Radiative heat transfers in fibrous insulations—Part I: Analytical study. *Journal of Heat Transfer, 105*, 70–75.

TransFresh Cooperation. (2011). Consumer acceptance study of California fresh strawberries [www.document]. http://www.transfresh.com/files/CQI_White_Paper_Final.pdf (accessed on 9th July 2025).

Tutar, M., Erdogu, F., & Toka, B. (2009). Computational modeling of airflow patterns and heat transfer prediction through stacked layer products in a vented box during cooling. *International Journal of Refrigeration, 32*, 295–306.

Tuval, A., Las, L., & Shilo-Benjamini, Y. (2018). Evaluation of injectable anesthesia with five medetomidine-midazolam based combinations in Egyptian fruit bats (*Rousettus aegyptiacus*). *Laboratory Animals, 52*(5), 515–525.

Unuigbe, O. M., & Onuoha, S. N. (2013). Assessment of impact damage to apple fruits. *Nigerian Journal of Technology, 32*(1), 137–140.

Van Zeebroeck, M., Darius, P., De Ketelaere, B., Ramon, H., & Tijskens, E. (2007a). The effect of fruit factors on the bruise susceptibility of apples. *Postharvest Biology and Technology, 46*, 10–19.

Vergano, P. J., Testin, R. F., & Newall, W. C. (1991). Peach bruising: Susceptibility to impact, vibration, and compression abuse. *Transactions of the ASAE (American Society of Agricultural Engineers), 34*(5), 2110–2116.

Vigneault, C., Thompson, J., & Wu, S. (2009). Designing container for handling fresh horticultural produce. In N. Benkeblia (Ed.), *Postharvest Technologies for Horticultural Crops* (Vol. 2, pp. 25–47). Kerale: Research Signpost.

Villahermosa, A. A. S., Bihn, L. N., Rolle, R. S., & Chonhenchob, V. (2011). *Packaging in Fresh Produce Supply Chain in Southeast Asia*. Bangkok: Food and Agriculture Organization of the United Nations.

Vursavuş, K., & Özgüven, F. (2004). Determining the effects of vibration parameters and packaging method on mechanical damage in Golden Delicious apples. *Turkish Journal of Agriculture and Forestry, 28*, 311–320.

Wang, D., Lai, Y., Zhao, H., Jia, B., & Yang, X. (2019). Numerical and experimental investigation on forced-air cooling of commercial packaged strawberries. *International Journal of Food Engineering, 15*, 1–14.

Wang, K., Yang, L., & Kucharek, M. (2020). Investigation of the effect of thermal insulation materials on packaging performance. *Packaging Technology and Science, 33*(6), 227–236.

Wang, L. J., Zhang, Q., Song, H., & Wang, Z. W. (2022). Mechanical damage of 'Huangguan' pear using different packaging under random vibration. *Postharvest Biology and Technology, 187*, 111847.

Wang, W., & Guan, S. (2017). Study on fabrication and properties of the aluminum foil. http://iccmcentral.org/Proceedings/ICCM21proceedings/papers/4353.pdf (accessed on 9th July 2025).

Wheeler, L., Kitinoja, L., & Barrett, D. M. (2015). Use of insulated covers over product crates to reduce losses in amaranth during shipping delays. *Agriculture, 5*(4), 1204–1223.

Yadav, A., Kumar, N., Upadhyay, A., Fawole, O. A., Mahawar, M. K., Jalgaonkar, K., Chandran, D., Rajalingam, S., Zengin, G., Kumar, M., & Mekhemar, M. (2022). Recent advances in novel packaging technologies for shelf-life extension of guava fruits for retaining health benefits for longer duration. *Plants, 11*(4), 547.

Ying-Chen, Z., Hong-Yan, W., & Yi-Ping, Q. (2010). Morphology and properties of hybrid composites based on polypropylene/polylactic acid blend and bamboo fiber. *Bioresource Technology, 101*(20), 7944–7950.

Yu, P., Li, C., Takeda, F., & Krewer, G. (2014). Visual bruise assessment and analysis of mechanical impact measurement in southern high bush blueberries. *Applied Engineering in Agriculture, 30*(1), 29–37.

Zarifneshat, S., Ghassemzadeh, H. R., Sadeghi, M., Abbaspour-Fard, M. H., Ahmadi, E., Javadi, A., & Shervani-Tabar, M. T. (2010). The effect of impact and fruit properties on the bruising of peach. *American Journal of Agricultural and Biological Sciences, 5*(2), 114–121.

Zeng, T., Jiang, H., & Hao, F. (2022). Study on the effect of aluminum foil on packaging thermal insulation performance in cold chain logistics. *Packaging Technology and Science, 35*(5), 395–403.

Zhang, Y., Duan, C., Bokka, S. K., He, Z., & Ni, Y. (2021). Molded fiber and pulp products as green and sustainable alternatives to plastics: A mini review. *Journal of Bioresources and Bioproducts*.

Zhou, R., Su, S., & Li, Y. (2008). Effects of cushioning materials on the firmness of Huanghua pears (*Pyrus pyrifolia* Nakai cv. Huanghua) during distribution and storage. *Packaging Technology and Science: An International Journal, 21*(1), 1–11.

Zhou, R., Su, S., Yan, L., & Li, Y. (2007). Effect of transport vibration levels on mechanical damage and physiological responses of Huanghua pears (*Pyrus pyrifolia* Nakai cv. Huanghua). *Postharvest Biology and Technology, 46*, 20–28.

CHAPTER 9

Nondestructive Techniques for Food Quality Evaluation

KRISHNA KUMAR PATEL,[1] ABHIMANYU KALNE,[2] and PANKAJ B. PATHARE[3*]

[1]*Department of Food Processing and Agricultural Structure, Baba Saheb Dr. Bhim Rao Ambedkar College of Agricultural Engineering and Technology (Etawah), Chandra Shekhar Azad University of Agriculture and Technology, Kanpur, Uttar Pradesh, India*

[2]*Department of Agricultural Process and Food Engineering, Indira Gandhi Agricultural University (IGAU), Raipur, Chhattisgarh, India*

[3]*Department of Soils, Water and Agricultural Engineering, College of Agricultural and Marine Sciences, Sultan Qaboos University, Muscat, Oman*

*Corresponding author

ABSTRACT

Quality of agricultural produce and food is vital from the point of consumer acceptance and effective marketing. At many instances, such a quality evaluation is done by destructive testing where only part of food is evaluated. On the other hand, many non-destructive methods have shown considerable potential in quality evaluation of food products. Short time needed for testing, less manpower engaged, and accuracy of tested samples are added advantages in non-destructive quality evaluation. Further, in non-destructive quality evaluation, each and every sample can be tested, and it is used for consumption after testing. In other words, no part of food is wasted in non-destructive quality testing. At present, many

Sustainable Approaches in Postharvest Handling and Management: Pankaj B. Pathare (Ed.)

DOI: 10.1201/9781779641076-9

non-destructive technologies are being applied to evaluate the intrinsic and extrinsic characteristics of agricultural produce as well as various food products. These technologies are well suited for real-time evaluation of external and internal quality attributes of agricultural produce and various food materials. This shows a promising future for non-destructive techniques in the food industry. Associated manpower with the use of these technologies is also needed to gather the basic knowledge of these innovative approaches for the efficient use of these technologies in the food industry. There are several non-destructive techniques that have now emerged potentially in the field of agriculture and the food sector, such as computer vision, X-ray and computed tomography, magnetic resonance imaging (MRI)/nuclear magnetic resonance (NMR), near-infrared, ultrasound, electronic nose and tongue, and so forth. These novel techniques, if properly applied to a variety of food materials, are a better alternative to conventional techniques for food quality assessment. This chapter, thus, discusses the basic concepts of non-destructive techniques, various components of these systems, as well as their applications and potential for quality (external and internal) assessment of postharvest agricultural produce and food products.

9.1 INTRODUCTION

Food provides the basic nutritional needs and energy for human beings to grow and develop, to stay active and healthy, to work and play, to think and learn, and even to stay alive. So, food is the first and foremost requirement of human beings after oxygen and water. Food demand is continuously increasing as the population of the world (i.e., about 8 billion in 2022) increases (Quddusi, 2018). Foods are the prime source of protein, fat, carbohydrate, vitamins, minerals, and so forth. The quality of food we consume, therefore, is vital, and consumers at present have put their focus on buying good quality food materials. In this modern era, artificial intelligence has the potential to evaluate the quality of food nondestructively using a variety of equipment/technology (Patel et al., 2022).

The quality of horticultural produce, in both the fresh food market as well as for the processed food industry, has always been one of the important areas to analyze the consumer's view and demand. Quality, which is meant as the degree of excellence (Kader, 1992) or superiority, can be characterized based on individual or a combination of various internal (flavor, texture, nutrition, defect, etc.), external (size, shape, color, defects, etc.), and other parameters such as mechanical, optical, sonic, electrical, electro-magnetic, thermal, hydro and aero dynamical, and so forth. These characteristics, attributes, and properties, individually or in combination, have a significant role during the assessment of quality and food safety, also.

Quality of food products, whether raw or processed, has always been a major area to analyze the consumer's demand and acceptance. Quality, that is, the degree of excellence (Kader, 1992), can be characterized based on individual parameters or combinations of various internal characteristics (flavor, texture, nutrition, internal anomalies, etc.) as well as external characteristics (size, shape, color, surface defects, etc.). These characteristics, individual or in combination, have significant contribution during the quality assessment process.

The quality of food can be assessed by destructive or non-destructive ways. Destructive techniques are the traditional methods which evaluate the quality of the food by following conventional ways such as cutting, crushing, and scrapping the food sample. This method needs to damage a sample, and the results of this test sample are correlated to the remaining batch of food. Another point of concern is that such a small test sample does not always represent the whole batch. On the other hand, non-destructive methods are rapid and accurate, and it is possible to monitor each sample. Furthermore, non-destructive methods are considered reliable, consistent, less laborious, and less costly than destructive methods. Non-destructive techniques are now gaining momentum with technological advancement (Patel et al., 2019).

Development of systems for inspecting internal quality parameters of food and agricultural produce is a challenging task. Many researchers have been working to find techniques for the evaluation of such interior quality characteristics, attributes, and properties non-destructively. As a consequence, several non-destructive technologies have now been developed and are available to use for various produce in horticultural and food industries. Among these techniques, X-ray (X-ray imaging and Computed Tomography: CT), optics (reflected, transmittance, absorbance, and laser spectroscopy), electromagnetic (magnetic resonance imaging: MRI), mechanics (sonic, ultrasonic, and vibrated excitation), and so forth, have been explored for non-destructive determination of the internal quality of a variety of agricultural and food products. For instance, the soluble solid content (SSC) of several fruits (apples, citrus, peach, pear, melon, watermelon, etc.) can be determined using NIR spectroscopy technique based on reflectance/transmittance. Similarly, maturity and defects in interior parts of melon and watermelon can be assessed non-destructively (Noh and Choi, 2006). Table 9.1 shows a list of non-destructive instruments for measurement of various parameters of agricultural produce along with their principle of operation (Jha et al., 2010).

TABLE 9.1 Nondestructive Instruments Along with Their Working Principle

Sl. No.	Instruments	Principles
1.	NIR spectroscopy	Reflection, Absorption, Refraction, Transmittance and Scattering
2.	Magnetic Resonance Imaging (MRI)	Absorption,
3.	X-ray Imaging	Absorption,
4.	Computed Tomography (CT)	Absorption,
5.	Ultrasound	Reflection
6.	Rheometers	Internal Resistance
7.	HPLC	Differential Adsorption
8.	Optical Density Measurement	Refraction
9.	Firmness Measurement	Internal resistance
10.	Glossiness Measurement	Reflection
11.	Impedance	Absorption

Nondestructive technology can be useful for various purposes when it comes to fruits and vegetables. In most horticultural produce, it is required to judge optimum harvesting time without inspecting its internal quality destructively. If harvested before the optimum maturity, fruits may not get fully ripe, and if harvested after maturity, fruits may get overripe, which degrades the quality of the produce. There may be some instances when it is required to check fruit quality internally without actually cutting it. Nondestructive techniques are thus suitable in such cases also where there may be the possibility of internal anomalies in fruits, such as internal water core damage in apples, spongy tissues in mangoes, black heart in potatoes, and so forth.

Considering the above facts, the main objective of this chapter is to provide fundamental knowledge of nondestructive technologies and their application in quality assessment of various food and agricultural products.

9.2 QUALITY ATTRIBUTES OF FRESH FRUITS AND VEGETABLES

Quality is the key factor for acceptance of the agricultural produce by the consumer. The quality of fruits and vegetables can be judged by a number of parameters. Acceptability is also usually dependent on subjective factors such as taste, smell, appearance, touch, and hearing (Noh and Choi, 2006). Consumers are interested in buying produce by observing external characteristics such as the appearance of fruits, size (i.e., weight, volume, and dimension), shape (i.e., diameter/depth ratio), being defect-free (i.e., bruise, stab, spots), color (i.e., uniformity, intensity), and so forth. Sometimes consumers may show interest in the internal quality characteristics of fruits/vegetables such as texture (firmness, crispness, juiciness, etc.), flavor (aroma, sweetness, sourness, astringency, etc.), taste, nutritional value (protein, fat, carbohydrate, vitamins, functional properties, etc.), being free from defects (watercore, internal cavity, rotten, etc.) (Jha et al., 2010; Noh and Choi, 2006; Patel et al., 2012). Though external characteristics can be monitored visually, judging internal quality parameters subjectively is not an easy task. Non-destructive quality evaluation techniques thus play a vital role in such circumstances. The advantage of non-destructive quality evaluation is that every fruit has to pass through inspection.

The quality of food products, however, is highly variable from product to product and is attributed to various factors such as cultivation methods, soil type, cultural practices, harvesting method, postharvest handling procedure, climatic conditions, and maturity at harvest. Both destructive and nondestructive methods can be used for the evaluation of quality characteristics of food products.

9.3 NONDESTRUCTIVE TECHNIQUES FOR FOOD QUALITY ATTRIBUTES

Quality attributes of agricultural produce, whether internal or external, are both important to detect quickly and within the time to avoid nutritional as well as economic losses. To assess the quality parameters of fresh fruits/vegetables and food products, the following techniques are the latest non-destructive techniques which are being used with promising results.

1. X-ray imaging and Computed tomography
2. Machine vision system
3. Hyperspectral imaging technology

4. Near infrared spectrometry (NIR)
5. Nuclear magnetic resonance imaging (NMRI) / magnetic resonance imaging (MRI)
6. Ultrasound technology
7. Electronic nose

While all techniques are important, they have their own limitations regarding computer image resolution, imaging duration, safe handling, sample-specific requirements, and other related properties such as surface color, texture, internal details, and so forth.

9.3.1 X-RAY IMAGING AND COMPUTED TOMOGRAPHY

In 1895, Wilhelm Conrad Rontgen was first introduced to X-ray radiation and reported that X-rays (wavelength range: 0.01 to 10 nm) can be generated by fast-moving electrons when bombarded on a metallic target of high melting point and high atomic weight (like tungsten, molybdenum, platinum, etc.), also known as Roentgen rays. X-ray performs as a subsurface technique. The X-ray imaging system has the following main components.

1. **X-Ray Source:** Radioactive substances or X-ray tubes, along with a power circuit (i.e., supplying the required potential to the X-ray tube), are the source for X-rays. An X-ray tube consists of a cathode (filament), an anode (i.e., a positive target with respect to the filament), a focal spot, a collimator, and tube housing. In X-ray tubes, X-rays are generated by bombarding the anode with electrons. X-ray tubes may have varying voltage, current, focal spot size, and so forth. When the filament is heated, a fine beam of electrons strikes the target, and mechanical energy is converted into radiant energy, producing X-rays. The intensity of X-rays may be controlled by controlling the current in the filament, while the penetrating power is controlled by controlling the voltage difference between the filament and target.

   High intensity means more X-ray radiation, and high penetrating power means X-rays can penetrate through many objects due to their high energy. The material properties (atomic number, density, etc.), however, affect the penetration of X-rays. Thus, when X-rays pass through an object, they undergo transmission, scattering, or absorbance. If I_0 (keV) is the intensity of incident

X-ray photons, 'T' is the thickness of the material through which X-rays pass, 'ρ' is the linear density (g/mm^3) of the material, and I (keV) is the intensity of X-ray photons after traversing a distance 'T,' then 'I' can be given as:

$$I = I_0 e^{-\mu_m m}$$

where, μ_m (= μ/ρ) is mass absorption coefficient or mass attenuation coefficient (mm^2/g), m (=ρT) is mass per unit area and 'μ' is linear absorption or attenuation coefficient defined as the fractional decrease in intensity of X-rays on traversing a unit length of material. So, 'I' can also be expressed as:

$$I = I_0 e^{-\mu T}$$

Since the attenuation coefficient is a function of material properties (atomic number, thickness, etc.), a different intensity of X-ray photons after transmitting through different materials is observed in the form of different contrast in a visual image.

2. **Imaging Medium:** X-ray imaging medium, also known as an X-ray image receptor, includes X-ray film/screen, computed radiography cassette (CR), and digital detectors. Earlier X-ray imaging was done on photographic films, which was similar to conventional film-based photography. However, with advances in technology, X-ray film/screens are being replaced by digital cassettes, which provide digital X-rays after reading the cassettes with an imaging plate in the system.

   The quality of X-ray images for various agricultural produce/food products depends on the selection of proper tube voltage and current because of the varying thickness and density of produce. Different types of detectors, including film, have different responses to X-ray exposure. To get clear radiographs, X-ray systems should be used at different energy and current settings, and the radiograph obtained should be inspected for quality. However, two types (soft and hard) of X-ray imaging are commonly used in food industries. The wavelength of soft X-rays, ranged between 1 nm and 100 nm, has low energy and less penetrating power, while the wavelength of hard X-rays, ranged between 0.1 and 1.0 nm, has low energy and more penetrating power than soft X-rays. Hard X-ray imaging, sometimes called X-ray computed tomography, is restricted to use in objects with high density.

9.3.1.1 COMPUTED TOMOGRAPHY (C-T SCAN)

CT imaging, based on mathematical principle radon transform introduced in 1917 by Johann Radon, is the technique of capturing 2D X-ray images of different slices of a biological object to give the visual information of inner cross-sections. It involves directing X-rays from multiple directions at an object and measuring the intensity reduction along a series of linear paths (Ketcham and Carlson, 2001). This decrease in the intensity of X-rays is characterized by Beer's Law. Beer's law describes the decrease in intensity as a function of the X-ray's energy, path length, and the linear attenuation coefficient (LAC) of the material. The main components of an X-ray tomography apparatus are an X-ray source (i.e., X-ray tube), an array of detectors, and a data acquisition system with rotational geometry with respect to the object being imaged. The detectors measure the intensity of X-rays that attenuated along the multiple beam paths. A special algorithm is used to reconstruct the distribution of X-ray attenuation in the volume being imaged. However, various configurations of these components can be used to create CT scanners optimized for imaging objects of different sizes and compositions.

9.3.1.2 APPLICATIONS OF RADIOGRAPHY AND CT-IMAGING

X-ray imaging or radiography is a well-known technique in the field of medical diagnostics. In addition, X-ray imaging has long been used for checking luggage at airports, inspecting industrial components, and so forth. The use of radiography, however, for the inspection of agricultural commodities is mentioned by some researchers. In recent years, X-ray inspection systems have increasingly been used for the detection of internal defects in horticultural produce. Many researchers have worked on X-ray-based non-destructive quality evaluation techniques for a variety of fruits and vegetables and reported the successes and limitations of this technique.

According to Diener et al. (1970), the X-ray scan line detection system could detect bruises on apples successfully when fruits are introduced to the scan line system with proper orientation. Kim and Schatzki (2000) used two-dimensional X-ray imaging to detect internal water core damage in apples. This system was able to correctly recognize apples into clean and severe categories within 5–8% false positive and negative ratios. The X-ray technique was also used for distinguishing peaches with split pits and peaches with normal pits by Han et al. (1992). He developed a method that could nondestructively distinguish split pit peaches and normal pit peaches with 98% success. But in this case, too, proper orientation of fruit is important during X-ray imaging. However, X-ray images and machine recognition can be used for identification of many, but not all, insect-infested pistachio nuts (Keagy et al., 1996).

Lenker and Adrian (1971) used a low-powered X-ray generator with a photodiode to differentiate between mature and immature lettuce heads. During this study, they concluded that the photodiode needs to be cooled on hot days to prevent changes in the sensitivity of the photodiode with temperature. In the case of detecting insect infestation in grains, Stermer (1972) conducted an experiment and concluded that a trained examiner could detect 100% insect infestation at medium and late larval stages by observing X-ray images. The accuracy for eggs and young larval stages was reported as 80–90%. In the case of quality analysis of wheat, Schatzki and Fine (1988) observed that manual analysis of radiographs was much slower, and only third and later instar hidden insects were visible. Beletskiy et al. (2021) studied methodological aspects of introscopy during the detection of internal defects of food grain during storage using X-ray imaging and reported that defective grains with hidden defects in wheat lots can be identified and quantified.

Further, dual-energy X-ray absorptiometry images were applied for the evaluation of tenderness of meat by Kroger et al. (2006). They reported that the tenderness of whole steak can be predicted using scans of DEXA images, with the shear forces having a coefficient of determination (R2) value of 0.69. So, it can be said that X-ray imaging is becoming more pronounced and practical day-by-day as a non-invasive technique for the quality evaluation of agricultural products.

Further, various quality parameters such as acidity, maturity, fat content, sugar content, defected tissues, and so forth, in food products can be investigated using X-ray computed tomographic imaging technology. For the evaluation of quality parameters, the CT number (i.e., the attenuation coefficient, which is calculated using water) of slice images is important. Its unit is Hounsfield (Hu) and can be given as:

$$\text{CT Number Hu} = (\mu\text{-}\mu_w / \mu_w) \times 1000$$

TABLE 9.2 Application of X-Ray and CT Scan in Food Quality Assessment

Produce	Quality Attribute	Output/Findings	Techniques Used	Reference
		X-Ray		
Apple	Bruises	• X-ray line scan detection system could detect bruises on apples. • Proper fruit orientation required before passing through the system to avoid any confusion among surface bruises, calyx and stem voids, etc.	Radiography	Diener et al., 1970
Lettuce	Mature/ immature lettuce heads	• Mature and immature lettuce heads can be differentiated with a low powered X-rays and a photodiode that sensed X-ray transmission through the heads.	Radiography	Lenker and Adrian, 1971
Wheat	Insect infestation	• Insect infestation in wheat can be successfully detected.	Radiography	Brayant, 1988
Peach	split pit and normal peaches	• Split peaches can be identified from normal pit peaches.	Radiography	Han et al. 1992
Mango	Seed weevil detection	• Presence of seed weevil in mango fruits can be detected.	Radiography	Thomas et al., 1995
Apple	Water core detection	• Water core damage in apples can be successfully detected.	Radiography	Kim and Schatzki, 2000
Wheat	Insect infestation	• Insect infestation in stored wheat can be successfully detected.	Radiography	Karunakaran et al., 2003
Apple	Internal imaging	• Imaging of interior regions of apples under varying moisture can be possible.	CT-imaging	Tollner et al., 1992
Mango	Density, moisture content, soluble solids, titrable acidity, pH	• Physico-chemical characteristics like density, moisture content, soluble solids, titrable acidity and pH of mangoes were related with X-ray absorption.	CT-imaging	Barcelon et al., 1999
Mango	Ripening changes	• Successfully observed internal changes associated with the ripening process of mango	CT-imaging	Barcelon et al., 2000

TABLE 9.2 *(Continued)*

Produce	Quality Attribute	Output/Findings	Techniques Used	Reference
Beef	Fat content	• Intramuscular fat content investigated. • Level of fat distribution assessed rapidly and more accurately	Micro CT-imaging	Frisullo et al., 2010
Apple Pears Eggplant Turnip	Porosity distribution	• Porosity differences based internal quality inspection • Different tissues, seeds and vascular bundles distinguished clearly.	CT-imaging	Bayu et al., 2019

where, μ and μ_m are the LAC of the sample and water, respectively. The approximate value of LAC of water is considered as 0.195 (Du et al., 2019; Donis-Gonzalez et al., 2014). This CT number is positively correlated to several parameters such as water content, density, acidity, and so forth, of agricultural products. Some applications of X-ray and CT scans in food quality assessment have been summarized in Table 9.2.

9.3.2 MACHINE VISION SYSTEM

Machine vision is the technology that is used in industry to provide image-based inspection. Machine vision combines mechanics, optical instrumentation, sensors, and image processing. This integrated system, which has a combination of mechanical, optical, electronic, and software systems, has a wider scope for inspecting, monitoring, and controlling numerous processes in a broad range of applications.

Machine vision is the substitution of the human visual sense in monitoring any process, such as the sorting of quality fruits. As machine vision is an objective process, possible human error can be eliminated, and consistent results can be obtained by using this system to perform an inspection task. Machine vision also reduces labor and saves time with accurate results.

9.3.2.1 COMPONENTS OF MACHINE VISION IMAGING

A complete machine vision system generally has the following basic processes: image acquisition (illumination chamber, lighting regime, and camera), frame grabber, image processing and image analysis software and hardware. An illumination chamber is a confined chamber to protect the object from interference from external light, and this chamber is commonly equipped with light sources, an object platform, and a digital camera setup. During image acquisition, a video signal is sent from the camera to the industrial computer, which is equipped with a frame grabber that captures the image and stores it in a suitable file format in computer hardware memory. Computer vision is, therefore, an electromechanical-cum-optical electronic device integrated into a single unit for advanced use in various sectors such as medical, security monitoring, surveillance, investigation of biological produce, and so forth.

The software can be used to control the camera settings, timing of image acquisition, and also extract features from captured images to make decisions. These may be regarding measuring object dimensions, detecting surface defects, and so forth. Frame grabbers can acquire digital or analog images depending on the type of camera used. Image analysis can offer broad information about a product being tested.

9.3.2.2 APPLICATIONS OF MACHINE VISION

Machine vision has a wide application for inspection or quality evaluation of a variety of fruits and vegetables. It is used for automatic sorting and grading of fruits, which not only results in labor saving but also saves time and reduces wastage. It has been used for such tasks as shape classification, defect detection, quality grading, and also variety classification of the fruits. Machine vision is normally used for external inspection of fruits, but pixel intensity can be correlated to the internal quality and freshness factor of fruits and vegetables (Patel et al., 2012a, b). Several research studies have been done under machine vision for quality inspection. Yang (1996) worked on apple grading where he assessed the feasibility of computer vision for the identification of apple stems and calyxes during automatic grading and coring.

Nagata et al. (1997) used a computer vision system for sorting fresh strawberries, based on the size and shape of the fruits. Leemans et al. (1998) mentioned the use of machine vision in defect detection in 'Golden Delicious' apples. For apples, a color machine vision system and Bayesian classification method were used for the segmentation of defects on the "Golden Delicious" apples by Leemans et al. (1999). Similarly, a real-time grading method based on features extracted from defects was also developed by Leemans and Destain (2004). Li et al. (2002) have also reported a computer vision-based system for the detection of defects on the surface of apples. An automatic image analysis system was used by Leiva-Valenzuela and Aguilera (2013) for the detection of orientation and diseases in blueberries to improve their postharvest storage quality. They used two best classifiers (SVM: Support Vector Machine and LDA: Linear Discriminant Analysis) in their study and reported that they distinguished the orientation of blueberries in 96.80% of the cases and classified the damages (fungally decayed, shriveled, and mechanically damaged) as 97%, 93%, and 86%, respectively. Further, a computer vision (CV) system was developed and applied for the nondestructive physical characterization of mangoes by using a color (RGB) camera (Patel et al., 2019b), a monochrome camera (Patel et al., 2020a), and an NIR camera (Patel et al., 2020b). In their research, they evaluated various physical/morphological properties for the sorting and grading of mango fruit.

Furthermore, Patel et al. (2019b) have used a color camera-based computer vision system to detect common external defects on the surface of mango fruit. In their study, they used a color (RGB) camera for image acquisition and LabView software for image processing and analysis of defects. They reported an overall accuracy and efficiency of the proposed algorithm for external defect detection of mango fruit as 88.60% and 93.30%, respectively. However, the accuracy (88.75%) and efficiency (97.88%) of the monochrome computer vision system defect detection algorithm were reported as a little better than the color (RGB) camera-based CV system (Patel et al., 2021). The computer vision-based reflected ultraviolet (Reflected-UV) image acquisition method can be used for the detection of defects (ruptures in cells) just underneath the peel. Bruises just below the peel of mango can be identified at a 400 nm wavelength bandpass filter (Patel et al., 2019a).

There are various studies that have been conducted to assess the quality of a number of food and agricultural products, such as strawberries (Bato et al., 2000), bayberries (Lu et al., 2011), pistachios (Pearson and Toyofuku, 2000), chestnuts (Donis-Gonzalez et al., 2013), olives (Riquelme et al., 2008; Wang et al., 2011), apples (De Belie et al., 1999; Xing et al., 2005), citrus (Lopez-Garcíaa et al., 2010), tomatoes (Lino et al., 2008; Monavar et al., 2011), plums (Kandi, 2010), potatoes (Wooten et al., 2010), and chili (Hahn and Sanchez, 2000), and so forth, using a color camera-based computer vision system. In addition, a CV system can also be applied for the evaluation of quality parameters of processed food, dairy products, and meat products. For instance, the required characteristics of cheddar and mozzarella cheese were analyzed by Wang and Sun (2002 a, b), and Ni and Gunasekaran (1998) measured cheese shred length using an image processing algorithm.

The CV system can also be applied for the assessment of meat and meat products. For example, Lu et al. (2000) investigated pork quality effectively using neural network modeling. Park and Chen (2001) identified the wholesomeness of chicken carcasses with 95.6% classification accuracy by using discriminant analysis.

9.3.3 HYPERSPECTRAL IMAGING TECHNOLOGY

Also known as imaging spectroscopy or imaging spectrometry, this is a combination of NIR spectroscopy and NIR imaging. This technique is more famously known as hyperspectral imaging and is a very promising technology applied in a wide variety of fields (mining, pharmaceutical, food, etc.). However, its application was initiated in 1980 by remote sensing areas, and now this technique is more prominent for assessing food quality and safety (Liu et al., 2008) and in the agricultural sector (Lawrence et al., 2003), also. This technology is more capable of directly assessing various quality factors simultaneously due to the incorporation of both spectroscopy and imaging techniques. The capability of location and identification of the spatial distribution of different components in tested products, food authentication, and nondestructive analysis are, thus, significant qualities of this technique. Hyperspectral imaging technique has been applied potentially for the detection of defects, classification, quality parameter determination, and other various quality assessment operations for food and agricultural produces.

HIS works on the basic principle that the difference in chemical composition or constituents, bonding, and structure of materials are the main factors for the distinctive reflection, emission, absorbance, and scattering of electromagnetic energy at different wavelengths, which is generally reported as a spectrum. These spectrums are generally used to identify, discriminate, and characterize the target products. The hyperspectral imaging system commonly receives three modes of light after interacting with the food materials, viz. reflectance mode (easy to use but level of light reasonably high relative to sample), transmittance mode (used for internal detection and carries more valuable information) (Schaare and Fraser, 2000), and interactance mode (i.e., combination of both reflectance and transmittance needs light seal so that no external light can interfere).

The main feature of the HIS system is that it contains hundreds of regularly spaced continuous bands in comparison to the multispectral imaging (MSI) system, which commonly consists of less than 10 bands. This is the reason why MSI does not show a real spectrum in every pixel, while HIS provides the full spectrum of every pixel (Ariana and Lu, 2008). The HIS data, also known as a hypercube (X, Y, λ), is a three-dimensional (3-D) data set having two spatial dimensions (X, Y) and one spectral dimension (λ). The push-broom HIS system is more consistent for the online analysis of food materials and comprises a camera (with a cooled 2D light detector), a spectrograph (wavelength dispersing unit: the heart of the HIS system), a lighting setup, a translational stage, and a computer as the main components of the HIS system. The light reflected, emitted, or transmitted in wavelength bands such as 200–400 nm (UV bands), 400–1000 nm (VIS/NIR bands), 900–1700 nm (NIR bands), and 1000–2500 nm (SWIR: short wavelength infrared bands) can be used to acquire the HS images, depending upon the type of detector.

However, the selection of the optimum wavelength, which reflects not only physical and/or chemical information but also maintains successive discrimination and classification efficiency without losing valuable information, is important (Liu et al., 2007). Conclusively, it can be said that there is a wide and potential application of such integrated technology (i.e., HIS) for food quality assessment and evaluation of quality parameters in meat, grains, fruits and vegetables, fish, and so forth. Some applications of HIS technique are discussed here.

9.3.3.1 APPLICATION

Prediction of meat and meat products tenderness using a CV system is not new, but using a HIS system is very efficient. In a study by Nagnathan et al. (2008a, b), they predicted the tenderness of cooked beef from 14-day aged beef using a push-broom HIS system in the VIS-NIR (400–900 nm) and NIR (900–1700 nm) range. They used HS images of rib eye steaks, using slice shearing force as tenderness reference methods. In pork meat, the microbial quality assessment (total viable count of bacteria) was done by Peng and Wang (2008). They predicted the total viable bacterial count using a support vector machine (SVM). Multi-linear regression in combination with a HIS system can also be used to detect and predict spoilage bacteria in beef (Peng et al., 2009). Chao et al. (2008) developed a hyperspectral imaging system for the differentiation between wholesome and unwholesome freshly slaughtered chickens and between wholesome and systemically diseased chickens. In their study, an online line-scan imaging system was used to scan 140 birds at a poultry processing plant. However, for wholesome and unwholesome testing, 100 K chickens were imaged on a commercial line, and it was reported that the wholesome and unwholesome accuracies achieved were 99% and 96%, respectively. The feasibility of an approach for determining the shelf life of rocket leaves was evaluated using hyperspectral imaging and multivariate accelerated shelf-life testing (MASLT), and it was reported that the 550–700 nm wavelength has great importance in the estimation of shelf life on the basis of appearance score (Chaudhry et al., 2018). A HIS data model was used for the prediction of pungent constituents in dried ginger by Samrat et al. (2022). In their study, they found that the combination of HIS and multivariate analysis has the capability to determine the 6-gingerol-shogoal ratio in the dried powder in real-time.

TABLE 9.3 Application of Hyperspectral Imaging for Quality Assessment of Food Produce

Sl. No.	Products	–	Quality Detection/ Assessment	References
1.	Meat and meat products	Pork meat	Spoilage (Total variable count of bacteria)	Peng and Wnag (2008)
			Tenderness	Tao et al. (2010)
		Beef	Tenderness	Wu et al. (2012)
		Lamb	Tenderness	Kamruzzaman et al. (2012)
2.	Fruit	Apple	Soluble solid content	Tian et al. (2022)
		Peaches	Soluble solid content	Yang et al. (2020)
		Banana	Color of ripe and unripe bananas	Chuanqi et al. (2018)
		Plum	Color, firmness and soluble solid content	Bo et al. (2018)
3.	Vegetable	lettuce cultivars	Nutrient content	Eshkabilov et al. (2021).
4.	Powder	Almond	Adulterants detection	Faqeerzada et al. (2020)
		Walnut	Detection of adulterants (whole wheat flour powder).	Zhao et al. (2018)
		Spices	Authentication	Kiani et al. (2019)
		Peanut	–	–

Similarly, walnut and peanut powders were detected in whole wheat flour using NIR hyperspectral imaging technique by Zhao et al. (2018). Kiani et al. (2019) have applied HS (hyperspectral) imaging as a novel system for the authentication of spices, and shortwave infrared hyperspectral imaging technologies were used by Faqeerzada et al. (2020) for the detection of adulterants in almond powder with a one-class classification method. They concluded that the proposed method can be applied for the development of a visual quality control procedure for powder authentication (nutmeg and almond). In apples, SSC can be detected using hyperspectral imaging in combination with a deep learning algorithm (Tian et al., 2022), while the SSC in peach was estimated using only deep features of hyperspectral imagery (Yang et al., 2020). Rapid detection of nutrients in hydroponically grown lettuce cultivars was carried out using HIS technique by Eshkabilov et al. (2021). Table 9.3 shows a summary of applications in food and agricultural commodities.

9.3.4 NEAR INFRARED SPECTROMETRY (NIRS)

NIR is an acronym for Near-Infrared spectroscopy, which is based on the absorption of electromagnetic radiation at wavelengths in the range of 780 to 2500 nm. NIR radiation interacting with a food product may be absorbed, transmitted, or reflected. When EM radiation interacts with food samples, the behavior of the food sample's molecules depends on the amount of energy it carries. The light interacts with the food, and the chemical components absorb the light energy as per the wavelength. The detector measures its transmittance and absorbance part of incident radiation, and spectrometers are used to test the collected spectra (El-Mesery et al., 2019). NIR is based on molecular overtone and combination vibrations. Besides medical and physiological diagnostics, applications of NIR are widely reported in the food quality field as a nondestructive quality assessment tool. Several researchers have applied NIRS for the quality assessment of food products due to the following advantages:

- Non-destructive and non-invasive method
- Rapid. Results emerges quickly
- High precision
- No or minimal need of sample preparation
- More environmentally friendly than other analytical methods,
- Can provide several analytical results
- Suitable for in-line use
- Useful for analyzing of biological materials

9.3.4.1 APPLICATION OF NIR SPECTROSCOPY

NIR spectroscopy has a wide application in food industries. Protein, fat, carbohydrates, carotenoids, chlorophylls, and so forth, are main internal quality parameters of food products that absorb the near-infrared wavelengths. NIRS can be applied for the nondestructive investigation of fats, firmness, dry matter, protein, total soluble solids (TSS), and so forth. For instance, the online determination of the sugar content in pears was carried out using visible and infrared spectroscopy by Schmilovitch et al. (2012). Visible and nNIR spectroscopy techniques can also be used for the prediction of soluble solids content and pH value in peaches (Shao et al., 2011). The soluble solids content and firmness of bell pepper was measured by Penchaiya et al. (2009) using NIR spectroscopy. Similarly, using NIRS in the wavelength range 750–1100 nm, the internal quality of mandarin fruit can be evaluated (McGlone et al., 2003), while SSC (soluble solids content) and acidity of mandarins can be evaluated using NIRS in the wavelength range 350–2500 nm (Bergaz et al., 2010). Flores et al. (2008) have reported that the quality of melon and watermelon can be assessed using the NIR spectra obtained in reflection mode in the wavelength range of 400–1700 nm.

In addition, intrinsic properties of fruits, so far, can be evaluated by NIR spectroscopy in the range of 1200–2200 nm (Jha et al., 2012, 2014). Jha et al. (2012) have predicted the sweetness of intact mangoes and the maturity of mangoes (Jha et al., 2014) nondestructively using NIR spectroscopy in this order. The best prediction model for the maturity index of mangoes was achieved in the wavelength range of 1600–1800 nm by them. Similarly, the potential of NIRS in the wavelength range of 900–1700 nm for the determination of sweetness (total soluble solids, TSS), sourness (acidity), and their ratio for 5 cultivars of apples was also studied by Jha and Garg.

9.3.5 MAGNETIC RESONANCE IMAGING (MRI)

MRI is also known as NMR. NMR was first introduced for medical purposes in the year 1977 by Mansfield (Mansfield, 1977). However, MRI is the combination of NMR (i.e., spectrometric) and imaging devoted to spatial codification of the signal intensity and produces 2D or 3D images. The basic principle of this technology is that it can identify the behavior of atoms (i.e., nuclear spin and magnetic moments) in a magnetic field. This concept, however, was first studied in the year about 1930 and comprised a spectrometer, which is composed of a magnet, radiofrequency oscillator, and radiofrequency detector. However, a large magnet (for generating a large, uniform, and constant external magnetic field), smaller electromagnetic coils with a controller and power-driven equipment (for generating a magnetic field gradient), a radio frequency (RF) producer or transmitter and receiver with receiving coils/ or antennae, and a computer software and hardware system for data storage are among the principle components of an MRI system (Ahmed et al., 2017; Patel et al., 2015). A single coil can be used for transmitting and receiving the signal, but for better signal-to-noise ratio (SNR), separate coils are generally used in commercial magnetic resonance systems. The SNR is often defined as the quantitative value that is used to describe the quality of an image to detect a true signal, and noise signals superimposed from the background (Yoshioka et al., 2009).

Initially, MRI (i.e., Magnetic: magnetization of spin within the body; Resonance: detection of spin; Imaging: spatial encoding of spin) has been used commercially in the field of medicine for the detection of tumors and other abnormalities in humans. But, the application of this nondestructive technology in food and agricultural produce for their quality detection is continuously increasing day by day and gaining momentum, so far. The presence of polar molecules (hydrogen and water) in food or biological materials causes angular momentum and creates bulk magnetic effects when placed in a strong external static magnetic field (B0), which is the fundamental principle of utilizing MRI as a nondestructive quality assessment tool (Kauten and McCarthy, 2005; Patel et al., 2015). At Larmor frequency (ω0), bulk magnet or magnetization rotates, and a radio frequency (RF) with the same frequency (as that of Larmor frequency) is applied to excite the magnetization and to obtain a resonant effect. When the RF coil is removed, the magnetization comes back to equilibrium (i.e., relaxation) and releases the energy/RF signal. This means that the RF signal, which is known as FID (free-induction decay), is received as an RF signal using the magnetic resonance (i.e., conductive field) coil which surrounds the object. The rate at which the reorientation (along the magnetic field) and returning of magnetic dipoles (natural) to their equilibrium position after excitation happens can be represented by two (longitudinal and transverse) relaxation times (T1 and T2). Associated computers process this input information and form the high-quality image of soft tissues inside the test sample. To get the spatial variation in this magnetization, a gradient field is applied, and spatial encoding is done according to spatial variation.

Further, radio signals detect small changes in the spin of polar nuclei, and the absorption and emission of radio signals or energies are analyzed by MRI tools. In the MRI system, a gradient coil encodes the spatial position of nuclear spins. Spatial encoding includes phase encoding and frequency encoding using gradient coils (x-gradient coil, y-gradient coil, and z-gradient coil). MRI uses strong magnetic fields (0.5 to 2.0 Tesla) to change the spin of atoms in an object. The object contains tissue (whether it is the human body in the case of medical diagnosis, or biological materials in the case of agricultural and food products), and tissue contains water and fat. Both water and fat have hydrogen nuclei. The hydrogen nucleus produces a significant magnetic resonance signal after imposing an external magnetic field (Brown and Semelka, 2010). This means that, due to the effect of imposing the magnetic field, the spins of nuclei of polar molecules get aligned in the direction of the external field. This effect is called the Larmor effect, and the frequency at this stage is termed Larmor frequency (Abdullah, 2008) and is proportional to the applied external magnetic field. The Larmor frequency at which net magnetization (M0) is induced within the system can be given as:

$$\omega_0 = \gamma B_0 \tag{1}$$

In MRI, in addition to large external magnetic fields a small magnetic field gradient (G). The resultant frequency ($\omega(r)$) of nuclear spin then become the function of their position (r) in space and can be given as:

$$\omega (r) = \gamma B_0 + \gamma G \bullet r \tag{2}$$

Where, γ is termed the gyromagnetic ratio (i.e., the ratio between magnetic momentum in a particle and its angular momentum), and G is the magnetic field gradient (Harding et al., 1997).

MRI is a collection of experimental techniques designed to allow one to measure the NMR properties of a sample as a function of spatial position (Kim et al., 1999). This means that MR imaging, based on the principles of NMR (a spectroscopic technique), can be used to obtain microscopic chemical and physical information regarding the molecules. However, a number of research groups are seeking to exploit the NMR-quality relationship on a commercial basis by developing low-cost NMR sensors for sorting and grading fruits and vegetables. A novel, low-cost online MRI prototype sensor has now been built and is being tested at the IFR in Norwich. It is, in principle, capable of monitoring the internal quality of horticultural products and has been designed to operate on an industrial conveyor belt and was used for grading and sorting postharvest fruit and vegetables (Marigheto et al., 2008).

In addition, MRI techniques have been used for examining agricultural products from biological and physiological points of view since the mid-1950s; however, small sample sizes and slow data processing have limited the usefulness of these studies in terms of in-line sorting. With the development of large magnets in medical applications, a variety of new types of magnets and radio frequency coils have become available for use in engineering applications of NMR (Kim et al., 1999). Nuclear magnetic resonance is sensitive to the existence of mobile water, oil, and sugar, which are major components of horticultural commodities.

Therefore, MRI has a better scope for use in internal-quality evaluation of horticultural produce due to its nondestructive nature. The NMR technique detects the concentration of hydrogen nuclei and is sensitive to variations in the concentration and state of free water and oil. Since NMR measures physical properties that are not observable by other techniques, NMR can detect quality factors that cannot be detected by other methods. Although its potential for detecting defects and other quality factors in fruits and vegetables has not been fully explored (Chen et al., 1993), MRI can therefore be used not only to detect internal damages, bruising, and invisible insects and pests, but also for the assessment of various internal quality parameters such as nutrition content, pH, moisture content, texture, fruit firmness, sensory attributes, seed detection, as well as physiochemical and microbiological properties in both industrial and commercial applications (Kamal et al., 2019). There are wide applications of MRI in food and agricultural produce. Some of them are discussed in subsection.

9.3.5.1 APPLICATIONS OF MRI

Mealiness in fruits like apples, peaches, and so forth, is an internal physiological disorder in sensory texture that can be assessed using MRI features. Barreiro et al. (1999, 2000) have assessed apples and peaches using the MRI technique. For apples, they reported that the value of T2 (transverse relaxation time) was significantly lower than in non-mealy apples. This means that a more desegregated structure and a lower juiciness content leads to a lower T2 signal. In addition, regional variation of contrast was obtained in T2 maps of mealy apples but not in non-mealy apples.

In the case of peach fruits, the results obtained for mealy apples, however, were not similar to those for woolly peaches. This observation indicates that there is a different underlying physiological change in both disorders. The application of MRI in peaches can be used to distinguish between woolly and non-woolly fruits (Barreiro et al., 2000). Table 9.4 has, however, summarized some applications of MRI/NMR in food and agriculture products.

Browning in apples is another internal disorder that can be identified using a low-cost, low-field magnetic resonance sensor (Chayaprasert and Stroshine, 2005). Low-field (0.088 Tesla) MRI is also useful for the detection of internal disease and mechanical damage. The spin echo sequence (SE), proton density, and T2 weighted varying echo time (TE) and repetition time (TR) features of an MRI system are considerable for this type of assessment (Suchanek and Olejniczak, 2008). The 2-D and 3-D NMR imaging was used to view the amelioration of watercore in Fuji apples by Clark et al. (1998a). They reported that the percentage of water-soaked tissues was found to be higher in the centrally located transverse and longitudinal image slices, while declining towards the fruit's boundaries. Watercore in apples is a well-known physiological disorder where intercellular spaces are filled with water and can be detected using 1H-MRI (Clark et al., 1998b). In another study, Clark et al. (1997) applied MRI for pre- and post-harvest studies of fruits and vegetables. In tomatoes, quantitative NMR was used to determine the structural aspect (Musse et al., 2009b), and quantitative MRI along with NMR relaxometry was used to monitor post-harvest ripening by (Musse et al., 2009a). Several internal parameters of meat were evaluated after correlating them with the chemical composition, carcass composition, connective tissue, muscle structure, and muscle type of meat, as determined by using MRI techniques. The MRI technique can also be applied, along with image processing, for the prediction of intracellular fat in beef (Lee et al., 2015). Muscle and fatty tissue can be discriminated using 1H-MRI images and longitudinal relaxation time (T1) features of MRI (Collewet et al., 2004). Since fat content has large longitudinal and transverse magnetization, the longitudinal relaxation time (T1) has a high correlation to the chemical analysis of fat content, which appears bright on a T1 weighted image (Kullberg et al., 2009).

TABLE 9.4 Application of MRI/NMR/ or Both in Food Quality Assessment

Agricultural Produce	Quality Attributes	Remarks/Finding	References
Avocado	Oil content	• Established a correlation between percentages of oil and dry matter. • Results of this study however were given only for dehydrated samples of avocado.	Chen et al. (1993)
Apple	Internal browning or defects	• Determine the effects of internal browning and watercore on the spin-spin relaxation (T_2) signal of whole apples.	Cho et al. (2008), Marigheto and Hills (2005)
		• Mealiness and watercore detection	–
Pears	Internal browning	• Developed a noninvasive procedure for on-line disorder identification	Hernandez et al. (2007)
Kiwifruits	Internal textural	• Identified effect of storage on texture quality. • Minimal texture damage using MR spectroscopy	Taglienti et al. (2009)
Corn kernels	Fat, moisture, and solid content	• T_2 values were related to fat and water content of corn kernels.	Persian and Rollwitz (1970)
Wheat	Moisture content	• Ratio between the two Free Induction Decay (FID) peaks could be used to determine the MC with an error range of + 0.2%.	Brusewitz et al. (1987)
Wheat	Viability loss	• Diffusion constant for water in embryo was evaluated. • Diffusion weighted MR imaging technique was applied. • Endosperm pore size and the embryo cell dimensions could also be achieved.	Gruwel et al. (2008)
Coffee	Free and bound water	• Determined free and bound water in coffee during the roasting process, • Compared the results with moisture mappings observed by MRI	Kino and Takagi, (1995), Toffanin et al. (2001), Takagi (1995)

9.3.6 *ULTRASOUND TECHNOLOGY*

The term ultrasound is used to describe sound waves with frequencies greater than 20 kHz, which is beyond the range of hearing capacity of an average adult human. According to Cho (2012), ultrasonic is nothing but a mechanical wave having a frequency beyond 20 kHz, piercing through a sample which, after reflecting, gives the inner characteristics of the sample. However, ultrasound provides information after the reflection or transmission of sound waves emitted by an external source, such as a piezoelectric crystal resonating between 1 MHz and 10 MHz. A transducer device is generally used to produce the ultrasound. This means that the transducer converts AC into ultrasound, as well as the reverse, sound into AC. Acoustic impedance (i.e., dependent on the density of objects and the speed of sound) and the frequency of emitted sound waves are the most important physical parameters for food quality assessment, significantly. Ultrasound technology can be applied very efficiently for various applications, such as cleaning, drying, low-temperature pasteurization, microbial inactivation, inactivation of enzymes, and so forth. In spite of various applications, ultrasound images provide three more common drawbacks, such as:

1. Low Spatial Resolution: Typically, of a few mm (millimeters) spatial resolution shares by the ultrasound images.
2. Low SNR (signal-to-noise ratio).
3. Many artifacts.

Some applications of ultrasound technique related to food quality assessment, however, are discussed here.

9.3.6.1 APPLICATIONS

Ultrasound technology has wide applications in the medical diagnostic field but also has uses in many industrial sectors in flaw detection and material characterization. In the case of any cracks or voids in material, the ultrasound technique showed a changed peak on the screen. Besides the use of ultrasound technology in medicine and industry, it has potential in the inspection of various food commodities in real-time as well as in laboratory experiments (Javanaud, 1988; Povey and McClements, 1988; Sarkar and Wolfe, 1983). Ultrasound technology is a promising tool for assessing the quality of food products as it is non-invasive in nature, rapid, and has a real-time approach. According to Simal et al. (2003), the protein, fat, moisture content, and other chemical parameters of meat and meat products can be predicted using ultrasonic velocity measurement. Similarly, Morlein et al. (2005) evaluated the fat content (intramuscular) of the *longissimus* muscle of pigs by means of spectral analysis of ultrasound echo-signals, while Camarena and Martinez-Mora (2005) evaluated the hydration and turgidity of orange peel, and thus they checked the potential of ultrasound technology. In another study by Gan et al. (2005) investigated the properties of food products using the high ultrasonic energy delivered by capacitive devices and PCL (pulse-compression technique) for signal recovery and analysis. The effect of high-power ultrasound on the physical chemical properties of polypropylene films for the packaging of food products was studied by Scetar et al. (2018). According to Chemat et al. (2011), there are three different methods upon which the application of ultrasound is based on viz. (1) direct application to the product, (2) coupling with device and (3) submergence in an ultrasonic bath.

9.3.7 ELECTRONIC-NOSE AND TONGUE

E-nose and e-tongue are artificial senses based on arrays of sensors. E-nose has arrays of gas sensors, but e-tongues are based on arrays of liquid sensors. Aroma, flavor, and taste, among the sensory values of food products, are the most significant attributes for their acceptability by consumers. Analyses of these attributes and sample characterization are, thus, very important and can be done using the e-nose and e-tongue non-destructively to avoid the traditional method (i.e., human senses).

As olfactory systems, among the five senses of human beings, are the most usable in our daily life and use the largest part of our brain, they can be used to smell and taste for the monitoring and judging of food products. An electronic nose consists of a sampling/aroma extraction system, a system of gas (chemical) sensor array, a control and measurement system, and a pattern recognition method or a computer with an appropriate pattern-classification algorithm capable of qualitative and/or quantitative analysis of samples (Lozano, 2006). There are different e-nose systems based on various types of gas sensors and combined with other technologies and data processing methodologies for the characterization and detection of food spoilage (Ghasemi-Varnamkhast et al., 2018). The sample type may be complex gases, vapors, odors, and so forth. The basic function of a working e-nose during odor recognition includes:

- **Heating of the Sample** for certain time for the generation of volatiles;
- **Transferring of Volatiles** to a device for detection, where the gas phase reacts to the presence of molecules
- **Classifying the Odor** using the several statistical calculation techniques reveals the differences in sensor reactions.

More than one class of sensors, known as heterogeneous sensor arrays, is commonly used for the construction of modern e-noses. Among these, quartz crystal microbalance, conductive polymer, composite polymer, colorimetric, surface acoustic wave, and so forth, are the more common types of sensors. The results obtained from the e-nose may be quantitative (intensity of odor, the concentration of molecules, etc.) and qualitative (good or bad, recognized, etc.) (Alpha, 2002). E-nose is, therefore, an instrument that comprises an array of electronic chemical sensors with partial specificity and an appropriate pattern recognition system, capable of recognizing simple or complex odors (Gardner and Bartlett, 1994).

E-tongue is a group of sensor chips capable of remitting real-time data to control the quality of liquid flows. E-tongue works by measuring dissolved compounds and taste substances in a liquid sample. Each taste sensation may correspond to a fingerprint signal induced by the differential activation of various taste receptors (Giese, 2001). As e-tongue is mostly applicable for the quality assessment of liquid food products, solid food products should be extracted in an electrolyte that can behave like a continuous phase and keep the electrode array in close contact (Lvova, 2016). The basic function of the working of e-tongue during taste recognition includes three levels, such as:

- **Receptors** (chemo-sensitive metal oxide sensors),
- **Transmission** (detectors and transducers),
- **Perception** (data analytics and chemometrics).

After automatic sampling and application of an array of sensors with different selectivity and sensitivity, chemometric software with a suitable algorithm is used for processing the signals from sensors and delivering the results. Precise information on the activity of food spoilage bacteria and enzymes is required, and an electronic tongue can be used for this (Ghasemi-Varnamkhasti et al., 2018; Kalit et al., 2014). It contains four different chemical sensors comprising very thin films of three polymers and small molecules containing rhodium ions. These materials are deposited onto gold electrodes hooked up to an electrical circuit.

9.3.8. APPLICATIONS OF E-NOSE AND E-TONGUE

There is enormous potential for e-noses and e-tongues in the quality evaluation, classification, authentication, and quality control of food. The application of e-noses in food safety is one of the prominent areas.

Kodogiannis et al. (2017) applied a portable e-nose coupled with the fuzzy-wavelet network for the detection of meat spoilage and reported that the proposed modeling could be considered a valuable detection methodology. Balasubramaniam et al. (2016) apply an e-nose for meat safety, while Boothe and Arnold (2002) applied an e-nose for the assessment of volatile compounds from poultry meat samples, fresh and after refrigerated storage.

In spite of having wide application in space stations and medicine/body function, e-tongues can be used in the detection of water impurities, low concentration detection of substances and compounds which are undetectable by humans, and in the discrimination of wines from two different years, areas, and from the same vintage but produced at different vineyards (Jiang et al., 2018; Legin et al., 2003). By following the process in the brewing industry, this tool can be applied for the monitoring of batch-to-batch variation of the beers (Giese, 2001). E-tongues are not only an important tool for the assessment of food and beverage quality and safety but also for the determination of compounds responsible for aroma decomposition, antibiotic residues, adulteration, and sample classification of dairy products. For instance, a multi-sensor system can be used to differentiate between clinically mastitis cow milk and control milk (Mottram et al., 2007). Similarly, the freshness of pork meat can be evaluated using potentiometric solid-state electrodes and putrescine and dimethyl sulfide during the initial stage of putrefaction on meat (Kaneki et al., 2004). In addition, rapid differentiation and detection of the flavor and chemical composition of different beef of different breeds can be done using e-tongues (Zhang et al., 2015).

9.4 CONCLUSION AND FUTURE PERSPECTIVES

This chapter has been an effort to review the non-destructive detection techniques for evaluation of the quality of horticultural produce and food products. The non-destructive quality evaluation for fruits/vegetables and other biological produce has its special advantage when compared to other instrumental analysis and chemical analysis/methods. As traditional quality evaluation methods often have some disadvantages, such as being time-consuming, laborious, and having a high cost, non-destructive techniques mentioned in this chapter can be used for better results in the field of quality evaluation in the agricultural and food industry.

With the fast-changing technology in electronics and digital gadgets, the future of using non-destructive technologies for evaluating the quality of food and agricultural/horticultural products seems promising and reliable. Results discussed in this chapter show that the measurement of internal quality characteristics of fruits and other produce can be possible in a more efficient manner. Precise imaging systems like machine vision techniques have a very promising future in the nondestructive quality evaluation of the horticultural segment. Though the initial cost for some systems/components is high at the present moment, with changing technology, it will be possible to reduce the cost in the near future. Developing portable systems based on these principles is also a possible future outcome by which nondestructive quality evaluation will possibly be used directly on the farm.

In this context, it is important for researchers and scientists from various fields to join hands and accept the challenges in nondestructive quality evaluation of agricultural and food products. With such mutual efforts, it would be possible to produce dedicated systems with defined process parameters suited for a variety of food and agricultural product quality evaluations.

KEYWORDS

- **agricultural produce**
- **food quality evaluation**
- **imaging technologies**
- **machine vision systems**
- **non-destructive testing**
- **postharvest assessment**

REFERENCES

Abdullah, M. Z. (2008). Image acquisition system. In: Sun D-W, editor, Computer vision technology for food quality evaluation-book, Elsevier Inc. Ch.1, p3–35.

Ahmed, R. M., Yasmin, J., Lee, W. H., Mo, C., & Cho, B. K. (2017). Imaging technologies for nondestructive measurement of internal properties of agricultural products: A review. *Journal of Biosystems Engineering, 42*(3), 2017.

Alpha MOS. (2002). Electronic nose technology overview. Technical note NO. N-P-01. Toulouse, France.

Ariana, D. P., & Lu, R. (2008). Detection of internal defect in pickling cucumbers using hyperspectral transmittance imaging. *Transactions of the ASABE, 51*, 705–713.

Balasubramanian, S., Amamcharla, J., & Shin, J. E. (2016). Possible application of electronic nose systems for meat safety: An overview. In *Electronic Noses and Tongues in Food Science* (pp. 59–71).

Barcelon, E. G., Tojo, S., & Watanabe, K. (1999). Relating X-ray absorption and some quality characteristics of mango fruit (*Mangifera indica* L.). *Journal of Agricultural and Food Chemistry, 47*, 3822–3825.

Barcelon, E. G., Tojo, S., & Watanabe, K. (2000). Nondestructive ripening assessment of mango using an X-ray computed tomography. *Agricultural Engineering Journal, 9*(2), 73–80.

Barreiro, P., Cabello, J., Fernandez-Valle, M. E., Ortiz, C., & Ruiz-Altisent, M. (1999). Mealiness assessment in apples using MRI techniques. *Magnetic Resonance Imaging, 17*(2), 275–281.

Barreiro, P., Ortiz, C., Ruiz-Altisent, M., Ruiz-Cabello, J., Fernandez-Valle, M. E., Recasens, I., & Asensio, M. (2000). Mealiness assessment in apples and peaches using MRI techniques. *Magnetic Resonance Imaging, 18*(9), 1175–1181.

Bato, P. M., Nagata, M., Cao, Q., Hiyoshi, K., Kitahara, T. (2000). Study on Sorting System for Strawberry Using Machine Vision (Part 2) Development of Sorting System with Direction and Judgement Functions for Strawberry (Akihime variety). *Journal of the Japanese Society of Agricultural Machinery, 62*(2), 101–110.

Beletskiy, S. L., Guryeva, K. B., & Haba, N. A. (2021). Methodological aspects of introscopic study by X-ray analysis of internal defects of food grain during storage. *AIP Conference Proceedings, 2356*, 020004. https://doi.org/10.1063/5.0054753 (accessed on 9th July 2025).

Bergaz, L. P., Ruiz, G. R., Gracia, L. M. N., Guimaraes, A. C., & Gil, J. G. (2010, August). Bakery products quality control using computer vision: Napolitalas case. In *Proceedings of the CIGR Workshop on Image Analysis in Agriculture, Budapest, Hungary* (pp. 26–27).

Bo, L. B., Cobo-Medina, M., Lecourt, J., Harrison, N., Harrison, R. J., & Cross, J. V. (2018). Application of hyperspectral imaging for nondestructive measurement of plum quality attributes. *Postharvest Biology and Technology, 141*, 8–15.

Boothe, D. D. H., & Arnold, J. W. (2002). Electronic nose analysis of volatile compounds from poultry meat samples, fresh and after refrigerated storage. *Journal of the Science of Food and Agriculture, 82*(3), 315–322.

Brown, M. A. & Semelka, R. C. (2010). MRI: basic principles and applications, 4th edn. Wiley-Blackwell.

Brusewitz, G. H. & Stone, M. L. (1987). Wheat moisture by NMR. *Trans ASAE 30*(3): 858–862

Brusewitz, G. H., & Stone, M. L. (1987). Wheat moisture by NMR. *Transactions of the ASAE, 30*(3), 858–0862.

Camarena, F., & Martínez-Mora, J. A. (2005). Potential of ultrasound to evaluate turgidity and hydration of orange peel. *Journal of Food Engineering, 75*(4), 503–507.

Chao, K., Yang, C. C., Kim, M. S., & Chan, D. E. (2008). High throughput spectral imaging system for wholesomeness inspection of chicken. *Applied Engineering in Agriculture, 24*(4), 475–485.

Chaudhrya, M. M. A., Amodio, M. L., Babellahi, F., de Chiara, M. L. V., Rubio, J. M. A., & Colelli, G. (2018). Hyperspectral imaging and multivariate accelerated shelf-life testing (MASLT) approach for determining shelf life of rocket leaves. *Journal of Food Engineering, 238*, 122–133.

Chayaprasert, W., & Stroshine, R. (2005). Rapid sensing of internal browning in whole apples using a low-cost, low-field proton magnetic resonance sensor. *Postharvest Biology and Technology, 36*(3), 291–301.

Chemat, F., Huma, Z., & Khan, M.K. (2011). Applications of ultrasound in food technology: Processing, preservation and extraction. *Ultrasonics Sonochemistry, 18*(4): 813–835.

Chen, P., McCarthy, M. J., Kauren, R., Sarig, Y., & Han, S. (1993). Maturity evaluation of avocados by NMR methods. *Journal of Agricultural Engineering Research, 55*(3), 177–187.

Cho, B. K., Chayaprasert, W. & Stroshine, R. L. (2008). Effects of internal browning and watercore on low field (5.4 MHz) proton magnetic resonance measurements of T2 values of whole apples. *Postharvest BiolTechnol* 47:81–89.

Cho, B. K. (2012). Ultrasonic technology. In S. N. Jha (Ed.), *Nondestructive Evaluation of Food Quality: Theory and Practice* (pp. 213–235). Springer: Heidelberg Dordrecht London New York.

Clark, C. J., Hockings, P. D., Joyce, D. C. & Mazucco, R. A. (1997). Application of magnetic resonance imaging to preandpost-harvest studies of fruits and vegetables. *Postharvest BiolTechnol* 11:1–21

Clark, C. J., MacFall, J. S., & Bieleski, R. (1998b). Loss of watercore from 'Fuji' apple observed by magnetic resonance imaging. *Scientia Horticultural, 73*(4), 213–227.

Clark, C. J., MacFall, J. S., & Bieleski, R. L. (1998a). Amelioration of watercore in 'Fuji' apple viewed by two- and three-dimensional nuclear magnetic resonance imaging. *Acta Horticultural, 464*, 91–96.

Collewet, G., Strzelecki, M., & Mariette, F. (2004). Influence of MRI acquisition protocols and image intensity normalization methods on texture classification. *Magnetic Resonance Imaging, 22*(1), 81–91.

De Belie N., Tu K, Jancsók P., De Baerdemaeker J. (1999) Preliminary study on the influence of turgor pressure on body reflectance of red laser light as a ripeness indicator for apples, Postharvest Biology and Technology, *16* (3): 279-284, https://doi.org/10.1016/S0925-5214(99)00025-3.

Diener, R. G., Mitchell, J. P. & Rhoten, M. L. (1970). Using an X-ray image scan to sort bruised apples. *AgricEng* 51:356–361

Donis-González, I. R., Guyer, D. E., Leiva-Valenzuela G. A., Burns, J. (2013). Assessment of chestnut (Castanea spp.) slice quality using color images, *Journal of Food Engineering, 115* (3): 407-414, https://doi.org/10.1016/j.jfoodeng.2012.09.017.

Donis-Gonzalez, I. R., Guyer, D. E., Pease, A., & Barthel, F. (2014). Internal characterisation of fresh agricultural products using traditional and ultrafast electron beam X-ray computed tomography imaging. *Biosystems engineering, 117*, 104–113.

Du, Z., Hu, Y., Ali Buttar, N., & Mahmood, A. (2019). X-ray computed tomography for quality inspection of agricultural products: A review. *Food Science & Nutrition, 7*, 3146–3160. https://doi.org/10.1002/fsn3.1179 (accessed on 9th July 2025).

El-Mesery, H. S., Mao, H., & Abd El-Fatah Abomohra, A. E. F. (2019). Applications of non-destructive technologies for agricultural and food products quality inspection. *Sensors, 19*, 846. https://doi.org/10.3390/s19040846 (accessed on 9th July 2025).

Eshkabilov, S., Lee, A., Sun, X., Lee, C. W., & Simsek, H. (2021). Hyperspectral imaging techniques for rapid detection of nutrient content of hydroponically grown lettuce cultivars. *Computers and Electronics in Agriculture, 181*. https://doi.org/10.1016/j.compag.2020.105968 (accessed on 9th July 2025).

Faqeerzada, M. A., Lohumi, S., Kim, G., Joshi, R., Lee, H., Kim, M. S., & Cho, B. K. (2020). Hyperspectral shortwave infrared image analysis for detection of adulterants in almond powder with one-class classification method. *Sensors (Basel), 20*(20). https://doi.org/10.3390/s20205855 (accessed on 9th July 2025).

Frisullo, P., Marino, R., Laverse, J., Albenzio, M., & Nolile, M. A. D. (2010). Assessment of intramuscular fat level and distribution in beef muscles using X-ray microcomputed tomography. *Meat Science, 85*, 250–255. https://doi.org/10.1016/j.meatsci.2010.01.008 (accessed on 9th July 2025).

Gan, Q., Wang, T., Cochrane, C., & McCarron, P. (2005). Modulation of surface charge, particle size and morphological properties of chitosan–TPP nanoparticles intended for gene delivery. *Colloids and Surfaces B: Biointerfaces, 44*(2–3), 65–73.

Gardner, J. W., & Bartlett, P. N. (1994).A brief history of electronic noses. *Sensors and Actuators B: Chemical, 18*(1–3), 210–211.

Ghasemi-Varnamkhasti, M., Apetrei, C., Lozano, J., & Anyogu, A. (2018). Potential use of electronic noses, electronic tongues and biosensors, as multisensory systems for spoilage examination in foods. *Trends in Food Science & Technology, 80*, 71–92.

Giese, J. (2001). Electronic tongues, noses and much more. *Food Technology, 55*(5), 74–81.

Graham, S., Kennedy, T., Chevallier, O., Gordon, A., Farmer, L., & Elliott, C. (2010). The application of NMR to study changes in polar metabolite concentrations in beef *longissimus dorsi* stored for different periods post mortem. *Metabolomics, 6*(3), 395–404.

Gruwel, M. L. H., Ghosh, P. K., Lata, P. & Jayas, D. S. (2008). On the diffusion constant of the water wheat. *J Agric Food Chem 56*, 59–62.

Hahn, F., Sanchez, S. (2000). Carrot volume evaluation using imaging algorithms. *J Agric Eng Res* 75:243–249.

Han, Y. J., Bowers, S. V., & Dodd, R. B. (1992). Nondestructive detection of split-pit peaches. *Transactions of the ASAE, 35*(6), 2063–2067.

Harding, S. G., Johns, M. L., Pugh, S. R., Fryer, P. J., & Gladden, L. F. (1997). Magnetic resonance imaging studies of diffusion in polymers. *Food Additives and Contaminants, 14*(6–7), 583–589.

Hatcher, D. W. (2001). In: Owens G (ed) Asian noodle processing. In cereal processing technology. *CRS Press, Wood head publishing Ltd, Cambridge*, pp 131–157.

Hernandez-Sanchez, N., Hills, B. P., Barreiro, P. & Marigheto, N. (2007). An NMR study on internal browning in pears. *Postharvest BiolTechnol 44*, 260–270.

Javanaud, C. (1988). Applications of ultrasound to food systems. *Ultrasonics, 26*, 117–123.

Jha, S. N., & Garg, R. (2010).Non-destructive prediction of quality of intact apple using near infrared spectroscopy. *Journal of food science and technology, 47*(2), 207–213.

Jha, S. N., Jaiswal, P., Narsaiah, K., Gupta, M., Bhardwaj, R. & Singh, A. K. (2012). Nondestructive prediction of sweetness of intact mango using near infrared spectroscopy. *ScientiaHorticulturae, 138*, 171–175.

Jha, S. N., Narsaiah, K. Sharma, A.D., Singh, M., Bansal, S. & Kumar R. (2010). Quality parameters of mango and potential of non-destructive techniques for their measurement– a Review. *Journal of Food Science and Technology, 47*(1), 1–14.

Jha, S. N., Narsaiah, K., Jaiswal, P., Bharadwaj, R., Gupta, M., Kumar, R. & Sharma, R. (2014). Nondestructive prediction of maturity of mango using near infrared spectroscopy. *J Food Engineering 124C*, 152–157, doi: 10.1016/j.jfoodeng.2013.10.012.

Jiang, H., Zhang, M., Bhandari, B. H. & Adhikari, B. (2018). Application of electronic tongue for fresh foods quality evaluation A review. *Journal Food Reviews International, 34*(8), 746-769.https//doi.org/10.1080/87559129.2018.1424184.

Kader, A. A. (1992). Quality and safety factors: Definition and evaluation for fresh horticultural crop. In *Postharvest Technology of Horticultural Crops* (Ch. 12, pp. 185–189). University of California, Division of Agriculture and Natural Resources.

Kalit, M., Marković, K., Kalit, S., Vahčić, N., & Havranek, J. (2014). Electronic nose and electronic tongue in the dairy industry. *Mljekarstvo, 64*(4), 228–244.

Kamal, T., Cheng, S., Khan, I. A., Nawab, K., Zhang, T., Song, Y. & Tan, M. (2019). Potential uses of LF-NMR and MRI in the study of water dynamics and quality measurement of fruits and vegetables. *Journal of Food Processing and Preservation, 43*(11), e14202.

Kamruzzaman, M., Barbin, D., ElMasry, G., Sun, D. W., & Allen, P. (2012a). Potential of hyperspectral imaging and pattern recognition for categorization and authentication of red meat. *Innovative Food Science & Emerging Technologies, 16*, 316–325.

Kandi S.G. (2010). Automatic Defect Detection and Grading of Single-Color Fruits Using HSV (Hue, Saturation, Value) Color Space, *J. Life Sci.*, *4*(7):39–45.

Kaneki, N., Miura, T., Shimada, K., Tanaka, H., Ito, S., Hotori, K., Akasaka, C., Ohkubo, S., & Asano, Y. (2004). Measurement of pork freshness using potentiometric sensor. *Talanta, 62*(1), 215–219.

Karunakaran, C., Jayas, D. S., & White, N. D. G. (2003). X-ray image analysis to detect infestations caused by insects in grain. *Cereal Chemistry, 80*(5), 553–557.

Kauten, R., McCarthy, M. J. (2005). Applications of NMR imaging in processing of foods. In: Gaonkar AG (ed) Food processing: recent developments. Elsevier Science BV, Netherlands, p 2

Keagy, P. M., Parvin, B., Schatzki, T. F. (1996). Machine recognition of navel orange worm damage in X-ray images of pistachio nuts. *LebensonWissTechnol 29*(1&2):140–145.

Ketcham, R. A., & Carlson, W. D. (2001). Acquisition, optimization and interpretation of X-ray computed tomographic imagery: Applications to the geosciences. *Computers and Geosciences, 27*, 381–400.

Kiani, S., van Ruth, S. M., van Raamsdonk, L. W. D., & Minaei, S. (2019). Hyperspectral imaging as a novel system for the authentication of spices: A nutmeg case study. *LWT, 104*, 61–69. https://doi.org/10.1016/j.lwt.2019.01.045 (accessed on 9th July 2025).

Kim, R. J., Fieno, D. S., Parrish, T. B., Harris, K., Chen, E. L., Simonetti, O. & Judd, R. M. (1999). Relationship of MRI delayed contrast enhancement to irreversible injury, infarct age, and contractile function. *Circulation, 100*(19), 1992–2002.

Kim, S., & Schatzki, T. F. (2000). Apple water-core sorting system using X-ray imagery: I. Algorithm development. *Transactions of the ASAE, 43*(6), 1695–1702.

Kodogiannis, V. S. (2017). Application of an electronic nose coupled with fuzzy-wavelet network for the detection of meat spoilage. *Food and Bioprocess Technology, 10*, 730–749.

Kroger, C., Bartle, C. M., West, J. G., Purchas, R. W., & Devine, C. E. (2006). Meat tenderness evaluation using dual energy X-ray absorptiometry (DEXA). *Computers and Electronics in Agriculture, 54*(2), 93–100. https://doi.org/10.1016/j.compag.2006.09.002 (accessed on 9th July 2025).

Kullberg, J., Brandberg, J., Angelhed, J. E., Frimmel, H., Bergelin, E., Strid, L., & Lonn, L. (2009). Whole–body adipose tissue analysis: Comparison of MRI, CT and dual energy X–ray absorptiometry. *British Journal of Radiology, 82*(974), 123–130.

Lawrence, K. C., Park, B., Windham, W. R., & Mao, C. (2003a). Calibration of a push broom hyperspectral imaging system for agricultural inspection. *Transactions of the ASAE, 46*(2), 513–521.

Lee, S., Lohumi, S., Lim, H. S., Gotoh, T., Cho, B. K., & Jung, S. (2015). Determination of intramuscular fat content in beef using magnetic resonance imaging. *Journal of the Faculty of Agriculture, Kyushu University, 60*(1), 157–162.

Leemans V., Destain, M. F. (2004). A real-time grading method of apple based on featuresextracted from defects. *J. Food Engg. 61*, 83–89.

Leemans V., H. Magein, M. F. (1999) Destain, Defects segmentation on "Golden Delicious" apples by using colour machine vision and Bayesian classification method. *Comput. Electron Agric. 23* (1), 43–53.

Leemans, V., Magein, H. & Destain, M. F. (1998). Defects segmentation on "Golden Delicious" apples by using colour machine vision. *Comput. Electron. Agric. 20* (2), 117–130 (1998).

Leiva-Valenzuela G.A. & Aguilera, J. M. (2013). Automatic detection of orientation and diseases in blueberries using image analysis to improve their postharvest storage quality. *Food Control 33*, 166–173 (2013).

Lenker, D. H. & Adrian, P. A. (1971). Use of soft X-rays for selecting mature lettuce heads. *Trans ASAE* 14:894–898

Legin, A., Rudnitskaya, A., Lvova, L., Vlasov, Y., Di Natale, C., & D'Amico, A. (2003). Evaluation of Italian wine by electronic tongue recognition, quantitative analysis and correlation with human sensory perception. *Analytica Chemical Acta, 484*(1), 33–44.

Li Q. Z., Wang M. H. & Gu W. K. (2002). Computer vision based system for apple surface defect detection. *Comput. Electron. Agric. 36*(2–3), 215–223.

Lino, A. C. L., Sanches. J. & Fabbro, I. M. D. (2008) Image processing techniques for lemons and tomatoes classification. *Bragantiacampinas 67*(3), 785–789.

Liu, M., Zhang, L., & Guo, E. (2008). Hyperspectral laser-induced fluorescence imaging for nondestructive assessing soluble solids content of orange. In *Computer and Computing Technologies in Agriculture, 1*, 51–59.

Liu, Z., Yu, H., & MacGregor, J. F. (2007). Standardization of line-scan NIR imaging systems. *Journal of Chemometrics, 21*, 88–95.

Lopez-Garcíaa F., Andreu-Garciaa, G., Blascob, J., Aleixosc, N. Valientea J. M. (2010). Automatic detection of skin defects in citrus fruits using a multivariate image analysis approach. *Comput.Electron. Agric. 71*: 189–197.

Lozano, J. (2006). New technology in sensing odors: From human to artificial noses. In J. A. Teixeira da Silva (Ed.), *Floriculture, Ornamental and Plant Biotechnology: Advances and Tropical Issues* (Vol. IV, pp. 152–161). London: Global Science Books.

Lu, H., Zheng, H., Hu, Y., Lou, H., & Kong, X. (2011). Bruise detection on red bayberry (MyricarubraSieb. &Zucc.)using fractal analysis and support vector machine. *Journal of Food engineering, 104*(1), 149–153.

Lu, J., Tan, J., Shatadal, P., & Gerrard, D. E. (2000). Evaluation of pork color by using computer vision. *Meat Sci 56*:57–60.

Lvova, L. (2016). Electronic tongue principles and applications in the food industry. In M. L. Rodríguez Méndez (Ed.), *Electronic Noses and Tongues in Food Science* (pp. 151–160). Academic Press.

Marigheto, N., & Hills, B. (2005). MRI as a potential on-line sensor of apple quality. In *Information and Technology for Sustainable Fruit and Vegetable Production, Frutic 05* (Montpellier, France, 16 September), pp. 455–464.

Marigheto, N., Venturi, L., & Hills, B. (2008). Two-dimensional NMR relaxation studies of apple quality. *Postharvest Biology and Technology, 48*(3), 331–340.

McGlone, V. A., Fraser, D. G., Jordan, R. B., & Künnemeyer, R. (2003).Internal quality assessment of mandarin fruit by vis/NIR spectroscopy. *Journal of Near Infrared Spectroscopy, 11*(5), 323–332.

Monavar H. M, Alimardani, R. & Omid M. (2011), Detection of red ripe tomatoes on stem using image processing techniques. *J. American Sci. 7*(7): 376–379.

Morlein, D., Rosner, F., Brand, S., Jenderka, K. V., & Wicke, M. (2005). Non-destructive estimation of the intramuscular fat content of the *longissimus* muscle of pigs by means of spectral analysis of ultrasound echo signals. *Meat Science, 69*, 187–199.

Mottram, T., Rudnitskaya, A., Legin, A., Fitzpatrick, J. L., & Eckersall, P. D. (2007). Evaluation of a novel chemical sensor system to detect clinical mastitis in bovine milk. *Biosensors and Bioelectronics, 22*(11), 2689–2693. https://doi.org/10.1016/j.bios.2006.11.006 (accessed on 9th July 2025).

Musse, M., Quellec, S., Cambert, M., Devaux, M. F., Lahaye, M., & Mariette, F. (2009a). Monitoring the postharvest ripening of tomato fruit using quantitative MRI and NMR relaxometry. *Postharvest Biology and Technology, 53*, 22–35.

Musse, M., Quellec, S., Devaux, M. F., Cambert, M., Lahaye, M., & Mariette, F. (2009b). An investigation of the structural aspects of the tomato fruit by means of quantitative nuclear magnetic resonance imaging. *Magnetic Resonance Imaging, 27*, 709–719.

Naganathan, G. K., Grimes, L. M., Subbiah, J., Calkins, C. R., Samal, A., & Meyer, G. E. (2008b).Visible/near-infrared hyperspectral imaging for beef tenderness prediction. *Computers and electronics in agriculture, 64*(2), 225–233. https://doi.org/10.1016/j.compag.2008.05.020

Naganathan, G. K., Grimes, L. M., Subbiah, J., Calkins, C. R., Samal, A., & Meyer, G. E. (2008a). Partial least squares analysis of near-infrared hyperspectral images for beeftenderness prediction. *Sensing and Instrumentation for Food Quality and Safety.* https://doi.org/10.1007/s11694-008-9051-3.

Nagata, M., Cao, Q., Bato, P. M., Shrestha, B. P. & Kinoshita, O. (1997). Basicstudy on strawberry sorting system in Japan. In: 1997 ASAEAnnual International Meeting Technical Papers, Paper No.973095, ASAE, 2950 Niles Road, *St. Joseph, Michigan* 49085–9659, USA

Ni, H., & Gunasekaran, S. (1998). A computer vision method for determining length of cheese shreds. *Artificial Intelligence Review, 12*(1), 27–37.

Noh, S. H., & Choi, K. H. (2006). Non-destructive quality evaluation technologies for fruits and vegetables. In *International Seminar on Enhancing Export Competitiveness of Asian Fruits.*

Nugraha, B., Verboven, P., Janssen, S., Wang, Z., & Nicolaï, B. M. (2019). Non-destructive porosity mapping of fruit and vegetables using X-ray CT. *Postharvest Biology and Technology, 150*, 80–88.

Park, B. & Chen, Y. R. (2001). Co-occurrence matrix texture features of multi spectral images on poultry carcasses. *J Agric Eng Res 78* (2):127–139.

Patel, K. K., Kar, A., Khan, M. A. (2019b). Common External Defect Detection of Mangoes using Color Computer Vision. *Journal of The Institution of Engineers (India): Series A. 100* (4), 559–568.

Patel, K. K., Kar, A., Khan, M. A. (2021). Rapid Assessment of Some Physical Parameters of Mangoes Using Monochrome Computer Vision. *Agric Res. 10*(3):464–482.

Patel, K.K. &Kar, A. (2022).Potential of NIR computer vision technique for the detection of mango's defects. *Journal of AgriSearch, 9*(4), 314–319.

Patel, K.K., Kar, A. & Khan, M.A. (2012b). Nondestructive food quality evaluation techniques: principle and potential. *Agricultural Engineering Today*, *36*(4), 29–34.

Patel, K.K., Kar, A. & Khan, M.A. (2019a). Potential of reflected UV imaging technique for detection of defects on the surface area of mango. *J Food Science and Technology, 56*(3), 1295–1301.

Patel, K. K., Kar, A. & Khan, M. A. (2020). NIR computer vision for rapid measurements of some physical properties of mangoes. *Journal of AgriSearch, 7*(4), 211–219.

Patel, K.K., Kar, A., Jha, S.N. & Khan, M.A. (2012a). Machine vision system: a tool for on-line sorting and grading of agricultural foods and produces. *J Food Science and Technolology*, *49*(2), 123–141

Patel, K.K., Khan, M.A. & Kar, A. (2015). Recent developments in applications of MRI techniques for foods and agricultural produce – an overview. *J Food Science and Technology*, *52*(1), 1–26.

Pearson, T., & Toyofuku, N. (2000).Automated sorting of pistachio nuts with closed shells. *Applied Engineering in Agriculture*, *16*(1), 91–94.

Penchaiya, P., Bobelyn, E., Verlinden, B. E., Nicolaï, B. M., & Saeys, W. (2009). Non-destructive measurement of firmness and soluble solids content in bell pepper using NIR spectroscopy. *Journal of Food Engineering, 94* (3–4), 267–273.

Peng, Y., & Wang, W. (2008). Prediction of pork meat total viable bacteria count using hyperspectral imaging system and support vector machines.In Food Processing Automation Conference Proceedings, 28–29 June 2008, Providence, Rhode Island (p. 35). American Society of Agricultural and Biological Engineers.

Peng, Y., Zhang, J., Wu, J., & Hang, H. (2009, April). Hyperspectral scattering profiles for prediction of the microbial spoilage of beef. In Sensing for agriculture and food quality and safety (Vol. 7315, pp. 156–167). SPIE.

Povey, M. J. W., & McClements, D. J. (1988). Ultrasonics in food engineering. Part I. Introduction and experimental methods. *Journal of Food Engineering, 8*, 217–245.

Quddusi, M. A. (2018). Importance of food in our daily life—How eating healthy affects our health? https://www.scientificworldinfo.com/2018/07/importance-of-food-in-our-daily-life.html (accessed on 9th July 2025).

Riquelme, M. T., Barreiro, P., Ruiz-Altisent, M., & Valero, C. (2008).Olive classification according to external damage using image analysis. *Journal of Food Engineering, 87*(3), 371–379.

Samrat, N. H., Johnson, J. B., White, S., Naiker, M., & Brown, P. (2022). A rapid non-destructive hyperspectral imaging data model for the prediction of pungent constituents in dried ginger. *Foods, 11*(5), 649.

Sarkar, N., & Wolfe, R. R. (1983). Potential of ultrasonic measurement in food quality evaluation. *Transactions of the ASAE, 26*, 624–629.

Ščetar, M., Kurek, M., Jambrak, A. R., Debeaufort, F., & Galić, K. (2018). Effect of high-power ultrasound on physical–chemical properties of polypropylene films aimed for food packaging: Structure and surface features. *Polymer Bulletin, 2018*, 1–15.

Schaare, P. N., & Fraser, D. G. (2000). Comparison of reflectance, interactome and transmission modes of visible-near infrared spectroscopy for measuring internal properties of kiwifruit (*Actinidia chinensis*). *Postharvest Biology and Technology, 20*, 175–184.

Schatzki, T. F., & Fine (Bryant), T. A. (1988). Analysis of radiograms of wheat kernels for quality control. *Cereal Chemistry, 65*(3), 233–239.

Shao, Y., Bao, Y., & He, Y. (2011). Visible/near-infrared spectra for linear and nonlinear calibrations: a case to predict soluble solids contents and pH value in peach. *Food and bioprocess technology, 4*(8), 1376–1383.

Simal, S., Benedito, J., Clemente, G., Femenia, A., & Roselló, C. (2003). Ultrasonic determination of the composition of a meat-based product. *Journal of Food Engineering, 58*(3), 253–257.

Stermer, R. A. (1972). Automated X-ray inspection of grain for insect infestation. *Trans ASAE* 1081–1085.

Suchanek, M., & Olejniczak, Z. (2008). Ocena jakości jabłek za pomocą niskopolowej tomografii magnetyczno-rezonansowej. *Acta Agrophysical, 12*(1), 183–190.

Taglienti, A., Massantini, R., Botondi, R., Mencarelli, F., & Valentini, M. (2009). Postharvest structural changes of Hayward kiwifruit by means of magnetic resonance imaging spectroscopy. *Food Chemistry, 114*(4), 1583–1589.

Thomas, P., Kannan, A., Degwekar, V. H., & Ramamurthy, M. S. (1995). Nondestructive detection of seed weevil-infested mango fruits by X-ray imaging. *Postharvest Biology and Technology, 5*(1, 2), 161–165.

Tian, Y., Sun, J., Zhou, X., Yao, K., & Tang, N. (2022). Detection of soluble solid content in apples based on hyperspectral technology combined with deep learning algorithm. *Journal of Food Processing and Preservation, 46*(4). https://doi.org/10.1111/jfpp.16414 (accessed on 9th July 2025).

Toffanin, R., Mlynarik, V., Russo, S., Szomolanyi, P., Piras, A., & Vittur, F. (2001). Proteoglycan depletion and magnetic resonance parameters of articular cartilage. *Archives of biochemistry and biophysics*, *390*(2), 235–242.

Tollner, E. W., Hung, Y. C., Upchurch, B. L., & Prussia, S. E. (1992). Relating X-ray absorption to density and water content in apples. *Transactions of the ASAE, 35*(6), 1921–1928.

Wang, C., Li, X., Wei, Wang, W., Feng, Y., Zhou, Z. & Zhan, H. (2011). Recognition of worm-eaten chestnuts based on machine vision. *Math. Comput. Model. 54,* 3–4 (August, 2011), 888–894, https://doi.org/10.1016/j.mcm.2010.11.012

Wang, H-H. & Sun D-W. (2002a). Melting characteristics of cheese: analysis of effects of cooking conditions using computer vision techniques. *J Food Eng 52*(3), 279–284.

Wang, H-H. & Sun, D-W. (2002b). Correlation between cheese meltability determined with a computer vision method and with Arnott and Schreiber. *J Food Sci 67*(2), 745–749.

Wu, J., Peng, Y., Li, Y., Wang, W., Chen, J., & Dhakal, S. (2012). Prediction of beef quality attributes using VIS/NIR hyperspectral scattering imaging technique. *Journal of Food Engineering, 109*(2), 267–273.

Xie, C., Chu, B., & He, Y. (2018). Prediction of banana color and firmness using a novel wavelengths selection method of hyperspectral imaging. *Food Chemistry, 245*, 132–140.

Xing, J., Linden, V. V., Vanzeebroeck, M. (2005). Josse De Baerdemaeker, Bruise detection on Jonagold apples by visible and near-infrared spectroscopy. *Food Control. 16* (4), 357–361, https://doi.org/10.1016/j.foodcont.2004.03.016.

Yang, Q. (1996). Apple stem and calyx identification with machine vision. *J Agric Eng Res 63*(3), 229–236.

Yang, X., Chen, J., Jia, L., Yu, W., Wang, D., Wei, W., Li. S., Tian, S. & Wu, D. (2020). Rapid and non-destructive detection of compression damage of yellow peach using an electronic nose and chemometrics. *Sensors, 20*(7), 1866.

Yoshioka, H., Schlechtyeg, P. M., Kose, K. (2009). Magnetic resonance imaging, chapter 3. In: BN Warren Weissman (ed) Imaging of arthritis and metabolic bone disease. *Elsevier Inc,* pp 34–48.

Zhang, X., Zhang, Y., Meng, Q., Li, N., & Ren, L. (2015). Evaluation of beef by electronic tongue system TS-5000Z: Flavor assessment, recognition and chemical compositions according to its correlation with flavor. *PLoS ONE, 10*(9).

Zhao, X., Wang, W., Ni, X., Chu, X., Li, Y. F., & Sun, C. (2018). Evaluation of near-infrared hyperspectral imaging for detection of peanut and walnut powders in whole wheat flour. *Applied Sciences, 8*(7). https://doi.org/10.3390/app8071076 (accessed on 9th July 2025).

Zhu, Q., Huang, M., Zhao, X., & Wang, S. (2013). Wavelength selection of hyperspectral scattering image using new semi-supervised affinity propagation for prediction of firmness and soluble solid content in apples. *Food Analytical Methods, 6*(1), 334–342.

CHAPTER 10

Internet of Things (IoT)-Enabled Blockchain for Traceability in the Fresh Produce Supply Chain

SANDEEP JAGTAP,[1,2,*] HANA TROLLMAN,[3] GUILLERMO GARCIA-GARCIA,[4] YANG LUO,[5] ABDO HASSOUN,[6] WAYNE MARTINDALE,[7] and SUMIT GUPTA[8]

[1]*Sustainable Manufacturing Systems Centre, Cranfield University, Cranfield, United Kingdom*

[2]*Division of Engineering Logistics, Lund University, Lund, Sweden*

[3]*School of Management, College of Business, University of Leicester, Leicester, United Kingdom*

[4]*Department of Chemical Engineering, Faculty of Sciences, University of Granada, Granada, Spain*

[5]*School of Intelligent Manufacturing Ecosystem, Xi'an Jiaotong-Liverpool University, Suzhou, Jiangsu, China*

[6]*Faculty of Agricultural Engineering, University of Aleppo, Aleppo, Syria; Sustainable AgriFoodtech Innovation & Research (SAFIR), Arras, France*

[7]*MPC Research Ltd, DMC, County Way, Barnsley, United Kingdom*

[8]*Department of Mechanical Engineering, Amity School of Engineering and Technology, Amity University, Noida, Uttar Pradesh, India*

*Corresponding author

Sustainable Approaches in Postharvest Handling and Management: Pankaj B. Pathare (Ed.)

DOI: 10.1201/9781779641076-10

ABSTRACT

With global food supply chains becoming more complex, the credibility of the food sector is under threat due to the loss of public trust with rising food fraud cases such as the horsemeat scandal, Chinese milk scandal, and so forth. Therefore, it has become essential to promote transparency and real-time visibility of the food supply chain from farm to fork to address the demand of all the stakeholders involved. This chapter aims to recognize opportunities to integrate Blockchain and the internet of things (IoT) in the fresh food supply chain to regain public trust by improving transparency and real-time visibility. This chapter includes a brief literature review and business cases to highlight the advantages, challenges, and recommendations for adopting Blockchain and IoT to improve traceability and transparency.

10.1 DEFINITION OF FOOD TRACEABILITY

The Codex Alimentarius Commission (CAC) and International Organization for Standardization (ISO) define food traceability as "the ability to follow the movement of food through specified stage(s) of production, processing, and distribution (Jakkhupan et al., 2015)."

ISO 22005:2007 systematically describes the principles and requirements for the design and implementation of a feed and food traceability system (Storøy et al., 2013). It permits organizations operating at any step of the food chain to:

1. Determine organization's position in the feed and food chain.
2. Track the flow of materials.
3. Identify necessary information and documentation for each stage.
4. Better perform coordination among all the actors involved.
5. Improve communication among all the involved entities.
6. Improve the correct use and reliability of information, effectiveness and productivity.

As per the EU law (No. 931/2011), traceability means "the ability to track any food, feed, food-producing animal, or substance that will be used for consumption, through all stages of production, processing, and distribution (Hu et al., 2013)."

10.2 CHARACTERISTICS OF FOOD TRACEABILITY

A food traceability system captures the data and operations that provide the desired information of the product; that is, it records and follows the movement of the product from its source until it reaches the end consumer (Aung and Chang, 2014). The basic characteristics of food traceability systems consist of the following steps:

- Identification of quantities and batches of all the fresh produce ingredients and products.
- Recording information about every action or movement that is, when and where quantities and batches are moved and processed.
- A platform or system to link all these data and transmitting all traceability information about the product processing.

Identification, information, and the links between supply chain partners are common, regardless of processes or products concerned. However, the traceability systems can vary based on the extent of information being recorded, that is, how far (backward or forward) and how much information is tracked, and at what accuracy the system can identify the movement of a food product (Olsen and Borit, 2018). In short, traceability systems are record-keeping systems to track products from source to consumers, as shown in Figure 10.1. Traceability systems also showcase information such as country of origin, species, and/or use-by dates linked with the product (Storøy et al., 2013). Traceability systems could range from a paper-based system to a system based on barcodes and radio frequency identification (RFID). However, the latter system, based on barcodes and RFID, is quicker and cheaper to operate (Jakkhupan et al., 2015).

As mentioned above, a traceability system can be characterized as follows (Smith et al., 2005):

- **Breadth:** Quantity of information collected.
- **Depth:** To what extent the information can be tracked both forward and backward.
- **Precision:** Level of accurate information of a food product and its movement in the supply chain.

10.3 BENEFITS OF TRACEABILITY IN FRESH PRODUCE CHAIN

Food safety is a basic right and the most important aspect of food provision, but we still encounter significant cases of breaches in food safety and scandals (Wiśniewska, 2023). Outbreaks caused by *Listeria*, *E. coli*, *Salmonella*, *C. botulinum*, and so forth, have resulted in significant numbers of people getting ill or even dying (Gourama, 2020). Also, incidents like the 2008 Chinese Milk Scandal and 2013 Horsemeat scandal in Europe have increased both public and private scrutiny. Before people completely lose trust in the food they are consuming, it is vital for all the entities involved in the supply chain to heighten the traceability of their products (Havinga et al., n.d.).

Fresh produce trade is on a continuous rise, partly due to an increase in population as well as consumers' desires to have fresh food available year-round (Jagtap et al., 2022). This has led to growth in production and expansion of the supply network (Padel and Foster, 2005). However, due to the increase in the number of entities, the supply chain has become more complex (Jagtap et al., 2024). Furthermore, uncertainty with supply and the perishable nature of fresh produce have increased the need for quality and safety assurance, thereby adding a need for traceability. Implementing robust traceability systems ensures the safety and quality of the food produced and supplied (Hassoun et al., 2023). It allows better management of risks and swift response to product recalls, quarantining, or safe disposal. Also, in case of outbreaks, it significantly reduces response time for all the supply chain partners, providing them with reliable and relevant information that helps in identifying the source and location of implicated products.

Thus, having a robust traceability system can reduce the recall of products, which further reduces waste happening due to the absence of traceability systems (Sterling et al., 2015).

10.4 INTERNET OF THINGS

Numerous IoT definitions are available in the literature. As IoT consists of two main words, that is, 'internet' and 'things,' it means both physical and virtual things that can communicate with each other and their surrounding environment over the internet (Jagtap, 2021; Jagtap et al., 2021). In terms of fresh produce, IoT can be defined as things that are

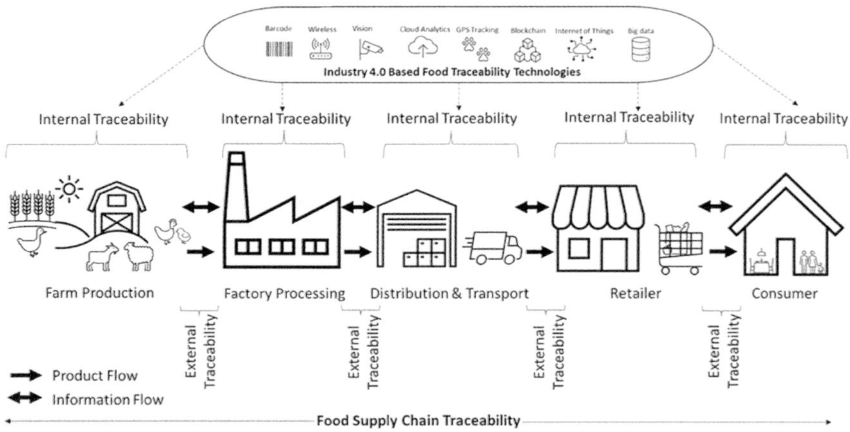

FIGURE 10.1 Food supply chain traceability in an industry 4.0 era.

interconnected to sense, monitor, and interact to provide visibility, transparency, tracking, and sharing to enhance planning, scheduling, control, and coordination of the supply chain partners and processes (Martindale et al., 2022).

According to academics and industrial experts, there is a growing trend of IoT technologies and their adoption in daily life as well as in the manufacturing sector (Echegaray et al., 2022). The widespread application of IoT in the fresh food industry is based on RFID (Ben-Daya et al., 2019). Based on the study conducted, it highlighted five IoT-based technologies that are essential in supply chains and are also relevant to fresh food supply chains (Aamer et al., 2021):

- **RFID:** It uses electromagnetic fields or radio waves to identify objects or things. It consists of tags attached to objects which transmit digital data when triggered by RFID readers. This tracking system could be used to track inventory goods in the fresh food warehouses, retailers, and so forth. It records every piece of information and stores it (Jones et al., 2004). RFID has five classes, as shown in Figure 10.2.

1. **Wireless Sensor Networks (WSN):** It consists of nodes where each node is connected to a set of sensors to monitor and track various parameters of fresh food supply chains, such as temperature, moisture, speed, pressure, location, and so

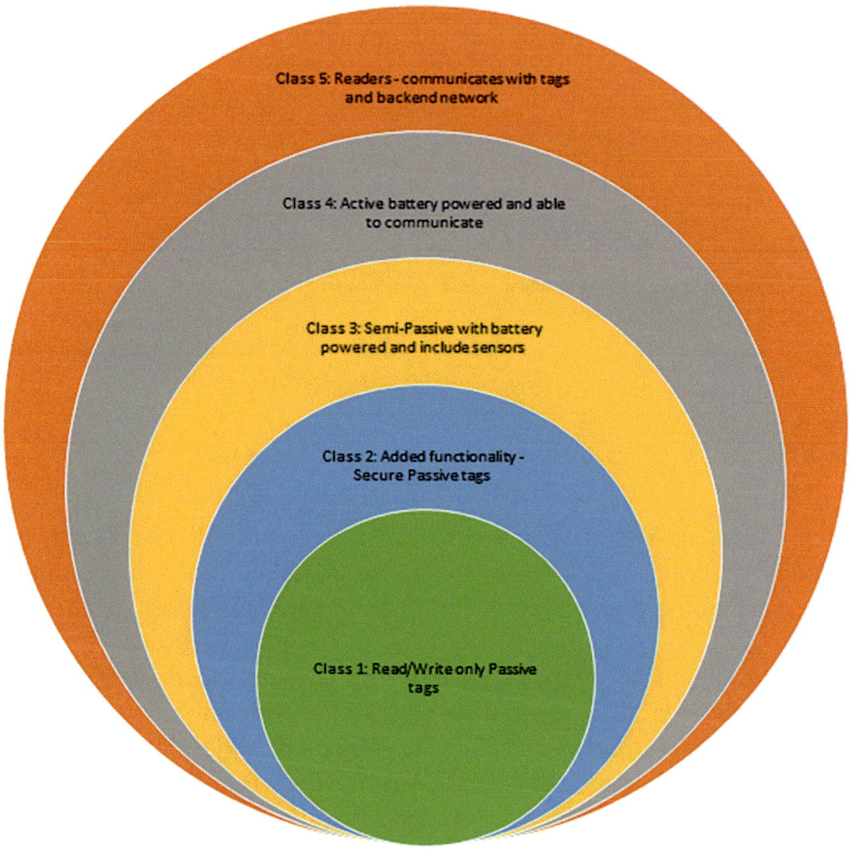

FIGURE 10.2 Classification of RFID tags.

forth. These sensors, when combined with RFID, can result in identification, tracking, and sensing, making the whole system intelligent and a good option for monitoring purposes (Poongodi et al., 2020).

2. **Middleware:** It is a service-oriented software that provides services to its users. It permits software developers to communicate with other devices like sensors, RFID, and so forth, which is crucial for quick messaging between various fresh food supply chain stakeholders (Al-Jaroodi and Mohamed, 2012).

3. **Cloud Computing:** It is an internet-powered computing platform that stores and processes large amounts of data.

This is very important since a large amount of data is generated by sensors installed in the fresh food supply chain. This data needs to be analyzed and presented to fresh food supply chain stakeholders in real-time. This could also enhance the security of the transmitted data (Sharma et al., 2017).

4. **Applications Layer:** It presents the data in a dashboard format wherein only the important information is displayed. The fresh food supply chain stakeholders can identify issues and action them in a real-time environment (Jagtap and Rahimifard, 2019b).

10.5 IOT ARCHITECTURE

IoT in fresh food supply chains is designed to connect various devices, machines, and other physical and virtual things over the network. This could be a very complex process, and therefore, an IoT architecture is needed to collect and transmit data securely. There are many architectures ranging from very simple ones with three layers to very detailed ones consisting of seven or more layers. However, when it comes to fresh food supply chains, the most suitable and widely used one has four layers: Sensing layer, Network layer, Service layer, and Application layer, as shown in Figure 10.3 (Jagtap and Rahimifard, 2019a).

1. **Sensing Layer:** Various crucial data with regards to the fresh food supply chain, such as temperature, moisture, location, pressure, and so forth, are collected using sensing devices such as sensors, cameras, RFID, and so forth. Some of the data is pre-processed, and the rest is transmitted to the Network layer.
2. **Network Layer:** Its function is to collect the data generated by the sensing layer and transmit it to the service layer by using technologies such as WiFi, Bluetooth, ZigBee, and so forth.
3. **Service Layer:** In this layer, the data collected from the Network layer is stored and processed to derive meaningful insights.
4. **Application Layer:** This layer showcases the data in a visual format, such as dashboards, graphs, and so forth. Also, based on who the user is, it will present only the data needed by that particular user.

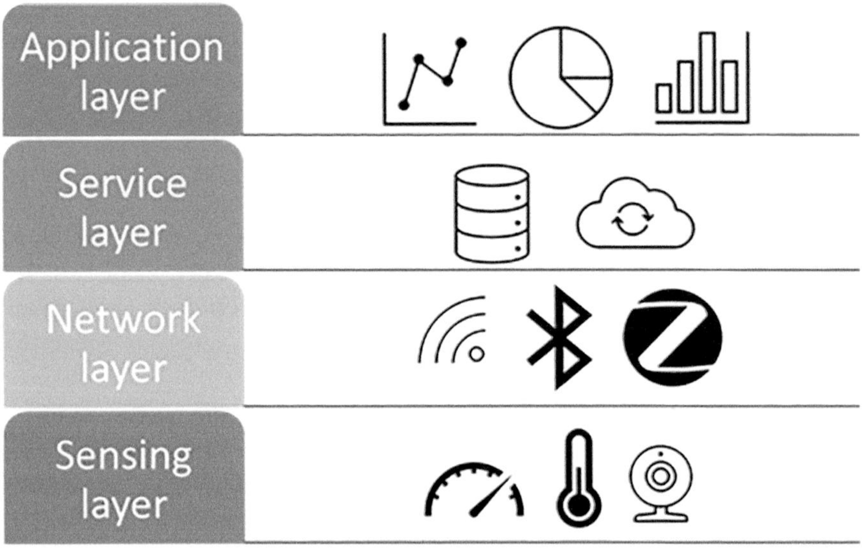

FIGURE 10.3 IoT architecture.

10.6 IOT APPLICATION IN FRESH FOOD SUPPLY CHAIN

IoT application in the fresh food supply chain allows virtualization of the whole supply chain. It allows all the stakeholders in the supply chain, that is, from farmers to the end consumer, to track and trace food products as they move through the supply chain. It enables the performance of quality control and planning in a real-time environment (Jagtap et al., 2021; Martindale et al., 2022).

The utilization of IoT in the fresh food supply chain offers significant opportunities. For instance, equipment and machines in the supply chain embedded with sensors can provide full visibility and real-time monitoring capability. It also supports improving operational control to enhance efficiencies, efficient resource utilization, and better planning and scheduling. Other than this, IoT can also be used for predictive maintenance, better connectivity of supply chains, and improving sustainability (Hassoun et al., 2023).

Fresh food delivery in the supply chain consists of warehousing, inventory management, and transportation. Most of the literature focuses on visibility during transportation of the food. Various IoT devices are used to improve the flexibility and efficiency of transportation operations.

For example, the global positioning system (GPS) is used to establish the exact location of food vehicles for better scheduling, planning, and optimized routing to reduce delivery times. Other conditions such as temperature, moisture, vibrations, handling, and so forth, can be monitored in order to improve in-transit traceability and visibility. Every minute-by-minute data can be analyzed on the cloud and stored for further analysis (Rahimifard et al., 2022).

IoT can also be used during reverse logistics. For instance, it can be used for tracking returnable goods such as packaging, pallets and trays, transport, non-saleable or damaged products, and storage. It can also be used to collect data during its consumption stage. This consumer behavior data can support better planning with regards to procurement, production, product recall, and pricing (Jagtap et al., 2020).

Food product data, such as nutritional information, recipes, cooking instructions, shelf-life, and so forth, can be relayed to the consumer by using smartphones to scan barcodes or quick response (QR) codes. This functionality is enabled by IoT technology. Overall, IoT application in the fresh food supply chain can be summarized by sharing information, monitoring, transparency, and traceability, which eventually leads to better food safety. Furthermore, IoT technology can be utilized to predict shelf-life, increase sales, and reduce wastage, enabling efficient use of resources and precision food production (Hassoun, Jagtap, Garcia-Garcia, et al., 2023).

10.7 BLOCKCHAIN TECHNOLOGY IN FRESH FOOD SUPPLY CHAIN

Blockchain technology was initially proposed and launched by Satoshi Nakamoto in 2008 as a central component of the cryptocurrency Bitcoin network (Srivastav et al., 2020). However, it did not remain limited to financial applications and cryptocurrencies but has expanded to other sectors such as pharma, manufacturing (automotive, aerospace, etc.), food supply chain, and even music. Many researchers see blockchain technology beyond its cryptocurrency application, and it is now more often used in supply chain transactions. Blockchain is a distributed ledger technology that provides high levels of transparency, integrity, and availability in a decentralized environment; therefore, it is becoming more popular. In this context, blockchain can be defined as a digital ledger of transactions consisting of blocks shared across many participating agents or network of computers so that the records are immutable (Babich and Hilary, 2019). Figure 10.4 shows an example of a blockchain process. Any new data or amendment will create a block, which will be shared with each computer or participating agent in the blockchain network. Each participating agent then approves or denies a block, and the new block is added to the chain, which is immutable.

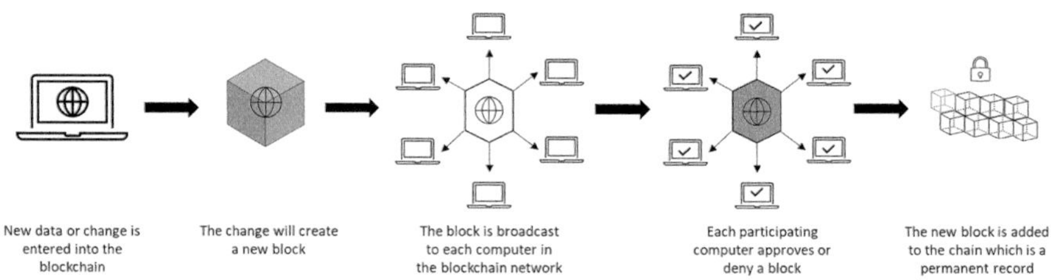

FIGURE 10.4 An example of blockchain.

1. **Decentralized Digital Database:** A decentralized digital database implies that every participating agent of the network has a copy of any transaction carried out in the blockchain. This allows every agent to have access to all the previous transactions made by any participant involved. All participants have their own local copies of each blockchain created, making it impossible to alter any existing information in the blockchain. To make any changes, the participant would have to change all the existing copies that have already recorded all the previous information, which is highly impossible. This is why the distributed ledger is more preferred, since it can improve transparency and authenticity of information (Benarous et al., 2022).
2. **Peer-to-Peer Transmission:** While executing transactions between two parties, both parties can directly communicate with each other without any involvement of a third party to verify the transactions. These are also termed as smart contracts since all the transactions are transparent and trustworthy because they are peer-to-peer transactions with no third party involved to approve or deny transactions (Benarous et al., 2022).

3. **Visibility:** The records in the blockchain are visible to all the entities in the network. This allows transparency and, at the same time, ensures anonymity by safeguarding the records behind crypto graphics (Benarous et al., 2022).
4. **Non-Alteration of Transactional Records:** Each change or new information is linked to all the previous transactions in a sequential order that is accessible to all the participating agents over the network. Hence, once any transaction is made and added into the blockchain, the information is immutable. Therefore, blockchain data can be trusted, consistent, timestamped, and authentic (Benarous et al., 2022).

10.8 BLOCKCHAIN ARCHITECTURE

IoT-enabled blockchain can improve transparency and trackability in the food supply chain (Jagtap et al., 2021). Figure 10.5 shows how the fresh food product and information flows in an IoT-based food supply chain system. All the activities of the supply chain actors, that is, from input suppliers to consumers, form part of the traceability system. The consumer will have access to all the information about the final product (Bhat et al., 2021). Blockchain transactions in the food supply chain mean every action is approved by all the participating agents in the network, such as farmers, processors, distributors, and retailers. All the food product information from all stages of the supply chain is stored in the cloud database with a unique cryptogram that cannot be altered once the block is created. All the entities involved in the network could use private or public keys to access only the relevant data, which creates a secure system.

10.9 BLOCKCHAIN IN FRESH FOOD SUPPLY CHAIN

In the food supply chain, end consumers are requesting better quality, origin, and sustainability of products (Hollands et al., 2018). Therefore, in order to gain consumers' trust, all the supply chain actors strive to improve the transparency and visibility of the supply chain. Blockchain technology, due to its distinctive features, can address most of the mentioned concerns and boost consumers' confidence in the product. For instance, Trabocca,

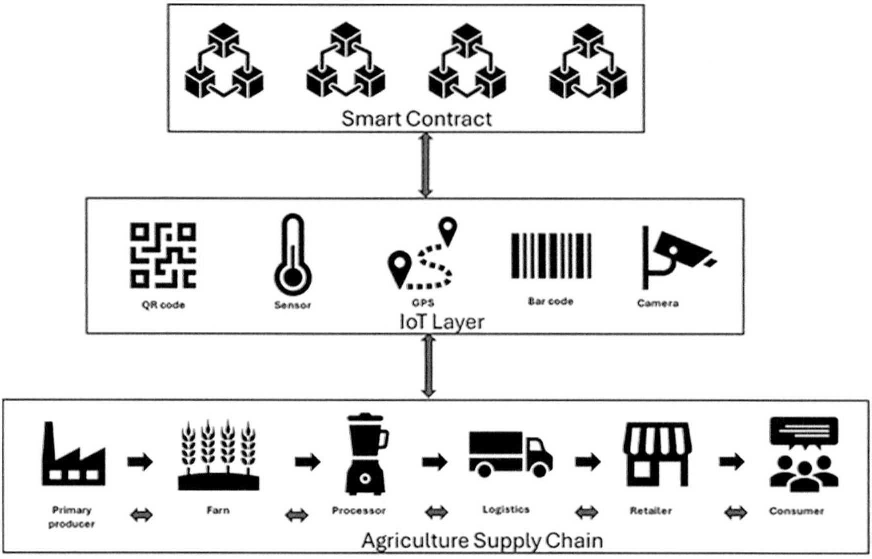

FIGURE 10.5 Blockchain architecture for fresh food supply chain.

a green coffee importer, employs Trace, a blockchain-based platform by Fairfood, to track and trace coffee from Ethiopia to consumers in Amsterdam, while Starbucks uses blockchain technology to trace the journey of their coffee, and consumers can simply scan the QR code or input the number on the back of bags to see the traceability data (Trollman et al., 2022).

Several research studies with regard to the implementation and application of blockchain technology in the food supply chain are being undertaken (Atlam and Wills, 2019). The sole purpose is to achieve transparency and authenticity of the food product. Various IoT-based sensors and devices are used to collect the food data, which is then stored in the blockchain network. This ensures that the quality of the product is maintained and not tampered with while moving along the food supply chain. For instance, food retailers are using blockchain technology to track and trace their food products in case of outbreaks or product recalls. Within a few seconds, they can identify the affected products and locate their whereabouts, reducing their product recall cost and improving food safety. For example, retailers like Walmart have associated with IBM's blockchain platform FoodTrust to address food safety issues (Yiannas, 2018). Barilla, the pasta manufacturer, uses blockchain technology to avoid any counterfeit products being distributed into the market, as well as to assure the quality of fresh Italian basil for its pesto (Nicoletti, 2018). Similarly, Nestle, JBS Foods, and Carrefour are using blockchain technology to improve the authenticity of their products (Yacoub and Castillo, 2022).

10.10 CASE STUDIES

10.10.1 IBM FOOD TRUST BLOCKCHAIN

The IBM Food Trust network enables collaboration among growers, processors, wholesalers, distributors, manufacturers, retailers, and regulators (Pavlić and Zaninović, 2020). Authorized users have immediate access to food supply chain data from farm to store. Stakeholders benefit from increased food safety due to enhanced visibility and accountability. Four main aspects of fresh food supply chains are addressed by the IBM Food Trust network (Köhler and Pizzol, 2020):

1. **Food Safety:** Increased supply chain visibility includes trustworthy information about the provenance, real-time location, and status of fresh food products. Should a food safety incident occur, impacts and actions are clear. Swift action may aid in preventing cross-contamination and the spread of foodborne illness.
2. **Food Fraud:** Increased accountability is accomplished by sharing security data among fresh food supply chain actors. These actors are less likely to commit food fraud due to the real-time traceability.
3. **Food Freshness:** The determination of the freshness of food results from knowledge of its location, shipping conditions, and current state. Fresh food supply chain actors equipped with this knowledge may better determine shelf life and make other proactive decisions.
4. **Food Sustainability:** Sustainability may be realized across the fresh food supply chain when shelf life and recall response are optimized, reducing food waste. Actors may also share audits, certificates, and other records that support their ethical and sustainable activities.

10.10.2 IBM FOOD TRUST OPERATION

To participate in IBM Food Trust online, fresh food supply chain actors select from the offered plans of the IBM Food Trust and upload their data, creating standardized, shareable records (Collart and Canales, 2022).

1. **Data Entry and Access:** The IBM Trust Connector API (application programming interface) enables the automated integration of legacy system data with network data. Existing databases containing records pertaining to inventory lists, order records, or vendor information may be imported automatically using solution software adapters. Four key elements may be uploaded or programmatically sent: supply chain events, transactions, master data, and certificate data (Raja and Muthuswamy, 2022).
2. **Trace and Recall:** After data relevant to fresh food and supply chain actors has been uploaded to the network, a trace and recall module is used, enabling user search for information about fresh food products, such as location and status. The information may vary from being general, such as region and time of production, to more specific, such as GTIN, batch, or lot number. Consequently, food safety and freshness may be immediately determined. The trace module can also reduce waste and increase supply chain efficiency (Raja and Muthuswamy, 2022).
3. **Certificates:** The certificate module may be used to verify relevant certifications or to access them as part of a safety inquiry. If a discrepancy or outdated certificate is located, both suppliers and buyers may be notified (Raja and Muthuswamy, 2022).

10.10.3 IBM MANGO CHAIN

Walmart identified a need for a blockchain-based food traceability system when it was found that tracing mangoes back to the farm from a local store took about seven days of calling and emailing distributors and suppliers. The distribution of mangoes is supported by global logistics, as these fruits are susceptible to *Listeria* and *Salmonella* contamination (Demestichas et al., 2020). Consequently, demonstrating transferability and accountability across borders would enhance public trust, which may be achieved across the supply chain by using blockchain and IoT technologies (Chang et al., 2019).

Implementing an effective traceability system based on blockchain and IoT technologies has reduced Walmart's farm tracking time to 2.2 seconds. Walmart can obtain information from the receipt of an affected customer about suppliers, how and where the mango was grown, and who undertook inspection from pallet to individual package (Kamath, 2018). This type of transparency improves customer loyalty whilst reducing risks and recall costs (Trollman et al., 2022).

Blockchain enables the storage and tracking of various data across the supply chain. In the production phase, blockchain together with IoT may monitor and capture data on fruit decay, surface defects, internal breakdown symptoms, chilling and heat injury, disorders during ripening, and other issues that mangoes are subject to (Kamath, 2018). In the logistics phase, perishable mangoes may be affected by temperature and moisture variations, influencing their freshness. In the distribution and aggregation phase, the shipment record, certificates, cargo and temperature deviations, and internal and external quality may be checked by importers (Kamath, 2018). Walmart decided to record supply chain data using IoT technology starting with mangoes on the tree, at harvest, at the packing shed, at wholesale markets, and finally at the retail outlet to identify their quality and marketability at each stage. For further accountability, actors collect and store data which may be accompanied by signatures and logs that are available with the status updates at each stage, reducing potential losses.

10.10.4 IBM COFFEE CHAIN

Conscientious consumers are demanding information about the coffee they consume, including place of origin and prices paid to farmers (Trollman et al., 2022). This is due to greater awareness that farmers frequently receive unfair compensation and delayed payments. Such consumers are willing to pay more to ensure coffee safety, quality, and fair and ethical sourcing (Trollman et al., 2022). It is estimated that 70%-80% of global coffee production comes from the 25 million smallholder farmers in developing countries (Bacon, 2005). Demand for coffee continues to grow, but despite being one of the world's top traded commodities, the complex coffee supply chain remains outdated and opaque. Consequently, the coffee industry, worth about $225.2 billion in 2015, is ready for a robust system of traceability and transparency to tackle the challenges of wholesale markets and regional distributors (Hellyer, 2020).

The world's first blockchain-traceable coffee originated in 2017 with Best360, a company that develops technologies in emerging economies by streamlining critical supply chains. Best360 partnered with Coda Coffee to trace coffee from Uganda to Denver, Colorado, using the bextmachine. The bextmachine was physically located in Kampala, Uganda, at the site of Great Lakes Coffee, a green coffee milling and export company. The bextmachine analyzes raw coffee beans deposited by smallholder farmers using optical recognition devices and sensors. Then, the platform's appraisal software receives live streams of data on the weight, size, and ripeness, as well as color and brightness, of the raw coffee beans to conduct a defect analysis. Coffee is scored according to these traits against industry standards, with a score of over 80 points being considered Specialty Grade (Kshetri, 2019).

Full transparency from the point of origin in Uganda to Coda Coffee in Denver, Colorado, is achieved by creating a text file based on individual farmers' coffee beans as processed by the bextmachine. Each step in the processing, including pulping, washing, fermenting, drying, milling, and shipping, is then recorded in the text file, which is hashed in the cloud layer to become an irreversible blockchain record. The machine produces a receipt for the farmer that may be taken to the Great Lakes Coffee company for immediate payment. This payment depends on the quality of the raw coffee beans, such that larger and riper ones are compensated more. The bextmachine links to special crypto tokens to record every step in the manufacturing process on the blockchain, providing complete visibility to end consumers. End consumers may scan a unique QR code printed on the package to access information from farm to washing and drying, milling, export, roasting, and retail (Kshetri, 2019).

10.11 ROADBLOCKS IN IOT-ENABLED BLOCKCHAIN IMPLEMENTATION IN THE FRESH PRODUCE SUPPLY CHAIN

In general, the primary obstacles to the broad adoption of blockchain and IoT are harmonized standards and interoperability, knowledge barriers, regulatory uncertainty, cost, technological impediments, and the issue of privacy.

Instead of a single blockchain-based system, the food supply chain comprises multiple private blockchains. This bolsters the need for standards and mutual agreements, especially with regards to the interoperability of blockchains (Berdik et al., 2021). A company's ability to successfully deploy blockchain and IoT could be hampered by the absence of standardized tools, methodologies, and indicators. For example, companies in a food supply chain may not regularly record and store the lot numbers of arriving items or cases. It may result in new lot numbers for items that do not match the arriving lot number for products which undergo processing at a facility. Different data capture, recording, storage, and sharing standards are therefore likely to result in miscommunication in the supply chain. In addition, the absence of standards for IoT technologies such as bar codes, RFID tags, and sensors might cause interoperability issues across supply chain actors. This might therefore reduce the effectiveness of supply chain information exchanges. The diversity in features of various supply chain actors is an additional factor contributing to the potential difficulty of standardizing. Therefore, the food supply chain faces the problem of enhancing standards and interoperability.

Despite the numerous potential advantages of implementing blockchain and IoT technologies, as evidenced by the plethora of research papers published on the subject, their use in the food supply chain remains in the nascent stages of development. It appears that familiarity with IoT is still mostly confined to academics and professionals. As a result, many enterprises and practitioners have yet to gain a comprehensive understanding of the potential business benefits that could be reaped from the integration of IoT and blockchain into their operations, which has emerged as a significant challenge. Consequently, there is a lack of uniform willingness among food supply chain partners to participate in the implementation of IoT and blockchain, particularly in developing countries. For instance, the failure of the Taiwan Agriculture and Food Traceability program, launched by the Taiwanese government in 2004, was primarily attributed to the lack of farmers' awareness of the traceability program (Liao et al., 2011). Thus, a lack of awareness may lead to organizations being resistant to change and hinder the adoption of IoT and blockchain technologies. Moreover, incorporating these technologies into the food supply chain necessitates the expertise to create and maintain the required applications, which is another barrier to adoption due to the limited technical expertise available (Kouhizadeh et al., 2021).

10.11.1 LEGISLATIVE AND REGULATORY OBSTACLES

The novelty of blockchain technology means that there is a lack of comprehensive policies at both the governmental and industry levels to provide guidance and support. Governments worldwide have yet to establish specific laws and regulations to facilitate the use of blockchain technology. Additionally, due to the global nature of the food supply chain, which involves various parties across borders, a consistent and unified regulatory framework is necessary to address disputes and resolve any uncertainties. In the absence of such regulations, issues such as ownership, data protection, and security can pose obstacles to the adoption of blockchain technology. Furthermore, some governments have released unfavorable policies regarding Bitcoin, which may have resulted in negative perceptions of blockchain and could impede its broader use in the food supply chain (Choi et al., 2020). Additionally, traceability legislation and quality management systems do not currently encompass the entire food supply chain, and different stages of the supply chain may have varying food safety standards. Consequently, one of the primary challenges to implementing blockchain and IoT to achieve traceability, transparency, and authenticity is developing comprehensive and equitable food safety standards (Trollman et al., 2022).

10.11.2 ECONOMIC BARRIERS

The implementation and development of IoT and blockchain in the food supply chain incur two types of costs: CAPEX and OPEX. This requires organizations to invest in expensive new hardware, software, data collection, sharing, and maintenance (Choi et al., 2020). The cost also varies depending on the type of ledger used, with a more secure ledger resulting in higher costs. Achieving traceability and transparency in the food supply chain requires the participation of all stakeholders. However, as most companies in the food supply chain are small and medium-sized enterprises, cost-effectiveness becomes a significant concern (Ali et al., 2021). For these organizations, the adoption of these technologies may not be economically viable. For example, some farmers in the upstream part of the supply chain may be unwilling to contribute to the costs of the system, and even wealthy farmers may prefer to invest in conventional aspects such as production and processing technology rather than in a management system of this kind (Weatherell et al., 2003). Additionally, the use of blockchain and IoT technologies requires a high level of computerization. Some developing and underdeveloped countries are not yet prepared to adopt IoT and blockchain due to economic constraints. Therefore, it is challenging to achieve complete traceability and transparency without the participation of all supply chain partners (Kshetri, 2019).

The blockchain system still lacks the maturity to handle scalability and a large volume of transactions (Xie et al., 2019). As the supply chain network requires increasingly more data, including information on processes and practices, scalability becomes a significant bottleneck. Managing immutable information is another challenge in the blockchain system. While the immutability of data enhances security, it can also result in erroneous records. Because of the trust mechanism, the data can be accepted without question, even if it is incorrect, and cannot be changed or deleted without agreement. Even if key owners can update the data with additional information, the mark of the erroneous record will always be present in the system. In this regard, blockchain can only ensure the authenticity of the information but not its accuracy (Fortuna and Risso, 2019). Additionally, the use of IoT technology brings about another concern because RFID and QR codes on product packaging do not always guarantee that the product corresponds to the label information. Although every participant is given the opportunity to verify transactions, collusion is still possible, making it difficult for participants to reach a consensus.

10.11.3 PRIVATE BARRIERS

Sharing information is a significant challenge in achieving transparency in the supply chain, as stakeholders are reluctant to share data with other participants and regulators (Nurgazina et al., 2021). In the traditional supply chain, it is difficult to achieve complete traceability, as proprietary tracking systems only provide traceability for a single step and rarely allow product life cycle traceability. However, with the implementation of blockchain and IoT technologies, it is possible to achieve complete transparency from the farm to the end consumer. Nevertheless, some organizations in the supply chain may not be willing to share certain information, such as contractors' identities, commercial data, price, and contract details, as they consider it a competitive advantage (Handfield and Bechtel, 2002). Thus, this may lead to reluctance from some participants to join the system.

10.12 CONCLUSION

Food traceability plays an important role in the food supply chain with regards to the safety of the food product. We presented various definitions of food traceability, its characteristics, and benefits. The one thing that was clear is that conventional paper-based traceability systems are inefficient and suffer from latency. With the advent of Industry 4.0 technologies, IoT-enabled blockchain technology can address the current issues faced by the food supply chain. IoT-enabled blockchain ensures real-time traceability, trackability, and authenticity. The case studies included in this chapter are examples of various food organizations that are involved in IoT-enabled blockchain food traceability initiatives. This work shows how all the stakeholders are interested in food traceability from farm to fork to improve food safety issues plaguing the supply chain. Although we discussed a limited number of barriers for implementing the IoT-enabled blockchain technology, such as harmonized standards and interoperability, knowledge barrier, regulatory uncertainty, cost, technological impediments, and the issue of privacy, there are other barriers as well. However, the ones discussed here are significant ones.

KEYWORDS

- **blockchain technology**
- **food safety**
- **food traceability**
- **industry 4.0**
- **internet of things**
- **supply chain transparency**

REFERENCES

Aamer, A. M., Al-Awlaqi, M. A., Affia, I., Arumsari, S., & Mandahawi, N. (2021). The internet of things in the food supply chain: Adoption challenges. *Benchmarking: An International Journal, 28*(8), 2521–2541. https://doi.org/10.1108/BIJ-07-2020-0371 (accessed on 9th July 2025).

Ali, M. H., Chung, L., Kumar, A., Zailani, S., & Tan, K. H. (2021). A sustainable Blockchain framework for the halal food supply chain: Lessons from Malaysia. *Technological Forecasting and Social Change, 170*, 120870. https://doi.org/10.1016/j.techfore.2021.120870 (accessed on 9th July 2025).

Al-Jaroodi, J., & Mohamed, N. (2012). Service-oriented middleware: A survey. *Journal of Network and Computer Applications, 35*(1), 211–220. https://doi.org/10.1016/j.jnca.2011.07.013 (accessed on 9th July 2025).

Atlam, H. F., & Wills, G. B. (2019). Intersections between IoT and distributed ledger (pp. 73–113). https://doi.org/10.1016/bs.adcom.2018.12.001 (accessed on 9th July 2025).

Aung, M. M., & Chang, Y. S. (2014). Traceability in a food supply chain: Safety and quality perspectives. *Food Control, 39*, 172–184. https://doi.org/10.1016/j.foodcont.2013.11.007 (accessed on 9th July 2025).

Babich, V., & Hilary, G. (2019). Blockchain and other distributed ledger technologies in operations. *Foundations and Trends® in Technology, Information and Operations Management, 12*(2–3), 152–172. https://doi.org/10.1561/0200000084 (accessed on 9th July 2025).

Bacon, C. (2005). Confronting the coffee crisis: Can fair trade, organic, and specialty coffees reduce small-scale farmer vulnerability in Northern Nicaragua? *World Development, 33*(3), 497–511. https://doi.org/10.1016/j.worlddev.2004.10.002 (accessed on 9th July 2025).

Benarous, L., Kadri, B., Bouridane, A., & Benkhelifa, E. (2022). Blockchain-based forgery resilient vehicle registration system. *Transactions on Emerging Telecommunications Technologies, 33*(10). https://doi.org/10.1002/ett.4237 (accessed on 9th July 2025).

Ben-Daya, M., Hassini, E., & Bahroun, Z. (2019). Internet of things and supply chain management: A literature review. *International Journal of Production Research, 57*(15–16), 4719–4742. https://doi.org/10.1080/00207543.2017.1402140 (accessed on 9th July 2025).

Berdik, D., Otoum, S., Schmidt, N., Porter, D., & Jararweh, Y. (2021). A survey on Blockchain for information systems management and security. *Information Processing & Management, 58*(1), 102397. https://doi.org/10.1016/j.ipm.2020.102397 (accessed on 9th July 2025).

Bhat, S. A., Huang, N. F., Sofi, I. B., & Sultan, M. (2021). Agriculture-food supply chain management based on Blockchain and IoT: A narrative on enterprise Blockchain interoperability. *Agriculture, 12*(1), 40. https://doi.org/10.3390/agriculture12010040 (accessed on 9th July 2025).

Chang, S. E., Chen, Y. C., & Lu, M. F. (2019). Supply chain re-engineering using blockchain technology: A case of smart contract-based tracking process. *Technological Forecasting and Social Change, 144*, 1–11. https://doi.org/10.1016/j.techfore.2019.03.015 (accessed on 9th July 2025).

Choi, D., Chung, C. Y., Seyha, T., & Young, J. (2020). Factors affecting organizations' resistance to the adoption of blockchain technology in supply networks. *Sustainability, 12*(21), 8882. https://doi.org/10.3390/su12218882 (accessed on 9th July 2025).

Collart, A. J., & Canales, E. (2022). How might broad adoption of blockchain-based traceability impact the U.S. fresh produce supply chain? *Applied Economic Perspectives and Policy, 44*(1), 219–236. https://doi.org/10.1002/aepp.13134 (accessed on 9th July 2025).

Demestichas, K., Peppes, N., Alexakis, T., & Adamopoulou, E. (2020). Blockchain in agriculture traceability systems: A review. *Applied Sciences, 10*(12), 4113. https://doi.org/10.3390/app10124113 (accessed on 9th July 2025).

Echegaray, N., Hassoun, A., Jagtap, S., Tetteh-Caesar, M., Kumar, M., Tomasevic, I., Goksen, G., & Lorenzo, J. M. (2022). Meat 4.0: Principles and applications of Industry 4.0 technologies in the meat industry. *Applied Sciences, 12*(14), 6986. https://doi.org/10.3390/app12146986 (accessed on 9th July 2025).

Fortuna, F., & Risso, M. (2019). Blockchain technology in the food industry. *Symphonya. Emerging Issues in Management, 2*, 151. https://doi.org/10.4468/2019.2.13fortuna.risso (accessed on 9th July 2025).

Gourama, H. (2020). *Foodborne Pathogens* (pp. 25–49). https://doi.org/10.1007/978-3-030-42660-6_2 (accessed on 9th July 2025).

Handfield, R. B., & Bechtel, C. (2002). The role of trust and relationship structure in improving supply chain responsiveness. *Industrial Marketing Management, 31*(4), 367–382. https://doi.org/10.1016/S0019-8501(01)00169-9 (accessed on 9th July 2025).

Hassoun, A., Jagtap, S., Garcia-Garcia, G., Trollman, H., Pateiro, M., Lorenzo, J. M., Trif, M., Rusu, A. V., Aadil, R. M., Šimat, V., Cropotova, J., & Câmara, J. S. (2023). Food quality 4.0: From traditional approaches to digitalized automated analysis. *Journal of Food Engineering, 337*, 111216. https://doi.org/10.1016/j.jfoodeng.2022.111216 (accessed on 9th July 2025).

Hassoun, A., Jagtap, S., Trollman, H., Garcia-Garcia, G., Abdullah, N. A., Goksen, G., Bader, F., Ozogul, F., Barba, F. J., Cropotova, J., Munekata, P. E. S., & Lorenzo, J. M. (2023). Food processing 4.0: Current and future developments spurred by the fourth industrial revolution. *Food Control, 145*, 109507. https://doi.org/10.1016/j.foodcont.2022.109507 (accessed on 9th July 2025).

Hassoun, A., Kamiloglu, S., Garcia-Garcia, G., Parra-López, C., Trollman, H., Jagtap, S., Aadil, R. M., & Esatbeyoglu, T. (2023). Implementation of relevant fourth industrial revolution innovations across the supply chain of fruits and vegetables: A short update on Traceability 4.0. *Food Chemistry, 409*, 135303. https://doi.org/10.1016/j.foodchem.2022.135303 (accessed on 9th July 2025).

Havinga, T., Casey, D., & van Waarden, F. (n.d.). Changing regulatory arrangements in food governance. In *The Changing Landscape of Food Governance* (pp. 3–18). Edward Elgar Publishing. https://doi.org/10.4337/9781784715410.00009 (accessed on 9th July 2025).

Hellyer, P. (2020). Time for a coffee break! *British Dental Journal, 228*(7), 519–519. https://doi.org/10.1038/s41415-020-1507-9 (accessed on 9th July 2025).

Hollands, T., Martindale, W., & Swainson, M. (2018). Blockchain or bust for the food industry? *Food Science and Technology, 32*(4), 40–45. https://doi.org/10.1002/fsat.3204_12.x (accessed on 9th July 2025).

Hu, J., Zhang, X., Moga, L. M., & Neculita, M. (2013). Modeling and implementation of the vegetable supply chain traceability system. *Food Control, 30*(1), 341–353. https://doi.org/10.1016/j.foodcont.2012.06.037 (accessed on 9th July 2025).

Jagtap, S. (2021). Utilizing the internet of things concepts to improve the resource efficiency of food manufacturing. https://doi.org/10.26174/thesis.lboro.11180456.v1 (accessed on 9th July 2025).

Jagtap, S., & Rahimifard, S. (2019a). Unlocking the potential of the Internet of Things to improve resource efficiency in food supply chains (pp. 287–301). https://doi.org/10.1007/978-3-030-02312-6_17 (accessed on 9th July 2025).

Jagtap, S., & Rahimifard, S. (2019b). The digitization of food manufacturing to reduce waste–Case study of a ready meal factory. *Waste Management, 87*, 387–397. https://doi.org/10.1016/j.wasman.2019.02.017 (accessed on 9th July 2025).

Jagtap, S., Bader, F., Garcia-Garcia, G., Trollman, H., Fadiji, T., & Salonitis, K. (2020). Food Logistics 4.0: Opportunities and challenges. *Logistics, 5*(1), 2. https://doi.org/10.3390/logistics5010002 (accessed on 9th July 2025).

Jagtap, S., Duong, L., Trollman, H., Bader, F., Garcia-Garcia, G., Skouteris, G., Li, J., Pathare, P., Martindale, W., Swainson, M., & Rahimifard, S. (2021). IoT technologies in the food supply chain. In *Food Technology Disruptions* (pp. 175–211). Elsevier. https://doi.org/10.1016/B978-0-12-821470-1.00009-4 (accessed on 9th July 2025).

Jagtap, S., Trollman, H., Trollman, F., Garcia-Garcia, G., & Martindale, W. (2024). Surviving the storm: Navigating the quadruple whammy impact on Europe's food supply chain. *International Journal of Food Science & Technology, 59*(6), 3652–3666. https://doi.org/10.1111/ijfs.17106 (accessed on 9th July 2025).

Jagtap, S., Trollman, H., Trollman, F., Garcia-Garcia, G., Parra-López, C., Duong, L., Martindale, W., Munekata, P. E. S., Lorenzo, J. M., Hdaifeh, A., Hassoun, A., Salonitis, K., & Afy-Shararah, M. (2022). The Russia-Ukraine conflict: Its implications for the global food supply chains. *Foods, 11*(14), 2098. https://doi.org/10.3390/foods11142098 (accessed on 9th July 2025).

Jakkhupan, W., Arch-int, S., & Li, Y. (2015). An RFID-based traceability system. *Telecommunication Systems, 58*(3), 243–258. https://doi.org/10.1007/s11235-014-9866-7 (accessed on 9th July 2025).

Jones, P., Clarke-Hill, C., Shears, P., Comfort, D., & Hillier, D. (2004). Radio frequency identification in the UK: Opportunities and challenges. *International Journal of Retail & Distribution Management, 32*(3), 164–171. https://doi.org/10.1108/09590550410524957 (accessed on 9th July 2025).

Kamath, R. (2018). Food traceability on blockchain: Walmart's pork and mango pilots with IBM. *The Journal of the British Blockchain Association, 1*(1), 1–12. https://doi.org/10.31585/jbba-1-1-(10)2018 (accessed on 9th July 2025).

Köhler, S., & Pizzol, M. (2020). Technology assessment of blockchain-based technologies in the food supply chain. *Journal of Cleaner Production, 269*, 122193. https://doi.org/10.1016/j.jclepro.2020.122193 (accessed on 9th July 2025).

Kouhizadeh, M., Saberi, S., & Sarkis, J. (2021). Blockchain technology and the sustainable supply chain: Theoretically exploring adoption barriers. *International Journal of Production Economics, 231*, 107831. https://doi.org/10.1016/j.ijpe.2020.107831 (accessed on 9th July 2025).

Kshetri, N. (2019). Blockchain and the economics of customer satisfaction. *IT Professional, 21*(1), 93–97. https://doi.org/10.1109/MITP.2018.2881299 (accessed on 9th July 2025).

Liao, P. A., Chang, H. H., & Chang, C. Y. (2011). Why is the food traceability system unsuccessful in Taiwan? Empirical evidence from a national survey of fruit and vegetable farmers. *Food Policy, 36*(5), 686–693. https://doi.org/10.1016/j.foodpol.2011.06.010 (accessed on 9th July 2025).

Martindale, W., Duong, L., & Jagtap, S. (2022). *Food Industry 4.0*. CABI. https://doi.org/10.1079/9781789248593.0000 (accessed on 9th July 2025).

Nicoletti, B. (2018). The future: Procurement 4.0. In *Agile Procurement* (pp. 189–230). Springer International Publishing. https://doi.org/10.1007/978-3-319-61085-6_8 (accessed on 9th July 2025).

Nurgazina, J., Pakdeetrakulwong, U., Moser, T., & Reiner, G. (2021). Distributed ledger technology applications in food supply chains: A review of challenges and future research directions. *Sustainability, 13*(8), 4206. https://doi.org/10.3390/su13084206 (accessed on 9th July 2025).

Olsen, P., & Borit, M. (2018). The components of a food traceability system. *Trends in Food Science & Technology, 77*, 143–149. https://doi.org/10.1016/j.tifs.2018.05.004 (accessed on 9th July 2025).

Padel, S., & Foster, C. (2005). Exploring the gap between attitudes and behavior. *British Food Journal, 107*(8), 606–625. https://doi.org/10.1108/00070700510611002 (accessed on 9th July 2025).

Pavlić Skender, H., & Zaninović, P. A. (2020). Perspectives of blockchain technology for sustainable supply chains (pp. 77–92). https://doi.org/10.1007/978-3-030-24355-5_5 (accessed on 9th July 2025).

Poongodi, T., Rathee, A., Indrakumari, R., & Suresh, P. (2020). IoT sensing capabilities: Sensor deployment and node discovery, wearable sensors, wireless body area network (WBAN), data acquisition (pp. 127–151). https://doi.org/10.1007/978-3-030-33596-0_5 (accessed on 9th July 2025).

Rahimifard, S., Brewer, S., Garcia-Garcia, G., & Jagtap, S. (2022). Digitalizing food manufacturing. *Food Science and Technology, 36*(3), 24–27. https://doi.org/10.1002/fsat.3603_5.x (accessed on 9th July 2025).

Raja Santhi, A., & Muthuswamy, P. (2022). Influence of blockchain technology in manufacturing supply chain and logistics. *Logistics, 6*(1), 15. https://doi.org/10.3390/logistics6010015 (accessed on 9th July 2025).

Sharma, N., Sawai, D., & Surve, G. (2017). Big data analytics: Impacting business in big way. *2017 International Conference on Data Management, Analytics and Innovation (ICDMAI)*, 111–116. https://doi.org/10.1109/ICDMAI.2017.8073494 (accessed on 9th July 2025).

Smith, G. C., Tatum, J. D., Belk, K. E., Scanga, J. A., Grandin, T., & Sofos, J. N. (2005). Traceability from a US perspective. *Meat Science, 71*(1), 174–193. https://doi.org/10.1016/j.meatsci.2005.04.002 (accessed on 9th July 2025).

Srivastav, R. K., Agrawal, D., & Shrivastava, A. (2020). A survey on vulnerabilities and performance evaluation criteria in blockchain technology. *ADCAIJ: Advances in Distributed Computing and Artificial Intelligence Journal, 9*(2), 91–105. https://doi.org/10.14201/ADCAIJ20209291105 (accessed on 9th July 2025).

Sterling, B., Gooch, M., Dent, B., Marenick, N., Miller, A., & Sylvia, G. (2015). Assessing the value and role of seafood traceability from an entire value-chain perspective. *Comprehensive Reviews in Food Science and Food Safety, 14*(3), 205–268. https://doi.org/10.1111/1541-4337.12130 (accessed on 9th July 2025).

Storøy, J., Thakur, M., & Olsen, P. (2013). The TraceFood Framework–Principles and guidelines for implementing traceability in food value chains. *Journal of Food Engineering, 115*(1), 41–48. https://doi.org/10.1016/j.jfoodeng.2012.09.018 (accessed on 9th July 2025).

Trollman, H., Garcia-Garcia, G., Jagtap, S., & Trollman, F. (2022). Blockchain for ecologically embedded coffee supply chains. *Logistics, 6*(3), 43. https://doi.org/10.3390/logistics6030043 (accessed on 9th July 2025).

Weatherell, C., Tregear, A., & Allinson, J. (2003). In search of the concerned consumer: UK public perceptions of food, farming and buying local. *Journal of Rural Studies, 19*(2), 233–244. https://doi.org/10.1016/S0743-0167(02)00083-9 (accessed on 9th July 2025).

Wiśniewska, M. (2023). Just culture and the reporting of food safety incidents. *British Food Journal, 125*(1), 302–317. https://doi.org/10.1108/BFJ-12-2021-1316 (accessed on 9th July 2025).

Xie, J., Yu, F. R., Huang, T., Xie, R., Liu, J., & Liu, Y. (2019). A survey on the scalability of blockchain systems. *IEEE Network, 33*(5), 166–173. https://doi.org/10.1109/MNET.001.1800290 (accessed on 9th July 2025).

Yacoub, G., & Castillo, M. (2022). Blockchain in your grocery basket: Trust and traceability as a strategy. *Journal of Business Strategy, 43*(4), 247–256. https://doi.org/10.1108/JBS-02-2021-0032 (accessed on 9th July 2025).

Yiannas, F. (2018). A new era of food transparency powered by blockchain. *Innovations: Technology, Governance, Globalization, 12*(1–2), 46–56. https://doi.org/10.1162/inov_a_00266 (accessed on 9th July 2025).

CHAPTER 11

Electronic Nose: Principles and Quality Indications of Agricultural and Food Products

MAHA AL KHALILI* and NASSER AL HABSI

Department of Food Science and Nutrition, College of Agricultural and Marine Sciences, Sultan Qaboos University, Al-Khod, Muscat, Oman

*Corresponding author

ABSTRACT

An electronic nose basically refers to a system operated by volatile compound sensors, signal dispensation, and a machine set of data (algorithms) for artificial olfaction recognition. This technique plays a key role in different applications. Sample preparation and the E-nose mechanism of use were discussed. In addition, several promising research directions were presented, such as ripening, decay detection, disease identification, grading, authenticity, and processing assessment. Despite decades of advances in this artificial intelligence technology, the stability and reliability of E-nose systems are still challenging. This is one of the major worries that prevents E-noses from large-scale deployment. However, increasing the number of sensors in the E-noses and using them in combination with other artificial sensory systems could potentially develop a better recognition of the food volatiles compounds in agricultural and food products.

Sustainable Approaches in Postharvest Handling and Management: Pankaj B. Pathare (Ed.)

DOI: 10.1201/9781779641076-11

11.1 INTRODUCTION

A growing demand for accurate and rapid quality inspection of agricultural and food products has been progressively witnessed due to hygiene and safety considerations and food adulteration concerns in the food processing and supply chains. However, the quality assessment of these products is still determined based on consumer routine visual preference inspection via subjective satisfaction level (Ali et al., 2020). The personal preference of consumers is usually dependent on the palatability and the food choice with regards to attributes like aroma, flavor, and taste. Each agricultural product is unique due to its different aromas and volatile organic compounds. McCrickerd and Forde (2016) indicated that food odor is a crucial sensory quality that can influence the integral entity of human flavor perception, which shapes the experience of taste and texture. In fact, many food manufacturers add tempting aromas to their products to satisfy consumers' preference (Ouyang et al., 2018). Therefore, the use of a smell indicator that can simulate the human nose would be a non-destructive sensing tool to better replace the conventional approaches.

Since the early eighties of the last century, the introduction of electronic nose technology experienced vast expansion, starting from technical to marketable aspects. The emergence of the electronic nose has made a distinct qualitative hurdle in evaluating the quality of agricultural and food products in a non-destructive manner, in addition to the prominent pros, which comprise ease of handling and cost-effectiveness. The capabilities of this tool provide a rapid assessment and analyses compared to the known traditional tools that require many stages and a longer duration of laboratory analyses (Jo et al., 2016). E-noses could be so sensitive and selective that they could evaluate the compositions of gases that are related to the physicochemical properties of the product while discriminating the gas mixtures as a whole chemical compound (Priyanka and Bhupinder, 2016). It could distinguish the organic sources, whether they were natural or synthetic, that releases volatile organic compounds in the form of gas from the surroundings (Ali et al., 2020).

Due to its comprehensive design with an array of sensors, the electronic nose technology is able to identify complex odors. It has been widely implemented in different domains such as the food industry

(Huang and Gu, 2022; Lee-Rangel et al., 2022; Lu et al., 2022; Yu et al., 2022), pharmaceuticals (Zorpeykar et al., 2022), and early health noninvasive inspection (Avian et al., 2022). The wide-ranging disciplines applying this technology indicate that the E-nose is a promising sensory device that is compatible with the traditional method of the human olfactory system.

Although the latest research validated the use and applications of electronic noses that mimic biological senses, it was elucidated along with other artificial sensory techniques. In addition, these studies tackle mostly a single type of food product (Calvini and Pigani, 2022; Kaushal et al., 2022; Munekata et al., 2023; Shi et al., 2021; Zaukuu et al., 2020). Thus, the objective of this review is to elucidate the basic definition and purpose of use, along with an assessment concept of operating the E-nose, and to classify the recent applications of E-nose under different qualities of detection.

11.2 THE ELECTRONIC NOSE

11.2.1 DEFINITION

The first accepted definition of an E-nose was presented by Gardner in 1994 as "an instrument which comprises an array of electronic chemical sensors with partial specificity and an appropriate pattern recognition system, capable of recognizing simple or complex odors" (Santos et al., 2017).

This definition limited the phrase E-nose to the classical types of sensor array systems used specifically to inspect odorous molecules in a similar way to the biological nose. The design of an E-nose, though, is pretty similar to multi-sensor systems that are used in the detection and quantification of individual components in a mixture of simple gas or vapor. This means that an E-nose is a sensitive gas sensor array that provides a response (fingerprint) to particular volatiles, which is then correlated to pattern recognition algorithms that perform discrimination and classification (Tan and Xu, 2020). In this sense, it will be difficult to have the same pattern in two different samples (Pineda and Pérez, 2017). Figure 11.1 represents an example handheld device E-nose design that is most widely used (Cyranose® 320).

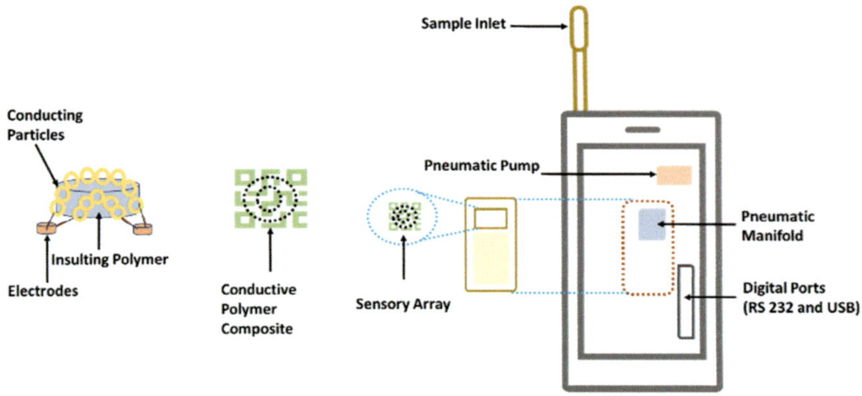

FIGURE 11.1 E-Nose product design (Cyranose), most widely used handheld device and has been for over 10 years in production.

The E-nose instruments were used for different purposes, such as in quality control laboratories, to ensure the conformity of raw materials, intermediate, and final products (Al-Dayyeni et al., 2021). Additionally, they were used to measure the consistency of batch to batch and for the recognition of contamination, spoilage, and adulteration (Peris and Escuder-Gilabert, 2016), as well as performing geographical origin or vendor selection (Al-Dayyeni et al., 2021) and monitoring food storage conditions (Chilo et al., 2016), and meat products quality (Wijaya et al., 2017).

11.2.2 SAMPLE PREPARATION AND MECHANISM

There are several considerations in the sample handling step (i.e., prior to E-nose device functioning). The volatile compounds will be generated in the headspace and then transformed to the E-nose sensors. Sample size, temperature, vial size, and the equilibrium time (i.e., when constant temperature and pressure are achieved between the sample and vapor phase) are the variables that need to be optimized. Figure 11.2 illustrates the basic principle of static headspace extraction. The sample is placed in a sealed vial that is temperature-controlled and thus creates an empty space on top of the sample. This empty space (i.e., headspace) is partly withdrawn after an equilibrium is achieved (Weggler et al., 2020). Different sampling methods were used for food and agricultural products. The most popular method is the static headspace method (SHS) due to its simplicity, where no special equipment is required and less time is needed for additional procedures (Burlachenko et al., 2016). Other methods include membrane introduction mass spectrometry (MIMS), purge and trap (P&T), inside-needle dynamic extraction (INDEX), solid-phase microextraction (SPME), and stir bar sorptive extraction (SBSE).

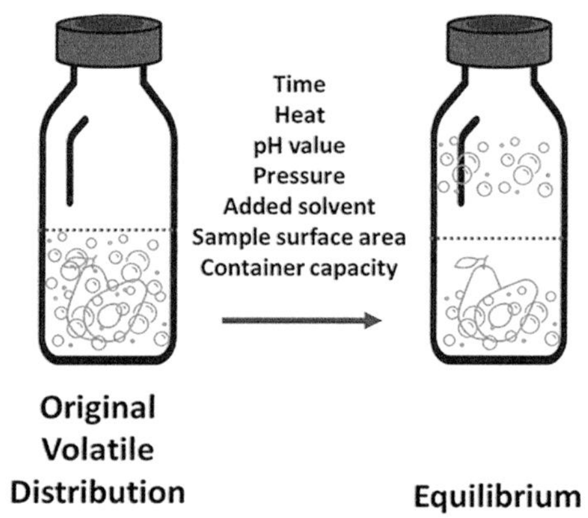

FIGURE 11.2 Static headspace (SHS) and factors affecting volatile formation.

However, SHS is relatively less sensitive due to the absence of a pre-concentration system to collect the volatile components. To enhance the achievement of equilibrium, sample preparation could be further developed. These techniques typically aim to increase free surface contact of the sample with the atmosphere (i.e., milling, homogenization for solid samples, and bubbling for liquids). The equilibrium could be achieved faster as well when procedures such as heating (due to a higher respiration rate) and lowering pressure are applied to promote transition of volatile substances to gaseous phase (Jalali et al., 2021).

The function of the electronic nose is based on imitating the structure and function of the human nose (Voss et al., 2020), both of which perform this function by going through the same stages of recognizing volatile odors (Figure 11.3). The principle of operating this device (i.e., like the human nose) is through interaction with volatile compounds, which are usually complex mixtures with appropriate receptors. These are the olfactory receptors in the biological nose and sensor arrays in the E-nose. Each receptor responds to many odors, which would cause an overlap recognition which affects their sensitivities, so that a single odor can be identified by several odor receptors. These signals are stored in the brain (in the case of the biological nose) or in the database of the pattern recognition (in the E-nose tool), which represents the learning phase that further identifies one of the smells being learned (the classification phase).

Rahman et al. (2018) indicated that using a higher number of replicates could remove the outliers from the data set before exploring the volatile features of a sample.

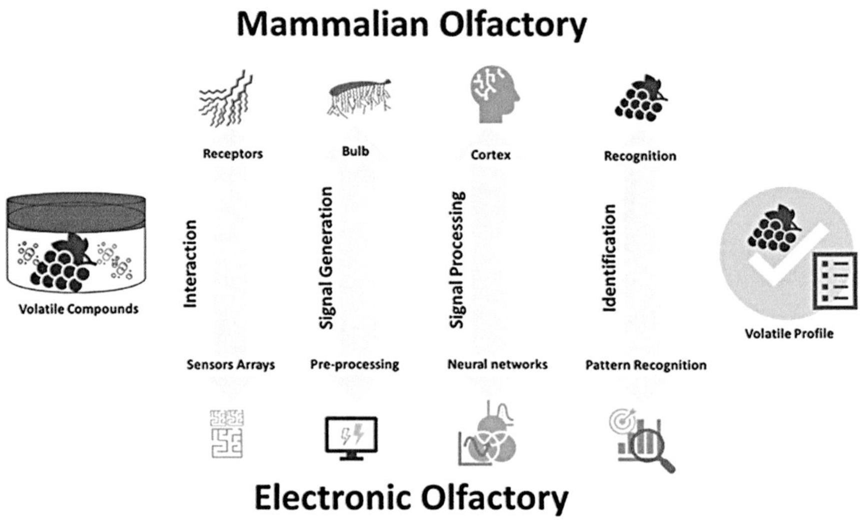

FIGURE 11.3 Structures of biological olfactory system in comparison to the E- nose.

11.2.3 ADVANTAGES AND LIMITATIONS OF E-NOSE

The impetus for developing this device lies in the fact that the human sense of smell as an odorant instrument has many limitations. This sense is highly subjective, which means that every person could identify the same product differently (bias). Additionally, it could get exhausted easily and is possibly difficult to interpret. Apart from that, the human nose cannot be relied on to detect poisonous gases (Tan and Xu, 2020). The human biological odor sense is very sensitive; however, E-noses have the pros of simple operation, relatively rapid and non-destructive measurement of headspace, and the possibility of real-time analysis. The required sample size of the E-nose is relatively small; however, the identification of individual compounds present in the food samples is challenging (Wei et al., 2023). Another key advantage of the E-nose, besides simple operating and construction, is the flexibility in the number of sensors used, durability, battery life, sensing technology, and tailoring sampling technique. Each version of the E-nose instrument could satisfy a specific purpose, which means that it could be manipulated (Esfahani et al., 2020). Moreover, the specs of biosensors could be developed by implementing the synthetic polypeptides for different food applications (Karakaya et al., 2020). The use of E-noses allows measuring the quality grading process of perishable food products in a shorter time, which reserves the quality of these products for a longer time before providing them to the market/consumers (Zou et al., 2022). It is worth mentioning that volatiles of wrapped and packed products such as fruit could still be measured by using the probes of E-nose systems inserted through the package, which means that the package will not be damaged due to the detection processes (Wei et al., 2018). However, the key drawback of this technique is that it only identifies volatile compounds under certain categories (not as a specific volatile compound). In addition, it could not assign quantitative data to trace differences or similarities in compounds among samples (Cellini et al., 2017). Another drawback of this technique is sensors' sensitivity to climate conditions, (mainly the humidity and temperature) (Liang et al., 2018; Liu et al., 2021).

11.3 QUALITY INDICATIONS OF THE E- NOSE

The aroma profile of fruit and vegetables varies with their life cycle, physiological changes (ripening), diseases, physical damages, and adulteration (Tyagi et al., 2023; Wilson, 2018). These factors may have many implications. In addition, food processing (cooking, canning) could change the odor characteristics of food products, which could indicate the quality and safety of manufacturing (Diez-Simon et al., 2019). Studies that implemented E-nose could be categorized under the following qualities: ripening, decay detection, disease detection, grading identification, authenticity, and processing assessment.

11.3.1 RIPENING

The quality inspection of maturation and growth of different crops is agriculture that predominates and depends on farmers' experience, thus susceptible to oversights (Chen et al., 2018). Aroma is a wide-ranging characteristic correlated to ripeness in fruits and vegetables. The aroma-related volatile substances from these crops change with the ripening time;

every variety in fruits and vegetables would have distinct aromas at the optimal ripe stage (Yahia and Carrillo-Lopez, 2018). In a study conducted by Wu and Li (2023), a portable E-nose was used to measure the accumulation headspace of bananas in simulated cold chain storage conditions. E-nose showed the capability to distinguish between yellow bananas with green necks and entirely yellow bananas while maintaining their biological activities. This could possibly detect the shelf life of bananas under these storage conditions. Similarly, the maturity of oranges, apples, grapes, bananas, and pomegranates was classified as unripe, ripe, and over-ripe with an average accuracy greater than 95% (Tyagi et al., 2023). A correlation analysis (based on the Pearson correlation coefficient, hierarchical clustering procedure) between an E-nose sensor and 57 volatile organic compounds distinguished the difference in ripeness level of strawberries (half-red and red), where the E-nose sensors generated distinctive signals to samples with different flavors (Palumbo et al., 2022). In the case of white and black berries, Aghilinategh et al. (2020) used E-nose to detect five ripeness grades with a precision range between 88.3 and 100%. In another instance, kiwifruits were incubated at the post-harvest stage at controlled natural conditions (i.e., 20°C, 70% relative humidity). They were stored for one week until they were fully ripe and edible. The response towards emitted volatiles from the kiwifruits within this week was detected by the E-nose as signals. Specific sensors were sensitive (increased) as the ripening days increased, which showed that E-nose signals showed potential correlations with the ripeness of kiwifruit. In a similar approach used by Macatangay et al. (2022), five specific sensors were used within 60 days for the unripe tomatoes to establish data acquisition. Three of which showed an increment at each ripeness stage. The overall accuracy of the attempt was 88%, which indicates that the method is reasonably accurate. This means that the E-nose device is used to predict the ripeness of kiwifruit (Du et al., 2019). In this sense, detecting ripeness attributes of the fruits and vegetables relaying on volatile compounds using E-nose techniques was investigated for different purposes like shelf-life evaluation, ripening stage classification, and ripping prediction.

11.3.2 DECAY DETECTION

Fruits and vegetables decay can be caused by exposure to non-ideal conditions in terms of humidity, air, temperature, light, and microbial growth (Leneveu-Jenvrin et al., 2020). Agricultural crops are vulnerable to decay naturally over time. However, identifying the development of crop spoilage at an early stage can avoid the occurrence of large losses of crop products and during the process of selling them. The potential of predicting the duration (days) before decay appeared in peach fruit was estimated using the electronic nose and the near-infrared spectroscopy (NIRS) (Huang et al., 2017). The best prediction (correct answer) of days before decay started in the fruit scored 82.3%. The combination of E-nose with the NIR spectroscopy showed higher accuracy compared by using them independently; thus, this model [is] considered promising to predict the days before the peach and other crops spoilage as well. E-nose was used to inspect 49 volatile compounds in different olives conditions (free of off-odors, off-flavors, without symptoms of ongoing alteration, abnormal fermentations) according to a previously developed protocol for the sensory classification. The detection (signals towards volatile compounds) showed higher values in the case of putrid defect and lowest towards butyric defect. These results reveal that E-nose could be used to differentiate olfactory sensors that agree with the tasting panel (Sánchez et al., 2021).

11.3.3 DISEASE DETECTION

The volatile profiles of the infected kiwifruits were studied to explore the presence of soft rot by using E-nose and headspace SPME coupled with gas chromatography–mass spectrometry (HS-SPME/GC–MS) Wang et al. (2023). The correlation was found significant ($p < 0.05$) between the physicochemical indices of the kiwifruits and their volatile profiles as obtained by the two methods. This means that the procedure could be used to detect the kiwifruits infected by soft rot. Similarly, Makarichian et al. (2022) examined the volatile profile of a fungal-infected garlic at early-stage storage conditions. They correlated the degradation rate of the garlic directly with the presence of infection. E-nose was used to detect a pathogen named Citrus Tristeza Virus in mandarin orange plants. The effective sensors (i.e., responding to the volatiles emitted by the virus infection) are thus identified and were considered as a base for custom developing a prototype with 95.30% precision. This implies that E-nose could differentiate between healthy and infected mandarin plants (Hazarika et al., 2020).

11.3.4 GRADING IDENTIFICATION

An optimized E-nose system was used to detect apple quality grading with a recognition accuracy (correct answer) of 96.5%. It showed higher efficiency in terms of training time and accuracy of classification compared to other traditional methods (Zou et al., 2022). However, as found by Tahri et al. (2017), E-nose was not sensitive enough to discriminate between the volatiles of different cumin cultivars picked from four different geographical regions (no distinct separation). This could be attributed to the similarity in cumin volatile compositions in different varieties.

11.3.5 AUTHENTICITY

The ripeness of apples was distinguished by the electronic nose technique, whether occurring naturally or artificially, with an accuracy that reached 98.3% (Qiao et al., 2022). The E-nose device was also used to detect the residues of diazinon (a toxic pesticide) used for sweet cherry in four ripeness grades. It was able to classify cherries as toxic and non-toxic with a precision of 100% (Nategh et al., 2021). Sanaeifar et al. (2021) combined an E-nose with confocal Raman microspectroscopy (CRM) to measure the pesticide (chlorpyrifos) residue in tea leaves. This setup, including both the spectral (i.e., molecular bond information) and an E-nose system (i.e., volatile information), was efficiently able to detect the pesticide residue at more than a 97% accuracy level. Likewise, Tatli et al. (2022) used E-nose as an inspection device to adjust the urea fertilizer application rates in cucumber in order to prevent nitrogen overfertilization. This was applied based on differences in signals in the sensor-array of the E-nose as a response to volatile emissions from the cucumber crop after different urea fertilizer treatments. Artificially colored safflower and artificially colored yellow styles of saffron were detected via electronic nose based on their aroma with an accuracy of 100%. Correlation coefficients of 0.95 and 0.97 were established between color and aroma (Kiani et al., 2017). A study aimed to detect the adulteration in cow ghee by using an E-nose system. The level of adulteration in the cow ghee with sunflower oil and cow body fat was between 10–50%. E-nose was able to detect the adulteration with an accuracy of 91.3% and 82.5% for sunflower oil and cow body fat, respectively (Ayari et al., 2018). Gan et al. (2016) measured the adulteration of honey syrup with corn syrup and rice syrup. The adulterant honey samples were in the concentration of 5–40% with pure honey. E-nose was used to measure volatile compounds, and it was combined with the e-tongue and Near Infrared spectrum. They were able to identify the pure honey from the adulterated honey with an accuracy above 96%. However, in another instance, Tahri et al. (2017) found E-nose inconclusive (unable to distinguish the pure and adulterated cumin). They proposed that the E-nose system could be more reliable as a routine methodology if it was supplemented with more sensors that could catch diversified signals.

11.3.6 PROCESSING ASSESSMENT

Gholami and Rabbani (2023) investigated the effect of storage conditions of mushrooms at two temperatures (4 and 25°C), two films (i.e., conventional polyethylene film and polyethylene film), and two injected gases (i.e., atmospheric gas and gas containing 5% oxygen and 5% carbon dioxide) by using the E-nose system. The E-nose was able to distinguish the volatile emissions in all samples, which were detectable by the E-nose. An electronic nose and computer vision were utilized to evaluate the cooking state of grilled chicken. The E-nose was able to distinguish the odor profile (volatile compounds) of the grilled chicken. The computer vision was used to detect the discoloration of the chicken. The odor profile, as indicated via the E-nose system, matches the detected water loss and sulfur-containing aromatic compounds during cooking. The approach was found comparable to the sensory evaluation that could better deconvolute the evaluation of food during cooking (Fedorov et al., 2021).

11.4 CHALLENGES AND CONCLUSION

Electronic nose technology has been applied recently in several detection methods in foods and agricultural products. These could include the detection of ripening, decay-freshness, and disease in these samples, or quality grading, processing assessment, and authenticity assurance. Hitherto, profiling odor types or quantifying aroma intensities under ambient conditions (i.e., nonlaboratory conditions) is still challenging. The reliability of this system could be improved by increasing the number of sensors (sensitivity and selectivity) that could distinguish volatile compounds more distinctively. Moreover, when comparing two or more similar food samples (e.g., cumin and coriander), volatile substance signals are likely to be obscured in the recognition phase, which requires a better understanding of the pattern recognition systems by developing statistical and intelligent pattern recognition methods. In addition, having a universal E-nose system for each of these food domain detections is not reasonable, which requires further development that is specially designed for each specific application. Combining E-nose with other artificial sensory systems like e-tongue and other spectrum techniques could develop a better understanding of food conditions with increased detection accuracy. Enhancing modeling, correlation between volatile compounds and sensor signals, along with advancements in algorithms of signal processing, could be validated for specific requirements.

KEYWORDS

- **artificial olfaction**
- **electronic nose**
- **food quality assessment**
- **pattern recognition algorithms**
- **postharvest monitoring**
- **volatile compounds detection**

REFERENCES

Aghilinategh, N., Dalvand, M. J., & Anvar, A. (2020). Detection of ripeness grades of berries using an electronic nose. *Food Science & Nutrition, 8*, 4919–4928.

Al-Dayyeni, W. S., Al-Yousif, S., Taher, M. M., Al-Faouri, A. W., Tahir, N. M., Jaber, M. M., Ghabban, F., Najm, I. A., Alfadli, I. M., & Ameerbakhsh, O. Z. (2021). A review on electronic nose: Coherent taxonomy, classification, motivations, challenges, recommendations and datasets. *IEEE Access, 9*, 88535–88551.

Ali, M. M., Hashim, N., Abd Aziz, S., & Lasekan, O. (2020). Principles and recent advances in electronic nose for quality inspection of agricultural and food products. *Trends in Food Science & Technology, 99*, 1–10.

Avian, C., Mahali, M. I., Putro, N. A. S., Prakosa, S. W., & Leu, J. S. (2022). Fx-Net and PureNet: Convolutional neural network architecture for discrimination of chronic obstructive pulmonary disease from smokers and healthy subjects through electronic nose signals. *Computers in Biology and Medicine, 148*, 105913.

Ayari, F., Mirzaee-Ghaleh, E., Rabbani, H., & Heidarbeigi, K. (2018). Detection of the adulteration in pure cow ghee by electronic nose method (Case study: Sunflower oil and cow body fat). *International Journal of Food Properties, 21*, 1670–1679.

Burlachenko, J., Kruglenko, I., Snopok, B., & Persaud, K. (2016). Sample handling for electronic nose technology: State of the art and future trends. *TrAC Trends in Analytical Chemistry, 82*, 222–236.

Calvini, R., & Pigani, L. (2022). Toward the development of combined artificial sensing systems for food quality evaluation: A review on the application of data fusion of electronic noses, electronic tongues and electronic eyes. *Sensors, 22*, 577.

Cellini, A., Blasioli, S., Biondi, E., Bertaccini, A., Braschi, I., & Spinelli, F. (2017). Potential applications and limitations of electronic nose devices for plant disease diagnosis. *Sensors (Basel), 17*.

Chen, L. Y., Wu, C. C., Chou, T. I., Chiu, S. W., & Tang, K. T. (2018). Development of a dual MOS electronic nose/camera system for improving fruit ripeness classification. *Sensors, 18*, 3256.

Chilo, J., Pelegri-Sebastia, J., Cupane, M., & Sogorb, T. (2016). E-nose application to food industry production. *IEEE Instrumentation & Measurement Magazine, 19*, 27–33.

Diez-Simon, C., Mumm, R., & Hall, R. D. (2019). Mass spectrometry-based metabolomics of volatiles as a new tool for understanding aroma and flavor chemistry in processed food products. *Metabolomics, 15*, 1–20.

Du, D., Wang, J., Wang, B., Zhu, L., & Hong, X. (2019). Ripeness prediction of postharvest kiwifruit using a MOS e-nose combined with chemometrics. *Sensors, 19*, 419.

Esfahani, S., Tiele, A., Agbroko, S. O., & Covington, J. A. (2020). Development of a tuneable NDIR optical electronic nose. *Sensors, 20*, 6875.

Fedorov, F. S., Yaqin, A., Krasnikov, D. V., Kondrashov, V. A., Ovchinnikov, G., Kostyukevich, Y., Osipenko, S., & Nasibulin, A. G. (2021). Detecting cooking state of grilled chicken by electronic nose and computer vision techniques. *Food Chemistry, 345*, 128747.

Gan, Z., Yang, Y., Li, J., Wen, X., Zhu, M., Jiang, Y., & Ni, Y. (2016). Using sensor and spectral analysis to classify botanical origin and determine adulteration of raw honey. *Journal of Food Engineering, 178*, 151–158.

Gholami, R., & Rabbani, H. (2023). Evaluation the effects of temperature and packaging conditions on the quality of button mushroom during storage using e-nose system. *Journal of Food Science and Technology*, 1–12.

Hazarika, S., Choudhury, R., Montazer, B., Medhi, S., Goswami, M. P., & Sarma, U. (2020). Detection of citrus tristeza virus in mandarin orange using a custom-developed electronic nose system. *IEEE Transactions on Instrumentation and Measurement, 69*, 9010–9018.

Huang, C., & Gu, Y. (2022). A machine learning method for the quantitative detection of adulterated meat using a MOS-based E-nose. *Foods, 11*, 602.

Huang, L., Meng, L., Zhu, N., & Wu, D. (2017). A primary study on forecasting the days before decay of peach fruit using near-infrared spectroscopy and electronic nose techniques. *Postharvest Biology and Technology, 133*, 104–112.

Jalali, A., Linke, M., Geyer, M., & Mahajan, P. (2021). Integrative programming for simulation of packaging headspace and shelf life of fresh produce. *MethodsX, 8*, 101514.

Jo, Y., Chung, N., Park, S. W., Noh, B. S., Jeong, Y. J., & Kwon, J. H. (2016). Application of E-tongue, E-nose, and MS-E-nose for discriminating aged vinegars based on taste and aroma profiles. *Food Science and Biotechnology, 25*, 1313–1318.

Karakaya, D., Ulucan, O., & Turkan, M. (2020). Electronic nose and its applications: A survey. *International Journal of Automation and Computing, 17*, 179–209.

Kaushal, S., Nayi, P., Rahadian, D., & Chen, H. H. (2022). Applications of electronic nose coupled with statistical and intelligent pattern recognition techniques for monitoring tea quality: A review. *Agriculture, 12*, 1359.

Kiani, S., Minaei, S., & Ghasemi-Varnamkhasti, M. (2017). Integration of computer vision and electronic nose as non-destructive systems for saffron adulteration detection. *Computers and Electronics in Agriculture, 141*, 46–53.

Lee-Rangel, H. A., Mendoza-Martinez, G. D., Díaz de León-Martínez, L., Relling, A. E., Vázquez-Valladolid, A., Palacios-Martínez, M., Hernández-García, P. A., Chay-Canul, A. J., Flores-Ramirez, R., & Roque-Jimenez, J. A. (2022). Application of an electronic nose and HS-SPME/GC-MS to determine volatile organic compounds in fresh Mexican cheese. *Foods, 11*, 1887.

Leneveu-Jenvrin, C., Charles, F., Barba, F. J., & Remize, F. (2020). Role of biological control agents and physical treatments in maintaining the quality of fresh and minimally-processed fruit and vegetables. *Critical Reviews in Food Science and Nutrition, 60*, 2837–2855.

Li, X., Yang, Y., Zhu, Y., Ben, A., & Qi, J. (2022). A novel strategy for discriminating different cultivation and screening odor and taste flavor compounds in Xinhui tangerine peel using E-nose, E-tongue, and chemometrics. *Food Chemistry, 384*, 132519.

Liang, Z., Tian, F., Yang, S. X., Zhang, C., Sun, H., & Liu, T. (2018). Study on interference suppression algorithms for electronic noses: A review. *Sensors, 18*, 1179.

Liu, H., Wu, R., Guo, Q., Hua, Z., & Wu, Y. (2021). Electronic nose based on temperature modulation of MOS sensors for recognition of excessive methanol in liquors. *ACS Omega, 6*, 30598–30606.

Lu, L., Hu, Z., Hu, X., Li, D., & Tian, S. (2022). Electronic tongue and electronic nose for food quality and safety. *Food Research International*, 112214.

Macatangay, E. C., Cruz, C. A. C. D., & Villaverde, J. F. (2022). Determination of tomato fruit stages using principal component analysis and fuzzy logic algorithm. *2022 IEEE International Conference on Artificial Intelligence in Engineering and Technology (IICAIET)*, 1–6. IEEE.

Makarichian, A., Chayjan, R. A., Ahmadi, E., & Zafari, D. (2022). Early detection and classification of fungal infection in *garlic (A. sativum)* using electronic nose. *Computers and Electronics in Agriculture, 192*, 106575.

McCrickerd, K., & Forde, C. (2016). Sensory influences on food intake control: Moving beyond palatability. *Obesity Reviews, 17*, 18–29.

Munekata, P. E., Finardi, S., de Souza, C. K., Meinert, C., Pateiro, M., Hoffmann, T. G., Domínguez, R., Bertoli, S. L., Kumar, M., & Lorenzo, J. M. (2023). Applications of electronic nose, electronic eye and electronic tongue in quality, safety and shelf life of meat and meat products: A review. *Sensors, 23*, 672.

Nategh, N. A., Dalvand, M. J., & Anvar, A. (2021). Detection of toxic and non-toxic sweet cherries at different degrees of maturity using an electronic nose. *Journal of Food Measurement and Characterization, 15*, 1213–1224.

Ouyang, Y., Behnke, C., Almanza, B., & Ghiselli, R. (2018). The influence of food aromas on restaurant consumer emotions, perceptions, and purchases. *Journal of Hospitality Marketing & Management, 27*, 405–423.

Palumbo, M., Cozzolino, R., Laurino, C., Malorni, L., Picariello, G., Siano, F., Stocchero, M., Cefola, M., Corvino, A., & Romaniello, R. (2022). Rapid and non-destructive techniques for the discrimination of ripening stages in Candonga strawberries. *Foods, 11*, 1534.

Peris, M., & Escuder-Gilabert, L. (2016). Electronic noses and tongues to assess food authenticity and adulteration. *Trends in Food Science & Technology, 58*, 40–54.

Pineda, D. M., & Perez, J. C. (2017). SENose: An under U $50 electronic nose for the monitoring of soil gas emissions. *Computers and Electronics in Agriculture, 133*, 15–21.

Priyanka, H., & Bhupinder, S. (2016). Electronic nose and their application in food industries. *Food Science Research Journal, 7*, 314–318.

Qiao, J., Su, G., Liu, C., Zou, Y., Chang, Z., Yu, H., Wang, L., & Guo, R. (2022). Study on the application of electronic nose technology in the detection for the artificial ripening of crab apples. *Horticultural, 8*, 386.

Rahman, M. S., Al-Farsi, K., Al-Maskari, S. S., & Al-Habsi, N. A. (2018). Stability of electronic nose (e-nose) as determined by considering date-pits heated at different temperatures. *International Journal of Food Properties, 21*, 850–857.

Sanaeifar, A., Li, X., He, Y., Huang, Z., & Zhan, Z. (2021). A data fusion approach on confocal Raman micro spectroscopy and electronic nose for quantitative evaluation of pesticide residue in tea. *Biosystems Engineering, 210*, 206–222.

Sánchez, R., Martín-Tornero, E., Lozano, J., Boselli, E., Arroyo, P., Melendez, F., & Martín-Vertedor, D. (2021). E-nose discrimination of abnormal fermentations in Spanish-style green olives. *Molecules, 26*, 5353.

Santos, J. P., Lozano, J., & Aleixandre, M. (2017). Electronic noses applications in beer technology. *Brewing Technology*, 177.

Shi, Y., Wang, X., Borhan, M. S., Young, J., Newman, D., Berg, E., & Sun, X. (2021). A review on meat quality evaluation methods based on non-destructive computer vision and artificial intelligence technologies. *Food Science of Animal Resources, 41*, 563.

Tahri, K., Tiebe, C., Bari, N. E., Hubert, T., & Bouchikhi, B. (2017). Geographical classification and adulteration detection of cumin by using electronic sensing coupled to multivariate analysis. *Procedia Technology, 27*, 240–241.

Tan, J., & Xu, J. (2020). Applications of electronic nose (e-nose) and electronic tongue (e-tongue) in food quality-related properties determination: A review. *Artificial Intelligence in Agriculture, 4*, 104–115.

Tatli, S., Mirzaee-Ghaleh, E., Rabbani, H., Karami, H., & Wilson, A. D. (2022). Rapid detection of urea fertilizer effects on VOC emissions from cucumber fruits using a MOS E-nose sensor array. *Agronomy, 12*, 35.

Tyagi, P., Semwal, R., Sharma, A., Tiwary, U. S., & Varadwaj, P. (2023). E-nose: A low-cost fruit ripeness monitoring system. *Journal of Agricultural Engineering.*

Va, B., Subramoniam, M., & Mathew, L. (2021). Noninvasive detection of COPD and lung cancer through breath analysis using MOS sensor array-based e-nose. *Expert Review of Molecular Diagnostics, 21*, 1223–1233.

Voss, H. G. J., Ayub, R. A., & Stevan, S. L. (2020). E-nose prototype to monitoring the growth and maturation of peaches in the orchard. *IEEE Sensors Journal, 20*, 11741–11750.

Wang, Y., Wang, D., Lv, Z., Zeng, Q., Fu, X., Chen, Q., Luo, Z., Luo, C., Wang, D., & Zhang, W. (2023). Analysis of the volatile profiles of kiwifruits experiencing soft rot using E-nose and HS-SPME/GC–MS. *LWT, 173*, 114405.

Weggler, B. A., Gruber, B., Teehan, P., Jaramillo, R., & Dorman, F. L. (2020). Chapter 5 – Inlets and sampling. In N. H. Snow (Ed.), *Separation Science and Technology* (pp. [insert page numbers if known]). Academic Press.

Wei, G., Dan, M., Zhao, G., & Wang, D. (2023). Recent advances in chromatography-mass spectrometry and electronic nose technology in food flavor analysis and detection. *Food Chemistry, 405*, 134814.

Wei, X., Zhang, Y., Wu, D., Wei, Z., & Chen, K. (2018). Rapid and non-destructive detection of decay in peach fruit at the cold environment using a self-developed handheld electronic-nose system. *Food Analytical Methods, 11*, 2990–3004.

Wijaya, D. R., Sarno, R., & Daiva, A. F. (2017). Electronic nose for classifying beef and pork using Naïve Bayes. *2017 International Seminar on Sensors, Instrumentation, Measurement and Metrology (ISSIMM)*, 104–108. IEEE.

Wilson, A. D. (2018). Applications of electronic-nose technologies for noninvasive early detection of plant, animal and human diseases. *Chemosensory, 6*, 45.

Wu, C., & Li, J. (2023). Portable FBAR based E-nose for cold chain real-time bananas shelf time detection. *Nanotechnology and Precision Engineering, 6*, 013004.

Yahia, E. M., & Carrillo-Lopez, A. (2018). *Postharvest Physiology and Biochemistry of Fruits and Vegetables*. Woodhead Publishing.

Yu, D. X., Guo, S., Wang, J. M., Yan, H., Zhang, Z. Y., Yang, J., & Duan, J. A. (2022). Comparison of different drying methods on the volatile components of ginger (*Zingiber officinale* Roscoe) by HS-GC-MS coupled with fast GC E-nose. *Foods, 11*, 1611.

Zaukuu, J. L. Z., Bazar, G., Gillay, Z., & Kovacs, Z. (2020). Emerging trends of advanced sensor-based instruments for meat, poultry and fish quality–A review. *Critical Reviews in Food Science and Nutrition, 60*, 3443–3460.

Zorpeykar, S., Mirzaee-Ghaleh, E., Karami, H., Ramedani, Z., & Wilson, A. D. (2022). Electronic nose analysis and statistical methods for investigating volatile organic compounds and yield of mint essential oils obtained by hydro distillation. *Chemosensory, 10*, 486.

Zou, X., Wang, C., Luo, M., Ren, Q., Liu, Y., Zhang, S., Bai, Y., Meng, J., Zhang, W., & Su, S. W. (2022). Design of electronic nose detection system for apple quality grading based on computational fluid dynamics simulation and K-nearest neighbor support vector machine. *Sensors, 22*, 2997.

CHAPTER 12

Sustainable Cold Chain Management for Postharvest Loss Reduction

RASAQ O. LAMIDI,[1] PANKAJ B. PATHARE,[2,*] and HAMEED B. MAHOOD[1]

[1]Centre for Sustainable Cooling, School of Chemical Engineering, University of Birmingham, Birmingham, United Kingdom

[2]Department of Soils, Water and Agricultural Engineering, College of Agricultural and Marine Sciences, Sultan Qaboos University, Muscat, Oman

*Corresponding author

ABSTRACT

More than half of fruits and vegetable produce is lost at post-harvest, mainly due to insufficient cold-chain infrastructure, namely both refrigerated (packhouse, store, vehicles, etc.) and non-refrigerated (technologies, software, etc.) activities, that link the harvested produce from farm to fork. The inequality of access to cold-chain logistics is a global challenge due to geographical differences and interdependency of nations on one another for food supply. A food cold chain is the inter-related processes carried out to ensure that temperature-sensitive food products are kept at the most-favorable temperature in the supply chain while moving from "farm to fork." Food and agricultural systems are among the most significant contributors to greenhouse gas (GHG) emissions, generating around 690 Mt CO_2-eq each year. They are also responsible for over 75% of the global freshwater withdrawal. Climate change, population expansion, food waste, and unsustainable consumer use are causing the world to edge closer to

Sustainable Approaches in Postharvest Handling and Management: Pankaj B. Pathare (Ed.)

DOI: 10.1201/9781779641076-12

food insecurity. Consequently, it is necessary to find ways to both make the infrastructure more sustainable and lower emissions from global food cold-chain systems. A change in perspective from a linear to a circular approach is necessary for a sustainable cold chain system. A long-term strategy with goals, interventions, and deadlines is needed to develop a sustainable cold chain. This includes not just moving to low-GWP refrigerants but also optimizing the requirements for cooling, optimizing energy efficiency, and switching to renewable energy systems.

12.1 INTRODUCTION

Postharvest loss (PHL) can be regarded as the quantifiable quantitative and qualitative food loss along the supply chain between harvesting and consumption (Kiaya, 2014). It encompasses interconnected processes from "farm to fork," including crop processing, transportation, marketing, food preparation, to the eventual choice by the consumer to consume or throw away the food. Qualitative food loss can lower the food's nutrients, texture, shape, or taste, cause seed viability loss, and commercial loss, while quantitative loss usually involves loss in weight or quantity of food along the food supply chain. PHL is more prominent at the beginning of the food supply chain in low- and middle-income countries, while it is predominant towards the end of the food value chain in developed countries (Food and Agricultural Organization, 2013). Depending on the region and crop, PHL can be as high as 50% for grains and up to 90% for fruits and vegetables (Adepoju, 2014; Kumar and Kalita, 2017).

Loss of food along the value chain has economic, social, and environmental implications. Infrastructural inadequacies such as refrigeration, lack of storage facilities, and poor road transport are responsible for PHL in developing countries. In contrast, PHL in developed countries is linked to spoilage or pest infestations. Agricultural activities are predominantly rain-fed in developing countries. Therefore, crop planting, maturation, and harvesting occur at the same time. As a result, many farmers sell their products at ridiculously low prices shortly after harvest—when prices are low due to oversupply—only to repurchase them at higher prices later (Lamidi, 2019). These phenomena play a pivotal role in impacting the lives of significant numbers of smallholder farmers by touching quantity, quality, as well as market values of the available food (Lamidi et al., 2019). The totality of food cultivated for human consumption but lost along the supply chain costs the global economy an estimated $936 billion a year, which may reach $1.5 trillion by 2030 (Gregoire, n.d.). Besides cost, about 25,000 people die daily from hunger, and 600 million sicknesses are linked to foodborne diseases, leading to around 420,000 (Nebehay, 2015) deaths annually. At the same time, the production of food which does not make it to market accounts for 8% of global greenhouse gas (GHG) emissions and consumes 250 km^3 of the world's freshwater, occupying about 30% of the world's agricultural land area as well as generating around 690 Mt CO_2eq emissions each year.

Production of food will need to increase substantially to feed the projected human population of 9.7 billion by 2050 (United Nations Population Fund, n.d.). This would involve closing the 56% "food gap" between global food supply and demand in reference to the 2010 baseline (Cooper, n.d.). Hence, feeding the global population would mean that the food produced does not go to waste. The conservative approach to the growth of food production areas is challenging due to the finitude of agricultural land and water resources. The alternative approach is reducing food losses in the supply chain from production to consumption.

Therefore, to prevent the above unintended consequences, and depending on the nature of food and intended use, several processes are being used along the food value chain to prevent food loss. A generic food chain, is presented in Figure 12.1, while some of the practices being used to prevent PHL are presented in further section.

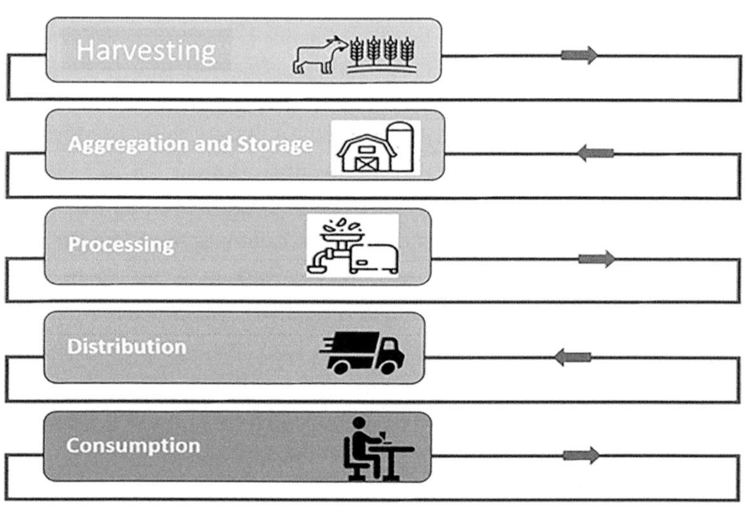

FIGURE 12.1 A generic food chain.

12.2 CURRENT PRACTICES TO REDUCE POSTHARVEST LOSSES

The increasing growth of the world population, proportional increase in the number of food-insecure households, and unpredictability of global food supply due to the finitude of land and water, as well as challenges posed by climate change, draw the attention of global policymakers and national governments to the reduction of PHL along the food supply chain. Different approaches are being adopted to reduce PHL, depending on the nature of food and stages along the food value chain.

12.2.1 HARVESTING

Harvesting is the most important phase of the food chain. This is because the subsequent PHL prevention methods can waste resources if this operation is not carefully and efficiently carried out. For example, if roots and tubers are bruised or damaged during harvesting, applying improved handling or packaging will be ineffective since early invasion with molds and viruses will appear, and decaying will have begun. Hence, poor harvesting practices and improper handling of tools predispose agricultural produce to PHL (Mutungi et al., 2022). Depending on crops, it can range between 1.5% for maize and groundnut and as high as 15% for vegetables (Kiaya, 2014). The first stage of postharvest management for fruit and vegetables is precooling. It is the first and most essential line of defense in reducing biological processes to preserve the quality of fruit and vegetables. For most fresh produce, an hour's delay at field temperature conditions of 35°C lowers shelf life by a day, even when it is subsequently stored at optimum temperature (Makule, Dimoso, and Tassou, 2022). Hence, the field heat should be eliminated as quickly as possible. Lack of pre-cooling immediately after harvesting to reduce field heat can also lead to increased deterioration, especially for fruits and vegetables. Loss at this stage is mainly due to the high cost and unavailability of pre-cooling facilities, insufficient training on pre-cooling technology, and lack of knowledge on the cost benefits of pre-cooling technology. Studies have indicated that commercial fruits and vegetables' postharvest losses reduce from 25–30% to only 5–10% without and with precooling, respectively (Duan et al., 2020). Therefore, current efforts at reducing PHL at the farm level are being directed towards providing good equipment and training farmers on good postharvest management practices (Kumar and Kalita, 2017).

12.2.2 AGGREGATION AND STORAGE

Agricultural produce skin, particularly roots and tubers, are a good hindrance to most of the opportunistic microorganisms that cause decay of the tissues. Besides, the breaking of the skin equally increases physiological deterioration and dehydration. Moreover, improper stacking, poor ventilation, and unsuitable storage conditions (temperature and relative humidity) (Atanda et al., 2011; Mutungi et al., 2022), also predispose agricultural produce to increased quality deterioration. It is also very pertinent to control pest infestation and diseases since damage triggered by pests (insects, rodents) and molds can lead to degeneration of storage facilities (e.g., mites in wooden storage) and subsequent loss in quality and quantity of food. Depending on the region and crop involved, loss due to poor storage could range from 20% for grains and 45% for fruits and vegetables (Mutungi et al., 2022). Santos et al. (2020) estimated a 30% loss in fruits and vegetables along the supply chain in Salvador, mainly at the handling and storage stages. Besides, the Food and Agricultural Organization (Al-Dairi et al., 2022; Mutungi et al., 2022) also suggests the pre-retail loss in fruits and vegetables is up to 60%, with severe loss in less developed countries. Therefore, the current post-harvest reduction initiatives are towards the reduction of infrastructural deficits and skill gaps in less developed countries, while institutional changes and consumer education are being favored in developed countries.

About 15% to 25% of postharvest loss is attributed to improper storage (Mutungi et al., 2022). This is equivalent to a loss of 150–200 kg/ton of harvested maize produce. This means that for an average maize farmer to meet up with the original intended quantity of food, maize farmers must use more resources—land, water, and other inputs.

12.2.3 DISTRIBUTION (TRANSPORTATION AND RETAILING)

The supply chain, particularly in the Global South, is currently characterized by poor road infrastructure, improper packaging, open transportation, use of unrefrigerated trucks, and so forth. In most of these countries, roads are inadequately designed for the transportation of fruits and vegetables. Transport vehicles and other modes of transportation are hardly sufficient, especially for the rural communities. Hence, agricultural produce is subjected to mechanical injury (compression, bruises, and improper handling) throughout transportation, thereby subjecting them to deterioration vulnerability (Al-Dairi et al., 2022). In a few cases, marketing organizations and cooperative societies have been able to procure transport vehicles but cannot solve poor road conditions (Kiaya, 2014). In Central and Southern Asia, transportation alone accounts for up to 25% of post-harvest loss of fruits and vegetables (Ewing-Chow, 2020), while loss during transportation can be up to 30% for tomatoes (Lamidi, 2019) and above 40% for cabbage (Zenda and Dyeyi, 2022). Retailing and marketing, which is dominated by "Pick and Pay" distribution centers/markets in the Global South, is also responsible for significant PHL. This stage of the supply chain is responsible for around 1.5% PHL in grains and an estimated 14.5% to 21.2% PHL in fruits and vegetables (Kiaya, 2014; Munhuweyi, 2012).

12.2.4 CONSUMPTION

PHL during the consumption stage of the food supply chain is mainly associated with decisions made at the household level, and it is generally regarded as food waste. Globally, food waste from households, retail establishments, and the food service industry totals 931 million tons, of which household food waste is 570 million tons each year (United Nations Environmental Programmed, 2021). Besides, household per capita food waste is similar regardless of country—middle- or low-income countries. The emission associated with food waste production and distribution is 170 million tons of CO_2 and consumes 261 million tons of resources. A study by Talia et al. (2019) indicated that consumers are largely unaware of the implications or environmental impact of food waste, with 45.07%, 26.29%, and 28.64% of respondents classified as non-aware, unaware but unwasteful, and conscious consumers, respectively. In the UK, around 70% of food waste occurs at the household level, and per capita food waste is 247 kg/household, costing an average UK family £470 per annum (WRAP, n.d.). A significant cause of these losses has been attributed to improper storage of food, such as storage at the wrong temperature, non-usage of the first-in-first-out principle, and purchase of unwanted food items during shopping. Hence, efforts at the reduction of PHL at the consumer stage are around consumer education, knowledge sharing, and policies to influence change in behavior towards food waste reduction.

12.3 IMPORTANCE OF COLD-CHAIN MANAGEMENT TO REDUCE LOSS

A cold chain is a temperature-controlled supply chain involving refrigerated production, storage, and distribution facilities supported by refrigerated equipment that can continuously preserve the required low-temperature range for temperature-sensitive agricultural products (Cold Chain Federation, 2022). It is an end-to-end temperature-controlled system from farm to fork involving pre-cooling, [primary refrigerated transportation to aggregation] and storage hub, [secondary refrigerated transportation] to processing facilities, tertiary refrigerated transportation to retail/distribution hub, and last-mile refrigerated transportation to consumers.

High temperatures result in increased rates of respiration, deterioration, and water loss in fresh produce, leading to reduced market value and decreased nutritional value. Extreme temperatures affect the postharvest period of horticultural perishables. For example, pulp temperatures for tomatoes in Rwanda were assessed at the farm, wholesale center, and pick-and-pay retail market and were observed to be 15.1, 7.1, and 8.4°C, respectively, higher than recommended temperatures (Hailu and Derbew, 2015). However, while cold chain management is well advanced in developed countries, it is either fragmented or not even available in developing countries. An estimated over 200 million tons of perishable food products are lost in developing countries due to insufficient cold chain facilities, while more than 90% of fruits and vegetables and 100% of meat and poultry products pass through refrigerated supply chains in developed countries (James and James, 2010). As a result of inadequate handling and a broken cold-chain system, it was reported that China lost about 12 million tons of fruits, 130 million tons of vegetables, and 6.9 million tons of meat, while about 8% and 25% of grains were lost at the storage and transportation stage every year in 2014. The disparity in refrigerated warehouse capacity of some selected countries is presented in Table 12.1. The table further revealed that the refrigeration development in indices (measured in cubic meters per urban residence) in countries like New Zealand, the United Kingdom, South Africa, and Kenya are 0.504, 0.441, 0.013, and 0.002, respectively (Salin, 2018). Importantly, lack of refrigeration directly led to the global loss of about 526 million tons of food in 2017 (United Nations Environmental Programmed, n.d.), while 3.1 billion people are unable to afford a healthy diet in 2019 (UNEP, 2022).

The lack of a cold-chain system results in the prevalence of pre-retail PHL along the supply chain in many developing countries. The resulting high PHL along the supply chain of perishable agricultural produce within these countries leads to poor turnover and impoverishment of farmers from low-income countries. This is because the per capita cold storage capacity and the turnover of cold chain freight have a strong relationship with economic development (Xie et al., 2022). Given the same level of refrigeration, developing countries could save about 144 million tons of food.

TABLE 12.1 Refrigerated Warehouse Capacities Per Country in 2018

Country	Refrigerated Warehouse Capacity (million m3)
Australia	5.083
Bangladesh	0.129
Belgium	2.720
Brazil	16.030
Canada	8.830
China	76.080
Egypt	3.250
France	15.300
Germany	23.950
Great Britain	24.646
India	130.720
Japan	32.650
Libya	0.230
Morocco	1.700
Namibia	0.130
Nigeria	0.040
United States	114.850
South Africa	0.323

Source: Adapted from Salin (2018).

Hence, a fully integrated cold chain has the potential to reduce food losses, it's connected carbon emissions and economic losses.

12.4 SUSTAINABLE COLD CHAIN MANAGEMENT

Conventional cold chains are energy intensive and heavily rely on diesel for transport and grid electricity for cold stores and warehouses, which in some countries are still currently being powered with coal or natural gas. The food cold chain also has impacts on worldwide climate change and the environment. Emissions associated with food loss and waste, which occurred due to insufficient refrigeration infrastructure, were estimated to be about 1 gigaton of carbon dioxide in 2017 (United Nations Environmental Programmed, n.d.).

Generally, the food cold chain is accountable for around 4% of total global GHG emissions, involving emissions from cold chain technologies (electricity, fuel, and refrigerant emissions) and from food loss and waste due to lack of refrigeration. Therefore, solutions are required to reduce emissions both from global food cold-chain systems as well as to make the infrastructure more sustainable. Such solutions must be holistic and must go beyond the current siloed system where, for instance, solar driven cold stores are procured and installed at farm-gate while agricultural products are evacuated from the same farmgate store and transported under ambient conditions during distribution. Hence, a sustainable cold chain system will require a paradigm shift from a linear to a circular approach. Such a system must involve an understanding of the interconnectedness and vigorous relationships within the whole system. The design must also be user-centric, using a bottom-up approach that considers country-level peculiarities, local economic, environmental, social, cultural, and political circumstances (UNEP, 2022). Hence, a sustainable cold chain system must have some of the features presented in Table 12.2.

TABLE 12.2 Considerations for Sustainable Cold Chain

Considerations	Features
Environmental considerations	• All stages, including pre-cooling, packaging/processing, transportation, warehousing, and last-mile delivery, must be designed with sustainability and circularity in mind.
	• Use less materials along the supply chain.
	• Use biodegradable materials where possible, and reuse is encouraged.
	• Efficient use of materials and resources along the supply chain.
	• Involve the use of natural refrigerants.
	• Seek to use renewable energy sources or technologies.
	• Data driven optimization of the logistic chain.
	• Improved data sharing and traceability to reduce waste along the supply chain.

TABLE 12.2 *(Continued)*

Considerations	Features
Social considerations	• Cold-chain design must be gender sensitive and encourage more women participation in design, technology uptakes, skill acquisition and opportunity sharing especially from the Global South. This is because women play significant roles in decision making on the adoption of cold-chain technologies at the farm level and consumption stage, especially in the Global South. Besides, the uptake of sustainable cold-chain systems can be fast-tracked with women's involvement. Due to family and cultural commitments, the mobility of women workers is less than that of men. Hence, training women as local engineers and technicians will mean the availability of and localization of trained personnel for the uptake of new technologies.
	• Must be designed to eliminate food waste while ensuring food security.
Economic considerations	• Agricultural system provides the highest employment in African and Asian countries where the cost of the ownership of cold chain equipment, maintenance and infrastructure requirements are problematic. Hence, the designed consideration in these countries must be innovative business models and solutions that can help adoption of cold chain. Such a model must focus on the affordability, availability and durability of technologies to enhance easy uptake and increased trust. Particularly, it must be designed to eliminate or reduce the initial cost of ownership.
Cultural considerations	• Cultural views and beliefs usually shape deeply held values related to consumption, trust and control and could be an impediment to the acceptability and uptake of sustainable cold technologies and solutions. For instance, socio-cultural barriers like objections towards using animal and human waste as raw material could be an impediment to the adoption of biogas-powered cold chain in some parts of the worldwide dietary rules and taboos, traditional food preparation methods, food taste preferences, and system rooted in tribal traditions of clans sharing resources could impede the uptake of cold-chain technologies (Muwanga, Mwiru, and Watundu, 2023; Sovacool and Griffiths, 2020).

12.5 CASE STUDIES OF SUSTAINABLE COLD CHAIN

There are currently no "one-size-fits-all" solutions that cover the entire cold chain from farm to fork. However, within the supply chain, there are few innovative technologies or business models addressing challenges at more than one stage of the supply chain. Some of these case studies are presented below:

1. **SunChill-Solar Powered Cooling for Horticultural Preservation (http://sunchill.no/)**
   i. **Issue:** Lack of pre-cooling to immediately remove field heat from horticultural produce accelerates deterioration and reduces shelf life.

ii. **Solution:** An inexpensive, off-grid, solar-powered system continuously produces chilled water at 10°C. Chilled water is then used to remove field heat from harvested vegetables.

iii. **Cold Chain Stage:** Precooling and packhouse

iv. **Impacts:** The technology reportedly generates increased horticultural production for consumption, resulting in extra income for smallholder farmers while also increasing access to nutritional fruits and vegetables.

2. **ColdHubs** (https://www.coldhubs.com/)

i. **Issue:** An estimated 45% of post-harvest waste in developing countries is attributed to lack of cold storage (United Nations Environmental Programmed, n.d.).

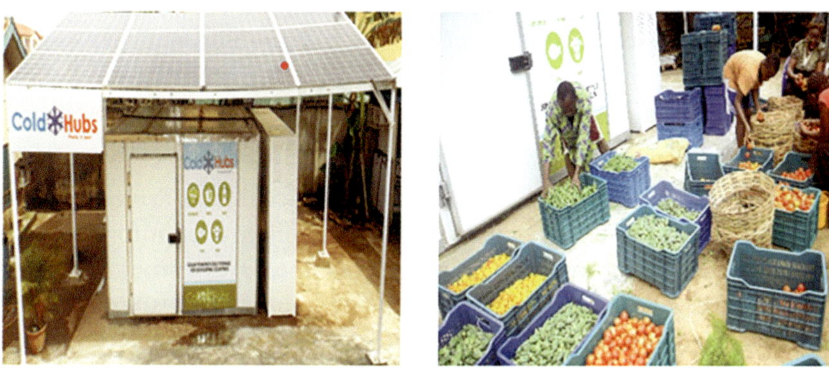

a b

FIGURE 12.2 ColdHub walk-in cold room.

ii. **Solution:** ColdHubs (Figures 12.2a and 12.2b) is a modular, solar-driven, no-prior-appointment cold store for non-grid-connected storage and preservation of temperature-sensitive agricultural produce. It addresses the challenges of post-harvest loss at farm-gate and distribution hubs. Roof-mounted solar PV generates electricity that powers the refrigeration compressor, and the remaining energy is stored in the battery to ensure continuous system running at night. Farmers are provided with plastic crates. Due to the high cost of equipment ownership, which is an impediment, a flexible pay-as-you-store subscription model is adopted. Farmers pay a daily fixed rate per crate of food they store.

iii. **Cold Chain Stage:** Storage and retail.

iv. **Impacts:** The shelf life of perishable produce can be extended from 2 to 21 days. Other impacts of the model include an 80% reduction in post-harvest waste and a 25% increase in the annual income of smallholder farmers.

3. **IBM Food Hubs** (https://www.scnsoft.com/blockchain/food-supply-chain)

   i. **Issues:** Consumers at the end of the food supply chain are increasingly interested in knowing the origin (food provenance tracking) and transparency of the food they consume. Food suppliers have a duty of care to have adequate information required for traceability of food along the cold food supply chain. This is very challenging due to the globalization of the food supply system and fragmented logistic system.

   ii. **Solution:** IBM Food Trust is a blockchain-driven solution. A blockchain stores a complete history of information on a food product's journey from the farm through aggregation, packaging, manufacturing, storage, transportation, and quality control processes to end consumers. Recorded food provenance data becomes immutable and can be accessed at any point.

   iii. **Cold Chain Stage:** All stages-from farm gate to consumer.

   iv. **Impacts:** According to Walmart, a global food retailer, the use of IBM Food Trust reduces goods provenance from 7 days to 2.2 seconds, and by 2021, Walmart relied on IBM Food Trust to trace 25+ food product groups.

4. **Sunswap (**https://sunswap.co.uk/)

   i. **Issue:** Refrigerated transport vehicles, especially trucks and trailers, use additional diesel power engines called auxiliary engines to power refrigeration units. Thus, emissions from food transport refrigeration can be as high as 40% of the GHG emissions from the vehicle's engine, and they vary between 14–43 ktCO_2-eq per year depending on vehicle size and operational usage (Cil, Abdurahman, and Cil, 2022). Moreover, the increasing costs of fossil fuels impose additional costs on temperature-controlled vehicle owners.

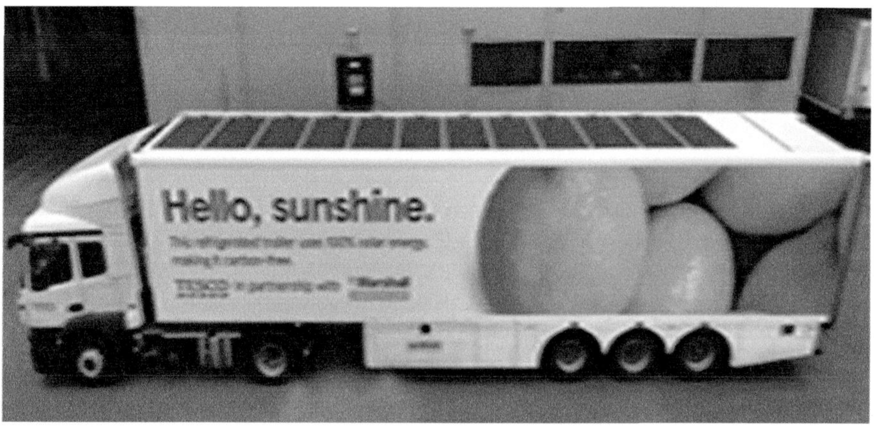

FIGURE 12.3 SunSwap solar rooftop refrigerated trailer.

- ii. **Solution:** The SunSwap Trailer (Figure 12.3) is a roof-mounted solar array that provides clean energy to run the refrigeration system and minimize charge time. Excess power is stored in a battery, while a cloud-based system provides real-time remote monitoring of the vehicle and refrigeration units.
- iii. **Cold Chain Stage:** Transportation and distribution.
- iv. **Impacts:** Compared to diesel-powered units, the solution promises 79–93% GHG emission savings, as well as a 20–50% reduction in the total cost of ownership.

5. **ELECRTRA Truck** (https://www.electracommercialvehicles.com/)

- i. **Issue:** Temperature-controlled vehicles have the twins' environmental burden from fuel use for traction and refrigeration units. Thus, transporting ingredients and food products accounts for about 20% of all carbon emissions in the food system, totaling 3.0 GtCO_2 equivalent in 2017 (Li et al., 2022).

ii. **Solution:** Electricity is produced via a hydrogen-powered fuel cell, and it is subsequently used to drive a vapor compression refrigeration system while also producing vehicle motive power. The 19-ton truck is powered with 4 by 5 kg type-three cylinders, making the total fuel capacity 20 kg of hydrogen at 350 bars.

iii. **Cold Chain Stage:** Transportation and distribution

iv. **Impacts:** The ELECTRA truck reportedly moves as long as 320 miles per day, saving an average of 314 kg of CO_2 emitted per day by a diesel truck making a similar trip.

6. **IcePoint Energy Storage** (Technology – (rebound-tech.com)

   i. **Issue:** Refrigeration systems in stores and retail outlets are mainly powered with grid-connected electricity. Adding renewable energy systems to the grid is challenging due to their intermittency, which affects the grid's resilience.

   ii. **Solution:** IcePoint is an embedded thermal energy storage system that helps improve grid resilience and demand response by storing energy in brine at –25°F. This energy can then be used whenever the need arises.

   iii. **Cold Chain Stage:** Retail and warehousing.

   iv. **Impact:** IcePoint thermal storage is 50% cheaper than battery storage and has a 2–3-year payback period compared to over 10 years for lithium battery storage.

7. **Greenlife Solar Powered Fridge** (GREEN LIFE – Home (greenlifesolution.in)

   i. **Issue:** An estimated 760.89 million people still lack access to electricity in 2019, predominantly from Sub-Saharan Africa, where access is as low as 7.4% in countries like South Sudan. This means there is no electricity to power household cooling devices like fridges and freezers, resulting in high domestic food waste.

ii. **Solution:** Greenlife is an off-grid, solar-powered DC combined fridge and freezer. The technology offers flexible temperature and humidity adjustments for the storage of various fruits and vegetables.

iii. **Cold Chain Stage:** Consumption stage

iv. **Impacts:** Reduction of food waste at the household level. The technology also promotes social inclusion and enhances food security.

12.6 FUTURE TRENDS

The food industry is rapidly expanding, resulting in increasing demand for cold-chain logistics. The international cold chain logistics market is projected to grow at 17.43%, reaching 358.49 billion from 2022 to 2027 (Technavio Research, 2023). However, the threat created by climate change, increased global political will to reduce GHG emissions, as well as continuous customer demand for the sustainability credentials of businesses, are drivers of new changes within cold chain logistics. Some of these changes within cold chain logistics center on digitalization, energy efficiency, renewable energy usage, and utilization of natural or low global warming potential refrigerants.

1. **Digitalization:** Traceability, increased regulatory requirements for transparency, and customers' growing demand for products' origin are drivers of digitalization being adopted within cold chain logistics. Hence, GPS-enabled sensors are being used in refrigerated containers to provide real-time temperature and humidity updates throughout the end-to-end journey of the commodities. Moreover, IoT-enabled technologies are strengthening the visibility of cold chain transportation, while blockchain technologies are being used for data sharing. Hence, to ensure compliance with the sector's quality management system, optimization of the journey, and prevention of businesses from incurring unnecessary costs, artificial intelligence, the Internet of Things, and machine learning are being deployed for the transportation of temperature-sensitive biological materials. These technologies will continue to shape operations of temperature-controlled logistics in the future (Cil, Abdurahman, and Cil, 2022; Loisel et al., 2021; Lin, Lin, and Wang, 2022).

2. **Low GWP Refrigerants:** The F-gases (hydrofluorocarbons, hydrofluoroolefins, hydrochlorofluoro-olefins, etc.) have high Global Warming Potentials, and without being checkmated, surface temperature warming from F-gases might have been as high as 0.3°C–0.5°C by 2100 (United States Environmental Protection Agency, N/A). Hence, the Montreal Protocol was established to control the continuous usage of F-gas and was amended in 2016 (Kigali amendment) to give an ambitious 80% phase down, which will prevent more than 80 billion metric tons of CO_2 equivalent emissions by 2050. Therefore, the commitments of nations to Kigali amendments are aiding the uptake of low GWP and environmentally friendly refrigerants, which will continue dominating the future trends of cold-chain refrigeration systems.
3. **Renewable Energy:** The cold chain is in transition to a sustainable, healthy, and inclusive food system. The transition is being driven by renewable energy, energy storage, and energy efficiency within the cold chain supply. Sustainability and energy security issues are drivers of Decentralised renewable energy systems across the globe, and many countries are now moving from fossil fuel grid systems to hydropower, wind, and nuclear systems. Grid-connected cold-chain units such as packaging and aggregation centers, warehousing, and retailing centers are benefiting from the renewable energy integrated grid systems. Besides, decentralized and off-grid systems mainly powered with renewable energy are increasingly being adopted in cold chain, for example, solar-powered cold storage (Gupta, 2021; Tizzaoui et al., 2020), hydrogen for refrigerated transport (Knegt, N/A), electric vehicles for last-mile distribution (Anosike et al., 2023; Gupta, N/A), and phase change materials for energy storage in refrigerated transportation (Oró et al., 2012; Villasmil, Fischer, and Worlitschek, 2019). Beside renewable energy and energy storage adoption, energy efficiency technologies and processes are increasingly being adopted within food cold chain logistics (Neusel and Hirzel, 2022; Xiaofeng and Xuelai, 2021). Therefore, these trends are expected to continuously shape the future of the cold chain.

12.7 CONCLUDING REMARK

A sustainable, healthy, and equitable food system is an important aspect of Sustainable Development Goals as well as a strategy to mitigate against climate change. However, the food cold chain may have twin challenges of fragmentation and improper attention from policymakers. The approach to the research and development within the cold chain is often siloed and with traditional attention to cold storage alone without other interlinks. There are currently scanty or non-existing specialized technology deployment mechanisms, such as feed-in tariffs, renewable heat incentives, green certificates, and so forth, for the food cold chain. Importantly, the food cold chain is predominantly under the control of private investors while little is being done by the government. Therefore, the full economic, social, health, and environmental opportunities of the food cold chain would be achieved if the sector is given adequate attention. Hence, government policies across the world must be targeted towards a robust and resilient food cold chain.

KEYWORDS

- **climate-resilient food systems**
- **cold chain logistics**
- **food cold chain**
- **greenhouse gas emissions**
- **postharvest losses**
- **sustainable infrastructure**

REFERENCES

Adepoju, A. O. (2014). Post-harvest losses and welfare of tomato farmers in Ogbomosho, Osun state, Nigeria. *Journal of Stored Products and Postharvest Research, 5*(2), 8–13. https://doi.org/10.5897/jsppr2014.0160 (accessed on 9th July 2025).

Al-Dairi, M., Pathare, P. B., Al-Yahyai, R., & Opara, U. L. (2022). Mechanical damage of fresh produce in postharvest transportation: Current status and future prospects. *Trends in Food Science & Technology, 124*, 195–207. https://doi.org/10.1016/j.tifs.2022.04.018 (accessed on 9th July 2025).

Anosike, A., Loomes, H., Udokporo, C. K., & Garza-Reyes, J. A. (2023). Exploring the challenges of electric vehicle adoption in final mile parcel delivery. *International Journal of Logistics Research and Applications, 26*(6), 683–707. https://doi.org/10.1080/13675567.2021.1978409 (accessed on 9th July 2025).

Atanda, S. A., Pessu, P. O., Agoda, S., Isong, I. U., & Ikotun, I. (2011). The concepts and problems of post-harvest food losses in perishable crops. *African Journal of Food Science, 5*(11), 603–613. http://www.academicjournals.org/AJFS (accessed on 9th July 2025).

Cil, A. Y., Abdurahman, D., & Cil, I. (2022). Internet of Things enabled real time cold chain monitoring in a container port. *Journal of Shipping and Trade, 7*(1). https://doi.org/10.1186/s41072-022-00110-z (accessed on 9th July 2025).

Cold Chain Federation. (2022). *Cold Chain Report–2022*. London.

Cooper, R. Changing our diet by 2050 is essential to achieving a sustainable future, new report reveals. *Climate Actions*. https://www.climateaction.org (accessed on 9th July 2025).

di Talia, E., Simeone, M., & Scarpato, D. (2019). Consumer behavior types in household food waste. *Journal of Cleaner Production, 214*, 166–172. https://doi.org/10.1016/J.JCLEPRO.2018.12.216 (accessed on 9th July 2025).

dos Santos, S. F., et al. (2020). Post-harvest losses of fruits and vegetables in supply centers in Salvador, Brazil: Analysis of determinants, volumes and reduction strategies. *Waste Management, 101*, 161–170. https://doi.org/10.1016/j.wasman.2019.10.007 (accessed on 9th July 2025).

Duan, Y., et al. (2020). Postharvest precooling of fruit and vegetables: A review. *Trends in Food Science & Technology, 100*, 278–291. https://doi.org/10.1016/j.tifs.2020.04.027 (accessed on 9th July 2025).

Ewing-Chow, D. (2020). Fruit and vegetable spoilage is a hidden contributor to underdevelopment. *Forbes*. https://www.forbes.com (accessed on 9th July 2025).

Food and Agricultural Organization. (2013). *Food Wastage Footprint: Impacts on Natural Resources, Summary Report* (p. 60). Food and Agricultural Organization, Rome. http://www.fao.org/docrep/018/i3347e/i3347e.pdf (accessed on 9th July 2025).

Gregoire, E. (n.d.). A coordinated global offensive can reduce annual food loss and waste by $700 billion. *The Boston Consulting Group*. https://www.bcg.com (accessed on 9th July 2025).

Gupta, A. (N/A). Future potential market of LEVs in last mile delivery industry in KSA: Ken Research. *Digital Journal*. https://www.digitaljournal.com (accessed on 9th July 2025).

Gupta, U. (2021). Solar-powered cold storage service. *PV Magazine, India*. https://www.pv-magazine-india.com (accessed on 9th July 2025).

Hailu, G., & Derbew, B. (2015). Extent, causes and reduction strategies of postharvest losses of fresh fruits and vegetables—A review, *5*(5). www.iiste.org (accessed on 9th July 2025).

James, S. J., & James, C. (2010). The food cold-chain and climate change. *Food Research International, 43*(7), 1944–1956. https://doi.org/10.1016/j.foodres.2010.02.001 (accessed on 9th July 2025).

Kiaya, V. (2014). *Post-Harvest Losses and Strategies to Reduce Them.*

Knegt, A. M. (N/A). Electra to show the first zero-emission refrigerated hydrogen HGV at the CV Show in a UK first. *Fleet Vision International*. https://fleetvisionintl.co.uk (accessed on 9th July 2025).

Kumar, D., & Kalita, P. (2017). Reducing postharvest losses during storage of grain crops to strengthen food security in developing countries. *Foods, 6*(1), 1–22. https://doi.org/10.3390/foods6010008 (accessed on 9th July 2025).

Lamidi, R. O. (2019). *Evaluation of Biogas Driven Poly-Generation System to Reduce Energy Poverty and Post-Harvest Loss* (Doctor of Philosophy thesis). Newcastle University, United Kingdom.

Lamidi, R. O., Jiang, L., Wang, Y. D., Pathare, P. B., & Roskilly, A. P. (2019). Techno-economic analysis of a biogas driven poly-generation system for postharvest loss reduction in a Sub-Saharan African rural community. *Energy Conversion and Management, 196*, 591–604. https://doi.org/10.1016/J.ENCONMAN.2019.06.023 (accessed on 9th July 2025).

Li, M., et al. (2022). Global food-miles account for nearly 20% of total food-systems emissions. *Nature Food, 3*(6), 445–453. https://doi.org/10.1038/s43016-022-00531-w (accessed on 9th July 2025).

Lin, H., Lin, J., & Wang, F. (2022). An innovative machine learning model for supply chain management. *Journal of Innovation & Knowledge, 7*(4), 100276. https://doi.org/10.1016/j.jik.2022.100276 (accessed on 9th July 2025).

Loisel, J., et al. (2021). Cold chain break detection and analysis: Can machine learning help? *Trends in Food Science & Technology, 112*, 391–399. https://doi.org/10.1016/j.tifs.2021.03.052 (accessed on 9th July 2025).

Makule, E., Dimoso, N., & Tassou, S. A. (2022). Precooling and cold storage methods for fruits and vegetables in Sub-Saharan Africa—A review. *Horticultural, 8*(9), 776. https://doi.org/10.3390/horticulturae8090776 (accessed on 9th July 2025).

Munhuweyi, K. (2012). *Postharvest Losses and Changes in Quality of Vegetables from Retail to Consumer: A Case Study of Tomato, Cabbage and Carrot* (Master of Science thesis). Stellenbosch University, Stellenbosch. http://scholar.sun.ac.za (accessed on 9th July 2025).

Mutungi, C., Abass, A., Fischer, G., & Kotu, B. (2022). Improved technologies for reducing post-harvest losses. In *Sustainable Agricultural Intensification: A Handbook for Practitioners in East and Southern Africa* (1st ed., pp. 91–105). CABI. https://doi.org/10.1079/9781800621602.0007 (accessed on 9th July 2025).

Muwanga, R., Mwiru, D. P., & Watundu, S. (2023). Influence of social-cultural practices on the adoption of Renewable Energy Technologies (RETs) in Uganda. *Renewable Energy Focus, 45*, 201–209. https://doi.org/10.1016/j.ref.2023.04.004 (accessed on 9th July 2025).

Nebehay, S. (2015). Food poisoning kills 420,000 people a year worldwide, says WHO report. *Independent*. https://www.independent.co.uk (accessed on 9th July 2025).

Neusel, L., & Hirzel, S. (2022). Energy efficiency in cold supply chains of the food sector: An exploration of conditions and perceptions. *Cleaner Logistics and Supply Chain, 5*, 100082. https://doi.org/10.1016/j.clscn.2022.100082 (accessed on 9th July 2025).

Oró, E., et al. (2012). Review on phase change materials (PCMs) for cold thermal energy storage applications. *Applied Energy, 99*, 513–533. https://doi.org/10.1016/j.apenergy.2012.03.058 (accessed on 9th July 2025).

Salin, V. (2018). *2018 GCCA Global Cold Storage Capacity Report*. Texas. http://AFCERC.tamu.edu (accessed on 9th July 2025).

Sovacool, B. K., & Griffiths, S. (2020). The cultural barriers to a low-carbon future: A review of six mobility and energy transitions across 28 countries. *Renewable and Sustainable Energy Reviews, 119*, 109569. https://doi.org/10.1016/j.rser.2019.109569 (accessed on 9th July 2025).

Technavio Research. (2023). Cold Chain Market size to grow at a CAGR of 17.43% from 2022 to 2027; Use of RFID in cold chain logistics expected to drive market growth- Technavio

Tizzaoui, M., et al. (2020). Solar PV power driven cold room storage for Saharan rural area. In *E3S Web of Conferences*. EDP Sciences. https://doi.org/10.1051/e3sconf/202015201004 (accessed on 9th July 2025).

UNEP. (2022). *Sustainable Food Cold Chains: Opportunities, Challenges and The Way Forward*. UNEP; FAO. https://doi.org/10.4060/cc0923en (accessed on 9th July 2025).

United Nations Environmental Programmed. (2021). *Food Waste Index Report 2021*.

United Nations Environmental Programmed. (n.d.). *Amid Food and Climate Crises, Investing in Sustainable Food Cold Chains Crucial*. UNEP. https://www.unep.org (accessed on 9th July 2025).

United Nations Population Fund. (n.d.). *Global Issues—Our Growing Population*. United Nations. https://www.unfpa.org (accessed on 9th July 2025).

United States Environmental Protection Agency. (N/A). *International Treaties and Cooperation About the Protection of The Stratospheric Ozone Layer*. EPA. https://www.epa.gov (accessed on 9th July 2025).

Villasmil, W., Fischer, L. J., & Worlitschek, J. (2019). A review and evaluation of thermal insulation materials and methods for thermal energy storage systems. *Renewable and Sustainable Energy Reviews, 103*, 71–84. https://doi.org/10.1016/j.rser.2018.12.040 (accessed on 9th July 2025).

WRAP. *Food waste – 2024 facts & statistics*. Waste and Resources Action Programmed. https://wrap.org.uk (accessed on 9th July 2025).

Xiaofeng, X., & Xuelai, Z. (2021). Simulation and experimental investigation of a multi-temperature insulation box with phase change materials for cold storage. *Journal of Food Engineering, 292*, 110286. https://doi.org/10.1016/j.jfoodeng.2020.110286 (accessed on 9th July 2025).

Xie, R., Huang, H., Zhang, Y., & Yu, P. (2022). Coupling relationship between cold chain logistics and economic development: An investigation from China. *PLoS One, 17*(2), e0264561. https://doi.org/10.1371/journal.pone.0264561 (accessed on 9th July 2025).

Zenda, M., & Dyeyi, M. (2022). Challenges in the supply chain of cabbage in Nelson Mandela Bay Metropolitan Municipality, Eastern Cape, South Africa. *South African Journal of Agricultural Extension (SAJAE), 50*(2), 42–56. https://doi.org/10.17159/2413-3221/2022/v50n2a11282 (accessed on 9th July 2025).

CHAPTER 13

Geothermal Energy for Drying of Fresh Produce

IMTIAZ HUSSAIN,[1,*] MUHAMMAD ABDUL RAHIM,[2] HUDDA AYUB,[3] AURBAB SHOUKAT,[3] LARAIB SHOUKAT,[4] FAIMA ATTA KHAN,[2] and SAADIA AMBREEN[5]

[1]*Department of Food Science and Technology, University of Poonch, Rawalakot, Pakistan*

[2]*Department of Food Science, Faculty of Life Sciences, Government College University, Faisalabad, Punjab, Pakistan*

[3]*National Institute of Food Science and Technology, University of Agriculture, Faisalabad, Punjab, Pakistan*

[4]*Department of Biochemistry, Faculty of Life Sciences, Government College University, Faisalabad, Punjab, Pakistan*

[5]*University Institute of Food Science and Technology, The University of Lahore, Lahore, Punjab, Pakistan*

*Corresponding author

ABSTRACT

In recent times, the energy crisis is affecting the whole world and demands finding alternative sources. Geothermal energy is a clean, sustainable, and renewable energy source that has gained attention in recent years due to its potential to reduce greenhouse gas (GHG) emissions and dependence on fossil fuels. It is being used as a promising alternative to fossil fuels in various applications, including drying fresh produce. Drying is an essential process in the food system, and it is a significant part of the energy

Sustainable Approaches in Postharvest Handling and Management: Pankaj B. Pathare (Ed.)

DOI: 10.1201/9781779641076-13

used in food production. This chapter presents an overview of the potential use of geothermal energy in drying fresh produce. Drying is a crucial step in preserving fresh produce and extending its shelf life. Traditionally, drying has been done using fossil fuels such as coal, gas, and electricity. However, the use of these fuels contributes significantly to environmental degradation, such as air pollution, and climate change. On the other hand, geothermal energy is a clean and renewable source of energy that can be used to dry fresh produce. In developed countries, geothermal energy is used to dry food products and has several benefits, including reduced energy costs, a reduced carbon footprint, and increased food quality and safety. It can be harnessed through several methods, including direct use and power generation. Geothermal energy is generated from the natural heat of the earth and is a sustainable energy source with a low carbon footprint. Additionally, geothermal energy can be used in remote areas, where access to traditional drying methods may be limited. In conclusion, the use of geothermal energy to dry food produce is a promising solution that can contribute to sustainable food production and reduce the environmental impact of the food industry. It is the need of the time to explore the potential of geothermal energy for drying different types of food production systems, optimizing the process, and developing cost-effective and efficient geothermal drying systems.

13.1 INTRODUCTION

In the current era, the energy requirements are enhanced day by day. Heat is the most convenient form of energy and is constantly present in our daily lives. It is not only produced from converting electricity and fossil fuels burning, but it is present naturally as Earth's internal heat. However, a massive quantity of heat is available in Earth, which is proved by surface appearances in different forms such as fumaroles, geysers, and hot springs, and so forth. Geothermal energy (heat energy present in the inner layers of Earth) is the cheapest source of energy, and it has temperatures ranging from 60°C–200°C (Yamamoto et al., 2001). Geothermal heat energy is produced by the constant decline of radioactive elements such as thorium and uranium since 4.6 billion years ago when the Earth was formed. The geothermal resources have different important features such as impermeable rock, a heat source, and an aquifer. Geysers and fumaroles are formed when hot water and steam outflow through cracks in the rock. So, this kind of energy can be utilized for multipurpose uses; one of them is power production through direct heating (Basaran and Ozegener, 2013).

Fresh produce, such as fish, meat, vegetables, fruits, and numerous agricultural commodities, are rich in water content, and water activity (a_w) is 0.98 to 0.99. This is the ideal condition for many types of microbial growth (Schmidt and Fontana, 2020). Fresh produce drying is beneficial because it assists in extending shelf life, minimizing packaging requirements, and reducing shipping weight. Fresh produce is highly perishable and extremely vulnerable to microbial decay, physical damage, and environmental factors because of high *aw* (Huang and Zhang, 2012). So, the drying of fresh produce is considered a key process for increasing shelf life, while end-product quality is the major factor during the drying process. The optimum drying conditions can evade the degradation of dried food and the production of undesirable products that induce changes in the structure of food (Miranda et al., 2009).

For instance, improper processing, such as drying with hot air at elevated temperatures, can speed up the oxidation of pigments and fats, cause a loss of nutrients and functional ingredients, and impair the natural micro- and macro-structuring. On the contrary, the industrial application of drying techniques has a major problem with the expenses of energy consumption and drying equipment. The ultimate drying techniques for developing new dried products would have many benefits, including high capacity, low environmental impact, low cost, safe operation, energy efficiency, and good product quality (Mujumdar and Law, 2010).

13.2 GEOTHERMAL ENERGY

Geothermal energy is not only associated with solar energy; it is eventually produced through radioactive decline of unstable atoms and gravitational energy. A larger quantity of heat is stored in the planet's body; it is sustainable because it cannot be exhausted by human usage. Sustainable utilization of renewed energy sources indicates that consumption rates may be equivalent to or below the renewal process rates. Renewable energy is defined as a process that can be rapidly renewed in terms of human timescale (Stober and Bucher, 2013).

13.2.1 GEOTHERMAL ENERGY SOURCES

Climate mostly regulates the subsurface temperatures in the upper layers of the crust. In temperate zones, the ground can freeze to a depth of one meter in winter, and it can be quite warm in summer. The sun's radiation provides direct heat input, and heat exchange with air and water absorbed during precipitation provides indirect heat input. Seasonal land temperature fluctuations decrease with depth. In the temperate zone, the yearly cycle vanishes at 10–20 m depth. At that depth, the temperature is persistent during the year and is nearly equal to the regional long-lasting mean external temperature (Stober and Bucher, 2013).

Previously, geothermal energy was associated with quite limited sources: usual earth temperature, where a ground source heat pump (GSHP) is used for heat extraction or dumping, and hot water or steam from hydrothermal vents. Another source of geothermal energy is the significant depth (approximately 4–5 km) beneath the surface of the ground, where it is possible to find high temperatures of about 200°C. In recent years, the utilization of this type of energy has increased. The fundamental method consists of drilling a subsurface injection and production well into a hot, broken rock mass. Injection wells are used for pumping water, which heats up by the hot, broken rock mass and eventually returns outward with the help of a production well. Then, the collected hot water is utilized to generate steam or explosive gases to move turbines for electricity production (Johnston et al., 2011).

Geothermal energy is a plentiful source of renewable energy, but its application is limited by its thermal properties (Gallup, 2009; Ramazankhani et al., 2016). For instance, low enthalpy geothermal energy (approximately 100°C) is extensively utilized for direct applications, medium enthalpy geothermal energy (about 100–150°C) mainly uses ORC technology for electricity generation, and high enthalpy geothermal energy (above 150°C) is primarily utilized for electricity generation (Kanoglu et al., 2010; Schuster et al., 2009). Major applications of geothermal energy consumption include cooling, agricultural crops drying, and electricity generation, and so forth (Kanoglu et al., 2007; Lund and Toth, 2021). This wide range of applications allows us to offer many possible product systems.

- **Advantages of Geothermal Energy**
  - **Environment Friendly:** It is more environment friendly than usual fuel resources.

- **Renewable:** it's a rich source of renewable energy resources that is generated by earth.
- **Huge Potential:** There will be more geothermal resources that can be used for energy production with ongoing industrial research and development.
- **Sustainable:** It is a sustainable energy resources because it is constantly available in contrast to solar and wind.
- **Trustworthy:** It is a trustworthy source for indicating the power output more accurately from geothermal plant.
- **Zero Fuel Requirement:** No need of fuel because geothermal energy is a natural resource (Svalova, 2018).

➢ **Disadvantages of Geothermal Energy**

- **Location Restricted:** The geothermal energy is the biggest drawback of geothermal energy is its location-specific.
- **Gas Emission:** The discharge of gases into environment due to digging process.
- **Earthquakes:** The risk of earthquakes will be increased due to geothermal energy.
- **High Cost:** High installation cost about $7 million for geothermal energy plant is also a limitation.

13.2.2 TYPES OF GEOTHERMAL ENERGY

Electricity is generated by geothermal power plants by harnessing the energy in the form of heat within the Earth. There are three main types of geothermal power plants:

13.2.2.1 DRY STEAM POWER PLANTS

Dry steam power plants are the first form of geothermal power plants. In this system, the hydrothermal fluids are utilized because they primarily comprise steam (Ngala et al., 2015). The term "hydrothermal fluid" means the chemical substances and gases are dissociated in water. Steam is produced inside the hydrothermal reservoir as a result of the hydrothermal fluid absorbing heat from the earth. Steam from the hydrothermal reservoir is transferred to the turbine within the dry steam power plant. The generator is coupled with the turbine, which is coupled to the generator, and is rotated by using the direct steam. Then, the steam is liquefied by lowering the temperature with the help of a condenser. The hydrothermal fluid in the reservoir is then pumped back by an injection well.

13.2.2.2 FLASH STEAM POWER PLANTS

Flash steam power plants are the second form of geothermal power plant. In this system, the hydrothermal reservoir situated deep within the innermost layer of ground is used for obtaining hydrothermal fluid or high-pressure hot water, which is then accumulated in the steam separator. High-pressure hot water travels up naturally into the separator, and pressure drops as it travels upward. Hot water is turned into steam due to pressure reduction and then isolated in the steam separator. The isolated steam is transferred to the turbine that is attached to the generator. The turbine is driven by using steam and gives power to the generator, producing electricity. Hydrothermal fluids must be heated to temperatures more than 182°C in flash steam geothermal power plants in order to produce electricity (Ngala et al., 2015).

13.2.2.3 BINARY CYCLE POWER PLANTS

Binary cycle power plants are the third form of geothermal power plant. In this method, hot water obtained from a hydrothermal reservoir generates heat energy, which is transmitted to a secondary fluid. The boiling point of the secondary fluid should be lower than that of the hot water. As a result, the secondary liquid is converted to steam due to the heat energy of the hot water, which is then used to drive the turbine. Hence, the lower operating temperature of this technique is one of its main benefits (Ngala et al., 2015). Since the boiling points of secondary liquids are lower than water, the operating temperature of hydrothermal fluid and water is minimal. It is a closed-loop system because the binary cycle emits almost nothing into the environment. However, no discharge of greenhouse gases (GHGs) is seen, and it has no impact on global warming (Kulasekara and Seynulabdeen, 2019).

13.3 IMPORTANCE OF FRUITS AND VEGETABLES DRYING

Fresh fruits and vegetables (FFVs) contain above 80% moisture content, whether in free or chemically bound form. Therefore, these fall into a highly perishable category and quickly decay (Sagar and Kumar, 2010). Inappropriate pre- and post-harvest handling of the raw material and a lack of processing and marketing facilities contribute to higher losses. It is estimated that almost 30–50% of fruit and vegetable losses occur from farm to fork. These losses are leading to excessively high levels of food insecurity worldwide (FAO, 2010, 2012). After harvest, different post-storage methods are needed to retain the product's freshness and maintain its nutritional profile. Worldwide, many storage methods are present which demand low temperatures to preserve raw materials (Sagar and Kumar, 2010); yet, their high price and unavailability in several places are the main drawbacks.

The conventional technique to extend the shelf life and maintain the quality parameters of fruits and vegetables is drying, which lessens the water content, halts the moisture-induced spoilage reactions, and inhibits reproduction and microbial growth (Mujumdar, 2014; Omolola et al., 2017). Drying can significantly lower the volume and weight of food and lead to advantages, including decreased storage, packaging, and shipping prices (Kamiloglu et al., 2016). Additionally, drying of agricultural items by reducing water content produces novel products with distinct physical and textural characteristics, like vegetable crisps.

Nowadays, dried fruits and vegetables have great demand due to the ease of manufacture and storage, comparatively reduced shipping and packaging price, and decreased moisture level, which prevents the growth of microbes that spoil the fresh produce (Camiloglu et al., 2016).

13.4 CONVENTIONAL DRYING METHODS

13.4.1 SUN DRYING

The most ancient method of preserving vegetables and fruits is sun drying (Misha et al., 2013). Smoky flames, air, and solar energy have been used throughout history to evaporate moisture content from meat, plants, fruits, and grains (Ahmed et al., 2013). Fruits have a high content of acid and sugar, so they are safe for sun drying, but vegetables are not suitable for sun drying because they have a low amount of acid content and sugar. Place the whole fruit or sliced pieces on trays on high boards and dry in open air until the desired dryness is obtained. Stainless steel, plastic, or Teflon-coated fiberglass screens are best. Optimum drying conditions are less than 60% relative humidity and a minimum temperature of 86°F (Ahmed et al., 2013). However, optimal sun-drying conditions may not be sufficient when certain fruits are ripe, which is one of its major drawbacks. Insect infestation, direct heating, contamination from debris and dust, quality degradation, long drying times, and low thermal conductivity due to evaporated moisture condensation are just a few of the major problems encountered in open air drying (Sontakke and Salv, 2015). Plums and raisins could be dried using this method.

13.4.2 SOLAR DRYING

Solar systems have qualities like ease of use, cost-effectiveness, and renewability. A variety of solar dryers with different designs, trays/racks, chambers, tunnels, and bins have been developed for agricultural produce (Fudholi et al., 2015). Solar dryers like liquid, spray, rack, tunnel, and cabinet dryers are convection dryers that dry food using air heated by radiant energy or sunlight energy, which is absorbed in the food with the help of a refractive medium, generally polyethylene or glass (Alamu et al., 2010). Short drying times decline mold growth and the risk of food spoilage. Even though solar drying manufactures a more qualitative product than sun drying, most solar dryers are less efficient than open-air drying. Some drying process complications are condensation of moisture inside the dryer, resulting in an increase in humidity. Solar dryers can dry food products like fruits, rosemary, mangoes, and bananas (Lingayat et al., 2017).

13.5 MODERN DRYING TECHNIQUES

Many traditional drying methods used to preserve vegetables and fruits result in a loss of nutritional value, texture, aroma, flavor, and color. Therefore, at present, the latest research is focused on the introduction of different drying technologies that are economical and maintain product quality.

13.5.1 FREEZE DRYING

Freeze-drying consists of these steps: freezing food, sublimating ice, and extraction of the water molecules bound in the food. At low temperature, reduced water or liquid content, and the freezing process leads to the production of qualitative final products and entirely inhibits mostly microbial-mediated reactions (Falade and Igbeka, 2007). Initially, the food is kept at –20°C to freeze, then controlled heat is applied in a vacuum to cause sublimation, where the ice turns directly into steam and then condenses into ice on a cooling coil, where it is usually stored at –55°C (Claussen et al., 2007). The most important property of freeze-drying agricultural products is their ability to rehydrate. The drawback of freeze-drying products is the high cost and amount of energy used during freezing, condensing, and drying. Due to prolonged freeze-drying time, the produce collapses, ending in an irregular product with poor rehydration and odor loss. It has been effective as an exotic vegetable and fruit, orange juice, mushroom, pulp of mango, soup ingredient, and other industrial applications. Although freeze-drying of onions using microwave ovens was optimized (Schossler et al., 2012), an integrated ultrasonic freeze-dryer was designed to dry bell peppers. By using ultrasonic technology, it was possible to reduce the drying rate by 11.5%.

13.5.2 VACUUM DRYING

When drying vegetables and fruits, vacuum technology is utilized in combination with drying methods like microwave ovens and freeze-drying. Flow driven by pressure is usually the most used form for moisture transfer during vacuum drying (Parikh, 2015). This is done at temperatures between 0.6 kPa to 101 kPa, where heat transfer is mostly by conduction. The drying time is reduced by boiling water due to pressure in a vacuum at a low temperature. In addition, enhanced product water circulation and mass transfer are obtained. Conversely, high pressure causes the product to darken.

13.5.3 OSMO-DEHYDRATION

Osmotic dehydration is a process of partially removing moisture from vegetables and fruits by submerging them in a hypertonic solution containing glycerol (a sugar with high osmotic pressure), salt, or sorbitol. When food is kept in a hypertonic solution, the vegetable and fruit tissues diffuse into the solutes of the solution (Mehta et al., 2013). The flavor, nutritional value, and color of food are preserved by the pretreatment with gentle heat treatment. Consequently, the energy requirement for the gross dehydration process is efficiently decreased. Difficulties in predicting the product taste and final chemical composition of the product, leaching of pigments, vitamins, minerals, acids, and carbohydrates, and unnecessary osmotic solution wastage are just a few problems to overcome. Kumar and Sagar (2014) reported that vacuum drying and osmotic treatment are more successful in combination for fruit drying.

13.5.4 MICROWAVE DRYING

Concerns about product cost and product quality have motivated researchers to develop production-based drying technologies. Electromagnetic radiation plays a vital role by generating heat inside and outside the raw material for rapid vegetable and fruit drying through microwave technology (Li et al., 2010; Wray and Ramaswamy, 2015). Microwave drying technology has a short drying time, good product quality, and the flexibility to dry a variety of dried value-added products, so it is more advantageous when used separately or in combination (Li et al., 2010). Conventional microwave drying has the disadvantage of uneven heating within the product (Li et al., 2011). The most employed technique for drying purposes in daily use is microwave-assisted techniques, which are more efficient for high sugar content products and improve the safety and quality attributes of the product (Ekezie et al., 2017).

13.5.5 INFRARED DRYING

Infrared drying of perishable raw materials has gained importance as the most appropriate method for drying many types of agricultural products (Doymaz, 2012). Infrared dryers are processed on the basic principle that radiation is applied to dry and heat materials containing moisture. Infrared rays penetrate the exposed material and increase the inside temperature (Motevali et al., 2011). It provides significant benefits over traditional dryers for agricultural products and can be considered energy-efficient (low energy consumption). It also provides uniformity of product temperature, minimizes the time period of drying, and maintains the quality parameters of the final product (Kocabiyik and Tezer, 2009).

13.5.6 OVEN DRYING

An oven drying oven is attached and a dehydrator. An oven can serve as a dehydrator with the combination of these factors: air flow, low humidity, and heat. The oven is great for occasionally drying fruit skins and banana chips, or storing excess produce such as mushrooms and celery. Ovens are needed for daily cooking, so they may not be sufficient to store the garden's abundant produce. Drying in a dehydrator is faster than drying in an oven because it does not contain fans for air movement. It takes twice as long to dry in an oven as compared with a dehydrator. Therefore, ovens are not as well-planned as dehydrators and consume more energy (Ahmed et al., 2013).

13.6 GEOTHERMAL ENERGY FOR DRYING OF FRESH PRODUCE

Geothermal energy can be employed as a heat source in the drying processes of agricultural produce. For a long time, the most commonly used method for drying agricultural products has been conventional methods, such as sun drying in the open air. This method has several disadvantages due to soil and dust contamination, and majorly the contamination by insects, so it is not suitable for drying spices and herbs. Some other drying processes are also used nowadays, like cabinet drying and tunnel drying, that show better drying because of the closed and controlled environment that maintains the quality of dried produce and decreases the time period of the drying process, but that uses a vast amount of electrical and thermal energy (Indiarto et al., 2021). Rather than the drying process, fossil fuels are mainly used in the food industry for generating energy, but fossil fuels are not environmentally friendly and cause disturbance in the ecosystem and pollution. Geothermal energy is the world's third energy source, which is potentially used in the food industry. Geothermal energy is a continuous source of energy; the geothermal fluids used can be used directly by constant flow rate and indirectly employing heat pumps and heat exchangers. For the drying of agricultural produce, geothermal energy can be used as both system cooling and heating systems (Calín-Sánchez et al., 2020).

Geothermal energy is a tremendous amount of energy under the earth's crust, demonstrated by different ways such as geysers and hot springs. The temperature of geothermal energy varies with the temperature range of 60–120. The continuous source of energy is the decay of radioactive materials such as uranium and thorium (Yamamoto et al., 2001). There are two major applications of using geothermal energy: first, the direct use of geothermal energy, and second, the indirect use of geothermal energy. The direct application includes fish farming, the use of geothermal energy in agriculture which includes greenhouse heating and drying of fresh produce, pasteurization of milk, and indirect application includes heating and cooling of space, generation of electricity, use of geothermal energy for extraction purposes in industries, and dehydration of food products. In general, geothermal fluid containing low temperatures is mostly used in the direct drying process rather than for electricity (Lund et al., 2005; Lund and Boyd, 2016).

13.6.1 OVERVIEW OF GEOTHERMAL DRYING TECHNOLOGY

Due to various human activities, including burning fossil fuels, forest destruction, and a rapid increase in population, the level of pollutants and harmful substances has increased in the atmosphere. These have caused deterioration of the air, water, and soil, endangering the diversity of life and the survival of the human race. Because of all that, renewable energy resources have acquired substantial importance in recent years. Apart from all these issues, improper handling and post-harvest processing of food from farm to the final product contributes to food wastage of up to more than 40%. The post-harvest losses of fruits and vegetables and roots and tubers are about 22% and 25%, respectively. The most common and widely used process for the preservation of food products is drying (Hasan et al., 2019).

The commercial food drying process, including drying drums and drying tunnels, requires a large amount of energy, which is about 25% of all industrial energy. Different conventional drying processes, along with their disadvantages, are explained in Figure 13.1. Many countries, especially developing countries, are facing serious energy crises; they are unable to employ conventional drying processes because of the limited amount of energy. So, sustainable energy resources such as geothermal energy have significant demand in the processing of post-harvest produce (Kumoro and Kristanto, 2003). The traditional drying technologies used for many years are divided into four categories: fossil fuel sources, electrical (ohmic heating), dielectric (microwave and radio frequency drying), and combined sources, which include dual and multi combinations. Because of the energy consumption of all the traditional drying processes and fossil fuels polluting the atmosphere, scientists and researchers have replaced these with renewable energy resources, which include biomass, air drying via heat pump, and geothermal drying processes. The biomass materials require intensive heat energy for combustion before drying the food. The drying done by air drying uses a heating pump, which has low drying efficiency. In renewable energy resources, geothermal drying is the most efficient and significant drying method in drying agricultural produce (Qu et al., 2022). Geothermal energy is used in several studies for drying purposes. Another scientist, Andritsos, conducted research on drying tomatoes by employing geothermal fluid energy that is used to heat the drying air in air-water heat exchangers. Geothermal energy requires low temperatures for efficient drying of agricultural produce (Andritsos et al., 2003).

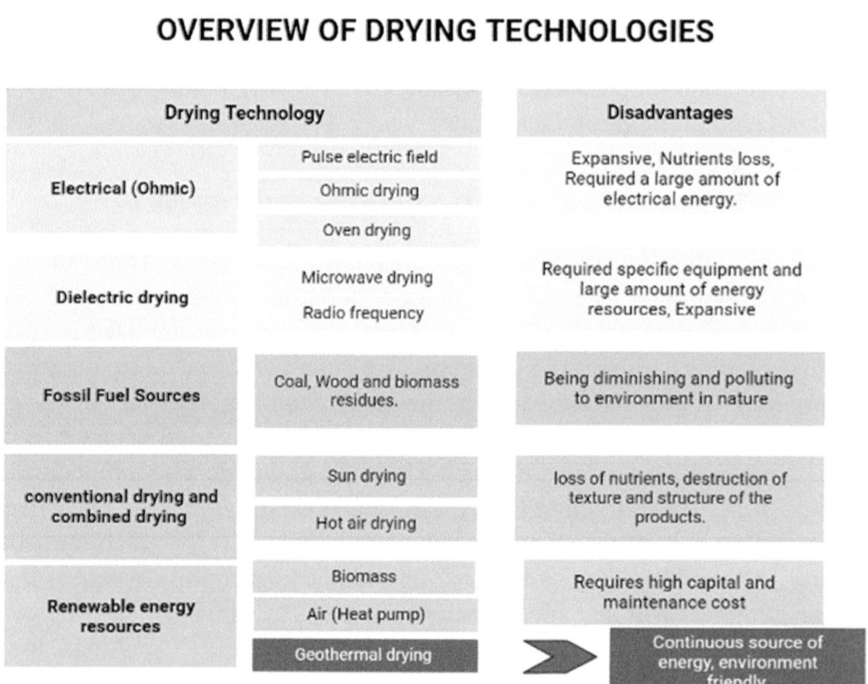

FIGURE 13.1 Briefly explains the different conventional mode of drying process along with their disadvantages.

Geothermal steam energy is used for the drying of tobacco leaves at different flow rates of steam. Increasing the steam velocity enhances the flow rates and drying efficiency. Since the primary goal of drying by geothermal energy is to remove the maximum amount of moisture by using the minimal amount of energy possible, the quality and quantity of produced energy are taken into account throughout the drying process (Helvacı and Akkurt, 2014).

13.6.2 GEOTHERMAL DRYING PROCESS AND EQUIPMENT

Food may rapidly deteriorate as a result of seasonal and environmental changes, and the existence of moisture content makes drying unsatisfactory since it is a discontinuous process. To improve the operation's outputs, constant drying requiring constant heat flow is needed (Reykdal, 2018).

For drying of agricultural produce, the most commonly used heat exchangers which works by increasing the temperature of air for drying purpose are as fellow:

1. Standalone Geothermal Food Drier
2. Geothermal Direct heat exchanger
3. Geothermal Food Dehydrator

13.6.2.1 STANDALONE GEOTHERMAL FOOD DRYER

It works by supplying constant hot drying energy at a constant flow rate via geothermal working fluid. In a standalone food drier, geothermal energy is used in an indirect way (Figure 13.2). Stainless steel trays are used for the drying of grains in the drying chamber. The fan blower is used for creating the pressure of geothermal water in the spray chamber. The fan blower is behind the heat exchanger, and hot air is blown over the food drying trays; waste gases are then moved through the outlet chamber. The temperature of air increases by extracting the heat from geothermal water. It is possible to determine accurate timings for the product quality by carrying out several testing runs. The system can be made commercially viable if the design complies with the specifications (Sumotarto, 2007).

Geothermal energy uses temperatures below 150°C and has low operational costs. Because of this, drying done by geothermal energy is highly suitable for drying agricultural produce. Geothermal fluid is used for the extraction of heat in the form of hot air or steam. This hot air or waste heat from geothermal power plants is used for the drying process at a continuous flow rate. The basic principle is that water is pumped via a blower fan and geothermal fluid inlet, as a heating source. The hot air is then passed onto the food in the drying chamber for the drying of produce. The food trays are stacked over each other in the drying chamber. The temperature of the drying chamber is kept below 40°C, and the moisture is reduced from 80% to 20% in the time period of 24 hours (Reykdal, 2018).

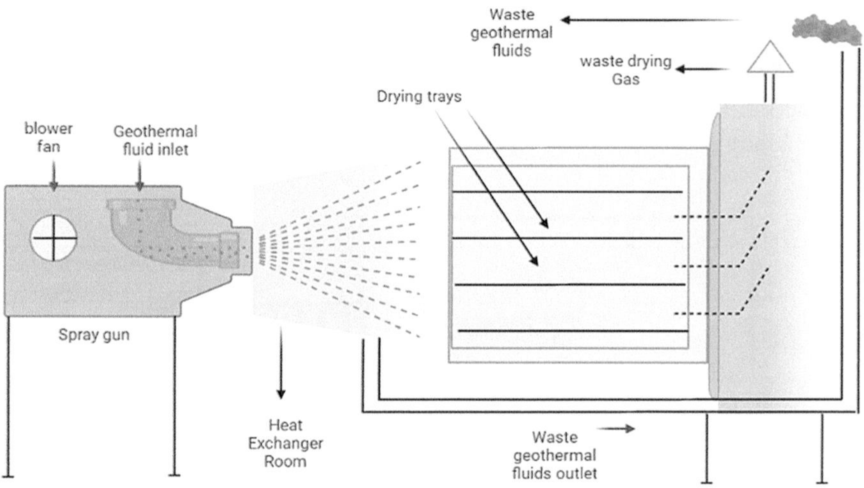

FIGURE 13.2 Explains the standalone geothermal food drier for the drying of agricultural produce.

13.6.2.2 GEOTHERMAL DIRECT HEAT EXCHANGER

Geothermal direct-use equipment is based on the characteristics of geothermal water and the conversion of this water into steam. The quality of geothermal water and its temperature must be considered. The peculiar chemistry of geothermal water may cause different problems, such as scaling and corrosion, to the operating instrument when it comes in contact with flowing geothermal water and steam (Lund et al., 2011). Fluid issues can usually be eliminated from the design of the system. One such instance is the lack of dissolved oxygen in most geothermal waters, with the possible exception of those with the lowest temperatures. Precautions should be made by making use of a proper storage tank in the direct heating of geothermal water by preventing the entry of atmospheric water in hot water (Lund, 2010).

Geothermal direct-use instruments work at low temperatures. The core components of the majority of geothermal direct heat systems include different types of heat extraction units, power units, circulation pumps, distribution and transmission pipes, and backup plants, as shown in Figure 13.3. To handle the highest load, a backup system and peaking system are required (Lund and Toth, 2021). The power unit increases the temperature of geothermal water and converts it into steam, which then goes into the heat exchange unit, which contains different trays for drying agricultural produce. Heat pumps are frequently used when the temperature of the geothermal water is hot (less than 50°C). Many different operational units are used in the equipment utilized in direct-use projects (Lund and Boyd, 2016; Mangi, 2012).

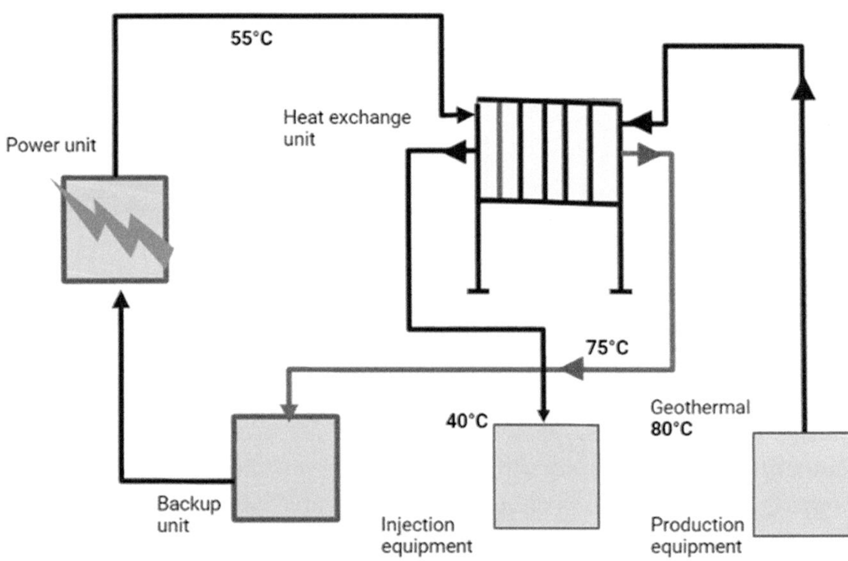

FIGURE 13.3 The equipment of direct geothermal heat exchanger.

13.6.2.3 GEOTHERMAL FOOD DEHYDRATOR

Most agricultural produce falls into the category of highly perishable fruits with a moisture content of 80%. To prevent postharvest losses and preserve the safety and quality parameters of fruits and vegetables without chemicals, dehydration and drying are extensively used. Due to their high moisture content, they are prone to microbial attack.

A geothermal food dehydrator is used for drying purposes (Figure 13.4). The optimum temperature range for bacterial growth is 25°C–45°C. The dehydrator maintains the temperature in the range of above 45°C–below 65°C (Vázquez et al., 1997). At temperatures above 65°C, the fruits and vegetables may perish, lose their texture, and vitamins and minerals are destroyed (Zanoni et al., 1998).

A plate heat exchanger is used to transfer thermal energy from low-enthalpy geothermal fluid (80°C) to water, which is subsequently reinjected into the well. In a finned tube heat exchanger that is positioned within a heating chamber, heated water (about 65°C) transfers heat to air. The air is heated to 55°C by passing through the heating chamber while it is drawn into the drying unit by a fan. Depending on the humidity of each fruit and the temperature of the air, the gradual elimination of moisture in food is a time-consuming process that can take up to 15 hours. When the ultimate moisture content is around 12%, the drying process is complete. Finally, a chimney is used for the removal of air from the drying chamber (Jiménez et al., 2016).

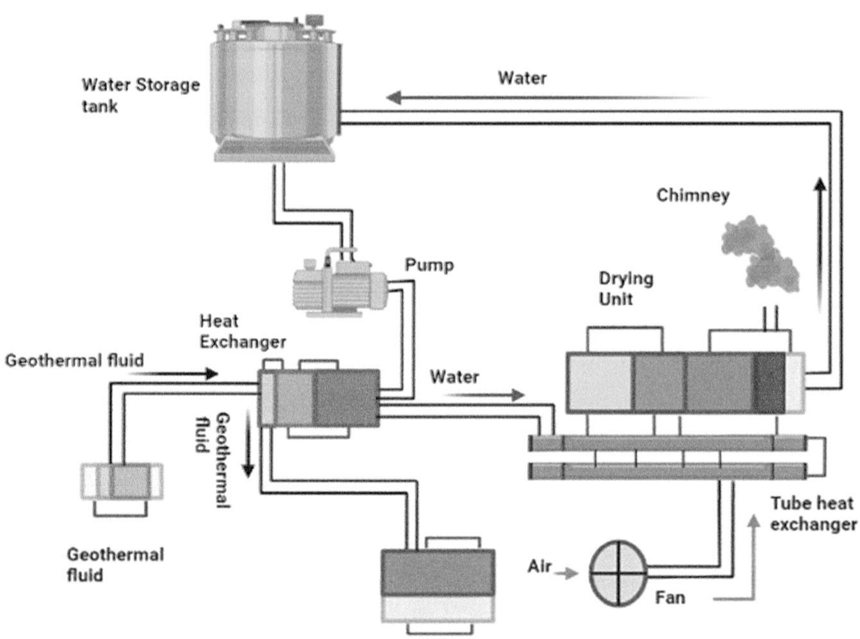

FIGURE 13.4 The equipment of geothermal food dehydrator and the drying mechanism.

Guava, orange, papaya, tomato, kiwi, apple, pineapple, pear, mango, prickly pear, strawberry, star fruit, watermelon, banana, and melon have all been dehydrated using the GFD. Four sensors were placed throughout the dryer at the same time to monitor the operation and maintain temperature and humidity (Khazaei et al., 2008). The trays filled with food are first placed inside the dehydrator, which has already been preheated to 50°C, to begin the dehydrating process. Air has a high level of relative humidity (70%) and an average ambient temperature of 21°C before it enters the heating chamber; after passing through the finned tube heat exchanger, the air's average temperature increases to 48°C, and its relative humidity drops to as low as 19%. The air has a relative humidity of 29% and a temperature of 41°C after exiting the drying chamber. When the humidity of the air entering the drying chamber and the humidity of the air leaving it, the operation is complete (García Torres, 2016; Jiménez et al., 2016).

13.7 ADVANTAGES OF GEOTHERMAL DRYING OF FRESH PRODUCE

Geothermal energy is used to enhance indoor drying technology using heat sources derived from renewable energy resources, an alternate strategy for solving the problem of food losses in the agricultural, livestock, and fishing industries (Abass et al., 2014). Geothermal drying is defined as the removal of water from food that would otherwise allow for the growth of microorganisms or chemical processes (Korese, 2016). On a dry basis, water content is always larger than on a wet basis, regardless of whether the basis is wet or dry. Depending on the kind of food product, the danger of food spoilage increases with increasing water activity (Mujumdar, 2006). Vegetables, fruits, and other grains have all been dried using geothermal energy. The drying of agricultural produce serves a crucial role in preventing waste and ensuring availability of nutrient-rich food throughout the year. Geothermal resources have the greatest potential for use in agricultural drying applications (Arason, 2003). Geothermal energy is the most advantageous method for agricultural processing, considering the significantly lower costs of employing hot water and steam, as opposed to using fossil fuels and electricity (Figure 13.6) (Lund et al., 2004). The estimated 500 MW generation deficit can be reduced by using renewable energy sources like geothermal energy as possible energy sources. However, establishing electricity generation on solar, wind, water, and biomass is inefficient since it depends on the weather. However, geothermal energy has a very high generation capacity and is not entirely reliant on the weather (Richter, 2011).

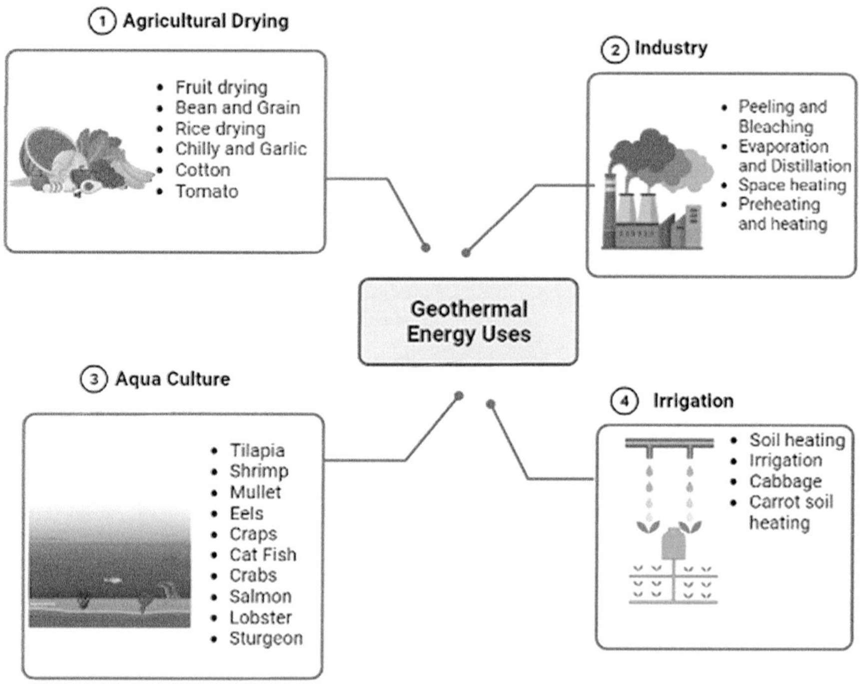

FIGURE 13.5 The possible applications of energy derived from geothermal resources in the agro-industrial sectors and agricultural sectors.

The geothermal energy in the temperature range of 20–150 is used for heating pumps, space heating, and industrial processing systems, while temperatures in the range of about 70–300 are more effective in the generation of steam and electricity. Geothermal energy applications can be classified into 4 different groups, including the heating of greenhouses, production of fish and algae, heating of soil, and agricultural processes (Bakos et al., 1999; Ogola, 2012). Geothermal energy is used in food processing for heating, preheating, evaporation, drying, sterilization, peeling, distillation, and blanching of food by means of geothermal water and geothermal steam in the temperature range of 90–150 (Minh et al., 2015).

Many food processing industries, such as confectionary and wine making, use evaporation and distillation and possess high processing temperatures in the range of 80–130 (Figure 13.7). Blanching and peeling is an important step in pre-processing that requires high temperatures in the range of 77–104. Geothermal hot water and steam are used for pasteurization, sterilization, and UHT treatment given for canning and preservation of food and dairy products, which requires high temperatures of 112–140 (Lund, 1996).

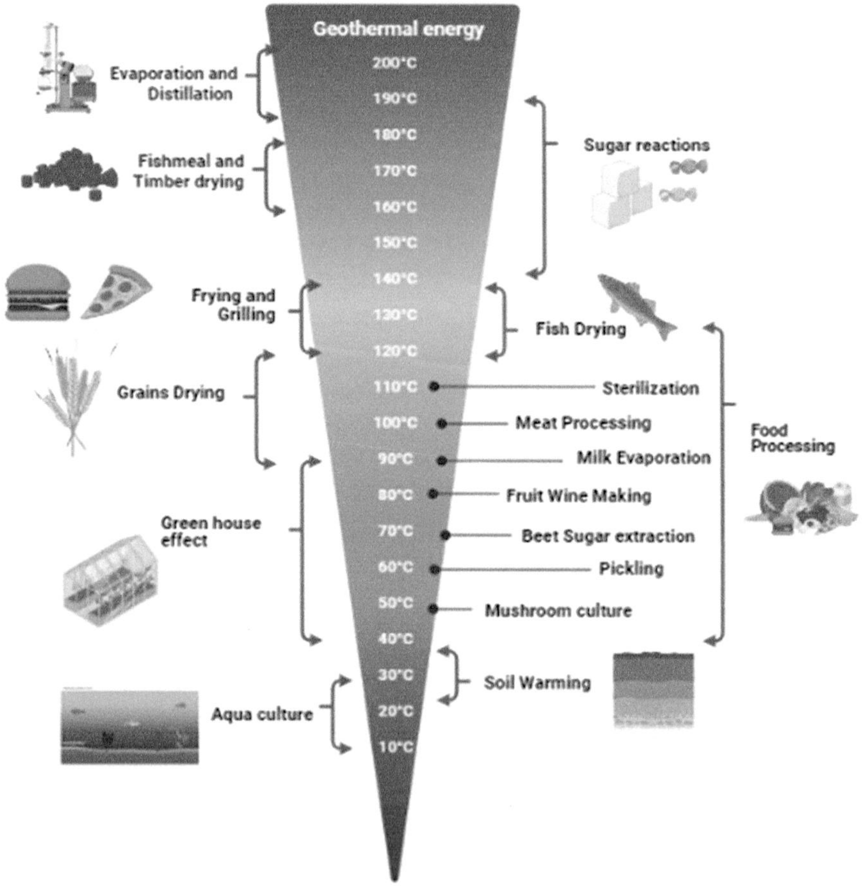

FIGURE 13.6 The geothermal temperature range from low to intermediate and high temperature ranges for agricultural and agro-industrial process.

13.8 CHALLENGES AND LIMITATIONS OF GEOTHERMAL DRYING OF FRESH PRODUCE

The major limitations and challenges to the use of geothermal energy in developing nations' agricultural and food sectors are:

i. Governmental and regulatory barriers
ii. Technical barriers
iii. Financial barriers

13.8.1 GOVERNMENTAL AND REGULATORY BARRIERS

Government policies and laws play a significant role in providing a conducive environment for geothermal investment and resource mobilization, as well as in stimulating both national and international investment from the private sector. Most underdeveloped nations lack the financial means to invest in geothermal exploration and usage (Omenikolo et al., N/A).

13.8.2 TECHNICAL BARRIERS

Technical understanding is required for the development of geothermal systems. It is necessary to have a critical mass of policy analysts, economic managers, engineers, and other experts. However, most emerging nations continue to face a skilled labor shortage. Infrastructure to support geothermal systems, such as transportation and communication networks, is frequently weak or inadequate (Mutumba et al., 2021; Omenikolo et al., N/A).

13.8.3 FINANCIAL BARRIERS

One of the major challenges to geothermal energy development is the high cost of geothermal energy systems. Most developing nations do not have the financial means to invest in the development of geothermal systems. Due to a lack of finance for key phases of geothermal energy deployment, investors are reluctant to take the critical first steps, such as energy resource evaluations or feasibility investigations for geothermal energy development projects (Omenikolo et al., N/A).

13.9 GEOTHERMAL DRYING OF FRUITS AND VEGETABLES

Fruit and vegetable dehydration (or drying) is the earliest means for the preservation of food. Fruits and vegetables are perishable foods with more than 80% moisture content. The drying process removes the bulk of the moisture content and reduces it to approximately 20% in dried fruits and vegetables. Dried fruits and vegetables are processed in the following ways: pre-drying treatments, post-drying treatments, and dehydration (Popovska-Vasilevska, 2003).

As shown in the schematic image Figure 13.8, the entire tomato dehydration process may be separated into three stages: pre-drying preparation (pretreatment), drying, and post-drying treatment. The raw tomatoes are prepared for the dehydration process by pre-drying. This stage begins with the selection of tomatoes based on maturity and soundness. The raw tomatoes are then placed in crates, cleaned to remove dust, dirt, plant pieces, and other debris, cut in half, and placed on stainless steel trays (Popovska-Vasilevska, 2003).

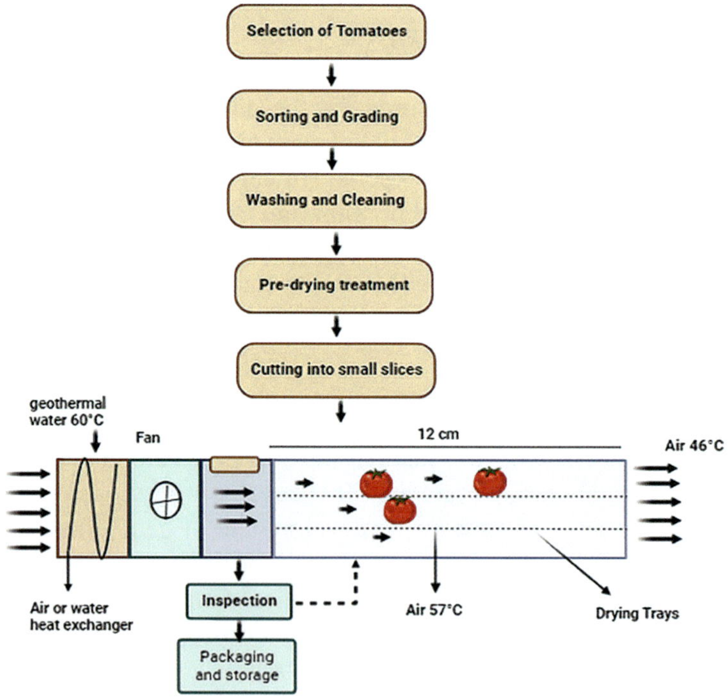

FIGURE 13.7 The systematic flow diagram of dehydration of tomatoes.

13.10 GEOTHERMAL DRYING OF FISH

There are several advantages to utilizing geothermal energy in the processing of fish instead of using other energy resources, which include oil and electricity. Geothermal energy has mostly been used in the fishing sector for drying salted fish, drying cod heads, stock fish, and other items indoors (Figure 13.9). The primary goals of drying processing are to prolong and extend the shelf life of produce and to enhance the time of preservation (Sircar et al., 2016). In most cases, food degradation is triggered by microorganisms, especially pathogenic microbes, and other chemical reactions. During the drying process, the oxidation process is delayed and eventually stopped. The drying time is generally separated into two periods: the first is the continuous and constant drying rate, and the other period is the decreasing drying rate. The drying of cod heads is done by indoor drying, which is divided into two distinct stages: primary drying of produce and secondary drying (Arason, 2003).

A conveyor-belt cabinet is used for primary drying. The best drying conditions are maintained by an 18–25°C temperature range, 20–50% relative humidity, and 3 m/s of air velocity, which is circulated over the produce. The period is around 24–40 hours. At the end of this stage, the moisture content of the heads is around 50–55%. The secondary drying of semi-dried cod heads is carried out in drying chambers of 1–2 m^3 volumes, on which hot air is thrown over them to achieve final drying. The most ideal conditions are: a temperature range of air 22–26°C, humidity 20–50%, and an air velocity of 0.5–1 m/s in a full container. After drying, the cod-heads have a water content of approximately 15% (Ragnarsson, 2005).

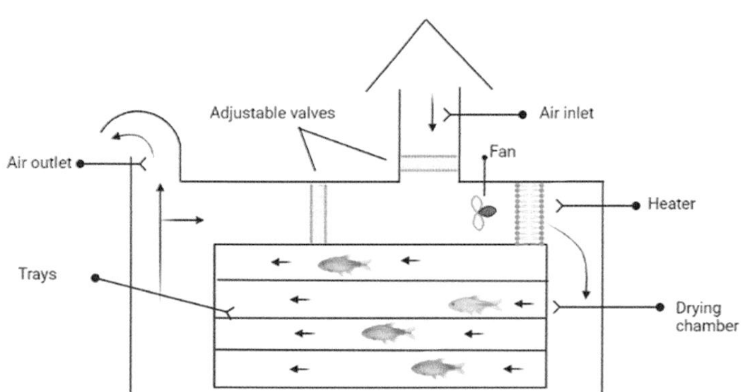

FIGURE 13.8 Geothermal drying chamber for drying of fish.

13.11 CONCLUSION

The most convenient application for drying agricultural produce is done by geothermal energy. This chapter deals with the overview of all drying technology, the advancement in geothermal drying of agricultural produce, the instrumentation, and further application in different food industries. Using geothermal resources replaces the expensive electricity usage and polluting fossil fuels for drying purposes. The drying uses of geothermal energy are confined to high and low temperature ranges for heating and drying agricultural produce. Geothermal energy produces a high-quality product without affecting the environment, reducing the pollution rate, and allowing the preservation of agricultural produce. Despite the numerous benefits of geothermal energy, such applications are currently extremely limited throughout the world.

KEYWORDS

- **fresh produce drying**
- **geothermal energy**
- **greenhouse gas reduction**
- **postharvest preservation**
- **renewable energy applications**
- **sustainable food processing**

REFERENCES

Abass, A. B., Ndunguru, G., Mamiro, P., Alenkhe, B., Mlingi, N., & Bekunda, M. (2014). Post-harvest food losses in a maize-based farming system of semi-arid savannah area of Tanzania. *Journal of Stored Products Research, 57*, 49–57.

Ahmed, N., Singh, J., Chauhan, H., Anjum, P. G. A., & Kour, H. (2013). Different drying methods: Their applications and recent advances. *International Journal of Food Nutrition and Safety, 4*(1), 34–42.

Alamu, O. J., Nwaokocha, C. N., & Adunola, O. (2010). Design and construction of a domestic passive solar food dryer. *Leonardo Journal of Sciences,* (16), 71–82.

Andritsos, N., Dalampakis, P., & Kolios, N. (2003). Use of geothermal energy for tomato drying. *Oregon Institute of Technology Geo-Heat Center Bulletin.*

Arason, S. (2003). The drying of fish and utilization of geothermal energy: The Icelandic experience. *International Geothermal Conference*. Citeseer.

Bakos, G. C., Fidanidis, D., & Tsagas, N. F. (1999). Greenhouse heating using geothermal energy. *Geothermics, 28*, 759–765.

Basaran, A., & Ozgener, L. (2013). Investigation of the effect of different refrigerants on performances of binary geothermal power plants. *Energy Conversion and Management, 76*, 483–498.

Calín-Sánchez, Á., Lipan, L., Cano-Lamadrid, M., Kharaghani, A., Masztalerz, K., Carbonell-Barrachina, Á. A., & Figiel, A. (2020). Comparison of traditional and novel drying techniques and its effect on quality of fruits, vegetables and aromatic herbs. *Foods, 9*, 1261.

Claussen, I. C., Ustad, T. S., Str⊘mmen, I., & Walde, P. M. (2007). Atmospheric freeze drying—A review. *Drying Technology, 25*(6), 947–957.

Doymaz, İ. (2012). Infrared drying of sweet potato (*Ipomoea batatas* L.) slices. *Journal of Food Science and Technology, 49*, 760–766.

Ekezie, F. G. C., Sun, D. W., Han, Z., & Cheng, J. H. (2017). Microwave-assisted food processing technologies for enhancing product quality and process efficiency: A review of recent developments. *Trends in Food Science & Technology, 67*, 58–69.

Falade, K. O., & Igbeka, J. C. (2007). Osmotic dehydration of tropical fruits and vegetables. *Food Reviews International, 23*(4), 373–405.

FAOSTAT. (2010 [2012]). Food and Agriculture Organization of the United Nations. http://faostat.fao.org/site/339/default.aspx (accessed on 9th July 2025).

Fudholi, A., Sopian, K., Bakhtyar, B., Gabbasa, M., Othman, M. Y., & Ruslan, M. H. (2015). Review of solar drying systems with air-based solar collectors in Malaysia. *Renewable and Sustainable Energy Reviews, 51*, 1191–1204.

Gallup, D. L. (2009). Production engineering in geothermal technology: A review. *Geothermic, 38*(3), 326–334.

García Torres, F. (2016). *Viabilidad De Un Proyecto De Aprovechamiento De Energía Geotérmica De Baja Entalpía Al Sector Industrial.*

Hasan, M. U., Malik, A. U., Ali, S., Imtiaz, A., Munir, A., Amjad, W., & Anwar, R. (2019). Modern drying techniques in fruits and vegetables to overcome postharvest losses: A review. *Journal of Food Processing and Preservation, 43*, e14280.

Helvacı, H. U., & Akkurt, G. G. (2014). Thermodynamic performance evaluation of a geothermal drying system. *Progress in Exergy, Energy, and the Environment*, 331–341.

Huang, L. L., & Zhang, M. (2012). Trends in development of dried vegetable products as snacks. *Drying Technology, 30*(5), 448–461.

Indiarto, R., Asyifaa, A. H., Adiningsih, F. C. A., Aulia, G. A., & Achmad, S. R. (2021). Conventional and advanced food-drying technology: A current review. *International Journal of Scientific & Technology Research, 10*, 99–107.

Jiménez, H. M. A., Pérez, P. S., Madrazo, O. V., González, E. P., & Rivera, A. J. (2016). Low-enthalpy geothermal food dehydrator. *Peach, 85*, 18.

Johnston, I. W., Narsilio, G. A., & Colls, S. (2011). Emerging geothermal energy technologies. *KSCE Journal of Civil Engineering, 15*, 643–653.

Kamiloglu, S., Toydemir, G., Boyacioglu, D., Beekwilder, J., Hall, R. D., & Capanoglu, E. (2016). A review on the effect of drying on antioxidant potential of fruits and vegetables. *Critical Reviews in Food Science and Nutrition, 56*(sup1), S110–S129.

Kanoglu, M., Bolatturk, A., & Yilmaz, C. (2010). Thermodynamic analysis of models used in hydrogen production by geothermal energy. *International Journal of Hydrogen Energy, 35*(16), 8783–8791.

Kanoglu, M., Dincer, I., & Rosen, M. A. (2007). Geothermal energy use in hydrogen liquefaction. *International Journal of Hydrogen Energy, 32*(17), 4250–4257.

Khazaei, J., Chegini, G. R., & Bakhshiani, M. (2008). A novel alternative method for modeling the effects of air temperature and slice thickness on quality and drying kinetics of tomato slices: Superposition technique. *Drying Technology, 26*, 759–775.

Kocabiyik, H., & Tezer, D. (2009). Drying of carrot slices using infrared radiation. *International Journal of Food Science & Technology, 44*(5), 953–959.

Korese, J. K. (2016). *Experimental and Modeling Studies of Forced Convection Storage and Drying Systems for Sweet Potatoes*.

Kulasekara, H., & Seynulabdeen, V. (2019). A review of geothermal energy for future power generation. In *2019 5th International Conference on Advances in Electrical Engineering (ICAEE)* (pp. 223–228). IEEE.

Kumar, P. S., & Sagar, V. R. (2014). Drying kinetics and physio-chemical characteristics of osmo-dehydrated mango, guava and aonla under different drying conditions. *Journal of Food Science and Technology, 51*, 1540–1546.

Kumoro, A. C., & Kristanto, D. (2003). Preliminary study on the utilization of geothermal energy for drying of agricultural product. *International Geothermal Conference*, 1–18.

Li, Z. Y., Wang, R. F., & Kudra, T. J. D. T. (2011). Uniformity issue in microwave drying. *Drying Technology, 29*(6), 652–660.

Li, Z., Raghavan, G. S. V., & Orsat, V. (2010). Optimal power control strategies in microwave drying. *Journal of Food Engineering, 99*(3), 263–268.

Lingayat, A., Chandramohan, V. P., & Raju, V. R. K. (2017). Design, development and performance of indirect type solar dryer for banana drying. *Energy Procedia, 109*, 409–416.

Lund, J. W. (1996). *Lectures on Direct Utilization of Geothermal Energy*. United Nations University Geothermal Training Programmed, Reykjavik, Iceland.

Lund, J. W. (2010). Direct utilization of geothermal energy. *Energies, 3*, 1443–1471.

Lund, J. W., & Boyd, T. L. (2016). Direct utilization of geothermal energy: 2015 worldwide review. *Geothermic, 60*, 66–93.

Lund, J. W., & Toth, A. N. (2021). Direct utilization of geothermal energy: 2020 worldwide review. *Geothermic, 90*, 101915.

Lund, J. W., Freeston, D. H., & Boyd, T. L. (2005). Direct application of geothermal energy: 2005 worldwide review. *Geothermic, 34*, 691–727.

Lund, J. W., Freeston, D. H., & Boyd, T. L. (2011). Direct utilization of geothermal energy: 2010 worldwide review. *Geothermic, 40*, 159–180.

Lund, J., Sanner, B., Rybach, L., Curtis, R., & Hellström, G. (2004). Geothermal (ground-source) heat pumps: A world overview. *Geo-Heat Center Quarterly Bulletin, 25*.

Mangi, P. (2012). Geothermal resource optimization: A case of the geothermal health spa and demonstration center at the Olkaria geothermal project. *Short Course VII on Exploration for Geothermal Resources*, UNU-GTP, GDC and KenGen, Lake Bogoria and Lake Naivasha, Kenya, October.

Mehta, B. K., Jain, S. K., Sharma, G. P., Doshi, A., & Jain, K. H. (2013). Response surface optimization of osmotic dehydration process parameters for button mushroom (*Agaricus bisporus*) Part I. *Focusing on Modern Food Industry, 2*(2), 91–102.

Minh, V. N., Arason, S., Gissurarson, M., & Pálsson, P. G. (2015). *Uses of Geothermal Energy in Food and Agriculture: Opportunities for Developing Countries*. Food and Agriculture Organization of the United Nations (FAO).

Miranda, M., Maureira, H., Rodríguez, K., & Vega-Gálvez, A. (2009). Influence of temperature on the drying kinetics, physicochemical properties, and antioxidant capacity of *Aloe vera* (*Aloe barbadensis* Miller) gel. *Journal of Food Engineering, 91*(2), 297–304.

Misha, S., Mat, S., Ruslan, M. H., Sopian, K., & Salleh, E. (2013). Review on the application of a tray dryer system for agricultural products. *World Applied Sciences Journal, 22*(3), 424–433.

Motevali, A., Minaei, S., Khoshtaghaza, M. H., & Amirnejat, H. (2011). Comparison of energy consumption and specific energy requirements of different methods for drying mushroom slices. *Energy, 36*(11), 6433–6441.

Mujumdar, A. S. (2006). *Handbook of Industrial Drying*. CRC Press.

Mujumdar, A. S. (2014). 15 Impingement drying. In *Handbook of Industrial Drying* (p. 371).

Mujumdar, A. S., & Law, C. L. (2010). Drying technology: Trends and applications in postharvest processing. *Food and Bioprocess Technology, 3*, 843–852.

Mutumba, G. S., Echegu, S., & Adaramola, M. S. (2021). Prospects and challenges of geothermal energy in Uganda. *Journal of Energy Research and Reviews, 9*, 47–58.

Ngala, G. M., Oumarou, M. B., & Oluwole, F. A. (2015). Review of geothermal energy technology and its potential for power generation in Borno Basin, Nigeria. *Annals of Borno, 25*(1), 81–90.

Ogola, P. F. (2012). The power to change: Creating lifeline and mitigation-adaptation opportunities through geothermal energy utilization (Doctoral dissertation) University of Iceland, Iceland.

Omenikolo, A. I., Obasi, I. B., & Nleonu, E. C. (2020). Application of geothermal energy in agriculture: a review. *Int J Eng Appl Sci Technol, 5*(1), 666–673.

Omolola, A. O., Jideani, A. I., & Kapila, P. F. (2017). Quality properties of fruits as affected by drying operation. *Critical Reviews in Food Science and Nutrition, 57*(1), 95–108.

Parikh, D. M. (2015). Vacuum drying: Basics and application. *Chemical Engineering, 122*(4), 48–54.

Popovska-Vasilevska, S. (2003). Drying of agricultural products with geothermal energy. *International Summer School on Direct Application of Geothermal Energy*.

Qu, H., Masud, M., Islam, M., Khan, M. I. H., Ananno, A. A., & Karim, A. (2022). Sustainable food drying technologies based on renewable energy sources. *Critical Reviews in Food Science and Nutrition, 62*, 6872–6886.

Ragnarsson, A. (2005). Geothermal development in Iceland 2000–2004. In *Proceedings* (pp. 24–29).

Ramazankhani, M. E., Mostafaeipour, A., Hosseininasab, H., & Fakhrzad, M. B. (2016). Feasibility of geothermal power assisted hydrogen production in Iran. *International Journal of Hydrogen Energy, 41*(41), 18351–18369.

Reykdal, Ó. (2018). Drying and storing of harvested grain: A review of methods. *Skýrsla Matís*, 05-18.

Richter, A. (2011). Private company exploring 200 MW project in Bangladesh. *Think GeoEnergy*. https://www.thinkgeoenergy.com (accessed on 9th July 2025).

Sagar, V. R., & Suresh Kumar, P. (2010). Recent advances in drying and dehydration of fruits and vegetables: A review. *Journal of Food Science and Technology, 47*, 15–26.

Schmidt, S. J., & Fontana Jr, A. J. (2020). E: Water activity values of select food ingredients and products. In *Water Activity in Foods: Fundamentals and Applications* (pp. 573–591).

Schössler, K., Jäger, H., & Knorr, D. (2012). Novel contact ultrasound system for the accelerated freeze-drying of vegetables. *Innovative Food Science & Emerging Technologies, 16*, 113–120.

Schuster, A., Karellas, S., Kakaras, E., & Spliethoff, H. (2009). Energetic and economic investigation of Organic Rankine Cycle applications. *Applied Thermal Engineering, 29*(8, 9), 1809–1817.

Sircar, A., Yadav, K., & Sahajpal, S. (2016). Overview on direct applications of geothermal energy. *International Advanced Research Journal in Science, Engineering and Technology, 3*, 128–137.

Sontakke, M. S., & Salve, S. P. (2015). Solar drying technologies: A review. *International Journal of Engineering Science, 4*(4), 29–35.

Stober, I., & Bucher, K. (2013). *Geothermal Energy*. Springer-Verlag Berlin Heidelberg. https://doi.org/10.1007/978-3-642-13352-7 (accessed on 9th July 2025).

Sumotarto, U. (2007). Design of a geothermal energy drier for beans and grains drying in Kamojang Geothermal Field, Indonesia. *GHC Bulletin, 28*, 13–18.

Svalova, V. (2018). Geothermal energy. In Bobrowsky, P. T., & Marker, B. (Eds.), *Encyclopedia of Engineering Geology*. *Encyclopedia of Earth Sciences Series*. Springer, Cham.

Vázquez, T., Arnéz, S., Fernández, M., & Fernández, J. (1997). *Manual De Secado Solar Técnico De Alimentos*. Energética.

Wray, D., & Ramaswamy, H. S. (2015). Novel concepts in microwave drying of foods. *Drying Technology, 33*(7), 769–783.

Yamamoto, T., Furuhata, T., Arai, N., & Mori, K. (2001). Design and testing of the organic Rankine cycle. *Energy, 26*, 239–251.

Zanoni, B., Peri, C., Nani, R., & Lavelli, V. (1998). Oxidative heat damage of tomato halves as affected by drying. *Food Research International, 31*, 395–401.

CHAPTER 14

Toward Sustainability Through Postharvest Value Addition

PREETINDER KAUR,[1,*] JAGBIR REHAL,[2] GAGANJYOT KAUR,[1] and GURJEET KAUR[1]

[1]Department of Processing and Food Engineering, Punjab Agricultural University, Ludhiana, Punjab, India

[2]Department of Food Science and Technology, Punjab Agricultural University, Ludhiana, Punjab, India

*Corresponding author

ABSTRACT

The processing of various fruits and vegetables generates a huge amount of waste, which invariably ends up in landfills or as animal feed. There is a rising demand to reduce post-harvest food loss and wastage to make the post-harvest value addition process highly sustainable. Efforts are being made by researchers to utilize these food wastes that are not only rich in bioactive components but also have high nutritional value. Protein is one such highly valuable component, which is in high demand owing to its ability to address the rampant malnutrition in underdeveloped and developing nations. The growing interest in newer and cheaper sources of protein that are non-animal based has given impetus to the global drive towards quality protein isolation from fruit and vegetable processing wastes. This chapter intends to focus on the technologies and processes for valorization of food processing waste through protein extraction for enhanced sustainability.

Sustainable Approaches in Postharvest Handling and Management: Pankaj B. Pathare (Ed.)

DOI: 10.1201/9781779641076-14

14.1 INTRODUCTION

The name "protein" comes from the word *proteois*, meaning "first place." Proteins constitute the most diverse group of molecules due to their structure and functions. They are polymers composed of amino acid monomers with a central carbon atom attached to an amino group ($-NH_2$) at one end, a carboxyl group (–COOH) at the other end, a hydrogen atom, and an R group. There are 20 different amino acid side groups, or R groups, ranging from a single hydrogen atom to complex carbon chains or rings. The difference in the side chains gives them their unique behavior and characteristics, differentiating them into different groups.

- Non-polar amino acids: Alanine, Valine, Leucine, Isoleucine, Glycine, Cysteine, Phenylalanine, Tryptophan, Methionine, proline.
- Uncharged polar amino acids: Serine, Threonine, Tyrosine, Asparagine, Glutamine
- Negatively charged (acidic) polar amino acids: Aspartic acid, Glutamic acid
- Positively charged (basic) polar amino acids: Lysine, Arginine, Histidine

The amino acid chains are linked together with peptide bonds to form proteins. Based on the protein structure, these are divided as primary, secondary, tertiary, and quaternary protein structures. The bioavailability of protein is primarily influenced by the nature of amino acids, peptide bonds, and its structure. They have an important role in maintaining the structure and function of the living system. Foods rich in protein, having appreciable amounts of essential amino acids, are needed to support growth and good health. Protein undernutrition has various implications, resulting in stunting, anemia, physical weakness, edema, vascular dysfunction, and impaired immunity; hence, adequate consumption of high-quality protein is essential for optimal growth, development, and health in humans (Wu, 2016). As per the estimates of WHO (2006), the requirement of protein for an average adult is 0.66 g/kg bodyweight/d, with a population safe level set at 0.83 g/kg bodyweight/d, provided that the protein source has a protein digestibility-corrected amino score of 1.0.

The world's population may exceed 9 billion by 2050 (FAO, 2009), and this will result in an increasing demand for food. In a major part of the world, malnutrition and micronutrient deficiency are still rampant.

To meet this increasing demand, alternate and sustainable sources of protein must be explored, like the plant waste materials and byproducts of the processing industries, which will also help to regulate and reduce food wastage. Proteins are sought after as food components not only for their nutritional value but also for the functionality they lend when incorporated into various foods. In order to make the harvesting of protein from the byproduct viable, it is important to know about the protein content as well as the protein value.

Alternate protein sources that aim to replace or substitute conventional plant and animal food sources are of growing interest in the research community for meeting the ever-growing global demand for proteins in a sustainable manner. The plant-based protein sources as an alternative to meats have invariably been soya bean and peas primarily (Schreuders et al., 2016). The abundant quantity of fruits and vegetables processing wastes, which are generated both in organized and unorganized sectors all over the world, are usually not effectively utilized and are often used as animal feed or landfills. According to Padayachee et al. (2015), about 50% of the original weight of fruits becomes waste during its post-harvest handling as peels, pomaces, seeds, and unripe or damaged fruits, which is not at all sustainable keeping in view the demand for good nutrition. One of the sustainable alternatives to meet the nutritional security of protein malnutrition is from the by-products of processing, which are rich in proteins.

Table 14.1 tabulates the percent of stones, kernels, and seeds constituted by various fruits and vegetables. These seeds are the plant's food reserve needed during its early growth period and are a storage source of nutrition consisting of proteins, peptides, lipids, and carbohydrates (Garcia et al., 2016). Table 14.2 deals with the amount of crude protein present in these fruit and vegetable by-products consisting of seeds.

For a waste material to be utilized as a source of protein, it should meet essentially 3 criteria's; have good protein content, have good quality protein (in terms of essential amino acids) and be devoid of toxic substances (Kamal et al., 2021).

As evident from the Table 14.2, the seeds and kernels are a rich source of protein with appreciable amounts of essential amino acids and can be utilized by extraction of proteins from the seeds or the seed cake/meal left after the oil extraction. Various conventional and modern techniques are being followed to do the same and are discussed further.

TABLE 14.1 Estimate of Percent Waste in Terms of Seed/Kernel

Commodity	% Waste Fruit Weight Basis		References
Guava	6–12		Mohamed et al. (2011)
Jackfruit seeds	8–15		Madruga et al. (2014)
Mango seed	20–60 (Kernel 45–75% of seed weight)		Diarra et al. (2014)
Orange seeds	Up to 10		Rosas et al. (2022)
Papaya seeds	6.5–15		Desai et al. (1995)
Prunus Family	Seed %	Kernel %	Kamel and Kakuda (1992)
Apricot	7.1	31.5	
Cherry	6.3	26.6	
Nectarine	7.6	7.3	
Peach	5.8	6.8	
Plum	2.8	9.1	
Tamarind seeds	34		Sarkar et al. (2018)

14.2 PROTEIN EXTRACTION

Protein extraction from plants, fruits, and vegetables, and their by-products and waste, requires disintegration of the tissues and cells for the release of proteins, peptide bonds, and amino acids. The presence of vacuoles, diversity in the nature of proteins, variability in the thickness of the tissue, cell wall, and presence of lipids, phenols, and other bioactive components poses hurdles in their extraction (González-García et al., 2014). To overcome these hurdles, different methods are reported for sample preparation and extraction techniques/methods (Figure 14.1).

Sample preparation is an important preliminary step, which includes drying, grinding, and sieving. These steps inhibit microbial activity, encourage the disintegration of tissues, and help achieve uniformity in particle size, respectively. Smaller particle size allows for a higher contact area, enabling higher extraction rates. Different methods are reported with variations in solvents, their concentrations, extraction times, and conditions. To further enhance the extraction yield of proteins, electric energy, ultrasound, and microwave-assisted extraction, and the use of nanomaterials are reported at the lab scale. The conventional methods, as well as advanced liquid – liquid extraction techniques, have been summarized in Table 14.3 and Table 14.4, respectively. The extraction of proteins can be classified based on the physical state of waste/by-products (insoluble/soluble).

TABLE 14.2 Protein Content and Amino Acid in Fruit Waste

Fruits (Scientific Name)	Commodity	g/100g Crude Protein	Amino Acids (mg/g Protein)	References
Apricot *(Prunus armeniaca)*	Kernels	14.6–49.3	Histidine, Isoleucine, Threonine, Tryptophan	Akhone et al. (2022); Kamel and Kakuda (1992); Özcan et al. (2010)
Apricot	Press cake	34.3–43.4	Histidine 29.0 Isoleucine 37.0 Leucine 70.0 Lysine 33.0 Phenylalanine 57.0 Methionine 6.0 Tryptophan 10.0 Valine 46.0	Ferreira et al. (2015); Yin et al. (2020)
Bitter gourd (*Momordica charantia*)	Seeds	25.0	Lysine 98.7 Isoleucine 30.7 Leucine 60.5 Methionine 23.6 Threonine 17.4 Valine 36.7 Histidine 40.9	Gayathry and John (2022); Saeed et al. (2018)
Cherry (*Prunus avium*)	Kernels	29.3–44.4	Histidine Isoleucine Threonine Tryptophan	Kamel and Kakuda, 1992
Palm (*Arecaceae*)	Defatted oil palm kernel meal	54.8	–	Kiat et al. (2014)
Orange (*Citrus sinesis*)	Defatted orange seed meal	17.9–26.5	–	Mahato et al. (2018); Rosas et al. (2022)
Cherry (*Prunus avium*)	Defatted sour cherry seed	42.1	Histidine 21.6 Isoleucine 40.3 Leucine 82.1 Lysine 11.2 Methionine 9.8 Phenylalanine 52.0 Threonine 59.2 Aspartic acid 117 Glutamic acid 273.7	Garcia-Aguilar et al. (2015)
Guava (*Psidium guayava*)	Seeds	7.6	Lysine 0.91 Isoleucine 4.05 Leucine 5.93 Methionine 3.52 Threonine 3.93 Valine 5.35 Histidine 2.02 Tryptophan 2.64	El Anany (2015); Prasad and Azeemoddin (1994)

TABLE 14.2 *(Continued)*

Fruits (Scientific Name)	Commodity	g/100g Crude Protein	Amino Acids (mg/g Protein)	References
Jack fruit (*Artocarpus heterophyllus*)	Seeds	16.01	Lysine 10.30 Isoleucine 8.61 Leucine 6.73 Methionine 4.82 Threonine 3.90 Valine 1.73 Histidine 1.92	Sultana et al. (2017)
Mango (*Mangifera indica*)	Kernel	10	Lysine 3.13 Isoleucine 3.23 Phenylalanine 4.46 Valine 3.8 Leucine 8.4 Tyrosine 3.17 lacks tryptophan g/100 g	Patel and Kheni (2018)
Mango (*Mangifera indica*)	Seeds	6–7.76	Leucine 6.9 Isoleucine 4.4 Methionine 1.2 Phenylalanine 3.4 Lysine 4.3 Threonine 3.4 Tyrosine 2.7 Valine 5.8 g/100 g protein	Abdalla et al. (2007)
Oil palm (*Elaeisguineensis*)	Kernels	12–16		Zahari and Alimon (2003)
Papaya (*Carica papaya*)	Seeds	24.9	Lysine 4.21 Isoleucine 3.09 Leucine 7.78 Methionine 1.30 Threonine 2.85 Valine 2.25 Histidine 2.21 g/100 g protein	Azevêdo et al. (2012); Dakare et al. (2011)
Peach (*Prunus persica*)	Kernels	43.0 42.2	Lysine 5.5 Isoleucine 5.65 Leucine 3.20 Methionine 0.21 Threonine 28.08 Valine 13.72 Histidine 4.23 Tryptophan 0.49 µg/g	Kamel and Kakuda (1992); Sun et al. (2022)
Plum (*Prunus domestica*)	Kernels	1.16	–	Ertekin et al. (2006)
Pumpkin (*Cucurbita maxima*)	Kernel cake	53.0	Leucine 34.5 Phenyl alanine 25.2 Valine 24.9 mg/g	Prandi et al. (2019)

TABLE 14.2 *(Continued)*

Fruits (Scientific Name)	Commodity	g/100g Crude Protein	Amino Acids (mg/g Protein)	References
Pumpkin (*Cucurbita maxima*)	Seeds	39.22	Limiting AA Methionine 1.83 Tryptophan 1.10 Sufficient AA Arginine 15.80, Glutamic acid 23.23 Aspartic acid 9.56 g/100 g protein	Alfawaz (2004)
Tamarind (*Tamarindus indica*)	Kernels	24.61	Rich in Isoleucine Leucine Lysine Histidine Methionine Phenylalanine Threonine, Tryptophan Valine	Sarkar et al. (2018); De Lumens et al. (1986)
Tomato (*Solanum lycopersicum*)	Seeds	27.4	Lysine Glutamic acid Aspartic acid	Dhillon et al. (2016); Baker et al. (2022)
Watermelon (*Citrullus lanatus*)	Meal	56.15	Arginine Glutamic acid Aspartic acid Leucine	Wani et al. (2008)
Watermelon (*Citrullus lanatus*)	Seeds	16.34	Arginine, Glutamic acid, Aspartic acid, Leucine	Wani et al. (2008)

*AA-Amino acids.

i. Insoluble waste comprises of pits, kernels, and peels.
ii. Soluble (recovery of components from the wastewater released from the processing units).

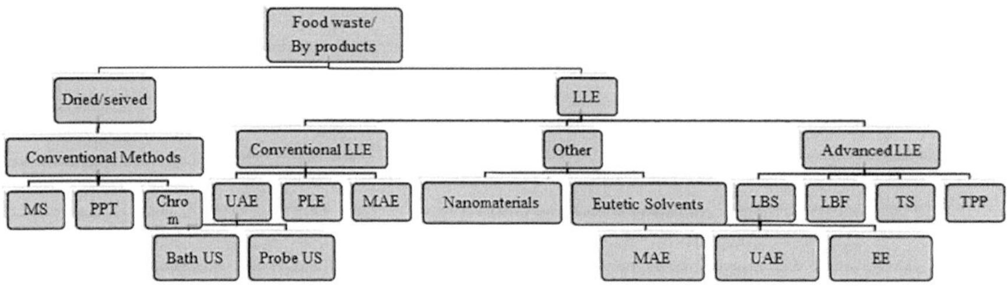

FIGURE 14.1 Different methods used for protein extraction from food waste and by-products.

*MembraneSeparation (MS), Precipitation (PPT), Chromatography (Chrom), Ultrasound Assisted Extraction (UAE), Pressurized Liquid Extraction (PLE), Microwave Ultrasound Assisted Extraction (MAE), Liquid Liquid Extraction (LLE), Liquid Biphasic System (LBS), LiquidBiphasic Flotation (LBF), Thermo-separation (TS), Three Phase Partitioning (TPP), Electric Energy (EE).

Liquid biphasic separation comprises of the advanced techniques to overcome the limitations of LLE by integrating various processes.

14.2.1 CHALLENGES IN THE USAGE OF CONVENTIONAL AND UNCONVENTIONAL EXTRACTION TECHNIQUES

The hydrophobic and aromatic amino acids are documented for imparting a bitter taste to protein, limiting its usage as an additive in food (Aluko, 2015). A wide range of solvents are reported for the extraction of proteins, including organic solvents, polluting reagents, and non-food grade solvents. This limits their future application in food processing/food enrichment. Additionally, the high extraction costs and lower yield limit the industrial application of the extraction processes (Galvan et al., 2020). Research on innovative extraction methods is important to minimize the costs and maximize their yield.

14.3 UTILIZATION OF PROTEINS EXTRACTED FROM FRUITS AND VEGETABLE PITS/SEEDS IN FOODS

In recent years, attempts have been made by researchers to incorporate nutritionally rich waste/by-products from fruit and vegetable industries

TABLE 14.3 Conventional Methods Used for the Separation of Proteins

Conventional Methods	Working Principle	Technologies Included / Particle Size	Advantages	Limitations
Membrane separation	Separation based on the particle size	Microfiltration Ultrafiltration Nanofiltration	Devoirs chemical usage Reduced energy consumption. Easy to scale up Require less space	Loading limits of membrane Emulsification on the membrane High investment Large solvent inventory
Precipitation	Introduction of salts, organic polymers, polar and non-polar solvents, allowing the separation of protein as precipitate	–	Can be applied to continuous process. Scalable Simple Storage stability	–
Chromatography	The separation of molecules occurs between the movement of stationery and mobile phase	Ionic Exchange Surface Adsorption Partition Size exclusion	–	Research is at nascent stage and needs further studies
Solvent Extraction (Liquid-liquid Extraction)	Based on the movement of the targeted analyte from one phase to another when two immiscible analytes come in contact	–	Simple Low cost Ease of scaling up Shorter time of phase separation Certified by regulatory bodies	Mostly related to recovery of proteins from the effluent/wastewater of food processing industry. Large volumes of reagents required. Involve multiple steps, large processing times. Formation of emulsion in habiting the process

TABLE 14.4 Advantages and Limitations of Advanced Liquid-Liquid Extraction Techniques

Advanced Liquid-Liquid Extraction Techniques	Working Principle	Advantages	Limitations
Liquid Biphasic System (LBS)	Employs water soluble polymers with either inorganic salt of polymer at the critical concentration.	High recovery of the proteins Satisfactory purification factor Potential recycling of the components Excellent results in partitioning the bioactive compounds	Difficulties in recycling the phase forming components. The yield and quality id dependent upon the pH, molecular weight of polymer, salt and polymer concentration, temperature
Liquid Biphasic Flotation (LBF)	–	Simple, fast and inexpensive Better selectivity, scale-up, process integration, continuous operations, high yield over LBS	–
Three phase partitioning (TPP)	Uses inorganic salt with crude protein and tert-butanol extract. The hydrophobic part of the protein binds to the tert-butanol, reducing the density which enables it to move up towards the denser mixture. Three layers are formed	High purity High recovery of proteins and enzymes Fewer steps Simple procedure	The formation of phases formed is dependent on the molecular weight and isoelectric point.

in different food formulations to enhance the nutritional value of foods. Bakery items have been chosen for this purpose as they are highly consumed worldwide. Other reasons for such wide popularity include being ready-to-eat, cheap, having good nutrition, a variety of tastes, and shelf-stability. However, they contain a high sugar content and low amounts of minerals and fibers, which makes them nutrition-deficient. Hence, incorporating a nutrient-rich ingredient in baked foods can be a perfect solution to enhance nutritional quality as well as to manage food processing waste.

Mango kernel, a waste generated after removal of mango pulp, is composed of 69.22–79.78% carbohydrates, 8.35–16.13% fat, 5.6–9.5% protein, 92% starch, and a fair amount of fiber (0.14%–2.95%). Legesse and Emire (2012) investigated mango seed kernel flour to prepare a value-added product by incorporating it in biscuit dough along with wheat flour. The formulations containing a blend of mango seed kernel flour (10, 20, 30%) and wheat flour (90, 80, 70%) indicated more protein content as compared to mango seed kernel flour. Maximum protein content (9.78 g/100 g) was reported for a blend having 10% mango seed kernel flour and 90% wheat flour, indicating that the major contributor of protein enhancement in prepared biscuits was wheat flour. Fig seeds are separated as waste during the production of ethyl alcohol, and they are considered unsuitable for consumption or further use. Bölek (2021) used fig seed powder (FSP), which was added to wheat flour at 5, 10, and 15% concentration levels, and biscuits were prepared. The quality analysis of biscuits revealed that the protein-rich fig seeds resulted in an enhancement of the protein content of biscuits, which ranged between 10.10–11.02%, along with increased dietary fiber, ash, total phenolic content, and antioxidant activity of the biscuits.

Another fruit processing waste with an impressive nutritional composition is pumpkin seed, and it is considered an attractive substitute for nutritional improvement of foods. Pumpkin seeds contain substantial amounts of protein (25 to 37%) and oil (37 to 45%) and are used as a protein supplement (whole or flour) for human consumption. Kaur and Sharma (2017) evaluated the nutritional composition of cookies prepared by incorporating pumpkin seeds in refined wheat flour. It substantially enhanced the protein content (8.29%) along with fat (28.97%), fiber, and ash content of cookies (2.50 and 2.52% respectively). Another bakery product, a muffin, was prepared by replacing cereal flours with pumpkin seed flour (5–30%) (Rana et al., 2022). The protein content was higher in pumpkin muffins supplemented with seed kernel flour (11.73%) compared to whole seed flour (9.76%). Öztürk and Turhan (2020) used pumpkin seed kernel (PSK) flour as an ingredient in meatballs. The physico-chemical analysis reported an increase in the protein content of meatballs from 16.78 to 20.28% as the concentration of PSK increased from 0 to 12%, indicating an improvement in the nutritional profile of meatballs.

Ferreira et al. (2015) prepared flour from solid residue obtained after juice extraction from fruits (orange, passion fruit, and watermelon) and vegetables (mint, rocket, lettuce, spinach, and taro), which presented 95.20 g/kg protein content. Biscuits and cereal bars prepared using this flour indicated maximum protein content in bittersweet biscuits (102.90 g/kg) and salty cereal bars (143.20 g/kg) due to a higher amount of flour. Hence, it has great potential to enhance the nutritional quality of baked goods. In a recent study, Yalcin et al. (2022) prepared muffins using whole wheat (*Triticum aestivum L.*), whole siyez wheat (*Triticum monococcum L.*), and whole oat (*Avena sativa L.*) flours formulated with 7.5 and 15% grape seed flour. The muffins had protein contents ranging from 7.86 (whole siyez wheat) to 9.65 g/100 g (whole wheat muffin cake with 15% GSF). The addition of GSF in all samples exhibited an increase by 12% in whole wheat muffins, 10% in whole siyez wheat muffins, and 7% in whole oat muffins by substituting these with 15% of GSF.

Watermelon (*Citrullus lanatus*) is one of the most under-utilized fruits grown in the tropical and subtropical areas (Koocheki et al., 2007). After consumption of juicy mesocarp, seeds are discarded as a waste. Anang et al. (2018)analyzed the use of this nutrient-rich seed (15–20%) to improve upon the nutritional value of bread. Proximate composition of bread indicated that defatted watermelon seed flour (WSF) had highest protein content (45%) due to oil removal and intensification of proteins and minerals followed by bread prepared from dough containing 25% WSF. Protein being an essential constituent for growth and development, its presence in bread in significant quantities (10%–14%) is a breakthrough in food formulation. A similar study on use of WSF in cookies as protein supplement have been conducted by Kausar (2020). The cookies formulated with 0, 10, 20, 30 and 40% WSF substitution with wheat flour indicated that cookies had 12.47, 11.21, 10.97, 9.73, 8.48% protein in cookies containing 40, 30, 20, 10, 0% WSF, indicating a positive influence of WSF addition on protein content of cookies.

By removal of the seed coat, a tamarind kernel is obtained, which is ground to a fine particle size to obtain tamarind kernel powder (TKP).

Presently, TKP is primarily being utilized as an important sizing material in the textile and jute industries for merchandising purposes. Its potential in food formulations was assessed by Rani Sarkar et al. (2018) by formulating instant chutney mixes made from coconut, groundnut, and coriander, added with 50 g of TKP. A significant improvement in the protein content (1.71–5.42 g/100 g) of the coriander chutney mix was recorded due to the addition of TKP. A similar trend was observed for the protein content of noodles prepared from TKP incorporated into wheat flour. As the tamarind kernel proportion varied from 50–20%, a parallel change in the protein content of noodles was observed, that is, 15.26–12.73% (Ananthu and Singh, 2018).

14.4 APPLICATIONS

The proteins derived from plant sources have the potential to fulfill various demands of both the food and non-food sectors (Figure 14.2). The proteins are used in foods due to their nutritional value, structural integrity, and presence of health-promoting compounds. The proteins in non-food applications are adopted as they contain non-protein impurities and anti-nutritional factors, which are undesirable in foods. The applications of plant proteins are discussed below.

14.4.1 FOOD SECTOR

14.4.1.1 NUTRITION

Plant proteins facilitate full nutrition to humans due to the presence of essential amino acids and vital macronutrients. A protein-rich diet offers a plethora of benefits to humans by supporting growth, muscle/bone metabolism, development of the nervous system, and agility in old age (Ranganathan Janet, 2016). Protein is obtained from different plant sources, viz., cereals, legumes, pseudo-cereals, nuts and almonds, and seeds. The quality of protein from different sources is measured in terms of the protein digestibility-corrected amino acid score (PDCAAS), which is >0.9 for animal proteins, whereas the plant protein sources, viz., gluten, sorghum, maize, and rice, have 0.25, 0.20–0.30, 0.46, and 0.47 PDCAAS scores, respectively. Thus, animal proteins are considered superior compared to plant proteins. To achieve better quality protein, protein isolates and concentrates are produced, which provide PDCAAS scores close to 1 (e.g., soy protein concentrate: 1, canola protein concentrate: 0.93). Thus, people having higher protein requirements for energy and protein synthesis adopt protein supplements in the form of isolates and concentrates. Moreover, the production of protein hydrolysates, concentrates, and isolates is an attractive step to mitigate waste management and cater to the demand for high-value products by the growing population worldwide (Venuste et al., 2013). The pumpkin seed residue obtained after oil extraction constitutes 70% protein, which is considered waste. Thus, the defatted residues containing a huge content of proteins and fibers have great potential to act as functional ingredients for human nutrition (Mattila et al., 2018). Similarly, canola meals obtained after oil extraction have around 50% proteins possessing a well-balanced amino acid profile for human nutrition. Rapeseed meal also holds good scope to enhance the nutrition of foods, as its defatted meal provides lysine and sulfur amino acid-rich protein (40%).

14.4.1.2 MEAT ANALOGS

Meat analogues (or meat substitutes) are plant-based products that imitate the appearance, flavor, and texture of animal meat. Despite the fact that animal proteins are nutritionally rich, a diet based on meat can be associated with health issues due to the presence of cholesterol and saturated fatty acids (Vang et al., 2008). Contrarily, plant-based foods exhibit a reduced risk towards cardiovascular disease, blood pressure, diabetes, and mortality (Mohamed et al., 2017; Springmann et al., 2018). Other factors, such as ethical and religious beliefs, also limit the intake of animal-based proteins (Dekkers et al., 2018). Thus, food processing industries are focusing on the development of meat-free products (nuggets, patties, sausages, etc.) from non-animal protein sources to substitute animal proteins (Boukid, 2021). A few years back, by-products of the oil extraction units, such as soy meals, were frequently used as animal feed. However, nowadays, these residues are finding their way to produce protein-rich meat analogues owing to their easy availability, low cost, balanced amino acid composition, and good properties such as gelling property and water-holding capacity (Röös et al., 2014). The utilization of soy, however, declined with time because of certain antinutritional factors and hence a negative effect on health (Nemecek et al., 2016). Another source, that is, gluten from wheat, is being used based on its unique film-forming property, which forms small fibers when used in meat analogues. Sunflower and rapeseed meals are also utilized as an ingredient to form meat analogues. In addition to this, many crops are evaluated for their protein content, and their derivatives in the form of concentrates or isolates are used in meat analogues (Röös et al., 2014).

14.4.1.3 GLUTEN REPLACEMENT

Celiac disease (CD) is a common enteropathy which is triggered by the consumption of grains, viz. wheat, barley, rye, and oats containing gluten. It is quite prevalent worldwide, affecting approximately 1% of the population (Deora et al., 2015).

To deal with it, the production of gluten-free products is in demand using non-gluten proteins. The addition of non-gluten proteins improves amino acid balance along with the enhancement of structural and textural properties of dough. Furthermore, the color and sensory characteristics of the final product also improve, which increases consumer acceptance. Among plant proteins, cereals such as zein and kaffirin have been used as an ingredient in gluten-free bread formulation (Deora et al., 2015; Pontieri et al., 2013). Andersson et al. (2011) reported improved dough rheology by the addition of corn protein in bread making, along with improved bread structure and loaf volume. Another gluten-free protein can be derived from legumes. Due to high lysine content, legumes are considered nutritionally superior to cereals, as lysine (a limiting amino acid) is absent in cereals. Most common proteins from this category are soy and pea protein isolates and concentrates. The addition of pea proteins in muffins provided a soft and elastic texture (Matos et al., 2014). However, excessive soy proteins negatively affect the quality of gluten-free products. Ribotta et al. (2004) reported better volume and structure of breads prepared by the addition of enzyme-active soybean flour over the flours with inactivated enzymes. Another protein, rapeseed protein, can also be utilized as a novel food ingredient to produce gluten-free foods. Korus et al. (2021) observed that the addition of rapeseed protein enhanced yellowness and limited staling of bread during storage.

14.4.1.4 FOOD FORMULATIONS

Apart from the utilization of proteins as supplements, gluten replacers, meat analogs, and so forth, the unique functional properties of proteins make these an interesting ingredient in different food formulations, viz., whipped creams, salad dressings, desserts, bakery, soups, and sauces. The functionality of proteins is attributed to the globular component, which affects their solubility due to the amphiphilic nature of molecules. Proteins contain both nonpolar (bounded inwardly) and polar (exposed outwardly) amino acid residues, which favor dipole-dipole bonding with the surrounding aqueous medium by twisting as well as unfolding these amino acid chains. Consequently, as the polar groups orient themselves at the surface, a developed network forms gels, holds water, absorbs fat, foams, emulsifies, and dissolves under various pH conditions (Aryee et al., 2017). These techno-functional characteristics of plant proteins have been reported for soybean, kidney bean, mung bean, lentils, sorghum (Sá et al., 2022). Wani et al. (2015) used watermelon seed cake to fortify cookies. A significant improvement was observed in dough stability and nutritional, textural, and sensory properties of cookies. The proteins isolated from rapeseed, soybean, pea, lupin, and chickpea indicated outstanding foaming properties (comparable to egg protein) due to high solubility, surface hydrophobicity, and net charge (Sun-Waterhouse et al., 2014).

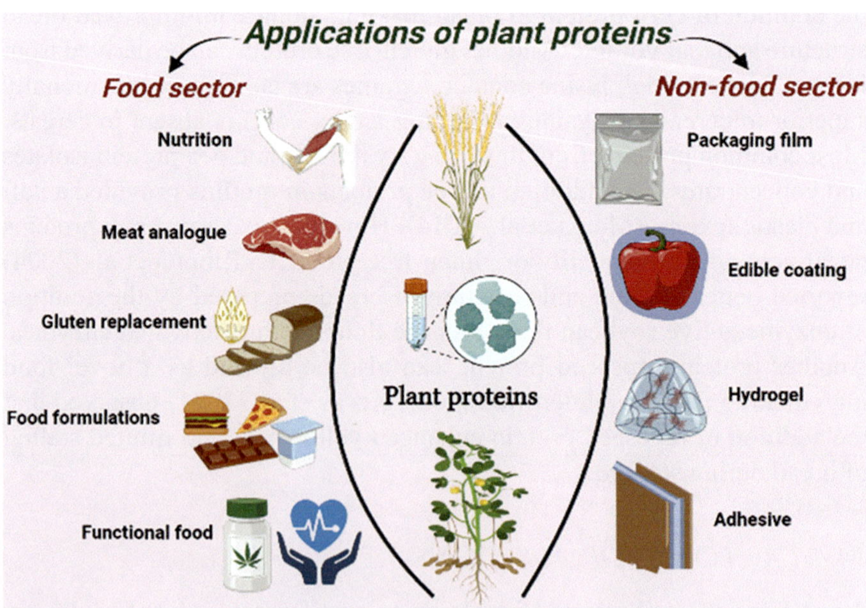

FIGURE 14.2 Applications of plant proteins in food and non-food sector.

Furthermore, the oil holding capacities (OHC) of peanut protein isolates were reported to be significantly better as compared to soybean protein isolates (He et al., 2014). A study on the analysis of rapeseed products reported poor gelation properties (Tan et al., 2011). Soybean protein isolate is serving as a gelling agent in semi-solid food products, especially for meat analogues (Bessada et al., 2019).

14.4.1.5 FUNCTIONAL FOODS

The plant proteins have been investigated for their potential as functional foods. The primary components of plants, such as carotenoids and flavonoids, provide several health benefits. Plant-based proteins also have shown health effects by acting as antitumor, antioxidant, ACE inhibitor, antimicrobial, hypoglycemic, and hypolipidemic agents (Luna-Vital et al., 2015; Luna-Vital and González de Mejía, 2018). It is evident from the studies that countries including a good amount of pulses reported less risk of type-2 diabetes, colorectal cancer, cardiovascular diseases, and other chronic diseases (Campos-Vega et al., 2010; Sánchez-Chino et al., 2015). The small peptides released because of enzymatic hydrolysis (by various proteases) provide bioactivities in pulse proteins (Awika and Duodu, 2017) and thus, are also used as foods, functional ingredients, and nutraceuticals. A review reported bioactive properties of proteins (pea, lupin, fava bean, rice, oat, hemp, and lentil) by examining blood glucose, insulin, and/or appetite-regulating hormones to assess their efficiency (Lonnie et al., 2020). Comparison of proteins from animal and plant sources provided heterogeneous results. Thus, elaborated studies on plant proteins as well as bioactive peptides are needed.

14.4.2 NON-FOOD SECTOR

14.4.2.1 PACKAGING FILMS

The prime objective of packaging film is to control the migration of vapor, moisture, and gases between food and its surroundings to improve quality and shelf life (Chen et al., 2019). Protein-based films present a poor moisture barrier due to their polar and hydrophilic nature, which limits their adoption as packaging. However, they have good oxygen barrier properties compared to films prepared from polysaccharides and lipids.

Soy protein-based films have oxygen permeability 500, 540, and 670 times lower than that of polyethylene, starch, and pectin, respectively. The commonly used plant-based proteins in food packaging are wheat gluten, zein, and soy protein, and so forth. Wheat gluten-based films have selective gas permeability and are successful in controlling respiratory gaseous exchange in packaged perishable foods (Murrieta-Martínez et al., 2018). Deepika et al. (2021) prepared a film using wheat gluten protein and polyvinyl alcohol (PVA) polymer and found that the incorporation of gluten enhanced the biodegradability and mechanical properties of packaging. Zein is hydrophobic and water-insoluble owing to its amino acid sequences. This unique structure leads to low water vapor permeability and water solubility. A film composed of zein and pomegranate peel extract offered an enhanced shelf life by exhibiting outstanding water barrier, strength, flexibility, antimicrobial, and antioxidant effects on Himalayan cheese (Mushtaq et al., 2018). Soy is the most analyzed protein in the packaging industry, and it can be solubilized in water by using heat and pH adjustment (Vieira et al., 2011). The soy protein-based film is an attractive approach for packaging due to its low cost and biodegradable nature. Another plant protein from lentil was used to prepare an edible film, which indicated high transparency and low water solubility, as reported by Aydogdu et al. (2018). Thus, these proteins could be considered an excellent component for edible film production.

14.4.2.2 EDIBLE COATING

An edible coating is applied in liquid form over the food surface to improve its efficiency to preserve foods by incorporating antimicrobial, antioxidant, and anti-browning agents (Garavand et al., 2022). Soy protein, being the extensively used component in packaging, was explored for edible coating along with thyme oil to preserve Barhi dates in cold storage (Yousef et al., 2020). This coating was successful in maintaining firmness and lowest pectinase enzyme activity. Mahfoudhi and Hamdi (2015) reported reduced ethylene production and respiration rate when cherries were coated with almond gum and Gum Arabic during storage at 2°C. The fruits' color, firmness, and weight loss also changed negligibly during storage. Mahfoudhi et al. (2014) worked on a novel coating from almond gum to preserve tomatoes. It was considered ideal, as the coating delayed ripening and weight loss of tomatoes. Another important protein, that is, zein, was used with chitosan by Salajegheh et al. (2020) to formulate an edible coating, applied to Mazafati dates. It was evident from the findings that the zein coating reduced the level of *Aspergillus Niger* fungi. Thus, the authors recommended the use of zein in food applications. Malt spent grain, a by-product from the brewing process, has a promising reuse potential as it contains a significant number of proteins, fibers, and phenolic compounds (Fărcaş et al., 2015). Moreover, it is a cheap and easily available alternative for the formation of biodegradable film with antioxidant activity.

14.4.2.3 HYDROGELS

Hydrogels are a polymeric network with a three-dimensional structure, which are hydrophilic in nature and tend to absorb fluids around 1000 times their weight. This unique structure is synthesized by crosslinking polymers induced by heat and cold setting of globular proteins. Hot set or cold set mechanisms denature proteins and expose their functional groups to the surrounding medium, which further interact with bioactive compounds through hydrogen-bonding and hydrophobic and electrostatic interactions. These interactions can be modified by controlling the structure and texture of the gel for carrying a specific compound (Egan et al., 2014). The structure of a protein contains acidic and basic groups which can accept or donate protons to change the gel structure and modulate the release behavior of the encapsulated component based on the pH of the target medium (Dan Ramdath et al., 2017). Hydrogels are now used in biosensors, regenerative medicines, pharmaceuticals, food additives, super absorbents, wound dressings, and regulated drug delivery (Raghavendra et al., 2015; Tang et al., 2012).

The most common plant proteins used in hydrogels are soybean protein (Abaee et al., 2017). Hydrogels from soybean protein isolates postulated poor riboflavin-transport due to a higher swelling ratio and rapid enzymatic degradation as compared to double-network hydrogels synthesized from corn fiber gum and soybean protein isolate. This reveals their suitability as an oral delivery medium for thermolabile bioactive compounds in the food industry (Yan et al., 2020).

14.4.2.4 ADHESIVES

The chemical-based adhesives can be replaced with proteins due to their structure. The unfolding of proteins resulting from denaturation exposes hydrophobic groups, which provide water-resistant protein-based adhesives. The active groups protein molecule surface reacts with crosslinking agents and form structures which act as adhesive agents. Although the adhesive properties of proteins are not equivalent to chemical adhesives, protein-based adhesives such as cottonseed protein or meal are suitable for the wood and particle board industry (Li et al., 2019). Liu et al. (2018) studied camelina-based protein for its application in the plywood industry as an adhesive. Camelina protein, a by-product after oil extraction, was used with polymeric amine epichlorohydrin as an adhesive. It generated small proteins which provided limited solubility due to increased hydrophobicity. Another study reported high resistance and shear strength offered by cottonseed proteins than soy proteins (Cheng et al., 2017).

14.5 INTERVENTIONS FOR ADOPTION OF PLANT-BASED PROTEINS

Animal proteins are considered of high quality due to the balanced proportion of essential and non-essential amino acids. However, the deficiency of some nutritional constituents in plant proteins limits their adoption as a protein source in diets. Other factors affecting the consumer choice about plant proteins are less bioavailability and digestibility, in contrast to animal proteins. Most grains lack lysine, and pulses have less methionine, cysteine, and tryptophan. Thus, to attract consumers toward plant proteins, a few strategies are being adopted to enhance the overall value of plant-based proteins, as follows:

- To achieve PDCAAS score 1 or close to 1, isolated plant-based proteins are made free from anti-nutritional compounds as in soybean.
- Fortification of plant proteins with the required amino acids is great option to perform protein synthesis with improved nutritional quality of plant protein. Fortification of soy proteins with leucine, isoleucine, and valine has reported an increased whole-body protein synthesis.

- Blending the accurate combination of proteins will also facilitate a complete source of amino acids. The proteins from peas and rice have a lower PDCAAS score, whereas a combined protein from these two represented a PDCAAS value of 1.00 (Day, 2013).

Thus, incorporation/fortification, blending, and modification are effective strategies to enhance the nutritional quality and welcome new growth opportunities for plant-based proteins in the food industry.

14.6 CONCLUSION AND FUTURE SCOPE

A rapid rise in population is also accompanying an increase in protein demand. Thus, food industries are actively looking for alternate protein sources. Animal proteins are considered the best source of nutrition; however, environmental, health, and ethical factors are motivating consumers to shift towards plant proteins. Agro-industrial waste and by-products hold exceptional perspective in the field of sustainable protein resources. These sources present a golden opportunity to fulfill nutritional requirements for humans. The diverse functions of proteins due to the structural arrangement within proteins make them suitable for food formulations by acting as emulsifying, gelling, and thickening agents due to water-holding, foaming, and fat absorption capacities. Proteins commonly used in food industries are nutrition supplementation, meat analogue formation, gluten replacement, functional ingredients, and modulating techno-functional properties. Apart from this, proteins also serve different non-food areas by developing edible films/coatings, hydrogels, adhesives, and so forth.

The documented literature on the utilization of proteins from plant waste is scarce in terms of nutritional composition and the prospect of their adoption in human nutrition. The increased concern about plant protein sources necessitates advanced processing and isolation techniques to achieve high-quality protein. Moreover, the techniques for adequate product formulation need improvement to achieve a nutritionally rich diet. These proteins derived from plants also contain some antinutritional factors which affect the bioavailability and absorption of minerals and proteins. The future use of proteins depends upon research innovations to remove these undesirable compounds and unpleasant flavors. The protein's structure study at the molecular level needs to be explored to understand the functionalities and formation of fibrous structures such as meat analogues which mimic meat texture. More research is demanded on the health benefits of plant proteins based on clinical trials and functionalities of plant proteins in terms of food ingredient/product development, compared with the proteins from other origins.

KEYWORDS

- **agro-industrial byproducts**
- **alternative protein sources**
- **food processing waste valorization**
- **plant-based proteins**
- **protein extraction technologies**
- **sustainable nutrition**

REFERENCES

Abaee, A., Mohammadian, M., & Jafari, S. M. (2017). Whey and soy protein-based hydrogels and nano-hydrogels as bioactive delivery systems. In *Trends in Food Science and Technology, 70*, 69–81. https://doi.org/10.1016/j.tifs.2017.10.011 (accessed on 9th July 2025).

Abdalla, A. E., Darwish, S. M., Ayad, E. H., & El-Hamahmy, R. M. (2007). Egyptian mango by-product 1. Compositional quality of mango seed kernel. *Food Chemistry, 103*(4), 1134–1140.

Akhone, M. A., Bains, A., Tosif, M. M., Chawla, P., Fogarasi, M., & Fogarasi, S. (2022). Apricot kernel: Bioactivity, characterization, applications, and health attributes. *Foods, 11*, 1–15.

Alfawaz, M. A. (2004). Chemical composition and oil characteristics of pumpkin (*Cucurbita maxima*) seed kernels. *Food Science and Agriculture, 2*(1), 5–18.

Anang, D. A., Pobee, R. A., Antwi, E., Obeng, E. M., Atter, A., Ayittey, F. K., & Boateng, J. T. (2018). Nutritional, microbial and sensory attributes of bread fortified with defatted watermelon seed flour. *International Journal of Food Science and Technology, 53*(6), 1468–1475. https://doi.org/10.1111/ijfs.13727 (accessed on 9th July 2025).

Ananthu, S., & Singh, J. K. (2018). Development and quality evaluation of noodles prepared from wheat flour supplemented with tamarind kernel powder. *International Journal of Scientific Research in Science and Technology, 7*(4), 285–293. www.ijsrst.com (accessed on 9th July 2025).

Andersson, H., Öhgren, C., Johansson, D., Kniola, M., & Stading, M. (2011). Extensional flow, viscoelasticity and baking performance of gluten-free zein-starch doughs supplemented with hydrocolloids. *Food Hydrocolloids, 25*(6), 1587–1595. https://doi.org/10.1016/j.foodhyd.2010.11.028 (accessed on 9th July 2025).

Aryee, A. N. A., Agyei, D., & Udenigwe, C. C. (2017). Impact of processing on the chemistry and functionality of food proteins. In *Proteins in Food Processing* (2nd ed., pp. 27–45). Elsevier. https://doi.org/10.1016/B978-0-08-100722-8.00003-6 (accessed on 9th July 2025).

Awika, J. M., & Duodu, K. G. (2017). Bioactive polyphenols and peptides in cowpea (*Vigna unguiculata*) and their health promoting properties: A review. *Journal of Functional Foods, 38*, 686–697.

Aydogdu, A., Kirtil, E., Sumnu, G., Oztop, M. H., & Aydogdu, Y. (2018). Utilization of lentil flour as a biopolymer source for the development of edible films. *Journal of Applied Polymer Science, 135*(23). https://doi.org/10.1002/app.46356 (accessed on 9th July 2025).

Azevêdo, J. A. G., Valadares Filho, S. C., Pina, D. S., Detmann, E., Pereira, L. G. R., Valadares, R. F. D., & Benedeti, P. B. (2012). Nutritional diversity of agricultural and agro-industrial by-products for ruminant feeding. *Arquivo Brasileiro de Medicina Veterinária e Zootecnia, 64*, 1246–1255.

Baker, P. W., Preskett, D., Krienke, D., Runager, K. S., Hastrup, A. C. S., Charlton, A., & Charlton, A. (2022). Pre-processing waste tomatoes into separated streams with the intention of recovering protein: Towards an integrated fruit and vegetable biorefinery approach to waste minimization. *Waste and Biomass Valorization, 13*(8), 3463–3473. https://doi.org/10.1007/s12649-022-01748-3 (accessed on 9th July 2025).

Bessada, S. M. F., Barreira, J. C. M., & Oliveira, M. B. P. P. (2019). Pulses and food security: Dietary protein, digestibility, bioactive and functional properties. *Trends in Food Science and Technology, 93*, 53–68. https://doi.org/10.1016/j.tifs.2019.08.022 (accessed on 9th July 2025).

Bölek, S. (2021). Effects of waste fig seed powder on quality as an innovative ingredient in biscuit formulation. *Journal of Food Science, 86*(1), 55–60. https://doi.org/10.1111/1750-3841.15548 (accessed on 9th July 2025).

Boukid, F. (2021). Plant-based meat analogues: From niche to mainstream. *European Food Research and Technology, 247*, 297–308. https://doi.org/10.1007/s00217-020-03630-9 (accessed on 9th July 2025).

Campos-Vega, R., Loarca-Piña, G., & Oomah, B. D. (2010). Minor components of pulses and their potential impact on human health. *Food Research International, 43*, 461–482. https://doi.org/10.1016/j.foodres.2009.09.004 (accessed on 9th July 2025).

Chen, H., Wang, J., Cheng, Y., Wang, C., Liu, H., Bian, H., Pan, Y., Sun, J., & Han, W. (2019). Application of protein-based films and coatings for food packaging: A review. *Polymers, 11*(12). https://doi.org/10.3390/polym11122039 (accessed on 9th July 2025).

Cheng, H. N., Ford, C., Dowd, M. K., & He, Z. (2017). Effects of phosphorus-containing additives on soy and cottonseed protein as wood adhesives. *International Journal of Adhesion and Adhesives, 77*, 51–57. https://doi.org/10.1016/j.ijadhadh.2017.03.008 (accessed on 9th July 2025).

Dakare, M. A., Ameh, D. A., & Agbaji, A. S. (2011). Biochemical assessment of daddawa food seasoning produced by fermentation of pawpaw (*Carica papaya*) seeds. *Pakistan Journal of Nutrition.*

Dan Ramdath, D., Padhi, E. M. T., Sarfaraz, S., Renwick, S., & Duncan, A. M. (2017). Beyond the cholesterol-lowering effect of soy protein: A review of the effects of dietary soy and its constituents on risk factors for cardiovascular disease. *Nutrients, 9*(4). https://doi.org/10.3390/nu9040324 (accessed on 9th July 2025).

Day, L. (2013). Proteins from land plants–Potential resources for human nutrition and food security. *Trends in Food Science and Technology, 32*(1), 25–42. https://doi.org/10.1016/j.tifs.2013.05.005 (accessed on 9th July 2025).

Deepika, K., Praveena, P. L., Srisugamathi, G., & Nisha, J. N. (2021). Development and evaluation study of polyvinyl alcohol with gluten film. *Materials Today: Proceedings, 45*, 597–602. https://doi.org/10.1016/j.matpr.2020.02.389 (accessed on 9th July 2025).

Dekkers, B. L., Boom, R. M., & van der Goot, A. J. (2018). Structuring processes for meat analogues. *Trends in Food Science and Technology, 81*, 25–36. https://doi.org/10.1016/j.tifs.2018.08.011 (accessed on 9th July 2025).

Deora, N. S., Deswal, A., & Mishra, H. N. (2015). Functionality of alternative protein in gluten-free product development. *Food Science and Technology International, 21*(5), 364–379. https://doi.org/10.1177/1082013214538984 (accessed on 9th July 2025).

Desai, U. T., Wagh, A. N., Salunkhe, D. K., & Kadam, S. S. (1995). *Handbook of Fruit Science and Technology: Production, Composition, Storage and Processing*. CRC Press.

Dhillon, G. S., Kaur, S., Oberoi, H. S., Spier, M. R., & Brar, S. K. (2016). Agricultural-based protein by-products: Characterization and applications. In *Protein Byproducts* (pp. 21–36). Academic Press.

Diarra, S. S. (2014). Potential of mango (*Mangifera indica* L.) seed kernel as a feed ingredient for poultry: A review. *World's Poultry Science Journal, 70*(2), 279–288.

Egan, T., O'Riordan, D., O'Sullivan, M., & Jacquier, J. C. (2014). Cold-set whey protein microgels as pH modulated immobilization matrices for charged bioactive. *Food Chemistry, 156*, 197–203. https://doi.org/10.1016/j.foodchem.2014.01.109 (accessed on 9th July 2025).

El Anany, A. M. (2015). Nutritional composition, antinutritional factors, bioactive compounds and antioxidant activity of guava seeds (*Psidium* Myrtaceae) as affected by roasting processes. *Journal of Food Science and Technology, 52*, 2175–2183.

Engelen, M. P., Rutten, E. P., De Castro, C. L., Wouters, E. F., Schols, A. M., & Deutz, N. E. (2007). Supplementation of soy protein with branched-chain amino acids alters protein metabolism in healthy elderly and even more in patients with chronic obstructive pulmonary disease. *The American Journal of Clinical Nutrition, 85*(2), 431–439.

Ertekin, C., Gozlekci, S., Kabas, O., Sonmez, S., & Akinci, I. (2006). Some physical, pomological and nutritional properties of two plum (*Prunus domestica* L.) cultivars. *Journal of Food Engineering, 75*(4), 508–514.

FAO. (2009). *How to Feed the World in 2050*. http://www.fao.org/fileadmin/templates/wsfs/docs/expert_paper/How_to_Feed_the_World_in_2050.pdf (accessed on 9th July 2025).

Fărcaş, A. C., Socaci, S. A., Dulf, F. V., Tofană, M., Mudura, E., & Diaconeasa, Z. (2015). Volatile profile, fatty acids composition and total phenolics content of brewers' spent grain by-product with potential use in the development of new functional foods. *Journal of Cereal Science, 64*, 34–42. https://doi.org/10.1016/j.jcs.2015.04.003 (accessed on 9th July 2025).

Ferreira, M. S. L., Santos, M. C. P., Moro, T. M. A., Basto, G. J., Andrade, R. M. S., & Gonçalves, É. C. B. A. (2015). Formulation and characterization of functional foods based on fruit and vegetable residue flour. *Journal of Food Science and Technology, 52*(2), 822–830. https://doi.org/10.1007/s13197-013-1061-4 (accessed on 9th July 2025).

Garavand, F., Cacciotti, I., Vahedikia, N., Rehman, A., Tarhan, Ö., Akbari-Alavijeh, S., Shaddel, R., Rashidinejad, A., Nejatian, M., Jafarzadeh, S., Azizi-Lalabadi, M., Khoshnoudi-Nia, S., & Jafari, S. M. (2022). A comprehensive review on the nanocomposites loaded with chitosan nanoparticles for food packaging. *Critical Reviews in Food Science and Nutrition, 62*(5), 1383–1416. https://doi.org/10.1080/10408398.2020.1843133 (accessed on 9th July 2025).

García, M. C., González-García, E., Vásquez-Villanueva, R., & Marina, M. L. (2016). Apricot and other seed stones: Amygdalin content and the potential to obtain antioxidant, angiotensin I converting enzyme inhibitor and hypocholesterolemia peptides. *Food & Function, 7*(11), 4693–4701.

García-Aguilar, L., Rojas-Molina, A., Ibarra-Alvarado, C., Rojas-Molina, J. I., Vázquez-Landaverde, P. A., Luna-Vázquez, F. J., & Zavala-Sánchez, M. A. (2015). Nutritional value and volatile compounds of black cherry (*Prunus serotina*) seeds. *Molecules, 20*(2), 3479–3495.

Gayathry, K. S., & John, J. A. (2022). A comprehensive review on bitter gourd (*Momordica charantia* L.) as a gold mine of functional bioactive components for therapeutic foods. *Food Production, Processing and Nutrition, 4*(1), 1–14.

He, X. H., Liu, H. Z., Liu, L., Zhao, G. L., Wang, Q., & Chen, Q. L. (2014). Effects of high pressure on the physicochemical and functional properties of peanut protein isolates. *Food Hydrocolloids, 36*, 123–129. https://doi.org/10.1016/j.foodhyd.2013.08.031 (accessed on 9th July 2025).

Kamal, H., Le, C. F., Salter, A. M., & Ali, A. (2021). Extraction of protein from food waste: An overview of current status and opportunities. *Comprehensive Reviews in Food Science and Food Safety, 20*(3), 2455–2475.

Kamel, B. S., & Kakuda, Y. (1992). Characterization of the seed oil and meal from apricot, cherry, nectarine, peach and plum. *Journal of the American Oil Chemists' Society, 69*, 492–494.

Kaur, M., & Sharma, S. (2017). Formulation and nutritional evaluation of cookies supplemented with pumpkin seed (*Cucurbita moschata*) flour. *Chemical Science Review and Letters, 6*(24). https://www.researchgate.net/publication/331400140 (accessed on 9th July 2025).

Kausar, T. (2020). Utilization of watermelon seed flour as protein supplement in cookies. *Pure and Applied Biology, 9*(1). https://doi.org/10.19045/bspab.2020.90024 (accessed on 9th July 2025).

Kiat, S., Ismail, A., & Yanagita, T. (2014). Biochemical characterization of the soluble proteins, protein isolates and hydrolysates from oil palm (*Elaeis guineensis*) kernel. *Food Bioscience, 7*, 1–10. https://doi.org/10.1016/j.fbio.2014.05.003 (accessed on 9th July 2025).

Koocheki, A., Razavi, S. M. A., Milani, E., Moghadam, T. M., Abedini, M., Alamatiyan, S., & Izadkhah, S. (2007). Physical properties of watermelon seed as a function of moisture content and variety.

Korus, J., Chmielewska, A., Witczak, M., Ziobro, R., & Juszczak, L. (2021). Rapeseed protein as a novel ingredient of gluten-free bread. *European Food Research and Technology, 247*(8), 2015–2025. https://doi.org/10.1007/s00217-021-03768-0 (accessed on 9th July 2025).

Legesse, M. B., & Emire, S. A. (2012). Functional and physicochemical properties of mango seed kernels and wheat flour and their blends for biscuit production. *African Journal of Food Science and Technology, 3*(9), 193–203.

Li, J., Jin, M., & Li, H. (2019). Exploring spatial influence of remotely sensed PM2.5 concentration using a developed deep convolutional neural network model. *International Journal of Environmental Research and Public Health, 16*(3). https://doi.org/10.3390/ijerph16030454 (accessed on 9th July 2025).

Liu, H., Bean, S., & Sun, X. S. (2018). Camelina protein adhesives enhanced by polyelectrolyte interaction for plywood applications. *Industrial Crops and Products, 124*, 343–352. https://doi.org/10.1016/j.indcrop.2018.07.068 (accessed on 9th July 2025).

Lonnie, M., Laurie, I., Myers, M., Horgan, G., Russell, W. R., & Johnstone, A. M. (2020). Exploring health-promoting attributes of plant proteins as a functional ingredient for the food sector: A systematic review of human interventional studies. *Nutrients, 12*(8), 1–29. https://doi.org/10.3390/nu12082291 (accessed on 9th July 2025).

Luna-Vital, D. A., Mojica, L., González de Mejía, E., Mendoza, S., & Loarca-Piña, G. (2015). Biological potential of protein hydrolysates and peptides from common bean (*Phaseolus vulgaris* L.): A review. *Food Research International, 76*(P1), 39–50. https://doi.org/10.1016/j.foodres.2014.11.024 (accessed on 9th July 2025).

Luna-Vital, D., & González de Mejía, E. (2018). Peptides from legumes with antigastrointestinal cancer potential: Current evidence for their molecular mechanisms. *Current Opinion in Food Science, 20*, 13–18. https://doi.org/10.1016/j.cofs.2018.02.012 (accessed on 9th July 2025).

Madruga, M. S., Albuquerque, F. S. M. de, Silva, I. R. A., Amaral, D. S. do, Magnani, M., & Queiroga, V. N. (2014). Chemical, morphological and functional properties of Brazilian jackfruit (*Artocarpus heterophyllus* L.) seeds starch. *Food Chemistry, 143*, 440–445.

Mahato, N., Sharma, K., Sinha, M., & Cho, M. H. (2018). Citrus waste derived Nutra-/pharmaceuticals for health benefits: Current trends and future perspectives. *Journal of Functional Foods, 40*, 307–316.

Mahfoudhi, N., & Hamdi, S. (2015). Use of almond gum and gum Arabic as novel edible coating to delay postharvest ripening and to maintain sweet cherry (*Prunus avium*) quality during storage. *Journal of Food Processing and Preservation, 39*(6), 1499–1508. https://doi.org/10.1111/jfpp.12369 (accessed on 9th July 2025).

Mahfoudhi, N., Chouaibi, M., & Hamdi, S. (2014). Effectiveness of almond gum trees exudate as a novel edible coating for improving postharvest quality of tomato (*Solanum lycopersicum* L.) fruits. *Food Science and Technology International, 20*(1), 33–43. https://doi.org/10.1177/1082013212469617 (accessed on 9th July 2025).

Matos, M. E., Sanz, T., & Rosell, C. M. (2014). Establishing the function of proteins on the rheological and quality properties of rice-based gluten-free muffins. *Food*

Hydrocolloids, 35, 150–158. https://doi.org/10.1016/j.foodhyd.2013.05.007 (accessed on 9th July 2025).

Mattila, P., Mäkinen, S., Eurola, M., Jalava, T., Pihlava, J. M., Hellström, J., & Pihlanto, A. (2018). Nutritional value of commercial protein-rich plant products. *Plant Foods for Human Nutrition, 73*(2), 108–115. https://doi.org/10.1007/s11130-018-0660-7 (accessed on 9th July 2025).

Mohamed, G. F., Mohamed, S. S., & Taha, F. S. (2011). Antioxidant, antimicrobial, and anticarcinogenic properties of Egyptian guava seed extracts. *Nature and Science, 9*(11), 32–41.

Mohamed, Z., Terano, R., Yeoh, S. J., & Iliyasu, A. (2017). Opinions of non-vegetarian consumers among the Chinese community in Malaysia toward vegetarian food and diets. *Journal of Food Products Marketing, 23*(1), 80–98. https://doi.org/10.1080/10454446.2017.1244795 (accessed on 9th July 2025).

Murrieta-Martínez, C. L., Soto-Valdez, H., Pacheco-Aguilar, R., Torres-Arreola, W., Rodríguez-Felix, F., & Márquez Ríos, E. (2018). Edible protein films: Sources and behavior. *Packaging Technology and Science, 31*(3), 113–122.

Musa, M. (2010). Properties of apricot kernel and oils as fruit juice processing waste. *Food and Nutrition Sciences, 2010*, 31–37. https://doi.org/10.4236/fns.2010.12006 (accessed on 9th July 2025).

Mushtaq, M., Gani, A., Gani, A., Punoo, H. A., & Masoodi, F. A. (2018). Use of pomegranate peel extract incorporated zein film with improved properties for prolonged shelf life of fresh Himalayan cheese (Kalari/Kradi). *Innovative Food Science and Emerging Technologies, 48*, 25–32. https://doi.org/10.1016/j.ifset.2018.04.020 (accessed on 9th July 2025).

Nemecek, T., Jungbluth, N., i Canals, L. M., & Schenck, R. (2016). Environmental impacts of food consumption and nutrition: Where are we and what is next? *The International Journal of Life Cycle Assessment, 21*, 607–620. https://doi.org/10.1007/s11367-016-1071-3 (accessed on 9th July 2025).

Öztürk, T., & Turhan, S. (2020). Physicochemical properties of pumpkin (*Cucurbita pepo* L.) seed kernel flour and its utilization in beef meatballs as a fat replacer and functional ingredient. *Journal of Food Processing and Preservation, 44*(9). https://doi.org/10.1111/jfpp.14695 (accessed on 9th July 2025).

Padayachee, A., Day, L., Howell, K., & Gidley, M. J. (2017). Complexity and health functionality of plant cell wall fibers from fruits and vegetables. *Critical Reviews in Food Science and Nutrition, 57*(1), 59–81.

Panigrahi, S., Bland, B., & Carlaw, P. M. (1989). The nutritive value of tamarind seeds for broiler chicks. *Animal Feed Science and Technology, 22*(4), 285–293.

Patel, G. N., & Kheni, J. (2018). Mango seed kernel, a highly nutritious food, should we continue to trash or use? *Journal of Pharmacognosy and Phytochemistry, 7*(4), 04–07.

Pontieri, P., Mamone, G., de Caro, S., Tuinstra, M. R., Roemer, E., Okot, J., de Vita, P., Ficco, D. B. M., Alifano, P., Pignone, D., Massardo, D. R., & del Giudice, L. (2013). Sorghum, a healthy and gluten-free food for celiac patients as demonstrated by genome, biochemical, and immunochemical analyses. *Journal of Agricultural and Food Chemistry, 61*(10), 2565–2571. https://doi.org/10.1021/jf304882k (accessed on 9th July 2025).

Prandi, B., Faccini, A., Lambertini, F., Bencivenni, M., Jorba, M., Van Droogenbroek, B., & Sforza, S. (2019). Food wastes from agrifood industry as possible sources of proteins: A detailed molecular view on the composition of the nitrogen fraction, amino acid profile and racemization degree of 39 food waste streams. *Food Chemistry, 286*, 567–575. https://doi.org/10.1016/j.foodchem.2019.01.166 (accessed on 9th July 2025).

Prasad, N. B. L., & Azeemoddin, G. (1994). Characteristics and composition of guava (*Psidium guajava* L.) seed and oil. *Journal of the American Oil Chemists' Society, 71*(4), 457–458.

Raghavendra, G. M., Varaprasad, K., & Jayaramudu, T. (2015). Biomaterials: Design, development and biomedical applications. In *Nanotechnology Applications for Tissue Engineering* (pp. 21–44). William Andrew Publishing.

Rana, S., Dhiman, A. K., & Kathuria, D. (2022). Formulation of antioxidant rich muffins using pumpkin (*Cucurbita moschata* Duchesne ex Poir.) pulp, seeds and different cereal flours. *Annals of Phytomedicine: An International Journal, 11*(2). https://doi.org/10.54085/ap.2022.11.2.66 (accessed on 9th July 2025).

Ranganathan, J., Vennard, D., Waite, R., Dumas, P., Lipinski, B., & Searchinger, T. (2016). Shifting diets for a sustainable future (p. 90). World Resources Institute.

Ribotta, P. D., Ausar, S. F., Morcillo, M. H., Pérez, G. T., Beltramo, D. M., & León, A. E. (2004). Production of gluten-free bread using soybean flour. *Journal of the Science of Food and Agriculture, 84*(14), 1969–1974. https://doi.org/10.1002/jsfa.1915 (accessed on 9th July 2025).

Röös, E., Ekelund, L., & Tjärnemo, H. (2014). Communicating the environmental impact of meat production: Challenges in the development of a Swedish meat guide. *Journal of Cleaner Production, 73*, 154–164. https://doi.org/10.1016/j.jclepro.2013.10.037 (accessed on 9th July 2025).

Rosas Ulloa, P., Ulloa, J. A., Ulloa Rangel, B. E., & López Mártir, K. U. (2022). Protein isolates from orange (*Citrus sinensis* L.) seeds: Effect of high-intensity ultrasound on its physicochemical and functional properties. *Food and Bioprocess Technology, 2*, 1–14.

Sá, A. G. A., Laurindo, J. B., Moreno, Y. M. F., & Carciofi, B. A. M. (2022). Influence of emerging technologies on the utilization of plant proteins. In *Frontiers in Nutrition, 9*. Frontiers Media S.A. https://doi.org/10.3389/fnut.2022.809058 (accessed on 9th July 2025).

Saeed, F., Afzaal, M., Niaz, B., Arshad, M. U., Tufail, T., Hussain, M. B., et al. (2018). Bitter melon (*Momordica charantia*): A natural healthy vegetable. *International Journal of Food Properties, 21*(1), 1270–1290.

Salajegheh, F., Tajeddin, B., Panahi, B., & Karimi, H. (2020). Effect of edible coatings based on zein and chitosan and the use of Roman aniseed oil on the microbial activity of Mazafati dates. https://doi.org/10.22059/jfabe.2020.306636.1058 (accessed on 9th July 2025).

Sánchez-Chino, X., Jiménez-Martínez, C., Dávila-Ortiz, G., Álvarez-González, I., & Madrigal-Bujaidar, E. (2015). Nutrient and nonnutrient components of legumes, and its chemo preventive activity: A review. *Nutrition and Cancer, 67*(3), 401–410. https://doi.org/10.1080/01635581.2015.1004729 (accessed on 9th July 2025).

Sarkar, B. R., Awasthi, P., & Joshi, H. (2018). Physical properties and nutritional composition of tamarind kernel powder and quality evaluation of instant chutney mix prepared incorporating tamarind kernel powder. *Journal of Pharmacognosy and Phytochemistry, 7*(6), 1342–1346.

Schreuders, F. K., Dekkers, B. L., Bodnár, I., Erni, P., Boom, R. M., & van der Goot, A. J. (2019). Comparing structuring potential of pea and soy protein with gluten for meat analogue preparation. *Journal of Food Engineering, 261*, 32–39.

Springmann, M., Wiebe, K., Mason-D'Croz, D., Sulser, T. B., Rayner, M., & Scarborough, P. (2018). Health and nutritional aspects of sustainable diet strategies and their association with environmental impacts: A global modelling analysis with country-level detail. *The Lancet Planetary Health, 2*(10), e451–e461.

Sultana, A., Amin, M. N., Miah, M. Y., Sarker, A. K., Rasel, M. M. A., Aziz, M. T., & Khanom, M. M. (2017). Determination of proximate composition and amino acid profile of jackfruit seed and utilization of its seed flour for development of protein enriched supplementary food. *Cell Biology, 5*(6), 57–65. https://doi.org/10.11648/j.cb.20170506.11 (accessed on 9th July 2025).

Sun, M., Zhao, B., Cai, Z., Yan, J., Ma, R., & Yu, M. (2022). Amino acid profiles in peach (*Prunus persica* L.) fruit. *Foods, 11*(12), 1718. https://doi.org/10.3390/foods11121718 (accessed on 9th July 2025).

Sun-Waterhouse, D., Zhao, M., & Waterhouse, G. I. (2014). Protein modification during ingredient preparation and food processing: Approaches to improve food processability and nutrition. *Food and Bioprocess Technology, 7*, 1853–1893.

Tan, S. H., Mailer, R. J., Blanchard, C. L., & Agboola, S. O. (2011). Canola proteins for human consumption: Extraction, profile, and functional properties. *Journal of Food Science, 76*(1). https://doi.org/10.1111/j.1750-3841.2010.01930.x (accessed on 9th July 2025).

Tang, C., Hackenberg, K., Fu, Q., Ajayan, P. M., & Ardebili, H. (2012). High ion conducting polymer nanocomposite electrolytes using hybrid nanofillers. *Nano Letters, 12*(3), 1152–1156. https://doi.org/10.1021/nl202692y (accessed on 9th July 2025).

Vang, A., Singh, P. N., Lee, J. W., Haddad, E. H., & Brinegar, C. H. (2008). Meats, processed meats, obesity, weight gain and occurrence of diabetes among adults: Findings from Adventist Health Studies. *Annals of Nutrition and Metabolism, 52*(2), 96–104. https://doi.org/10.1159/000121365 (accessed on 9th July 2025).

Venuste, M., Zhang, X., Shoemaker, C. F., Karangwa, E., Abbas, S., & Kamdem, P. E. (2013). Influence of enzymatic hydrolysis and enzyme type on the nutritional and antioxidant properties of pumpkin meal hydrolysates. *Food and Function, 4*(5), 811–820. https://doi.org/10.1039/c3fo30347k (accessed on 9th July 2025).

Vieira, M. G. A., da Silva, M. A., dos Santos, L. O., & Beppu, M. M. (2011). Natural-based plasticizers and biopolymer films: A review. *European Polymer Journal, 47*(3), 254–263. https://doi.org/10.1016/j.eurpolymj.2010.12.011 (accessed on 9th July 2025).

Wani, A. A., Kaur, D., Ahmed, I., & Sogi, D. S. (2008). Extraction optimization of watermelon seed protein using response surface methodology. *LWT–Food Science and Technology, 41*(8), 1514–1520. https://doi.org/10.1016/j.lwt.2007.10.001 (accessed on 9th July 2025).

Wani, A. A., Sogi, D. S., Singh, P., & Khatkar, B. S. (2015). Influence of watermelon seed protein concentrates on dough handling, textural and sensory properties of cookies. *Journal of Food Science and Technology, 52*(4), 2139–2147. https://doi.org/10.1007/s13197-013-1224-3 (accessed on 9th July 2025).

World Health Organization. (2007). *Protein and Amino Acid Requirements in Human Nutrition.* https://apps.who.int/iris/bitstream/handle/10665/43411/WHO_TRS_935_eng.pdf?ua=1 (accessed on 9th July 2025).

Wu, G. (2016). Dietary protein intake and human health. *Food & Function, 7*(3), 1251–1265.

Yalcin, E., Ozdal, T., & Gok, I. (2022). Investigation of textural, functional, and sensory properties of muffins prepared by adding grape seeds to various flours. *Journal of Food Processing and Preservation, 46*(5). https://doi.org/10.1111/jfpp.15316 (accessed on 9th July 2025).

Yan, W., Zhang, B., Yadav, M. P., Feng, L., Yan, J., Jia, X., & Yin, L. (2020). Corn fiber gum–soybean protein isolates double network hydrogel as oral delivery vehicles for thermosensitive bioactive compounds. *Food Hydrocolloids, 107*, 105865. https://doi.org/10.1016/j.foodhyd.2020.105865 (accessed on 9th July 2025).

Yin, M., Wuyun, T., Jiang, Z., & Zeng, J. (2020). Amino acid profiles and protein quality of Siberian apricot (*Prunus sibirica* L.) kernels from Inner Mongolia. *Journal of Forestry Research, 31*(4), 1391–1397. https://doi.org/10.1007/s11676-019-00882-4 (accessed on 9th July 2025).

Yousef, A. R., El-Moniem, E. A. A. A., & Mahmoud, T. S. M. (2020). Edible coating of soy protein or gelatin as a carrier of thyme oil for maintaining quality of 'Barhee' dates fruits during cold storage. *Plant Archives, 20*(2), 9311–9322.

Zahari, M. W., & Alimon, A. R. (2003). Use of palm kernel cake and oil palm by-products in compound feed. *Palm Oil Developments, 40*, 5–9.

CHAPTER 15

Postharvest Fruit and Vegetable Wastage and the Economic and Environmental Impacts

IKECHUKWU KINGSLEY OPARA,[1] OLANIYI AMOS FAWOLE,[2,3] and UMEZURUIKE LINUS OPARA[1,3,*]

[1]*Faculty of AgriSciences, Africa Institute for Postharvest Technology, South African Research Chair in Postharvest Technology, Stellenbosch University, Stellenbosch, Western Cape, South Africa*

[2]*Department of Botany and Plant Biotechnology, South African Research Chairs Initiative in Sustainable Preservation and Agroprocessing Research, Postharvest and Agroprocessing Research Centre, University of Johannesburg, Auckland Park, Gauteng, South Africa*

[3]*UNESCO International Centre for Biotechnology, Nsukka, Enugu, Nigeria*

*Corresponding author

ABSTRACT

The issue of postharvest losses and waste of fruits and vegetables represents a complex global challenge that hinders the achievement of various Sustainable Development Goals (SDGs). This wastage occurs throughout the food value chain, manifesting in different ways in the developing and developed countries. Several factors contribute to this problem, including inadequate handling and storage practices, inefficient transportation systems, stringent marketing standards that prioritize appearance over

Sustainable Approaches in Postharvest Handling and Management: Pankaj B. Pathare (Ed.)

DOI: 10.1201/9781779641076-15

quality, and consumer behaviors that often lead to waste. In developing countries, the challenges are often rooted in inadequate infrastructure, which can impede the effective storage and transportation of fresh produce. On the other hand, in developed countries, the focus tends to be on market demands and consumer preferences, which lead to high levels of waste due to the rejection of perfectly edible produce that does not meet cosmetic standards. Therefore, this study used a descriptive approach to examine the intricacies of postharvest wastage within the global fruit and vegetable sector. It aims to identify the predominant types of waste and assess the underlying causes. Additionally, the impacts of postharvest wastage are highlighted, emphasizing their critical ramifications on the socioeconomic and health dynamics within societies. The study emphasizes that the consequences of fruit and vegetable wastage extend beyond economic loss, but also environmental degradation, exacerbating food insecurity, climate change, and nutritional deficiencies. Fruit and vegetable wastage represents the unsustainable exploitation of natural resources, leading to the misuse of resources that could otherwise serve beneficial purposes.

15.1 INTRODUCTION

Food security has been a topical issue among researchers and experts in the food system, with a recent focus on nutritional security, owing to the FAO 1996 definition of food security, which gave cognizance to nutritional security and food preference. Nutrient-rich diets contain a healthy, high-quality range of food commodities in appropriate proportion. According to the WHO (2016), about 2 billion people do not have sufficient intake of micronutrients. This could present a serious concern with the projection of over 9 billion people to live in the world during the next 30 years (UN, 2011).

Fruit and vegetables contain essential micro- and macronutrients that are necessary for a healthy life. Fruit and vegetables contribute enormously to good health and wellbeing, and there has been a strong correlation between fruit and vegetable consumption and good health outcome (Keatinge et al., 2011). Fruit and vegetables contain essential nutrients that are necessary for adequate nutrition and wellbeing, such as vitamins, amino acids, minerals, calories, and fiber (Keatinge et al., 2010). A strong correlation was found for fruit and vegetable consumption with cardiovascular disease protection, reduced risk of pancreas diseases, low risk of depression, cancer, and stroke protection (Angelino et al., 2019). Also, there is evidence of fruit and vegetable consumption in improving mental and cognitive health in older adults (Gehlich et al., 2019). These benefits are a result of essential nutritional contents such as phytochemicals and antioxidants (Opara and Al-Ani, 2010), including phenolic compounds and bioactive compounds that exhibit anti-inflammatory and antitumoral properties (Viuda-Martos, Fernández-López, and Pérez-Álvarez, 2010).

Historically, insufficient availability of fruit and vegetables has persisted due to postharvest wastage despite the health benefits (Mason-D'Croz et al., 2019). This presents a serious food and nutritional security challenge. Globally, fruit and vegetables wastage is as high as 37–55% (Gustavsson et al., 2011) and accounts for about $750 billion (FAO, 2013). The incidence of fruit and vegetables postharvest wastage in South Africa is estimated at 4.2 million tons, accounting for 47% of the total food losses and waste in the country (Oelofse and Nahman, 2013). This high level of losses constitutes severe negative impacts on the environment and economic losses to farmers and the actors along the value chain.

The global production and trade of fruit and vegetables have a significant economic contribution to the gross domestic product (GDP) of many countries. For example, in 2013, vegetables contributed about $25.25 billion and $6.25 billion to the revenue of China and India, respectively (Produce Marketing Association, 2016). Fruit production in China amounted to 260 million tons in 2014, and the total export accounted for 4.1% of global fruit export (Produce Marketing Association, 2016). India produced 179 million tons of fruit and vegetables in 2011, accounting for 21.2% of total global fruit and vegetable production (Mahajan, 2020). The annual value of fruit and vegetable production globally is estimated at $1 trillion (Schreinemachers, Simmons and Wopereis, 2018). In South Africa, fruit alone contributed an estimated revenue of about $1.8 billion in 2015, with deciduous fruit contributing $835 million, citrus contributing $834 million, and other selected subtropical fruit contributing $205 million (Louw, 2016). The fruit industry in the country helps to curtail the rising unemployment rate by employing people who work on farms and along the value chain. The deciduous fruit sector employs an estimated 75,657 permanent staff, the citrus fruit sector about 95,690, while some subtropical selected fruit employs about 24,375 persons (Louw, 2016). Louw (2016) indicated that these estimates are only for in-farm employment. The job opportunities created down the value chain were not included as the system at the value chain is more complex, with multiple activities and complexities at a different level that makes it difficult for a comprehensive estimate.

Reducing postharvest wastage of fruit and vegetables has been argued by recent studies as the most sustainable means to mitigate food and nutritional insecurity and improve the local economy, especially in developing countries (Ellis, Kwofie and Ngadi, 2020; Louw, 2016; Nshizirungu and Kitinoja, 2019). Postharvest wastage in developing countries due to inefficiency at the production and handling stages can be as high as 40–50% (Nshizirungu and Kitinoja, 2019). Hence, assessing the amount of postharvest wastage and identifying the hotspot for losses and waste is as important as food production itself. This is because it does not make economic sense only to increase production to solve food and nutritional security problems if a third of what is produced goes to waste. Therefore, there is consensus among researchers, development practitioners, and policy experts that reducing postharvest waste should be one of the strategies to increase food and nutrition security amid the increasing world population (Opara, 2010). The objective of this review is to discuss the causes and impacts of fruit and vegetable wastage in relation to economic loss, unsustainable use of resources, and nutritional security. Many studies have been done on postharvest wastage of fruit and vegetables in different countries and regions. However, these studies focused on quantitative loss, environmental impacts, and reduction strategies with little or no attention to nutritional loss due to postharvest wastage. For example, Porat, Lichter, Terry, Harker, and Buzby (2018) assessed the magnitude and causes of fruit and vegetable losses during retail and consumption and the emerging technologies and strategies to prevent wastage at retail and home. Kasso and Bekele (2016) assessed the factors causing quality deterioration and postharvest wastage of horticultural crops in the Dire Dawa region of Ethiopia. McKenzie, Singh-Peterson, and Underhill (2017) quantified postharvest wastage of tomatoes using weight and volume in two commercial, domestic supply chains in Queensland, Australia. The drivers and factors contributing to postharvest losses were qualitatively identified and analyzed. Underhill, Joshua, and Zhou (2019) assessed postharvest losses of horticultural produce in roadside markets and municipal markets in Guadalcanal, Solomon Islands, using short semi-structured interviews. The factors contributing to postharvest losses were also discussed.

Kitinoja, Tokala, and Brondy (2018) did a comprehensive review of 268 postharvest losses and waste studies, including assessment methodologies. The study discovered that out of the 268 postharvest wastage studies reviewed, interviews and questionnaires were the most used method to measure quantitative losses, and direct measurement was the least method used. The review also revealed that most of the postharvest wastage studies provided data on quantitative losses, while few studies included information on qualitative and economic loss measurements. Only 5 out of the 268 studies provided information on nutritional losses as an impact of postharvest wastage. Kummu, De Moel, Porkka, Siebert, Varis et al. (2012) estimated postharvest losses and the impacts on natural resources and other production inputs at the global food supply chain level. There is a gap in the literature on information about nutritional losses due to postharvest wastage of fruit and vegetables. Therefore, this review would provide information on postharvest wastage of essential nutrients that could benefit people by improving health and wellbeing.

To conduct this study, a search was conducted on databases to make sure that the study did not replicate previous research. Searches on Google Scholar and Scopus were done to obtain articles in academic journals, and no evidence of duplicate results was seen. Special attention was given to articles to ensure that most of them were obtained from peer-reviewed and reputable journals. The search was done using the following keywords and phrases: "food losses," "food waste," "food losses and food waste," "fruit losses," "vegetable losses," "fruit and vegetable losses," "quantifying fruit losses and waste," "postharvest losses," "postharvest waste," "understanding fruit losses and waste," and "environmental impacts of food losses and waste." The results of the review were summarized under the following sub-topics: (a) an overview of postharvest wastage in the global fruit and vegetable industry; (b) types of postharvest wastage of fruit and vegetables; (c) causes of postharvest wastage of fruit and vegetables; and finally (d) an overview of the impacts of postharvest wastage of fruit and vegetables.

15.2 POSTHARVEST WASTAGE IN THE GLOBAL FRUIT AND VEGETABLE INDUSTRY – AN OVERVIEW

Postharvest wastage in the value chain can be reasonably large in the fruit and vegetable industry. About 45% of the total food losses globally are fruit and vegetables (FAO, 2011), of which an estimated 50% occur at production, handling, and storage, and 46% occur during processing, distribution, and final consumption. Postharvest wastage of fruit and vegetables is a challenge both in developed and developing countries (Musasa et al., 2013). In developed countries, fruit and vegetable waste occurs mainly at the retail and consumer levels (Porat et al., 2018). In contrast, in developing countries, losses and waste occur mostly in production and processing (Kasso and Bekele, 2016; Porat et al., 2018). Louw (2016) reported that an estimated 32% of the total production is lost in the fruit and vegetable industry in developing countries. Despite the high amount of fruit and vegetable lost annually (Table 15.1), only less than 5% of research funding is allocated for postharvest research globally (Louw, 2016). This makes it challenging to invest in postharvest research and innovation needed to cost-effectively reduce the losses and waste. For example, in South Africa, handling, storage, processing, and packaging are still ranked the highest among the contributors of waste in the food value chain (Oelofse and Nahman, 2013). However, there has been an improvement in postharvest packaging, shelf life, transportation, storage, and disease and pest control before access to the market (Louw, 2016).

The magnitude of fruit and vegetables postharvest wastage varies significantly among types of fruit and vegetables, production area, and seasons. The estimation of fruit and vegetable wastage became popular in the 1960s and 1970s (Ceponis and Butterfield, 1973). One of the early estimations was done by the US Department of Agriculture, Consumer and Marketing Services (C&MS, 1970), which revealed that in 1969, the value of fresh fruit and vegetables at wholesale wasted in New York alone was $450 million and which was projected to reach $750 million in retail value. In the UK, an estimated 3 million tons of fruit and vegetables are wasted annually (WRAP, 2009). However, there has been a reduction recently to 1.6 million tons, amounting to over $4.8 billion (WRAP, 2019), as a result of the vigorous effort by the government and food businesses to reduce food waste. These wastes are due to grading, customer behavior, and inconsistencies in the value chain. However, it was noted that losses due to natural causes, such as environmental conditions, could not totally be controlled (WRAP, 2011).

The FAO (2011) estimated that the losses and waste of fruit and vegetables in developing countries was 37–55%. Recent studies have estimated postharvest wastage of fruit and vegetables in developing countries as high as 60% (Yahia, 2019; Yahia, Fonseca and Kitinoja, 2019). The reasons for this include inadequate skilled personnel, inadequate cold storage and transport facilities, and the generally poor state of postharvest technology (Hodges et al., 2011; Porat et al., 2018). On the other hand, higher wastage of fresh produce (including fruit and vegetables) from retail to consumption was reported in the developed countries (FAO, 2011; Yahia, 2019), which can be attributed to high market grade and preference, as well as economic prosperity (WRAP, 2019). Hence, people tend to buy more than they can consume. This defeats the argument of increasing production to feed the anticipated increase in world population in the future. Table 15.1 presents the postharvest wastage magnitude of some fruit and vegetables in some developing countries.

TABLE 15.1 Estimated Postharvest Wastage of Fruit and Vegetables in Several Developing Countries

Country	Commodity	Wastage %	Hotspot	References
Ethiopia	Tomato	45.32	Harvesting and marketing	Kasso and Bekele (2016)
	Mango	43.53		
	Coffee	15.75		
Oman	Fresh produce	3–19	Supermarket	Opara (2003)
Fiji	Fruit and vegetables	0.07–2.44 4.07–10	Municipal markets	Underhill and Kumar (2014)
Fiji	Tomato	32.9	Supply chain	Underhill and Kumar (2015)
Zimbabwe	Orange	40	Villages	Musasa et al. (2013)
South Africa	Fruit	50	Fruit market	Mashau, Moyane and Jideani (2012)
Solomon Island	Fruit and vegetable	7.9–9.5 2.6–7	Municipal and roadside markets	Underhill. Joshua and Zhou (2019)
South Africa	Cabbage	12–46	Retail to consumer	Munhuweyi et al. (2016)
South Africa	Pomegranate	15.3–20.1	Farm	Opara et al. (2021a)
South Africa	Pomegranate	6.74–7.69	Packhouse	Opara et al. (2021b)

The challenge of postharvest wastage of fruit and vegetables in Sub-Saharan Africa is complex, as there is variation in magnitude at different stages of occurrence (Table 15.2). Fruits and vegetables in Sub-Saharan Africa have the highest percentage of loss compared to other crops, totaling a staggering 51% of total production (Table 15.2). The losses occur more during processing and distribution, mainly because of mechanical damage such as bruises and excessive trimming (Fadiji et al., 2016; Hussein, Fawole and Opara, 2019a; Opara and Fadiji, 2018).

TABLE 15.2 Food wastage by type of crop in Sub-Saharan Africa

Location	Fruits and Vegetables (%)	Roots and Tubers (%)	Oilseeds and Pulses (%)	Cereals and Grains (%)
Production	10.00	14.00	12.00	6.00
Handling and storage	8.00	15.00	7.00	8.00
Processing	20.00	11.00	6.00	3.00
Distribution	10.00	3.00	2.00	2.00
Consumption	3.00	1.00	1.00	1.00
Total	51.00	44.00	28.00	20.00

Source: FAO (2011).

15.3 TYPES OF POSTHARVEST WASTAGE OF FRUIT AND VEGETABLES

Reasons for postharvest fruit and vegetable loss vary according to the activities at each stage of the food value chain. Therefore, the type of loss is determined by the causative factors and the type of defect on the fruit and vegetables. There are two main types of postharvest fruit and vegetable losses common in the mainstream literature, namely, quantitative losses and qualitative loss. Each of these types of losses occurs along the food value chain (Aulakh and Regmi, 2013; Gardas et al., 2018).

15.3.1 QUANTITATIVE LOSS

Quantitative fruit and vegetable loss refers to the loss in weight and volume, which are usually measured through scientific investigation (Batu, 2004; Munhuweyi et al., 2016). This is measured by weighing the fruit and vegetables along the value chain and comparing it with the original weight at the point of departure (farm or packhouse) (Matare, 2012). However, a quantitative loss can also manifest through changes in physical appearances, such as shriveling (shrinking) (Fawole and Opara, 2013a) and through water loss, which affects pomegranate and other fruit and vegetables (Lufu, Ambaw and Opara, 2020). The reduction in weight is caused by factors like changes in temperature and relative humidity, which leads to a loss in moisture content and change in chemical composition (Lufu et al., 2020). Since the appearance of the fruit and vegetables is affected, the commodity becomes less appealing for consumption, which downgrades the commercial value (Aulakh and Regmi, 2013). There is also variation in quantitative loss, which includes partial and total loss (Prusky, 2011). Partial loss is described as loss due to respiration and the peeling off of some of the edible parts of fruit and vegetables due to damage or spoilage, leaving a portion good for consumption. A situation where the whole fruit and vegetables are unfit for consumption or industrial use and discarded is described as a total loss. The consideration of weight loss as a factor to determine quantitative food loss is argued to be unsatisfactory in some postharvest situations (Aulakh and Regmi, 2013), such as drying, which is a required postharvest process to preserve the quality and safety of grain and cereal foods as well as dried fruit and vegetable products. Under this consideration, such weight loss cannot be categorized as a loss.

15.3.2 QUALITATIVE LOSS

Qualitative fruit and vegetable loss occurs because of unwanted factors that affect the perception of the food and its market value, such as a change in texture, taste, and color (Buzby and Hyman, 2012). Qualitative loss can occur due to several factors ranging from the incident of pests and rodents to poor handling systems, contamination by pesticides, and insect damage (Aulakh and Regmi, 2013). Fruit and vegetable losses due to qualitative loss are mainly based on grading and market criteria to meet local and international marketing requirements and standards (Kader, 1983). This means that the fruit and vegetables are sorted according to how appealing they look to the customers and the final consumers. This type of grading is made to have an acceptable minimum required standard of quality, which helps to determine the market value of fruit and vegetables since they are susceptible to loss due to moisture content (Munhuweyi et al., 2016).

Both quantitative and qualitative losses are subject to customer and final consumer appeal, which are determined by the type of market, the minimum acceptable standard, and culture. Revenue is lost when these losses occur along the value chain, and this affects the local economy and the market price. However, higher postharvest losses may create scarcity, which causes an unexpected price increase (Sudheer and Indira, 2007), but this does not guarantee an increase in revenue, as the spike in price affects the affordability of the commodity. To reduce losses and waste, it is important to analyze the factors causing losses and waste of fruit and vegetables at each phase of the value chain to improve their quality and shelf life (dos Santos et al., 2020).

15.3.3 CAUSES OF POSTHARVEST WASTAGE OF FRUIT AND VEGETABLE

Fruit and vegetables are susceptible to postharvest spoilage; therefore, they have a very short shelf-life and account for up to 37–55% of the food that is wasted globally (Gustavsson et al., 2011). This accounts for about 40% of financial losses to farmers, distributors, retailers, and various actors in the food value chain (Gardas et al., 2018; Porat et al., 2018). Factors contributing to postharvest losses mostly originate from practices along the food value chain, such as handling, processing, production practices, transportation facilities and infrastructures, and general production practices (Aulakh and Regmi, 2013). Also, losses occur because of pests and diseases, which are spread by pathogens (Yahaya and Mardiyya, 2019). Price stability in the marketing system is also a contributing factor (Macheka et al., 2018). Environmental conditions such as relative humidity and temperature, especially during storage, contribute to causing fruit and vegetables to be susceptible to microbial and pathological attacks (Yahaya and Mardiyya, 2019). Yahaya and Mardiyya (2019) also suggested that among all the causes of postharvest wastage, pathological and mechanical damage are the most severe causes of the wastage of fruit and vegetables. These factors that cause postharvest wastage are categorized into two main types, namely, primary causes and secondary causes (Table 15.3), with a distinction made according to how and when the wastage occurs (FAO, 1989).

TABLE 15.3 Classification of Causes of Postharvest Fruit and Vegetable Wastage

Primary Causes	Secondary Causes
Mechanical damage	Inadequate equipment and tools
Physiological damage	Poor facility and machinery maintenance
Pathological deterioration	Poor production and management practices
Environmental and physical condition	Inadequate transportation facilities
Microbiological damage	Inadequate storage facilities
Biological damage	Poor packaging
Chemical and biochemical damage	Lack of technological skills
	Legislation, quality standards, and marketing system

Source: Hussein, Fawole and Opara (2019a); Opara and Pathare, (2014); Atanda, Pessu, Agoda, Isong, and Ikotun, (2011).

15.3.4 PRIMARY CAUSES OF FRUIT AND VEGETABLE WASTAGE

The primary causes of postharvest wastage of fruit and vegetables are mainly due to technical factors and are direct in how they affect fruit and vegetables. They are major because of microbial, physiological, mechanical, and environmental factors (Atanda et al., 2011). These factors are complementary in the way they affect fruit and vegetables, as damage caused by microbial factors is usually a result of previous mechanical or physical damage, which reduces the fruit or vegetable's defense mechanism by creating injury, thereby making it susceptible to bacteria and fungi attacks (Munhuweyi, 2012). Following is the description of the primary causes of fruit and vegetables postharvest wastage.

15.3.4.1 MECHANICAL DAMAGE

Mechanical damage occurs along the value chain and has become a major factor that reduces the market value and quality of fruit and vegetables (Opara and Pathare, 2014). Mechanical damage occurs in three ways: compression, vibration, and impact during harvesting and postharvest handling (Hussein, Fawole and Opara, 2019b). Damage may also occur because of thrust and pressure during packaging and transportation (Yahaya and Mardiyya, 2019). Mechanical damage is mainly due to machinery and operational processes and is visible in the form of bruises, injuries, and excessive trimming of fruit and vegetables, causing loss (Atanda et al., 2011; Hussein et al., 2019a; Opara, 2003; Opara and Pathare, 2014).

Sometimes, the impact of mechanical damage is not visible, as the damage to fruit and vegetables is internal by way of ruptured cells and tissues, which make the fruit and vegetables prone to faster deterioration during senescence (when chemical reactions are weak, which results in ageing and death of tissues) (Yahaya and Mardiyya, 2019). Mechanical damage also occurs during the processing of fruit and vegetables. Processing operations cause damages such as abrasion and excessive polishing (Bourne, 1977; Yahaya and Mardiyya, 2019). During packaging, defective seals and storage units also cause mechanical damage. Mechanical damages cause injuries which result in loss of moisture and an increase in respiratory activities, leading to qualitative loss.

15.3.4.2 PHYSIOLOGICAL DAMAGE

Physiological damage is a result of prolonged storage, leading to aging. It is evident in senescence in fruit and vegetables and other natural reactions caused by respiration and transpiration (Lufu, Ambaw and Opara, 2019). Respiration and transpiration cause significant weight loss, as heat is also generated during this process (Atanda et al., 2011). Changes because of this natural process result in terminating dormancy, causing fruit and vegetables to sprout and increasing susceptibility to pathogen infection. This leads to qualitative loss, making fruit and vegetables lose appeal to customers (Buzby and Hyman, 2012).

15.3.4.3 PATHOLOGICAL DETERIORATION

Pathological deterioration is caused by microorganisms like bacteria and fungi (Salunkhe and Desai, 1984). Fruit and vegetables are high in moisture content and are succulent, making them susceptible to microbial attack and damage. The rate of pathological deterioration is dependent on many environmental factors, such as the velocity of the air, relative humidity, and atmospheric composition (Mukama, Ambaw and Opara, 2020). If the environmental factors are favorable to the pathogens, they thrive and cause damage to fruit and vegetables.

15.3.4.4 ENVIRONMENTAL AND PHYSICAL CONDITION

Environmental and physical conditions play an important role in the quality of fruit and vegetables along the value chain. Such conditions are temperature, relative humidity, and the composition and proportion of gases in atmospheric controlled storage (Mukama et al., 2020; Nshizirungu and Kitinoja, 2019; Yahaya and Mardiyya, 2019). While insufficient or improper atmosphere affects the shelf life of fruit and vegetables (Miguel et al., 2004), high temperature and relative humidity encourage the growth of microorganisms that cause damage to fruit and vegetables (Yahaya and Mardiyya, 2019). Also, high temperature increases the rate of respiration of fruit and vegetables, causing a breakdown of internal tissues resulting in qualitative loss (Lufu et al., 2019). Therefore, optimum temperature and relative humidity are required for storing fruit and vegetables according to their biochemical and biological composition.

According to Yahaya and Mardiyya (2019), the role of relative humidity is as important as that of temperature. This is because, during storage, the effect of temperature and relative humidity is similar on fruit and vegetables (Yahaya and Mardiyya, 2019). Therefore, air distribution in a storage unit is required; this operation allows heat transfer from fruit and vegetables to cold air, which reduces their temperature and physiological response (Opara and Fadiji, 2018). The movement of air in storage units has a direct effect on temperature and relative humidity, and such could make fruit and vegetables susceptible to diseases and decay if air movement is inadequate. This is because fruit and vegetables have different temperature and relative humidity requirements for cold storage along the value chain. Although many deciduous fruits have similar temperature and relative humidity requirements for cold storage (Table 15.4), it is important to note that some of the environmental requirements for storage and quality maintenance can vary according to the type of cultivar and growing location. In this case, to minimize qualitative loss, adequate storage condition is required according to the specific fruit and vegetable cultivar. Excessive heat supply, the inappropriate composition of atmospheric gases in storage, and inappropriate cold storage temperature and relative humidity all contribute to postharvest wastage. These environmental factors cause fruit and vegetable tissue damage, which manifests in the form of changes in texture, taste, and color. Therefore, it affects the perception of fruit and vegetables and their market value (Buzby and Hyman, 2012).

TABLE 15.4 Recommended Storage Temperature and Relative Humidity for Selected Deciduous Fruit

Fruit Name	Storage Temperature (°C)	Relative Humidity (%)	Storage Period (Weeks)
Pomegranate	5–7	90–95	–
Plum	varies	95	2–4
Apple	0.5	95	16–32
Peach	0.5	95	–
Grape	0.5	95	6–8
Nectarine	0.5	95	–
Pear	0.5	95	10–40
Apricots	0.5	95	4

Source: Adapted from DAFF (2017).

15.3.4.5 MICROBIOLOGICAL DAMAGE

The succulent nature of fruit and vegetables makes them susceptible to microbial attack. Microorganisms like microbes, bacteria, and fungi damage fruit and cause losses (Atanda et al., 2011; Nshizirungu and Kitinoja, 2019). Microbes eat small portions of fruit and vegetables, which usually damages them, making them unacceptable to the market and sometimes unfit for consumption due to defects. Microbial infection happens rapidly and causes an extensive breakdown of fruit and vegetables, and sometimes affects entire fruit and vegetable batches, leading to total loss (Yahaya and Mardiyya, 2019). The source of microbial infection is mostly from the farm. Also, fruit and vegetable contact with infected equipment, unclean water used for washing, and an untidy storage environment leads to microbiological infestation (Atanda et al., 2011).

According to Yahaya and Mardiyya (2019), the common fungi causing rot in fruit and vegetables are *Phomopsis*, *Penicillium*, *Botrytis*, and *Fusarium*. Bacteria are *Pseudomonas*, *Erwinia*, and other microbes. Substances that are toxic, like carcinogens and patulin, which are mycotoxins produced by mold and fungi, are harmful, thereby causing affected fruit and vegetables to be unfit for consumption and lost (Atanda et al., 2011).

15.3.4.6 BIOLOGICAL DAMAGE

Biological damage occurs from the consumption of fruit and vegetables by rodents, insects, birds, and even large animals (Atanda et al., 2011). This causes partial or total loss of fruit and vegetables (Prusky, 2011). Atanda et al. (2011) asserted that, in some cases, fruit and vegetable contamination by the feathers of birds, hair of furry animals, and animal excreta are to the extent that the fruit and vegetables are unfit for consumption, resulting in a total loss. Biological damage to fruit and vegetables can also occur through webbing and deposit of substances that release unpleasant smells by animals, hence affecting the quality of fruit and vegetables (Atanda et al., 2011).

15.3.4.7 CHEMICAL / BIOCHEMICAL DAMAGE

The chemical makeup of some stored fruit and vegetables naturally reacts to cause discoloration, loss of texture and flavor, and even loss of nutritional content (Atanda et al., 2011; Nshizirungu and Kitinoja, 2019). An example of such a reaction is the Maillard reaction, which causes discoloration, especially in dried fruit (Atanda et al., 2011). In the process of handling, there could be an incident of contamination of fruit and vegetables with toxic substances such as chemicals or pesticides that makes the fruit and vegetables unfit for consumption, thereby resulting in the qualitative loss (Aulakh and Regmi, 2013). Also, biochemical enzyme-related reactions occur in stored fruit and vegetables, causing them to soften with undesirable taste (Atanda et al., 2011; Nshizirungu and Kitinoja, 2019).

There are cases where losses occur due to more than just one of the primary causes. In this case, the primary causative factor may work at the same time or one after the other (Bourne, 1977). For example, there could be an insect attack and the growth of mold simultaneously. On the other hand, the growth of mold first, before enzyme or biochemical reaction, causing discoloration and soft texture.

15.3.5 SECONDARY CAUSES OF FRUIT AND VEGETABLE WASTAGE

Secondary causes of loss are described by Kader (1983) as socio-economic factors that lead to conditions that enable primary causes of loss to occur. These factors are indirect and are described by the way they affect postharvest wastage (Hodges et al., 2011). They are mostly a result of unavailability, poor, or inadequate postharvest facilities that ensure that the quality of fruit and vegetables are maintained along the value chain (Atanda et al., 2011; Hodges et al., 2011).

Inadequate or unavailability of the necessary facilities and equipment and poor maintenance of infrastructure results in a huge loss of fruit and vegetables along the value chain (Cardoen et al., 2015; Kasso and Bekele, 2016; Murthy et al., 2009). Also, the lack of enhanced production and management practices contributes to postharvest losses, especially in developing countries (Hodges et al., 2011; Porat et al., 2018). This is evident in the FAO (2011) study, which was carried out at local and international levels, and postharvest wastage compared in developed and developing countries. For example, poor transportation networks, inadequate storage facilities, inadequate packaging, and lack of processing facilities are among the major causes of postharvest wastage in Ethiopia (Kasso and Bekele, 2016). A similar situation was observed in the value chain of selected fruit and vegetables in India, where fruit and vegetable losses amount to $34 billion annually (Cardoen et al., 2015; Murthy et al., 2009).

Most times, fruit and vegetable handlers (in harvesting, packing, packaging, and transportation) have inadequate knowledge of how to maintain fruit and vegetable quality along the value chain in developing countries due to limited training and low skill. The lack of technical skills required at each stage of the value chain to maintain the quality of fruit and vegetables can be a huge source of postharvest wastage. This is because fruit and vegetables are susceptible to spoilage due to their high moisture content and succulent nature. Kader (1983) asserted that in developing countries, cold chain transportation is not available in some transportation modes or is inadequate where available, thereby making their demand more than the supply. This leads to a delay between harvesting and preservation by cooling, which causes qualitative loss, such as a change in texture, taste, and color (Buzby and Hyman, 2012). Additionally, poor maintenance of packhouses, inadequate packing space, late repairs on facilities, and other poor management decisions affect the quality of fruit and vegetables.

Legislation and marketing systems could also be an indirect source of postharvest wastage. Laws, grading, and standards about consumption are contributing factors in determining the quantity of food consumed in a community and what is wasted (Atanda et al., 2011; FAO, 1989). Also, the extent of government influence and control in the marketing system, especially on pricing and the middlemen along the value chain, contribute to losses (Kasso and Bekele, 2016; Murthy et al., 2009). This is because multiple middlemen would mean a longer time for the fruit and vegetables to get to the retail stores and the final consumer. Because fruit and vegetables are perishable commodities, a long time along the value chain makes them susceptible to quality loss. Irrespective of the causes, postharvest wastage of fruit and vegetables has a detrimental impact on the farmer and value chain actors, as well as the natural environment and, ultimately, human health.

15.3.6 IMPACTS OF POSTHARVEST WASTAGE OF FRUIT AND VEGETABLES – AN OVERVIEW

Transitioning to a more sustainable future has, at its core, the transformation of the food system to minimize food wastage and ensure food and nutrition security (Atanda et al., 2011). If the goals of research organizations, policymakers, and various actors in the food industry are to be met in terms of a sustainable food system (with minimal impact on the environment, economy, and society), conditions that encourage postharvest wastage must be reduced. According to FAO (2011), over 45% of the total food lost annually is fruit and vegetables. This comes with huge impacts on the farmers and the food system actors along the value chain. For example, the total loss of pomegranate fruit at the packhouse level in South Africa in 2016 and 2019 were estimated at 13% and 6%, respectively (POMASA, 2016, 2019). This may sound acceptable, but it was without a record of the losses and waste at the farm level. The amount of fruit losses at the farm level could spike the figures and reveal the actual percentage of loss of pomegranate fruit in 2016 and 2019. Postharvest wastage impact is enormous in terms of financial (economic) loss, negative impact on the environment (GHG emission, freshwater use, and cropland use), and negative impact on food security in terms of nutritional loss.

15.3.6.1 ECONOMIC

The economic impact of postharvest wastage is mostly in terms of financial loss that farmers and food actors along the value chain incur as a result of loss and waste. Postharvest losses also impact the consumers directly as much as they impact the farmers (Gustavsson et al., 2011; Murthy et al., 2009). For example, a food-insecure household would have an improved livelihood if they cut down on the amount of food they waste, as this simply means that more money would be spared to purchase other household items other than food. For farmers, the losses will result in a direct loss of production inputs in monetary terms. The cost of global food waste was about \$750 billion, with vegetables accounting for 23% of the total cost and fruit 19% (FAO, 2013). This is due to the high susceptibility of fruit and vegetables to postharvest wastage, especially in developing countries.

A study in three different counties in Kenya revealed that, on average, the economic loss due to postharvest wastage of African nightshade plants amounted to over \$2.7 million (Gogo et al., 2017). At the macro level in India, which is the second fruit and vegetable producing country in the world, annual fruit and vegetable wastage was estimated at \$1.8 billion, which was based on 30% loss (Murthy et al., 2009). In South Africa, on average, about 21,950 tons of cabbage valued at $973,147 is lost at the retail level annually (Munhuweyi et al., 2016). The losses represent a loss of production input and investments at all levels and an impact on food security in these countries. The amount of postharvest wastage impacts the price of food available in the market, thereby causing food insecurity. This is because market prices impact access to food as poor households do not have the purchasing power to get sufficient and nutritional food (Papargyropoulou et al., 2014). Another form of the economic cost of postharvest wastage is that the resources used to produce wasted food would have otherwise been used for other activities, such as providing ecosystem services. For example, land used to produce wasted foods could be used for recreational parks to generate revenue.

In economic terms, reducing postharvest wastage could be a way of lowering food prices, thereby making it possible for the poor and food insecure to afford healthy food that meets their nutritional requirements. Also, the reduction in postharvest wastage results in saving costs, which is not only linked to reduced food prices in the market but also the cost of waste disposal (EPA, 2012). The cost of waste disposal by the government at all levels is reduced with minimized postharvest wastage, and this makes more funds available for developmental projects in other sectors of the economy. According to UNEP (2011), minimizing postharvest wastage not only saves the cost of production but helps agricultural businesses identify new business areas to boost employment and competitiveness in the larger economy. Again, economic investments made to reduce postharvest losses and waste are less expensive for farmers and agricultural businesses than increasing production (which seems conventional) to affect food security (Gogo et al., 2017).

15.3.6.2 ENVIRONMENTAL

Literature suggests that studies have been conducted to quantify the environmental impacts of food losses and waste (Bais-Moleman, Goossens et al., 2019; Heard et al., 2019; Kashyap and Agarwal, 2020; Kummu et al., 2012; Schulp and Verburg, 2019). These studies focused on how postharvest wastage results in unsustainable use of natural resources. The environmental impact of postharvest wastage is of serious concern because, as the world population grows, the demand for food increases with resultant postharvest wastage. Also, the increase in demand for food further puts pressure on the environment for agricultural food production. This usually leads to unsustainable use of resources, which are currently depleting and increasing the risk of climate change, which is currently a global issue (Beretta et al., 2013; Munhuweyi et al., 2016; Ridoutt et al., 2010; Willersinn et al., 2017).

The environmental impacts of postharvest wastage can be assessed by five different factors: greenhouse gas emission (GHG), freshwater use, cropland use, biodiversity disruption, and landfill (FAO, 2013). Resources such as freshwater used for irrigation, cropland, energy, fertilizer, and other agricultural inputs are limited in nature and, as such, require sustainable utilization in food production and consumption.

15.3.6.3 GREENHOUSE GAS (GHG) EMISSION

GHG is made up of methane, nitrous oxide, and carbon dioxide. According to Robertson, Paul, and Harwood (2000), the radiative force of the atmosphere of the Earth is increasing due to the increase in the emission of GHG. Due to mechanization in farming and the processing of agricultural produce, agriculture is known to be a significant contributor to GHG. The GHG attributed to agriculture is estimated at 22% of the total GHG emission (FAO, 2013). Food waste has a significant contribution to agricultural-related GHG emissions. The FAO has reported that food waste would be third if put into the country ranking of GHG emitters, with only China and the US coming first and second, respectively (FAO, 2013). This amount of GHG from food waste is more than that of Turkey, South Africa, Spain, and Ukraine put together according to FAO estimation. This means that food losses and waste are huge contributors to global warming and climate change. Postharvest wastage of fruit and vegetables is significant in terms of their impact on climate change because of the amount of waste they generate due to their moisture content and susceptibility to waste (Beretta, Stucki, and Hellweg, 2017). The GHG emission attributed to fruit and vegetables is linked to their harvesting, processing, storage, transportation, and ultimately, waste disposal in landfills. Fruit and vegetables contribute a combined 27% of carbon footprint (Table 15.5) as compared to other food commodities.

TABLE 15.5 Comparing Commodity Contribution to Food Wastage and Carbon Footprint

Food Commodity	Wastage (%)	Carbon Footprint (%)
Cereals	25.00	34.00
Starchy roots	18.00	5.00
Oil crops and pulses	3.00	2.00
Fruit	16.00	6.00
Meat	4.00	21.00
Fish and sea food	2.00	4.00
Milk and egg	7.00	7.00
Vegetables	24.00	21.00

Source: FAO (2013).

Agricultural GHG emissions are also directly generated by the addition of fertilizer to the soil and the application of pesticides (Beretta et al., 2017). This is because fertilizers and pesticides contain chemical compounds that diffuse into the atmosphere and contribute to global warming. In developed countries where fruit and vegetable farming are extensively mechanized, the onsite (farm) GHG emission is more because of farming activities that involve the use of various machines and the application of fertilizers. However, agricultural GHG emission is relatively low in countries where fruit and vegetable farming are not mechanized or where the country depends on importation for most of its fruit and vegetable supply. For example, in the UK, the agricultural sector is considered a low GHG emitter because energy use for agricultural purposes in relation to fruit and vegetable production is relatively low (Garnett, 2006). This is because most fruit and vegetables are imported as opposed to Spain and the US, which grow most of their fruit and vegetables (Garnett, 2006). Germany has a heavily mechanized agricultural and food production system and produces 2.7 tons of GHG emissions per capita/year (Eberle and Fels, 2016). In Australia, 79% of agricultural GHG emission is from primary production (farm level) (Reutter et al., 2017). In Sweden, the emission attributable to food waste is estimated at 25% of the food consumed (Reutter et al., 2017). Following this analogy, if a third of the food produced is wasted (according to the FAO estimates), the environmental impact of food waste could be higher than estimated in the studies. This is because the embedded GHG already emitted along the value chain before the food gets to the final consumption phase was not accounted for in the studies.

The impact of GHG emissions on the Earth's atmosphere directly triggers climate change, which is an environmental problem affecting the whole world but especially developing countries. The effect of climate change was described as "a unique and involuntary exposure to many societies, and therefore represents possibly the largest health inequity of our time" (Patz, Gibbs, Foley, Rogers and Smith, 2007:397). This is because the effects of climate change are most felt in poor societies, which have contributed less to it and are already experiencing many health challenges associated with the rise in temperature (Patz et al., 2007). Climate change has also caused severe natural disasters such as flooding, wildfire, and pollution (Anbumozhi, 2020). The majority of these devastating effects of GHG emissions can be mitigated by reducing postharvest wastage of food.

15.3.6.4 BIODIVERSITY LOSS

There have been estimations of how much additional food production is required to meet the global food need in the future. However, one of the pitfalls of this idea is the further degradation of biodiversity and loss of the natural habitat of animals. Loss of natural habitats results in the depletion of microorganisms and higher animals and consequently leads to their extinction. Commercial agriculture involves the use of chemical fertilizers and heavy mechanization, which causes soil nutrient imbalances and disrupts soil formation, respectively (Blakeney, 2019; Cardoen et al., 2015). The nutrient elements in chemical fertilizers, such as urea, leach to contaminate underground water bodies and are harmful to several microorganisms (Cardoen et al., 2015). In India, for example, the loss of nitrogen from fertilizers is up to 60–80% (Cardoen et al., 2015), and this comes with huge consequences for the natural environment.

Furthermore, the production of fruit and vegetables uses the most amount of pesticides (Zhang, Jiang and Ou, 2011). For example, in the US, 80% of fruit and vegetables are produced using fungicides (Zhang et al., 2011). This high use of pesticides has huge, devastating effects on humans and biodiversity (Pimentel and Burgess, 2014). Pesticides and their residue find their way to rivers, the atmosphere, and the soil, which results in the gathering of harmful substances that are harmful to biodiversity and human health (Rani et al., 2020). According to a survey of the Chinese fruit and vegetable markets, 41 out of 81 samples of vegetables showed the presence of pesticide residue (Zhang et al., 2011). Cabbage and leek showed residues of more than 60% and 80%, respectively, of the Chinese minimum acceptable standard (Zhang et al., 2011). Richter (2002) reports that globally, about 26 million people suffer from pesticide poisonings, resulting in an estimated 220,000 deaths in a year. This means that the combined number of microorganisms and animals affected by using chemical fertilizers and pesticides for fruit and vegetable production would be higher. Therefore, postharvest losses of fruit and vegetables also mean losses of biodiversity and a huge threat to human life.

15.3.6.5 LANDFILL CHALLENGES

Landfill waste disposal has a serious environmental impact on postharvest wastage. It poses a serious challenge both in developed and developing countries, as wasted food usually ends up in landfills (Blakeney, 2019). The disposed food waste decomposes to produce noxious gases, which contributes to global warming (Nahman et al., 2012). Postharvest wastage contributes to GHG emissions from the energy used during production, distribution, and storage and produces methane, which is known to trap heat 21 times more than carbon dioxide (Adhikari, Barrington and Martinez, 2006). In the US, for example, about 25% of methane emissions are from landfills where municipal waste is disposed of, and only about 3% of the waste along the value chain is converted to compost (Gunders and Bloom, 2017). Landfill is a significant contributor to methane in the US and in other developed countries (Blakeney, 2019). In the UK, it is reported that if food waste were removed from all landfills, the GHG emission mitigation would be equal to removing one-fifth of cars in the country from the roads (Gunders and Bloom, 2017).

Furthermore, carbon dioxide and litter are produced from landfills and pollute the surrounding environment with an offensive odor that has a significant negative impact on human health (Nahman et al., 2012). Leachate is another problem associated with landfills, as the liquid produced by the breakdown of food waste permeates into the soil to pollute the groundwater and soil (Blakeney, 2019; Nahman et al., 2012; Osei et al., 2011). So, reducing postharvest wastage means reducing the area of land used as a landfill and mitigating its environmental consequences in terms of GHG emission, environmental pollution, and leachate.

15.3.6.6 NATURAL RESOURCES

15.3.6.6.1 Freshwater use

Water is one of the essential commodities upon which plants and animals depend for life. According to the Summary Report of the FAO on the footprint and impact of food wastage on natural resources in 2013, water resources accounting is either by withdrawal or consumption. Water withdrawal was described as the withdrawal of water from either surface or groundwater sources, while water consumption entails the water used by plants by transpiration, consumed by animals, or consumed in another form (FAO, 2013). Agricultural water use is consumptive in nature and accounts for about 92% of the total water footprint of humans (Hoekstra and Mekonnen, 2012). There have been suggestions that global water demand will be about 6900 billion m^3/year by 2030 (Blakeney, 2019). Table 15.6 presents the global freshwater use by region and indicates that the freshwater loss per capita/year due to lost and wasted food is high in developed countries. This could be attributed to the high food wastage at retail and consumption levels in these countries (Yahia, 2019).

TABLE 15.6 Total Global Freshwater Use Per Region

Region	Total Freshwater Use (m3/cap/year)	Used for Lost and Wasted Food (m3/cap/year)
Sub-Saharan Africa	52.00	12.00 (22%)
Europe	59.00	18.00 (31%)
Industrialized Asia	74.00	19.00 (25%)
Latin America	65.00	22.00 (34%)
North Africa and West-Central Asia	258.00	86.00 (33%)
North America and Oceania	120.00	42.00 (35%)
South and Southeast Asia	161.00	30.00 (18%)
Global	111.00	27.00 (24%)

Source: Adapted from Kummu et al. (2012).

Hoekstra and Mekonnen (2012) suggest that the majority of the water usage in agriculture is at the production level. Estimates suggest that the total freshwater used to produce food crops that are lost and wasted along the value chain is about 24% (27 m^3/cap/year) (Kummu et al., 2012).

In the UK, avoidable food waste amounts to about 6% of the water footprint per person (Blakeney, 2019). Water use in Germany seems even more, as 14 m^3 of freshwater is used for agricultural production purposes per person, and water used for food production amounts to one-third of the household's water use (Eberle and Fels, 2016). To differentiate the process of freshwater use in fruit and vegetable production, Ridoutt et al. (2010) classified freshwater use into two–orchard operations and postharvest operations. Freshwater use in orchard pomegranate production operations, for instance, is intensive, with irrigation accounting for about 23% of the capital cost of production (POMASA, 2019). This is important to note because, in South Africa, pomegranate is mainly grown in the Western Cape Province, which has a history of water scarcity. Water scarcity and agricultural water usage have remained major challenges in many regions of the world (Wada, Van Beek and Bierkens, 2011). The study by Ridoutt et al. (2010) on the water footprint of fresh mangoes grown in Australia reported that from production to consumption, an annual average of 26.7 Gl (gigalitres) of rainfall water and 16.6 Gl of irrigation water is wasted. In general, water associated with food waste in Australia is estimated at 8980 Gl, which accounts for 9.1% of the total water use in the country (Reutter, Lant, Reynolds and Lane, 2017). In another study, Liu, Lundqvist, Weinberg and Gustafsson (2013) reported that the water footprint of China associated with fruit and vegetables is estimated at 14% of the total water footprint. In the US, it was estimated that about 34% (1237 kcal/cap/day) of food was lost in 2015, with 90 km^3/y (cubic kilometers/year) of water footprint attributable to this loss (Mekonnen and Fulton, 2018). At the retail level, fruit and vegetables accounted for 18% of the water footprint of the lost food (Mekonnen and Fulton, 2018).

From the FAO estimation (Table 15.7), fruit and vegetables account for a combined 26% of the irrigation water footprint of food losses and waste (FAO, 2013). Irrigated agriculture poses serious environmental challenges such as waterlogging, causing soil degradation, salinization, and groundwater depletion (Aldaya, Allan and Hoekstra, 2010). Therefore, postharvest wastage of fruit and vegetables not only represents an unnecessary waste of freshwater that could have been used for other purposes but also causes degradation of the natural environment.

TABLE 15.7 Comparing Commodity Contribution to Food Wastage and Irrigation Water Footprint

Food Commodity	Wastage (%)	Irrigation Water Footprint (%)
Cereals	26.00	52.00
Starchy roots	19.00	2.00
Oil crops and pulses	4.00	6.00
Fruit	16.00	18.00
Meat	5.00	8.00
Milk and egg	8.00	8.00
Vegetables	25.00	8.00

Source: FAO (2013).

15.3.6.6.2 Cropland use

Land is a natural resource which is scarce in supply in the sense that humans cannot create more of it. Land for crop cultivation occupies an estimated 1.53 billion hectares of the total earth landmass (Foley et al., 2011). The cultivation of crops comes with severe consequences and impacts on biodiversity, animal habitats, soil condition, and carbon sequestration. These impacts on the natural environment disrupt the enjoyment of ecosystem services that come from the natural environment. Furthermore, the use of fertilizers for crop production also depletes resources like phosphorous (Dawson and Hilton, 2011). Also, there are problems of GHG associated with food losses and waste (Garnett and Wilkes, 2014). Challenges associated with cropland usage due to postharvest wastage can be huge in some countries. For example, in the US, up to 40% of the food produced goes to waste (Gunders and Bloom, 2017).

Table 15.8 shows that the total global cropland area used for lost and wasted food along the value chain accounts for 23%, which translates to 198 Mha/yr (Kummu et al., 2012). This amount of land used for farming wasted food could be used to plant trees and build parks for the enjoyment of ecosystem services. This is particularly important given that a significant part of the Amazon forest in Brazil, which is referred to as the Earth's lungs, got burnt in 2019.

TABLE 15.8 Total Global Cropland Uses Per Region

Region	Total Cropland Use (m^2/cap/year)	Used for Lost and Wasted Food (m^2/cap/year)
Sub-Saharan Africa	1950.00	431.00 (22%)
Europe	1282.00	334.00 (26%)
Industrialized Asia	948.00	232.00 (25%)
Latin America	1475.00	361.00 (24%)
North Africa and West-Central Asia	1473.00	407.00 (28%)
North America and Oceania	1611.00	498.00 (31%)
South and Southeast Asia	1298.00	237.00 (18%)
Global	1334.00	305.00 (23%)

Source: Adapted from Kummu et al. (2012).

15.3.6.7 FOOD AND NUTRITION SECURITY

The health status of a community is determined by the lifestyle choices and nutritional security of its people (Paul and Shaha, 2004). Whether a community is food secure or not is a function of what people consume and the impact on their health. Until 1996, food security was defined as "access by all people to enough food to live a healthy and productive life" (Pinstrup-Anderson, 2009). The World Food Summit of the FAO in 1996 modified this definition to incorporate nutritional security and preferences. The FAO definition states that food security is achieved when "all people, at all times, have physical and economic access to sufficient, safe, and nutritious food to meet their dietary needs and food preferences for an active and healthy life" (FAO, 1996). The definition has gained more attention owing to the numerous health-related and pharmaceutical benefit discoveries about fruit and vegetables. Fruit and vegetables are an important part of human dietary need as they contain essential vitamins that help to maintain nutritional security (Liu, 2003). Also, fruit and vegetables add color and flavor to foods and serve as a source of dietary fiber, minerals, and energy (Kader and Barrett, 1996).

However, despite all the benefits derived from fruit and vegetable consumption, fruit and vegetables are still the most wasted food commodities globally (FAO, 2013). Efforts to advance food security and feed the world's teeming population are undermined by postharvest wastage of fruit and vegetables. This is because food security does not only entail the availability of food but also the availability of the right nutritional content (FAO, 1996). This supports the argument of Pinstrup-Andersen (2009) that having enough calories in a diet does not mean that the diet is healthy and nutritional.

15.3.6.7.1 What nutrients are in wasted fruit and vegetables?

Fruit and vegetables contain essential minerals that help to maintain a healthy life. Minerals are inorganic substances that are required by an organism in small quantities for the maintenance of important processes essential for life (Paul and Shaha, 2004). Examples of macro and micro minerals are calcium, iron, potassium, zinc, magnesium, sodium, phosphorus, and copper, while vitamins include ascorbic acid, riboflavin, and thiamine (Table 15.9). Also, dietary fibers, phenolic compounds, organic acids, and sugar derivatives are richly available in fruit and vegetables (Sagar et al., 2018). Tables 15.9 and 15.10 present some nutrients, vitamins, and mineral content of selected fruit and vegetables.

TABLE 15.9 Selected Nutrient and Vitamin Contents of Some Fruit and Vegetables

Fruit	Fiber ($g100^{-1}g$)	Carbohydrate ($g100^{-1}g$)	Thiamine ($mg100^{-1}g$)	Ascorbic Acid ($mg100^{-1}g$)
Pomegranate	0.50	9.90	0.06	15.00
Tomato	5.00	14.90	0.10	30.00
Orange	0.30	6.00	0.12	62.00
Pineapple	8.60	23.50	0.20	35.00
Lemon	1.60	10.80	0.02	37.00
Blackberry	0.60	16.00	0.12	30.00
Plum	–	8.90	0.04	10.00
Litchi	0.50	18.90	0.14	39.00

Source: Adapted from Paul and Shaha (2004).

The deficiency of essential calories, vitamins, and micro and macro mineral elements fosters the development of disease and results in an overall decline in physical health and the ability of the body to protect itself from diseases (WHO-FAO, 2005). For example, according to Bender (2003), a 10 mg intake of vitamin C is required per day to prevent deficiency, and 20 mg is required to heal wounds. Fruits such as citrus and berries contain more than 20 mg of vitamin C in less than 100 g of fruit tissue (Matare, 2012).

Also, the consumption of fruits and vegetables ensures the intake of vital nutrients such as antioxidant vitamins, polyphenols, and other nutrients, which are essential in lowering the risk and development of chronic diseases (Kerch, 2015). The phytochemicals in fruits and vegetables help to prevent oxidative stress, thereby preventing diseases like cancer, diabetes, and cardiovascular diseases (Li et al., 2014; Opara and Al-Ani, 2010). This makes fruits and vegetables important in solving the global micronutrient deficiency crisis. Consumption of fruits and vegetables serves as the most sustainable source of micronutrients in foods.

TABLE 15.10 Selected Mineral Content of Some Fruit and Vegetables

Fruit	Calcium ($mg100^{-1}g$)	Magnesium ($mg100^{-1}g$)	Sodium ($mg100^{-1}g$)	Phosphorus ($mg100^{-1}g$)	Potassium ($mg100^{-1}g$)
Pomegranate	30.00	12.00	4.00	30.00	171.00
Tomato	27.00	17.00	5.50	28.00	275.00
Orange	25.50	16.20	28.00	24.20	99.40
Pineapple	15.00	42.00	2.90	20.90	228.00
Lemon	70.00	12.00	1.50	10.00	148.00
Blackberry	21.50	49.80	3.50	18.50	130.00
Plum	20.00	9.80	4.10	20.00	129.00
Litchi	9.80	22.50	0.80	17.20	89.90

Source: Adapted from Paul and Shaha (2004).

Postharvest nutritional loss is mostly related to factors such as temperature, light, moisture, oxygen, and duration of exposure to heat (Matare, 2012). The loss of nutrients, especially vitamins C, through postharvest wastage of fruit and vegetables reduces the health benefits obtained from consuming fruit and vegetables. This is because vitamin C, which is the most important vitamin in the human diet, is mainly supplied by fruit and vegetables (Lee and Kader, 2000). Therefore, according to Opara and Al-Ani (2010), inadequate intake of fruit and vegetables contributes to micronutrient deficiencies that have devastating effects, such as a weakened immune system and even birth defects. Postharvest wastage of fruit and vegetables means loss of nutrients that could have been consumed to ensure food security and maintain a healthy life. So, reducing postharvest wastage of fruit and vegetables means having more micronutrients available to ensure food and nutritional security.

15.3.6.7.2 Impact on nutrition security

The impact of postharvest losses on food and nutritional security cannot be overemphasized. A report by the US Department of Agriculture's Economic Research Service estimates that about 141 trillion calories/year, which amounts to 1249 calories/per capita/day, in the food value chain in 2010 was wasted (Buzby, Farah-Wells and Hyman, 2014). In 2012, the amount of wasted food at the retail and consumer levels in the US contained 1216.5 calories/capita/day (Table 15.11). Given that the daily calorie intake for healthy living is 2000 cal/capita/day for adult women, these amounts of calories wasted per year could meet the daily requirement of not less than 1.3 million women in a year. Regrettably, fruit and vegetables consist of 19% of the contributing food commodities (Buzby et al., 2014). Also, Gunders and Bloom (2017) reported that reducing food wastage by only 15% would save enough food requirements for over 25 million people in the US every year, given that one in every six Americans does not have an adequate food supply. Additionally, Kummu et al. (2012) found that about 614 kcal/cap/day, which accounts for about a quarter of the produced food supply, is lost along the value chain. Table 15.11 demonstrates the magnitude of nutrient loss in food commodities in the US in 2012 at retail and consumer levels only.

TABLE 15.11 The Magnitude of Nutrient Loss in Wasted Food at the Retail and Consumer Levels in the US in 2012 Compared to the Daily Nutritional Requirement for Adult Women

Nutrition	Recommended Daily Intake (Adult Women)	Nutrient Loss (Daily/Capita)	Equivalent Number of Recommended Intakes (Millions of Adults/Capita/Day)
Energy (kcal)	2000.00	1216.50	190.90
Dietary fiber (g)	25.00	5.90	73.60
Magnesium (mg)	310.00	85.00	86.00
Vitamin C (mg)	75.00	35.40	148.00
Calcium (mg)	1000.00	286.10	89.80
Potassium (mg)	4700.00	880.20	58.80
Vitamin E (mg)	15.00	3.60	75.90
Iron (mg)	18.00	5.30	92.60
Vitamin A (mcg)	700.00	308.30	138.30
Vitamin D (mcg)	15.00	1.70	36.60

Source: Adapted from Spiker et al. (2017).

In Africa, where poor households in remote villages depend on agriculture for survival (Opara, 2010), nutritional insecurity deepens as fresh fruit and vegetables are wasted (Kitinoja and Kader, 2015). For example, nutritional loss in the common beans value chain in the district of Luwingu, Northern Province of Zambia, is enough to meet the recommended daily allowance for 49 people (Ellis, Kwofie and Ngadi, 2020). Matare (2012) and Munhuweyi (2012) discussed the proximate composition of some fruit and vegetables and the magnitude of postharvest wastage of commodities at the national level in South Africa in 2011. The studies reported the nutritional loss of fruit per 100 g loss (Table 15.12). Matare (2012) reported the annual wastage of peach, pear, and tangelo at the retail level to be an estimated 7240 tons, 418 tons, and 1000 tons, respectively. Carrot, cabbage, and tomato annual wastage during the same period were estimated at 15,250 tons, 24,470 tons, and 15,250 tons, respectively (Munhuweyi, 2012). The nutritional loss from the wasted fruit and vegetables could meet the daily nutritional requirement of at least 25,000 people per capita/year in South Africa.

TABLE 15.12 Nutrient Loss per 100 g in Lost Fruit and Vegetables at the Retail Level in South Africa in 2011

Commodity	Protein (g)	Crude fat (g)	Dietary Fiber (g)	Carbohydrate (g)	Energy (kJ)	Annual Wastage (tons)
Peach	2.50	0.05	1.13	10.95	202.33	7240.00
Pear	2.45	0.05	0.95	9.82	111.67	418.00
Tangelo	3.21	0.07	2.43	23.83	–	1000.00
Carrot	1.11–1.20	–	2.04–2.3	22.12–36.05	18.96–30.56	15,250.00
Cabbage	1.06–1.20	0.03	–	4.39–5.32	92.18–110.38	24,470.00
Tomato	0.78–0.80	0.01–0.02	0.96–1.13	3.43–3.77	71.18–73.77	15,250.00
Total						63,628.00

Source: Adapted from Matare (2012); Munhuweyi (2012).

Reducing postharvest wastage means reducing the waste of energy used for the production and transportation of fruit and vegetables, and consequently reducing pollution because of transportation. Postharvest wastage represents a significant loss of production output and loss of investment, loss of scarce resources, nutritional loss, lost labor, and all farm inputs. This means a gross financial loss to farmers when equated in monetary terms and perpetuates poverty and micronutrition deficiency, especially in developing countries. Therefore, reducing postharvest wastage calls for sustainable handling, distribution, and utilization of food supplies to enhance food and nutritional security (Opara, 2010). To emphasize the role of the value chain in reducing postharvest losses and enhancing the availability of perishable foods such as fruit and vegetables, Adam and Gollin (2015) suggested that sophisticated and highly streamlined processing and a real-time value chain to link farmers and consumers is necessary.

15.3.6.7.3 Impact on food availability

There is a persistent concern about satisfying the demand for food currently, and this could be worse if the world attains the over 9 billion population estimated to live in the world by 2050 (Swilling and Annecke, 2012; UN, 2011). There has been a suggestion about increasing food production by 70% to alleviate food insecurity and to feed the world's teeming population (FAO, 2009). Nevertheless, more food is currently produced to feed the world, yet 925 million people are food insecure (FAO, 2010). This flaws the suggestion of increased food production because it does not make sense to produce more food when postharvest wastage persists. Therefore, conscious efforts should be made to improve technology and innovation, and skills at food production and distribution levels, especially in developing countries where facilities to maintain the quality of food along the value chain are inadequate (Atanda et al., 2011; Hodges et al., 2011). Also, behavioral changes towards food are necessary for developed countries, where food wastage is high at the retail and consumption levels (FAO, 2011; Kadar, 2005).

The nutritional content and overall quality of food, especially fruit and vegetables, are retained when an adequate and proper storage and handling system is in place along the value chain, given their susceptibility to spoilage due to high moisture content (Kader, 1983; Munhuweyi et al., 2016). But in developing countries where value chain facilities are inadequate, postharvest losses persist, deepening the problem of fruit and vegetable availability for consumption. It is estimated that losses and waste amount to up to 31% of total fruit and vegetable production in developing countries (Oelofse and Nahman, 2013), thereby contributing to food insecurity by reducing fruit and vegetable availability.

Furthermore, an increase in population in developing countries also means an increase in urbanization (Swilling and Annecke, 2012), which means that more people are moving away from the areas of primary production of fruit and vegetables, leading to longer time along the value chain before the fruit and vegetables reach the final consumer. This reduces the availability of the commodities because the more time it takes for the fruit and vegetables to reach the consumer, the more they are susceptible to postharvest loss (Kader, 1983). At the same time, the need to meet the demand of the rising population in urban areas continues to increase. Postharvest wastage occasioned by physical, biological, and environmental factors impacts the nutritional value of fruit and vegetables. Literature suggests that postharvest losses in storage are more significant with higher temperatures and prolonged storage periods. For example, the management of temperature and storage condition of citrus fruit impact the retention of vitamin C in such fruit (Lee and Kader, 2000). Also, leafy vegetables tend to lose nutrients in conditions that favor the loss of moisture content (Kerch, 2015; Lee and Kader, 2000).

15.4 CONCLUSIONS

Postharvest wastage of fruit and vegetables is a global challenge and must be mitigated if the food and nutritional security of over 9 billion people living in the world by 2050 will be met. Literature reveals that postharvest wastage occurs both in developed and developing countries; however, the difference is that wastage occurs more during production and along the value chain in developing countries and at retail and consumption in developed countries. This is understood to be because of the poor and inadequate postharvest storage and handling facilities in developing countries and consumer behavior in developed countries. Therefore, the nutritional impacts of postharvest wastage in developed and developing countries are similar, as demonstrated by the amount of food and nutrition loss in the US and UK as compared to countries like Zambia and Ethiopia.

The major inconsistency in literature is the definition of 'food losses' and 'food waste.' Some authors defined them according to the stage of the food value chain, while others defined them according to what happened to the food material. But all agreed that despite where and how losses occur, they impact farmers and food value chain actors and affect the environment negatively. The types and causes of fruit and vegetable postharvest wastage are similar in literature. Quantitative losses are mostly internal and evident in weight loss and other internal damages, while qualitative losses are mostly physical losses that affect the appearance and perception of the food, leading to downgrading. Postharvest wastage due to mechanical, environmental (especially in storage), and handling damage are more profound in the way they affect the quality of fruit and vegetable along the value chain.

The impacts of postharvest wastage reflect economic loss, environmental degradation, and food and nutritional insecurity. These impacts of postharvest wastage manifest in unsustainable utilization of natural resources, which results in the loss of resources that could have been put to other beneficial use. The continuous unsustainable use of energy, water, cropland, and other production inputs as occasioned by postharvest wastage of food means that it makes no sense to increase food production if postharvest wastage is not reduced. Also, nutritional insecurity and micronutrient deficiency could be mitigated by reducing postharvest wastage and increasing postharvest technology and innovation, especially in developing countries.

KEYWORDS

- **food supply chain efficiency**
- **food system sustainability**
- **fruit and vegetable losses**
- **micronutrient deficiency**
- **nutritional security**
- **postharvest wastage**

REFERENCES

Adam, C., & Gollin, D. (2015). Editors' introduction: The economics of the global food and agriculture system. *Oxford Review of Economic Policy, 31*(1), 1–7.

Adhikari, B. K., Barrington, S., & Martinez, J. (2006). Predicted growth of world urban food waste and methane production. *Waste Management & Research, 24*(5), 421–433.

Aldaya, M. M., Allan, J. A., & Hoekstra, A. Y. (2010). Strategic importance of green water in international crop trade. *Ecological Economics, 69*(4), 887–894.

Anbumozhi, V. (2020). Improving the resilience of regional food value chains against climate change and natural disasters. In M. Breiling & V. Anbumozhi (Eds.), *Vulnerability of Agricultural Production Networks and Global Food Value Chains Due To Natural Disasters* (pp. 153–167). Economic Research Institute for ASEAN and East Asia.

Angelino, D., Godos, J., Ghelfi, F., Tieri, M., Titta, L., Lafranconi, A., Marventano, S., Alonzo, E., Gambera, A., Sciacca, S., & Buscemi, S. (2019). Fruit and vegetable consumption and health outcomes: An umbrella review of observational studies. *International Journal of Food Sciences and Nutrition, 70*(6), 652–667.

Atanda, S. A., Pessu, P. O., Agoda, S., Isong, I. U., & Ikotun, I. (2011). The concepts and problems of post–harvest food losses in perishable crops. *African Journal of Food Science, 5*(11), 603–613.

Aulakh, J., & Regmi, A. (2013). *Postharvest Food Losses Estimation—Development of Consistent Methodology*. FAO.

Bais-Moleman, A. L., Schulp, C. J., & Verburg, P. H. (2019). Assessing the environmental impacts of production- and consumption-side measures in sustainable agriculture intensification in the European Union. *Geoderma, 338*, 555–567.

Batu, A. (2004). Determination of acceptable firmness and color values of tomatoes. *Journal of Food Engineering, 61*(3), 471–475.

Bender, D. A. (2003). *Nutritional Biochemistry of The Vitamins*. Cambridge University Press.

Beretta, C., Stoessel, F., Baier, U., & Hellweg, S. (2013). Quantifying food losses and the potential for reduction in Switzerland. *Waste Management, 33*(3), 764–773.

Beretta, C., Stucki, M., & Hellweg, S. (2017). Environmental impacts and hotspots of food losses: Value chain analysis of Swiss food consumption. *Environmental Science & Technology, 51*(19), 11165–11173.

Blakeney, M. (2019). *Food Loss and Food Waste: Causes and Solutions*. Edward Elgar Publishing.

Bourne, M. (1977). Postharvest food losses–The neglected dimension in increasing the world food supply. *Cornell International Agriculture Mimeograph 53*. Cornell University, Ithaca, New York.

Buzby, J. C., & Hyman, J. (2012). Total and per capita value of food loss in the United States. *Food Policy, 37*(5), 561–570.

Buzby, J. C., Farah-Wells, H., & Hyman, J. (2014). *The Estimated Amount, Value, And Calories of Postharvest Food Losses at The Retail and Consumer Levels in the United States*. USDA-ERS Economic Information Bulletin, 121.

Cardoen, D., Joshi, P., Diels, L., Sarma, P. M., & Pant, D. (2015). Agriculture biomass in India: Part 2. Postharvest losses, cost and environmental impacts. *Resources, Conservation and Recycling, 101*, 143–153.

Ceponis, M. J., & Butterfield, J. E. (1973). *The Nature and Extent of Retail and Consumer Losses in Apples, Oranges, Lettuce, Peaches, Strawberries, And Potatoes Marketed in Greater New York*. US Department of Agriculture. Marketing Research Report No. 996.

Dawson, C. J., & Hilton, J. (2011). Fertilizer availability in a resource-limited world: Production and recycling of nitrogen and phosphorus. *Food Policy, 36*, 14–22.

Department of Agriculture, Forestry and Fishery (DAFF). (2017). *Fresh Food Trade SA*. https://www.daff.gov.za (accessed on 9th July 2025).

dos Santos, S. F., Cardoso, R. D. C. V., Borges, Í. M. P., e Almeida, A. C., Andrade, E. S., Ferreira, I. O., & do Carmo Ramos, L. (2020). Postharvest losses of fruits and vegetables in supply centers in Salvador, Brazil: Analysis of determinants, volumes and reduction strategies. *Waste Management, 101*, 161–170.

Eberle, U., & Fels, J. (2016). Environmental impacts of German food consumption and food losses. *The International Journal of Life Cycle Assessment, 21*(5), 759–772.

Ellis, E., Kwofie, E. M., & Ngadi, M. (2020). Economic and nutritional implications of losses and contributing factors along the bean value chain. *Journal of Stored Products Research, 87*, 101582, 1–13.

Fadiji, T., Coetzee, C., Chen, L., Chukwu, O., & Opara, U. L. (2016). Susceptibility of apples to bruising inside ventilated corrugated paperboard packages during simulated transport damage. *Postharvest Biology and Technology, 118*, 111–119.

Fawole, O. A., & Opara, U. L. (2013). Effects of storage temperature and duration on physiological responses of pomegranate fruit. *Industrial Crops and Products, 47*, 300–309.

Foley, J. A., Ramankutty, N., Brauman, K. A., Cassidy, E. S., Gerber, J. S., Johnston, M., Mueller, N. D., O'Connell, C., Ray, D. K., West, P. C., & Balzer, C. (2011). Solutions for a cultivated planet. *Nature, 478*, 337–342.

Food and Agriculture Organization of the United Nations (FAO). (1989). *Prevention of Postharvest Food Losses: Fruits, Vegetables, And Root Crops. A Training Manual*. Rome, Italy.

Food and Agriculture Organization of the United Nations (FAO). (1996). *Declaration on World Food Security*. World Food Summit. Rome, Italy.

Food and Agriculture Organization of the United Nations (FAO). (2009). *High Level Expert Forum–How to Feed the World in 2050*. Economic and Social Development Department. http://www.fao.org/fileadmin/templates/wsfs/docs/Issues_papers/HLEF2050_Global_Agriculture.pdf (accessed on 9th July 2025).

Food and Agriculture Organization of the United Nations (FAO). (2010). *The State of Food Insecurity in The World: Addressing Food Insecurity in Protracted Crises*. Rome, Italy.

Food and Agriculture Organization of the United Nations (FAO). (2011). *Global Food Losses and Food Waste–Extent, Causes and Prevention*. Rome, Italy.

Food and Agriculture Organization of the United Nations (FAO). (2013). *Food Wastage Footprint: Impacts on Natural Resources*. Rome, Italy.

Gardas, B. B., Raut, R. D., & Narkhede, B. (2018). Evaluating critical causal factors for postharvest losses (PHL) in the fruit and vegetables supply chain in India using the DEMATEL approach. *Journal of Cleaner Production, 199*, 47–61.

Garnett, T. (2006). *Fruit and Vegetable and UK Greenhouse Gas Emissions: Exploring the Relationship*. A working paper produced as part of the work of the Food Climate Research Network 06-01.

Garnett, T., & Wilkes, A. (2014). *Appetite for Change: Social, Economic and Environmental Transformations in China's Food System*. Food Climate Research Network. http://www.ccjc-beijing.com/manage/images/2014619213033.pdf (accessed on 9th July 2025).

Gehlich, K. H., Beller, J., Lange-Asschenfeldt, B., Köcher, W., Meinke, M. C., & Lademann, J. (2019). Fruit and vegetable consumption is associated with improved mental and cognitive health in older adults from non-Western developing countries. *Public Health Nutrition, 22*(4), 689–696.

Gogo, E. O., Opiyo, A. M., Ulrichs, C., & Huyskens-Keil, S. (2017). Nutritional and economic postharvest loss analysis of African indigenous leafy vegetables along the supply chain in Kenya. *Postharvest Biology and Technology, 130*, 39–47.

Goossens, Y., Berrens, P., Custers, K., Van Hemelryck, S., Kellens, K., & Geeraerd, A. (2019). How origin, packaging and seasonality determine the environmental impact of apples, magnified by food waste and losses. *The International Journal of Life Cycle Assessment, 24*(4), 667–687.

Gunders, D., & Bloom, J. (2017). *Wasted: How America is Losing Up to 40 Percent of Its Food from Farm to Fork to Landfill*. Natural Resources Defence Council.

Gustavsson, J., Cederberg, C., Sonesson, U., Van Otterdijk, R., & Meybeck, A. (2011). *Global Food Losses and Food Waste* (pp. 1–38). Rome: FAO.

Heard, B. R., Bandekar, M., Vassar, B., & Miller, S. A. (2019). Comparison of life cycle environmental impacts from meal kits and grocery store meals. *Resources, Conservation and Recycling, 147*, 189–200.

Hodges, R. J., Buzby, J. C., & Bennett, B. (2011). Postharvest losses and waste in developed and less developed countries: Opportunities to improve resource use. *The Journal of Agricultural Science, 149*, 37–45.

Hoekstra, A. Y., & Mekonnen, M. M. (2012). The water footprint of humanity. *Proceedings of the National Academy of Sciences, 109*, 3232–3237.

Hussein, Z., Fawole, O. A., & Opara, U. L. (2019b). Harvest and postharvest factors affecting bruise damage of fresh fruits. *Horticultural Plant Journal, 6*(1), 1–13.

Hussein, Z., Fawole, O. A., & Opara, U. O. (2019a). Bruise damage of pomegranate during long-term cold storage: Susceptibility to bruising and changes in textural properties of fruit. *International Journal of Fruit Science*, 1–20.

Kader, A. A. (1983). Postharvest quality maintenance of fruits and vegetables in developing countries. In *Postharvest Physiology and Crop Preservation* (pp. 455–470). Springer.

Kader, A. A. (2005). Increasing food availability by reducing postharvest losses of fresh produce. *International Postharvest Symposium, 682*, 2169–2176.

Kader, A. A., & Barrett, D. M. (1996). Classification, composition of fruits, and postharvest maintenance of quality. In *Processing Fruits: Science and Technology* (Vol. 1, pp. 1–24).

Kashyap, D., & Agarwal, T. (2020). Food loss in India: Water footprint, land footprint and GHG emissions. *Environment, Development and Sustainability, 22*(4), 2905–2918.

Kasso, M., & Bekele, A. (2016). Postharvest loss and quality deterioration of horticultural crops in Dire Dawa Region, Ethiopia. *Journal of the Saudi Society of Agricultural Sciences, 17*(1), 88–96.

Keatinge, J. D. H., Yang, R. Y., Hughes, J. D. A., Easdown, W. J., & Holmer, R. (2011). The importance of vegetables in ensuring both food and nutritional security in attainment of the Millennium Development Goals. *Food Security, 3*(4), 491–501.

Keatinge, J. D., Waliyar, F., Jamnadas, R. H., Moustafa, A., Andrade, M., Drechsel, P., Hughes, J. D. A., Kadirvel, P., & Luther, K. (2010). Relearning old lessons for the future of food—By bread alone no longer: Diversifying diets with fruit and vegetables. *Crop Science, 50*, 51–62.

Kerch, G. (2015). Chitosan films and coatings prevent losses of fresh fruit nutritional quality: A review. *Trends in Food Science and Technology, 46*(2), 159–166.

Kitinoja, L., & Kader, A. A. (2015). Measuring postharvest losses of fresh fruits and vegetables in developing countries. *PEF White Paper, 15*-02.

Kitinoja, L., Tokala, V. Y., & Brondy, A. (2018). A review of global postharvest loss assessments in plant-based food crops: Recent findings and measurement gaps. *Journal of Postharvest Technology, 6*(4), 1–15.

Kummu, M., De Moel, H., Porkka, M., Siebert, S., Varis, O., & Ward, P. J. (2012). Lost food, wasted resources: Global food supply chain losses and their impacts on freshwater, cropland, and fertilizer use. *Science of the Total Environment, 438*, 477–489.

Lee, S. K., & Kader, A. A. (2000). Preharvest and postharvest factors influencing vitamin C content of horticultural crops. *Postharvest Biology and Technology, 20*(3), 207–220.

Li, A. N., Li, S., Zhang, Y. J., Xu, X. R., Chen, Y. M., & Li, H. B. (2014). Resources and biological activities of natural polyphenols. *Nutrients, 6*(12), 6020–6047.

Liu, J., Lundqvist, J., Weinberg, J., & Gustafsson, J. (2013). Food losses and waste in China and their implication for water and land. *Environmental Science & Technology, 47*(18), 10137–10144.

Liu, R. H. (2003). Health benefits of fruit and vegetables are from additive and synergistic combinations of phytochemicals. *The American Journal of Clinical Nutrition, 78*(3), 517–520.

Louw, D. (2016). *An Impact Evaluation Study of The Postharvest Innovation Programmed: A Final Report for the OABS Development*. Paarl, South Africa.

Lufu, R., Ambaw, A., & Opara, U. L. (2019). The contribution of transpiration and respiration processes in the mass loss of pomegranate fruit (cv. *Wonderful*). *Postharvest Biology and Technology, 157*, 110982, 1–10.

Lufu, R., Ambaw, A., & Opara, U. L. (2020). Water loss of fresh fruit: Influencing pre-harvest, harvest and postharvest factors. *Scientia Horticultural, 272*, 109519, 1–16.

Macheka, L., Spelt, E. J., Bakker, E. J., van der Vorst, J. G., & Luning, P. A. (2018). Identification of determinants of postharvest losses in Zimbabwean tomato supply chains as basis for dedicated interventions. *Food Control, 87*, 135–144.

Mahajan, P. (2020). Agriculture trade scenario in India and its global comparisons. *International Journal of Agricultural Economics, 5*(3), 63–70.

Mashau, M. E., Moyane, J. N., & Jideani, I. A. (2012). Assessment of postharvest losses of fruits at Tshakhuma fruit market in Limpopo Province, South Africa. *African Journal of Agricultural Research, 7*(29), 4145–4150.

Mason-D'Croz, D., Bogard, J. R., Sulser, T. B., Cenacchi, N., Dunston, S., Herrero, M., & Wiebe, K. (2019). Gaps between fruit and vegetable production, demand, and recommended consumption at global and national levels: An integrated modelling study. *The Lancet Planetary Health, 3*(7), 318–329.

Matare, T. (2012). *Postharvest Losses and Changes in Physic-Chemical Properties of Fruit (Peaches, Pears and Oranges) At Retail and During Post-Purchase Storage* (Unpublished MSc thesis). Stellenbosch University, South Africa.

McKenzie, T. J., Singh-Peterson, L., & Underhill, S. J. (2017). Quantifying postharvest loss and the implication of market-based decisions: A case study of two commercial domestic tomato supply chains in Queensland, Australia. *Horticultural, 3*(3), 2–15.

Mekonnen, M. M., & Fulton, J. (2018). The effect of diet changes and food loss reduction in reducing the water footprint of an average American. *Water International, 43*(6), 860–870.

Miguel, G., Fontes, C., Antunes, D., Neves, A., & Martins, D. (2004). Anthocyanin concentration of "Assaria" pomegranate fruits during different cold storage conditions. *BioMed Research International, 5*, 338–342.

Mukama, M., Ambaw, A., & Opara, U. L. (2020). Advances in design and performance evaluation of fresh fruit ventilated distribution packaging: A review. *Food Packaging and Shelf Life, 24*, 100472, 1–14.

Munhuweyi, K. (2012). *Postharvest Losses and Changes in Quality of Vegetable from Retail to Consumer: A Case Study of Tomato, Cabbage and Carrot* (Unpublished MSc thesis). Stellenbosch University, South Africa.

Munhuweyi, K., Lennox, C. L., Meitz-Hopkins, J. C., Caleb, O. J., & Opara, U. L. (2016). Major diseases of pomegranate (*Punica granatum* L.), their causes and management—A review. *Scientia Horticultural, 211*, 126–139.

Munhuweyi, K., Opara, U. L., & Sigge, G. (2016). Postharvest losses of cabbages from retail to consumer and the socio-economic and environmental impacts. *British Food Journal, 118*(2), 286–300.

Murthy, D. S., Gajanana, T. M., Sudha, M., & Dakshinamoorthy, V. (2009). Marketing and postharvest losses in fruits: Its implications on availability and economy. *Indian Journal of Agricultural Economics, 64*, 259–275.

Musasa, S. T., Mvumi, B. M., Manditsera, F. A., Chinhanga, J., Musiyandaka, S., & Chigwedere, C. (2013). Postharvest orange losses and small-scale farmers' perceptions on the loss causes in the fruit value chain: A case study of Rusitu Valley, Zimbabwe. *Food Science and Quality Management, 18*, 1–8.

Nahman, A., De Lange, W., Oelofse, S., & Godfrey, L. (2012). The costs of household food waste in South Africa. *Waste Management, 32*(11), 2147–2153.

Nshizirungu, R., & Kitinoja, L. (2019). *Tomato Postharvest Management in Rwanda*. PEF White No. 19-04. La Pine, Oregon, USA: The Postharvest Education Foundation.

Oelofse, S. (2013). *Food Waste in South Africa*. Africa: Opportunities and challenges. Pretoria: Council for Scientific and Industrial Research (CSIR).

Opara, I. K., Fawole, O. A., & Opara, U. L. (2021b). Postharvest losses of pomegranate fruit at the packhouse and implications for sustainability indicators. *Sustainability, 13*(9), 5187, 1–19.

Opara, I. K., Fawole, O. A., Kelly, C., & Opara, U. L. (2021a). Quantification of on-farm pomegranate fruit postharvest losses and waste, and implications on sustainability indicators: South African case study. *Sustainability, 13*(9), 5168, 1–20.

Opara, L. U. (2003). Postharvest losses at the fresh produce retail chain in the Sultanate of Oman. *Australian Postharvest Horticulture Conference*, Brisbane, Australia, 1–3 October 2003; 248–249.

Opara, U. L. (2010). High incidence of postharvest food losses is worsening global food and nutrition security. *International Journal of Postharvest Technology & Innovation, 2*(1), 1–3.

Opara, U. L., & Al-Ani, M. R. (2010). Antioxidant contents of pre-packed fresh-cut versus whole fruit and vegetables. *British Food Journal, 112*(8), 797–810.

Opara, U. L., & Fadiji, T. (2018). Compression damage susceptibility of apple fruit packed inside ventilated corrugated paperboard package. *Scientia Horticultural, 227*, 154–161.

Opara, U. L., & Pathare, P. B. (2014). Bruise damage measurement and analysis of fresh horticultural produce—A review. *Postharvest Biology and Technology, 91*, 9–24.

Osei, J., Osae, S. K., Fianko, J. R., Adomako, D., Laar, C., Anim, A. K., Ganyaglo, S. Y., Nyarku, M., & Nyarko, E. S. (2011). The impact of Oblogo landfill site in Accra-Ghana on the surrounding environment. *Research Journal of Environmental and Earth Sciences, 3*(6), 633–636.

Papargyropoulou, E., Lozano, R., Steinberger, J. K., Wright, N., & bin Ujang, Z. (2014). The food waste hierarchy as a framework for the management of food surplus and food waste. *Journal of Cleaner Production, 76*, 106–115.

Patz, J. A., Gibbs, H. K., Foley, J. A., Rogers, J. V., & Smith, K. R. (2007). Climate change and global health: Quantifying a growing ethical crisis. *Eco Health, 4*(4), 397–405.

Paul, D. K., & Shaha, R. K. (2004). Nutrients, vitamins and minerals content in common citrus fruits in the northern region of Bangladesh. *Pak J Biol Sci, 7*(2), 238–242.

Pimentel, D., & Burgess, M. (2014). Environmental and economic costs of the application of pesticides primarily in the United States. In *Integrated Pest Management* (pp. 47–71). Springer, Dordrecht.

Pinstrup-Andersen, P. (2009). Food security: Definition and measurement. *Food Security, 1*(1), 5–7.

Pomegranate Producers Association of South Africa (POMASA). (2016). *Pomegranate Industry Overview: Statistics and Information* (online). https://www.sapomegranate.co.za/statistics-and-information/pomegranate-industry-overview/ (accessed on 9th July 2025).

Pomegranate Producers Association of South Africa (POMASA). (2019). *Pomegranate Industry Overview: Statistics and Information* (online). Available: https://www.sapomegranate.co.za/statistics-and-information/pomegranate-industry-overview/ (accessed on 9th July 2025).

Porat, R., Lichter, A., Terry, L. A., Harker, R., & Buzby, J. (2018). Postharvest losses of fruit and vegetables during retail and in consumers' homes: Quantifications, causes, and means of prevention. *Postharvest Biology and Technology, 139*, 135–149.

Produce Marketing Association (PMA). (2016). *Exporting Fresh Fruit and Vegetables to China: A Market Overview and Guide for Foreign Suppliers*. M.Z. Marketing Communications, PMA China Market Development Representative.

Prusky, D. (2011). Reduction of the incidence of postharvest quality losses, and future prospects. *Food Security, 3*(4), 463–474.

Rani, A., Saghir, A., Usman, S., Ch, K. M., & Ali, S. (2020). Residual effects of pesticides on human health as perceived by farmers in Tehsil Faisalabad Sadar, Punjab, Pakistan. *The Professional Medical Journal, 27*(2), 395–402.

Reutter, B., Lant, P., Reynolds, C., & Lane, J. (2017). Food waste consequences: Environmentally extended input-output as a framework for analysis. *Journal of Cleaner Production, 153*, 506–514.

Richter, E. D. (2002). Acute human pesticide poisonings. In *Encyclopedia of Pest Management*. New York: Marcel Dekker, Inc.

Ridoutt, B. G., Juliano, P., Sanguansri, P., & Sellahewa, J. (2010). The water footprint of food waste: Case study of fresh mango in Australia. *Journal of Cleaner Production, 18*, 1714–1721.

Robertson, G. P., Paul, E. A., & Harwood, R. R. (2000). Greenhouse gases in intensive agriculture: Contributions of individual gases to the radiative forcing of the atmosphere. *Science, 289*(5486), 1922–1925.

Sagar, N. A., Pareek, S., Sharma, S., Yahia, E. M., & Lobo, M. G. (2018). Fruit and vegetable waste: Bioactive compounds, their extraction, and possible utilization. *Comprehensive Reviews in Food Science and Food Safety, 17*(3), 512–531.

Salunkhe, D. K., & Desai, B. B. (1984). *Postharvest Biotechnology of Fruits: Volume I.* Boca Raton, FL: CRC Press.

Schreinemachers, P., Simmons, E. B., & Wopereis, M. C. (2018). Tapping the economic and nutritional power of vegetables. *Global Food Security, 16*, 36–45.

Spiker, M. L., Hiza, H. A., Siddiqi, S. M., & Neff, R. A. (2017). Wasted food, wasted nutrients: Nutrient loss from wasted food in the United States and comparison to gaps in dietary intake. *Journal of the Academy of Nutrition and Dietetics, 117*(7), 1031–1040.

Sudheer, K. P., & Indira, V. (2007). *Postharvest Technology of Horticultural Crops* (Vol. 7). New India: New India Publishing.

Swilling, M., & Annecke, E. (2012). *Just Transitions: Explorations of Sustainability in An Unfair World.* Cape Town: UCT Press.

Underhill, S. J. R., & Kumar, S. (2015). Quantifying postharvest losses along a commercial tomato supply chain in Fiji: A case study. *Journal of Applied Horticulture, 17*(3), 199–204.

Underhill, S. J. R., Joshua, L., & Zhou, Y. (2019). A preliminary assessment of horticultural postharvest market loss in the Solomon Islands. *Horticultural, 5*(1), 1–14.

Underhill, S. J., & Kumar, S. (2014). Quantifying horticulture postharvest wastage in three municipal fruit and vegetable markets in Fiji. *International Journal of Postharvest Technology and Innovation, 4*, 251–261.

United Nations (UN). (2011). *World Population Prospects: The 2010 Revision, Volume I.* https://www.un.org/en/development/desa/population/publications/pdf/trends/WPP2010/WPP2010_Volume-I_Comprehensive-Tables.pdf (accessed on 9th July 2025).

United Nations Environmental Programmed (UNEP). (2011). *Decoupling Natural Resource Use and Environmental Impacts from Economic Growth.* Paris. https://wedocs.unep.org/bitstream/handle/20.500.11822/9816/Decoupling_FReport_EN.pdf?sequence=1&isAllowed=y (accessed on 9th July 2025).

United States Department of Agriculture, Consumer and Marketing Service. (1970). *Fresh Fruit and Vegetable Unloads in Eastern Cities.* U.S. Dept. Agr., Consum. and Mktg. Serv. (C&MS) Bulletin. https://archive.org/search.php?query=creator%3A%22United+States.+Consumer+and+Marketing+Service.+Fruit+and+Vegetable+Division.+Market+News+Branch%22 (accessed on 9th July 2025).

United States Environmental Protection Agency (EPA). (2012). *Putting Surplus Food to Good Use.* Washington, DC. https://archive.epa.gov/wastes/conserve/tools/rogo/web/pdf/food-guide.pdf (accessed on 9th July 2025).

Viuda-Martos, M., Fernández-López, J., & Pérez-Álvarez, J. A. (2010). Pomegranate and its many functional components as related to human health: A review. *Comprehensive Reviews in Food Science and Food Safety, 9*(6), 635–654.

Wada, Y., Van Beek, L. P. H., & Bierkens, M. F. (2011). Modelling global water stress of the recent past: On the relative importance of trends in water demand and climate variability. *Hydrology and Earth System Sciences, 15*(12), 3785–3805.

Waste Resources Action Programme (WRAP). (2019). *Evidence and Insights Informing Updated Guidance Aimed at Reducing Fresh Produce Waste and Plastic Packaging.*

(online). Available: https://wrap.org.uk/sites/files/wrap/Evidence_informing_guidance_on_fresh_produce.pdf (accessed on 9th July 2025).

Waste Resources Action Programmed (WRAP). (2009). *Household Food and Drink Waste in the UK.* https://www.wrap.org.uk/sites/files/wrap/Household%20food%20and%20drink%20waste%20in%20the%20UK%20-%20report.pdf (accessed on 9th July 2025).

Waste Resources Action Programmed (WRAP). (2011). *Fruit and Vegetable Resource Maps: Mapping Fruit and Vegetable Waste Through the Wholesale Supply Chain.* (online). Available: https://www.wrap.org.uk/retail (accessed on 9th July 2025).

WHO–FAO. (2005). *Fruits and Vegetables for Health: Report of The Joint FAO/WHO Workshop, 1–3 Sept., Kobe, Japan.* https://apps.who.int/iris/handle/10665/43143 (accessed on 9th July 2025).

Willersinn, C., Möbius, S., Mouron, P., Lansche, J., & Mack, G. (2017). Environmental impacts of food losses along the entire Swiss potato supply chain–Current situation and reduction potentials. *Journal of Cleaner Production, 140*, 860–870.

World Health Organization (WHO). (2016). *Database on Anemia, Vitamin and Mineral Nutrient Information System (VMNIS).* https://www.who.int/vmnis/database/anaemia/en/ (accessed on 9th July 2025).

Yahaya, S. M., & Mardiyya, A. Y. (2019). Review of post-harvest losses of fruits and vegetables. *Biomedical Journal of Scientific & Technical Research, 13*(4), 10192–10200.

Yahia, E. M. (2019). *Postharvest Technology of Perishable Horticultural Commodities.* Woodhead Publishing.

Yahia, E. M., Fonseca, J. M., & Kitinoja, L. (2019). Postharvest losses and waste. In *Postharvest Technology of Perishable Horticultural Commodities* (pp. 43–69). United Kingdom: Woodhead Publishing.

Zhang, W., Jiang, F., & Ou, J. (2011). Global pesticide consumption and pollution: With China as a focus. *Proceedings of the International Academy of Ecology and Environmental Sciences, 1*(2), 125.

Index

F

P

Q

R

X

Y

Z

For Product Safety Concerns and Information please contact our EU representative GPSR@taylorandfrancis.com Taylor & Francis Verlag GmbH, Kaufingerstraße 24, 80331 München, Germany